Drugs During Pregnancy and Lactation

Drug	Embryonic period (until week 12 after LMP)	Fetal period (from week 13 after LMP)	Peripartum	Pregnancy, see page	Lactation	Lactation, see page
Gestagenes (weigh critical progesterone during pregnancy; gestagene contraceptives during lactation tolerable)	S	C	C	405	1	755
Glibenclamide	2	2	T	401	2	754
Glucocorticoids, systemical	2	2	2	392	2	752
Glucocorticoids, topical	1	1	1	447	1	752
Glyceryl trinitrate	2	2	2	222	2	691
Gold compounds	2	2	2	44	2	630
Griseofulvin	2	2	2	142	2	669
Haloperidol	2	2	1	301	2	724
Heparins	1	1	T	239	1	695
(Di-)Hydralazine	1	1	1	198	1	682
Hydrochlorothiazide	2	2	2	224	2	690
Hydroxy ethyl starch	1	1	1	250	1	691
Ibuprofen	1	T/S	T/S	38	1	628
Imipramine	1	1	T	289	1	712
Indomethacin	1	T/S	T/S	38	S	628
Insulin (human)	1	1	1	399	1	754
Iodine supplementation	1	1	1	388	1	751
Isoniazid + vitamin B6	1	1	1	152	1	666
Isotretinoin	C	C	C	452	C	765
Itraconazole	2	2	2	139	2	668
Ketoconazole	2	2	2	138	2	668
Lamotrigine (as antiepileptic)	1	1	1	274	2	704
Lindane (topical)	T	T	T	458	T	764
Lithium salts	T	2	T	305	T	727
Local anesthetics	1	1	1	431	1	632
Loratadine	1	1	1	58	1	639
Mebendazole	2	1	1	162	1	669
Meclozine	1	1	1	85	1	656
Mefloquine	2	2	2	145	2	667
Mesalazine	1	1	T	110	1	653
Metamizol	2	T	T	32	T	629
Metformin	2	2	2	401	2	754
Methimazole	2	2	2	390	2	750
α-Methyldopa	1	1	1	195	1	682
Methylergometrine	C	C	T	372	T/S	747
Metoclopramide	2	2	2	85	2	650
Miconazole (topical)	2	2	2	137	2	668
Misoprostol	C	C	1	369	T	649
Morphine	2	2	T	33	2	625
Nifedipine	2	1	1	200	1	683
Nitrendipine	2	2	2	201	1	683
Nitrofurantoin	2	2	2	132	2	662
Norfloxacin	2	2	2	131	2	663
Nystatin	1	1	1	137	1	668
Olanzapine, and other sufficiently tested atypical neuroleptics	2	2	T	302	2	725
Omeprazole	1	1	1	98	1	649
Opiates/opioids	2	2	T/S	33	2/S	625
Oxytocin	C	C	1	371	1	747
Paracetamol	1	1	1	28	1	623
D-Penicillamine	T	T	T	44	2	630
Penicillins	1	1	1	124	1	660
Pentazocine	2	2	T	37	2	627
Pethidine (meperidine)	2	2	T	34	2	625
Phenobarbital (as antiepileptic)	T	2	T	263	1	701
Phenothiazine-neuroleptics	1	1	T	300	1	720
Phenprocoumon	T	T	C	242	2	696
Phenylbutazone	2	T	T	41	2	629
Phenytoin	T	T	T	266	1	702
Prazosin	2	2	2	210	2	685
Primidone	T	2	T	263	1	701
Probenecid	1	1	1	48	1	635
Proguanil	1	1	1	144	1	667
Propylthiouracil	1	1	1	390	1	750
Prostaglandins	C	C	S	368	T	758
Pyrethrum (topical)	1	1	1	458	1	580
Pyrimethamine	2	2	T	146	1	668
Pyrviniumembonate	1	1	1	163	1	669
Radiopharma-ceuticals	T	T	T	508	T	781
Ranitidine	1	1	1	97	1	649
Rifampicin	1	1	1	153	1	666
Roxithromycin	2	2	2	126	1	661
Sertraline	1	1	T	291	1	717
Spironolactone	2	2	2	226	2	690
Sulfasalazine	1	1	1	109	1	653
Testosterone	C	C	C	408	C	757
Tetracyclines	2	C	C	128	2	662
Thalidomide	C	C	C	329	C	
Theophylline	1	1	1	68	1	642
Thiamazol	2	2	2	390	2	750
Thyroxine (L-)	1	1	1	389	1	749
Tinidazole	2/S	2/S	2/S	135	2/S	665
Tramadol	2	2	T/S	37	2/S	627
Tretinoin (topical)	T	T	T	454	2	765
Valproic acid	T	T	T	269	1	702
Verapamil	2	1	1	200	1	689
Vitamin A (10 000 U/d or less)	1	1	1	468		
Warfarin	T	T	C	242	2	696

Drugs During Pregnancy and Lactation

Treatment options and risk assessment

Second edition

Edited by
Christof Schaefer, Paul Peters, and Richard K. Miller

ELSEVIER

AMSTERDAM • BOSTON • HEIDELBERG • LONDON • NEW YORK • OXFORD
PARIS • SAN DIEGO • SAN FRANCISCO • SINGAPORE • SYDNEY • TOKYO
Academic Press is an imprint of Elsevier

Academic Press is an imprint of Elsevier
84 Theobald's Road, London WC1X 8RR, UK
30 Corporate Drive, Suite 400, Burlington, MA 01803, USA
525 B Street, Suite 1900, San Diego, California 92101-4495, USA

First edition 2001
Second edition 2007

Notice
No responsibility is assumed by the publisher for any injury and/or damage to persons
or property as a matter of products liability, negligence or otherwise, or from any use
or operation of any methods, products, instructions or ideas contained in the material
herein. Because of rapid advances in the medical sciences, in particular, independent
verification of diagnoses and drug dosages should be made

British Library Cataloguing in Publication Data
A catalogue record for this book is available from the British Library

Library of Congress Catalog in Publication Data
A catalog record for this title is available from the Library of Congress

ISBN: 978-0-444-52072-2

For information on all Academic Press publications visit
our web site at http://books.elsevier.com

Typeset by Charon Tec Ltd (A Macmillan Company), Chennai, India
www.charontec.com
Printed and bound in Great Britain

07 08 09 10 11   10 9 8 7 6 5 4 3 2 1

Contents _____

1   General commentary on drug therapy and drug risks in pregnancy

Richard K. Miller, Paul W. Peters, and Christof E. Schaefer

2   Specific drug therapies during pregnancy

3 General commentary on drug therapy and drug risk during lactation
Ruth Lawrence and Christof Schaefer

4 Specific drug therapies during lactation
Christof Schaefer and Ruth Lawrence

List of contributors

MATITIAHU BERKOVITCH
Drug Information Center, Assaf Harofeh Medical Center, 70300
Zerifin, Israel

HANNEKE GARBIS
Teratology Information Service, National Institute of Public
Health and Environment, PO Box 1, 3720 BA Bilthoven,
The Netherlands

LEE H. GOLDSTEIN
Internal Medicine Department C, Haemek Medical Center, Afula
18101, Israel

HENRY M. HESS
Department of Obstetrics and Gynecology, University of Rochester,
School of Medicine and Dentistry, 2255 Clinton Avenue,
Rochester, NY, 14618, USA

RUTH LAWRENCE
Lactation Research Center, Department of Pediatrics, University
of Rochester, School of Medicine and Dentistry, 601 Elmwood
Avenue, Rochester, NY, 14642-8777, USA

PATRICIA McELHATTON
The National Teratology Information Service (NTIS),
Regional Drug & Therapeutics Centre, Claremont Place,
Newcastle-upon-Tyne, NE2 4HH, UK

RICHARD K. MILLER
PEDECS, NY Teratogen Information Service, Department of
Obstetrics and Gynecology, University of Rochester, School of
Medicine and Dentistry, 601 Elmwood Avenue, Rochester, NY,
14642-8668, USA

ASHER ORNOY
Israel Teratogen Information Service, Jerusalem Child
Developmental Center, Rechov Yafo 157, Jerusalem, Israel

PAUL PETERS
University Medical Centre Utrecht, Department of Obstetrics,
Karel Doormanlaan 150, 3572 NR Utrecht, The Netherlands

MINKE REUVERS
Teratology Information Service, National Institute of Public Health
and Environment, PO Box 1, 3720 BA Bilthoven, The Netherlands

ELISABETH ROBERT-GNANSIA
Agence Française de Sécurité Sanitaire de l'Environnement et du
Travail, 253 Avenue du Général Leclerc, 94701 Maisons-Alfort
Cedex, France

ELVIRA RODRIGUEZ-PINILLA
Servicio de Informacion sobre Teratogenos (SITTE), Sección de
Teratología Clínica,
Centro de Investigacion sobre, Anomalias Congenitas (CIAC),
Instituto de Salud Carlos III, c/ Sinesio Delgado 6 (Pabellon 6),
28029 Madrid, Spain

MARGREET ROST VAN TONNINGEN
Teratology Information Service, National Institute of Public Health
and Environment, PO Box 1, 3720 BA Bilthoven, The Netherlands

CHRISTOF SCHAEFER
Pharmakovigilanz- und Beratungszentrum für Embryonaltoxikologie,
Berlin Institute for Clinical Teratology and Drug Risk Assessment
in Pregnancy, Spandauer Damm 130, Haus 10, 14050 Berlin,
Germany

HERMAN VAN GEIJN
Department of Obstetrics and Gynaecology, VU University
Medical Center, PO Box 7057, 1007 MB Amsterdam,
The Netherlands

CORINNA WEBER-SCHÖNDORFER
Pharmakovigilanz- und Beratungszentrum für Embryonaltoxikologie,
Berlin Institute for Clinical Teratology and Drug Risk Assessment
in Pregnancy, Spandauer Damm 130, Haus 10, 14050 Berlin,
Germany

Preface

Physicians and all health care providers who care for women in their reproductive years are frequently asked by concerned women who are planning a pregnancy, are pregnant or breastfeeding about the risk of medicinal products for themselves, their unborn or breastfed infant. These Dermatologists, Family Medicine physicians, Internists, Obstetricians, Pediatricians, Pharmacists, Midwives, Nurses, Lactation consultants, Medical geneticists, Psychiatrists, Psychologists, Toxicologists to name but a few should be well-informed in regard to acceptable treatment options and be capable of assessing the risk of an inadvertent or required treatment/exposure.

All aspects of drug counseling are inadequately supported by various sources of information such as the *Physicians Desk Reference*, package leaflets or general pharmacotherapy handbooks. Formal drug risk classifications or statements such as "contraindicated during pregnancy" may lead to a simplified perception of risk, e.g. an overestimation of the risk or simple fatalism, and withholding of essential therapy or the prescription of insufficiently studied and potentially risky drugs may result. This simplified perception of risk, can lead to unnecessary invasive prenatal diagnostic testing or even to a recommendation to terminate a wanted pregnancy. During lactation, misclassification of drug risk may lead to the advice to stop breastfeeding, even though the drug in question is acceptable or alternatives appropriate for the breastfeeding period are available.

This book is based on a survey of the literature on drug risks during pregnancy and lactation, as yet unpublished results of recent studies, and current discussions in professional societies dealing with clinical teratology and developmental toxicology. The book reflects accepted "good therapeutic practice" in different clinical areas. It is written for clinical decision-makers. Arranged according to treatment indications, the book provides an overview of the relevant drugs in the referring medical area available on the market today that might be taken by women of reproductive age. The book's organization facilitates a comparative risk approach, i.e., identifying the drugs of choice for particular diseases or symptoms. In addition, recreational drugs, diagnostic procedures (X-ray), vaccinations, poisoning, workplace and environmental contaminants, herbs, supplements and breastfeeding during infectious diseases are discussed in detail.

The second edition has had major revisions throughout, most sections were completely rewritten. The content has been adapted for an international readership. Two additional editors were enlisted;

he number of contributing authors has increased and reflects expert-se in a range of clinical specialties, e.g. dermatology, obstetrics, pedi-trics, internal medicine, psychiatry and many others. Moreover, most uthors are active members of the teratology societies including the Organization of Teratogen Information Specialists (OTIS) and Euro-pean Network of Teratology Information Services (ENTIS). The for-mat is completely different and last but not least the price is much ower – making the book available to far greater readership.

It is important to realize that the origin of this book lies in a book published in German last year in its 7th edition. The success of the atter (more than 50 000 copies sold) can be described as a best-eller – a strange term – for a book giving pertinent medical infor-mation. This also demonstrates the need to be informed in this difficult area of pharmacotherapeutics during pregnancy.

We are grateful to Kirsten Funk, publishing editor, from Elsevier/Academic Press for providing support and advice for this project o thrive. We thank Sue Armitage for copy editing and Claire Hutchins from Elsevier for overseeing production. The editors truly appreciate the many hours of work each contributor has performed n the development of their chapters and with the suggested edito-ial revisions. Finally, the editors wish to express our appreciation o our families for providing the time and support to develop this volume.

May the reader use this volume to examine treatment options for pecific diseases not only during pre-pregnancy but also before the woman becomes pregnant. By providing prepregnancy counseling, he editors and authors hope that inappropriate therapeutic, occu-pational and/or environmental exposures will be minimized.

Richard K Miller, Rochester, New York, USA
Christof Schaefer, Berlin, Germany
Paul Peters, Utrecht, Netherlands
May 2007

Notice

Medical knowledge is constantly changing. Standard safety precautions must be followed, but as new research and clinical experience broaden our knowledge, changes in treatment and drug therapy may become necessary or appropriate. The Authors and Editors have expended substantial effort to ensure that the information is accurate; however, they are not responsible for errors or omissions or any consequences from the application of the information in this educational publication and make no warranty, expressed or implied, with respect to the currency, completeness or accuracy of this publication.

Readers are advised to check the most current product information provided by the manufacturer of each drug to be administered to verify the recommended dose, the method and duration, adverse drug effects, and interactions. Application of the content of this volume for a particular situation remains the professional responsibility of the practitioner. It is ultimately the responsibility of the practitioner, relying on experience and knowledge of the patient, to determine dosages and the best treatment or intervention for each individual patient. Neither the Publisher, the Editors nor the Authors assume any liability for any injury and/or damage to persons or property arising from this publication.

General commentary on drug therapy and drug risks in pregnancy

1

Richard K. Miller, Paul W. Peters,
and Christof E. Schaefer

1.1   Introduction

Most prescribers and users of drugs are familiar with the precautions given concerning drug use during the first trimester of pregnancy. These warnings were introduced after the thalidomide disaster in the early 1960s. However, limiting the exercise of caution to the first 3 months of pregnancy is both shortsighted and effectively impossible – first, because chemicals can affect any stage of pre- or postnatal development; and secondly, because when a woman first learns that she is pregnant, the process of organogenesis has already long since begun (for example, the neural tube has closed). Hence, the unborn could already be inadvertently exposed to maternal drug treatment during the early embryonic period (Figure 1.1).

This book is intended for practicing clinicians, who prescribe medicinal products, to evaluate environmental or occupational exposures in women who are or may become pregnant. Understanding the risks of drug use in pregnancy has lagged behind the advances in other areas of pharmacotherapy. Epidemiologic difficulties in establishing causality and the ethical barriers to randomized clinical trials with pregnant women are the major reasons for our collective deficiencies. Nevertheless, since the recognition of prenatal vulnerability in the early 1960s, much has been accomplished to identify potential developmental toxicants such as medicinal products and to regulate human exposure to them. The adverse developmental effects of pharmaceutical products are now recognized to include not only malformations, but also growth restriction, fetal death and functional defects in the newborn.

The evaluation of human case reports and epidemiological investigations provide the primary sources of information. However, for

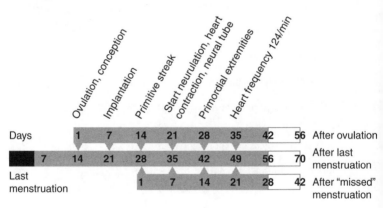

Figure 1.1 Timetable of early human development.

many drugs (and even more so in the case of chemicals) experience with human exposure is scarce, and animal experiments, *in vitro* tests, or information on related congeners provide the only basis for risk assessment. The FDA has mandated that medications potentially used in pregnant women must now be followed via pregnancy registries.

This book presents the current state of knowledge about the use of drugs during pregnancy. In each chapter, the information is presented separately for two different aspects of the problem: first, seeking a drug appropriate for prescription during pregnancy; and secondly, assessing the risk of a drug when exposure during pregnancy has already occurred.

1.2   Development and health

The care of pregnant women presents one of the paradoxes of modern medicine. Women usually require little medical intervention during an (uneventful) pregnancy. Conversely, those at high risk of damage to their own health, or that of their unborn, require the assistance of appropriate medicinal technology, including drugs. Accordingly, there are two classes of pregnant women; the larger group requires support but little intervention, while the other requires the full range of diagnostic and therapeutic measures applied in any other branch of medicine (Chamberlain 1991). Maternal illness demands treatment tolerated by the unborn. However, a normal pregnancy needs to avoid harmful drugs – both prescribed and over-the-counter, and drugs of abuse, including cigarettes and alcohol – as well as occupational and environmental exposure to potentially harmful chemicals. Obviously, sufficient and well-balanced nutrition is also essential. Currently, this set of positive preventive measures is by no means broadly guaranteed in either developing or industrial countries. When such primary preventive measures are neglected, complications of pregnancy and developmental disorders can result. Furthermore, nutritional deficiencies and toxic effects during prenatal life predispose the future adult to some diseases, such as schizophrenia (St Clair 2005), fertility disorders (Elias 2005), metabolic imbalances (Painter 2005), diabetes, and cardiovascular illnesses, as demonstrated by Barker (1998), based upon epidemiological and experimental data.

1.3   Reproductive stages

The different stages of reproduction are, in fact, highlights of a continuum. These stages concern a different developmental time-span, each with its own sensitivity to a given toxic agent.

1 General commentary on drug therapy and drug risks in pregnancy

1

Pregnancy

Table 1.1. Reproductive stages: organs and functions potentially affected by toxicants

Reproductive stage	Female	Male	Possible endpoints
Germ cell formation	Oogenesis (occurs during fetal development of mother) Gene replication Cell division Egg maturation Hormonal influence on ovary Ovulation	Spermatogenesis Gene replication Cell division Sperm maturation Sertoli cell influence Hormonal influence on testes	Sterility, subfecundity, damaged sperm or eggs, chromosomal aberrations, menstrual effects, age at menopause, hormone imbalances, changes in sex ratio

Fertilization	Oviduct
	  contractility
	  secretions
	Hormonal influence on secretory and muscle cells
	Uterus
	  contractility
	  secretions
	Nervous system
	  behavior
	  libido
		Accessory glands
		Sperm motility and nutrition
		Hormonal influence on glands
		Nervous system
		  erection
		  ejaculation
		  behavior
		  libido
			Impotence, sterility, subfecundity, chromosomal aberrations, changes in sex ratio, reduced sperm function
			
			Impotence, sterility, subfecundity, chromosomal aberrations, changes in sex ratio, reduced sperm function

Implantation	Changes in uterine lining and secretions Hormonal influence on secretory cells		Spontaneous abortion, embryonic resorption, subfecundity, stillbirths, low birth weight

1

Pregnancy

Stage		Effects

Embryogenesis	Uterus
	  yolksac
	  placenta formation
	Embryo
	  cell division,
	  tissue differentiation,
	  hormone production,
	  growth
		Spontaneous abortion, other fetal losses, birth defects, chromosomal abnormalities, change in sex ratio, stillbirths, low birth weight

Organogenesis	Placenta
	  nutrient transfer
	  hormone production
	  protection from toxic agents
	Embryo
	  organ development and
	  differentiation
	  growth
	Maternal nutrition
		Birth defects, spontaneous abortion, fetal defects, death, retarded growth and development, functional disorders (e.g. autism), transplacental carcinogenesis

Perinatal	Fetus
	  growth and development
	Uterus
	  contractility
	  Hormonal effects
	  on uterine muscle cells
	Maternal nutrition
		Premature births, births defects (particularly nervous system), stillbirths, neonatal death, toxic syndromes or withdrawal symptoms in neonates

Postnatal	Infant survival Lactation	Mental retardation, infant mortality, retarded development, metabolic and functional disorders, developmental disabilities (e.g. cerebral palsy and epilepsy)

1 **General commentary on drug therapy and drug risks in pregnancy**

Primordial germ cells are present in the embryo at about 1 month after the first day of the last menstruation. They originate from the yolksac-entoderm outside the embryo, and migrate into the undifferentiated primordia of gonads located at the medio-ventral surface of the urogenital ridges. They subsequently differentiate into oogonia and oocytes, or into spermatogonia. The oocytes in postnatal life are at an arrested stage of the meiotic division. This division is restarted much later after birth, shortly before ovulation, and is finalized after fertilization with the expulsion of the polar bodies. Thus, all-female germ cells develop prenatally and no germ cells are formed after birth. Moreover, during a female lifespan approximately 400 oocytes undergo ovulation. All these facts make it possible to state that an 8-weeks' pregnant mother of an unborn female is already prepared to be a grandmother!

The embryonal spermatogenic epithelium, on the contrary, divides slowly by repeated mitoses, and these cells do not differentiate into spermatocytes and do not undergo meiosis in the prenatal period. The onset of meiosis in the male begins at puberty. Spermatogenesis continues throughout (the reproductive) life.

When the complexity of sexual development and female and male gametogenesis is considered, it becomes apparent that pre- and postnatal drug exposure is a special toxicological problem having different outcomes. The specificity of the male and female developmental processes also accounts for unique reactions to toxic agents, such as drugs, in both sexes.

After fertilization of the oocyte by one of the spermatozoa in the oviduct, there is the stage of cell divisions and transport of the blastocyst into the endocrine-prepared uterine cavity. After implantation, the bilaminar stage is formed and embryogenesis starts. The next 7 weeks are a period of finely balanced cellular events, including proliferation, migration, association and differentiation, and programmed cell death, precisely arranged to produce tissues and organs from the genetic information present in each conceptus. During this period of organogenesis, rapid cell multiplication is the rule. Complex processes of cell migration, pattern formation and the penetration of one cell group by another characterize the later stages.

Final morphological and functional development occurs at different times during fetogenesis, and is mostly only completed after birth. Postnatal adaptation characterizes the passage from intra- into extra-uterine life with tremendous changes in, for example, circulatory and respiratory physiology (see also Table 1.1; Miller 2005).

1.4   Reproductive and developmental toxicology

Reproductive toxicology is the subject area dealing with the causes, mechanisms, effects and prevention of disturbances throughout the entire reproductive cycle, including fertility induced by chemicals. Teratology (derived from the Greek word τερας which originally meant *star*; later meanings were *wonder, divine intervention* and, finally, *terrible vision, magic, inexplicability*) is the science concerned with the birth defects of a structural nature. However, the terminology is not strict, since literature recognizes also "functional" teratogenic effects without dysmorphology.

Reproductive toxicity represents the harmful effects by agents on the progeny and/or impairment of male and female reproductive functions. Developmental toxicity involves any adverse effect induced prior to attainment of adult life. It includes the effects induced or manifested in the embryonic or fetal period, and those induced or manifested postnatally. Embryo/fetotoxicity involves any toxic effect on the conceptus resulting from prenatal exposure, including the structural and functional abnormalities of postnatal manifestations of such effects. Teratogenicity is a manifestation of developmental toxicity, representing a particular case of embryo/fetotoxicity, by the induction or the increase of the frequency of structural disorders in the progeny.

The rediscovery of Mendel's laws about a century ago, and the knowledge that some congenital abnormalities were passed from parents to children, led to attempts to explain abnormalities in children based on genetic theory. However, Hale (1933) noticed that piglets born to sows fed a vitamin A-deficient diet were born without eyes. He concluded that a nutritional deficiency leads to a marked disturbance of the internal factors which control the mechanism of eye development. During a rubella epidemic in 1941, the Australian ophthalmologist Gregg observed that embryos exposed to the rubella virus often displayed abnormalities, such as cataracts, cardiac defects, deafness and mental retardation (Gregg 1941). Soon after it was discovered that the protozoon *Toxoplasma*, a unicellular parasite, could induce abnormalities such as hydrocephaly and vision disturbances in the unborn. These observations proved undeniably that the placenta is not an absolute barrier against external influences.

Furthermore, in the early 1960s maternal exposure to the mild sedative *thalidomide* appeared to be causing characteristic reduction deformities of the limbs, ranging from hypoplasia of one or more digits to the total absence of all limbs. An example of the thalidomide embryopathy is phocomelia: the structures of the hand and feet may be reduced to a single small digit, or may appear virtually normal but protrude directly from the trunk, like the flippers of a seal (phoca). This discovery by Lenz (1961) and McBride (1961) independently led to a worldwide interest in clinical teratology.

Fifty years after the thalidomide disaster, the risk of drug-induced developmental disorders can be better delimited; to date there has

Pregnancy

1 General commentary on drug therapy and drug risks in pregnancy

been no sudden confrontation by a medicinal product provoking, as in the case of thalidomide, such devastating disorders. Drugs that nevertheless caused birth defects, such as retinoids, were known and expected, based upon animal experiments, to cause these conditions. Moreover, the prevalence of birth defects (3–4 percent) has not increased in the last half century, although substantially more substances have been marketed during these years.

Contrary to the assessment of drug-induced disorders, it is more difficult to indicate a risk from occupational chemical and physical exposure. In such situations an individual risk assessment is nearly impossible since the information necessary for a pertinent evaluation is lacking, although Occupational Exposure Limits (OELs) or Threshold Limit Values (TLVs) and occupational precautions have their effect (see Chapter 2.23).

An essential aim of public health is prevention. Primary prevention of developmental disorders can be defined as an intervention to prevent the origin of a developmental disorder – for example, by rubella vaccination, or by correction of an aberrant lifestyle such as alcohol abuse. Moreover, primary prevention of developmental disorders can be achieved when a chemical substance is identified as a reproductive toxicant and either is not approved for marketing, or is approved with specific pregnancy labeling, restricted in use or removed from the market. This is in contrast to secondary prevention of developmental disorders, which means the prevention of the birth of a child with a developmental defect – usually by abortion. In this context, tertiary prevention indicates an early detection of a metabolic disorder so that, for example, in the case of phenylketonuria (PKU) as an intervention a special diet low in phenylanaline is indicated to prevent mental retardation (phenylpyruvic oligophrenia).

When thalidomide was recognized as being the causal factor of phocomelia, the removal of the drug from the market resulted in the disappearance of the embryopathy. This event was also accompanied by a transient drastic avoidance of general drug intake by pregnant women.

Healthcare professionals and pregnant women must continue to develop a more critical attitude to the use of drugs and exposure to chemicals, not only during pregnancy but also before pregnancy – or, even better, during the entire fertile period. Such a critical attitude could result in avoiding many unnecessary and unknown risks.

These remarks imply that health professionals, couples planning to have children, and pregnant women must be informed about drugs proven to be safe, and the risks of wanted or unwanted exposures to chemicals.

1.5   Basic principles of drug-induced reproductive and developmental toxicology

Drugs that have the capacity to induce reproductive toxicity can be identified to a large extent before being marketed, based upon the outcome of laboratory animal experiments. The final conclusions can only become available through epidemiological studies after the product has been on the market for some time. The determination of whether a given medicinal product has the potentiality or capability to induce developmental disorders is essentially governed by four established fundamental principles (Wilson 1977). It can be stated that an embryo- and fetotoxic response depends upon the exposure to: (1) a specific substance in a particular dose, (2) a genetically susceptible species, and (3) a conceptus in a susceptible stage of development; and (4) by the mode of action of reproductive toxic drugs.

Principle 1

As in other toxicological evaluations, reproductive toxicity is governed by dose–effect relationships; the curve, however, is generally quite steep. The dose–response is of the utmost importance in determining whether there is a true effect. Moreover, nearly every reproductive toxic drug that has been realistically tested or was clinically positive has been shown to have a threshold, a "no-effect", level. Another aspect worth mentioning here is the occasionally highly specific nature of the substance – for instance, thalidomide is a clear-cut teratogen in the human and specific species, in contrast to its analogs, which were never proven to be developmental toxicants. Moreover, not only is the daily dose of importance to result in a potential embryo/fetotoxic concentration of the drug, but also the route of exposure.

Principle 2

Not all mammalian species are equally susceptible or sensitive to the reproductive toxic influence of a given chemical. The inter- and intraspecies variability may be manifested in several ways: a drug that acts in one species may have little or no effects in others; a reproductive toxicant may produce similar defects in various species, but these defects will vary in frequency; a substance may induce certain developmental disorders in one species that are entirely different from those induced in others. The explanation is that there are genetic differences such as in pharmocokinetics and in receptor sensitivity that influence the teratogenic response. This may be further modified by environmental factors.

Principle 3

There exists a sensitive period for different effects, i.e. the developmental phase, during which originating, proliferating and differentiating cells and organs become susceptible to a given drug. This period may not be related to critical morphogenetic periods, but may, for example, be related to the appearance of specific receptors. This explains how, at an early period of development, dysmorphology is induced by a substance which, at the opposite end of the developmental timetable, induces functional disorders such as those of the central nervous system.

Principle 4

The pathogenesis and the final effects of developmental toxicity can be studied rather well. Knowledge about the early onset or the mechanism of this process of interference of agents with development is practically absent. Mechanistic information is, however, essential to understanding how chemicals can disturb development, and is a critical component of risk evaluation. To improve the understanding of the mode of action of toxicants, including early repair mechanisms, critical molecular targets of components of developmental processes should be identified. These targets are, among others: evolutionary conserved pathways of development; conserved molecular-stress and checkpoint pathways; and conserved toxicokinetic components such as those involved in the transport and metabolism of toxicants. About 18 different signaling pathways that operate in the development of the organs of model animals, such as the fruitfly, roundworm and zebrafish, also operate in the development of mammalian organs. Therefore, the effects of medicinal products on fundamental processes such as signaling can be detected. Because the same signaling pathways operating in the various kinds of organ development in mammals are partially known, and will soon be better known, a chemical's toxicological impact on these pathways can be predicted on the basis of the results in non-mammalian organisms and tested in mammals (Committee on Developmental Toxicology 2000).

1.6   Effects and manifestations

A wide variety of responses characterizes developmental toxicity. Infertility, chromosomal and genetic disorders, spontaneous abortion, intrauterine death, prematurity, low birth weight, birth defects and functional disorders are the effects of such drug interference with the developmental and reproductive processes. The manifestation of a developmental or reproductive toxicant can either be seen immediately after exposure, or will be expressed at a much later date. Interfering with male or female germ cell development might result in infertility, decreased sperm activity and/or libido, and impaired gametogenesis. The effects on the pre-implantation stage will cause early embryonic death, extra-uterine implantation, or delayed transport of the fertilized zygote.

A critical phase for the induction of structural malformations usually occurs during the period of organogenesis. In humans, this critical period extends from about 20–70 days after the first day of the last menstruation period, or from 1 week before the missed menstruation until the woman is 44 days overdue. It may be unwise to rely absolutely on this time period. With physical agents such as X-rays used in laboratory animals, exposure can be limited exactly to a period of minutes to discover the exact sensitive period for inducing a specific disorder. However, with drugs and other chemicals, we are unsure about the time courses of absorption, metabolism and excretion. In addition, the actual proximate teratogen may be a metabolite rather than the compound administered. If the moment of final differentiation of a particular organ is known with certainty, then a teratogen must have been present prior to that time, if it is presumed to be the causal agent of the malformation.

During the fetal period, the manifestations from toxicological interference are growth restriction, some forms of structural malformations, fetal death, functional impairment, and transplacental carcinogenesis. The period of organ and system maturation extends beyond the period of organogenesis, and even beyond the prenatal period. Therefore, the susceptible period for the induction of insults that may lead to functional deficits is much longer than that for the induction of gross structural defects. Functions shown to be affected by pre- and early postnatal exposure to chemicals include behavior, reproduction, endocrine function, immune competence, xenobiotic metabolism, learning capacity, and various other physiological functions.

Fetal tissues are intrinsically highly vulnerable to carcinogens because of their high rate of cellular proliferation. This phenomenon has been demonstrated in rats, mice, hamsters, rabbits, pigs, dogs, and monkeys. About 25 compounds and groups of chemicals and 10 industrial processes have been shown to induce carcinogenic effects in human beings. However, there is convincing epidemiological evidence of transplacental tumor-induction in humans for only one compound – i.e. diethylstilbestrol (DES). Exposure to DES *in utero* leads to the development of clear-cell adenocarcinoma of the vagina or cervix in about 1 in 1000 of those at risk. Moreover, DES is now a recognized female genital tract teratogen. The effects of exposure to DES *in utero* for males are known (e.g. short phallus); however, others (e.g. infertility) remain controversial.

Pregnancy

1 General commentary on drug therapy and drug risks in pregnancy

1.7 Pharmacokinetics in pregnancy

Metabolism and kinetics of medicinal products are more complicated in pregnancy than otherwise. In general, the effective concentration of a drug or its metabolites is influenced by the following:

- the uptake, distribution, metabolism and excretion by the mother (changes during pregnancy of some physiologic parameters influencing the metabolism of chemicals are summarized in Table 1.2)
- the passage and metabolism through the yolk sac and the placenta
- the distribution, metabolism and excretion by the embryo or fetus
- re-absorption and swallowing of substances by the unborn from the amniotic fluid.

Pregnancy induces many maternal physiological changes and adaptations, which can lead to clinically important reductions in the blood concentrations of certain medicinal products. The total

Table 1.2. Changes during pregnancy of the pharmacokinetics of drugs

Resorption	
Gastrointestinal motility	↓
Lung function	↑
Skin blood circulation	↑
Distribution	
Plasma volume	↑
Body water	↑
Plasma protein	↓
Fat deposition	↑
Metabolism	
Liver activity	↑ ↓
Excretion	
Glomerular filtration	↑

Source: Loebstein (1997).

body water increases by as much as 8 l during pregnancy, which provides a substantially increased volume in which drugs can be distributed. During pregnancy, the intestinal, cutaneous and inhalatory absorption of chemicals changes due to a decreased peristalsis of the intestines and an increase in skin and lung blood flow. However, this has no consequences for the uptake of medicines from the intestinal tract. Serum proteins relevant to drug binding undergo considerable changes in concentration. Albumin, which binds acidic drugs and chemicals (such as phenytoin and aspirin), decreases in concentration by up to 10 g/l. The main implication of this change is in the interpretation of drug concentrations. The increased production of female hormones activates enzymes in the maternal liver, and this may result in a modified inactivation of medicinal and environmental agents. The renal plasma flow will have almost doubled by the last trimester of pregnancy, and drugs that are eliminated unchanged by the kidney are usually eliminated more rapidly; this change in renal clearance has been clinically important in only a few cases, and does not require adaptation of the dose of drugs in general (Loebstein 1997). Some drugs, such as anticonvulsants and theophylline derivatives, can undergo changes in distribution and elimination, which lead to ineffective treatment because of inadequate drug concentrations in the blood (Lander 1984).

1.8 Passage of drugs to the unborn and fetal kinetics

Most studies of drug transfer across the maternal and embryonic/ fetal barrier are concerned with the end of pregnancy. Little is known about the transport of substances in the early phases of pregnancy, in which, morphologically and functionally, both the yolk sac and the placenta develop and change in performance (Miller 2005, Carney 2004, Garbis-Berkvens 1987). This is not a major issue with single doses, but becomes a matter of concern with long-term therapy. The placenta is essentially a lipid barrier between the maternal and embryonic/fetal circulations, like the lipid membrane of the gastrointestinal tract, allowing fat-soluble medicines to cross more easily than water-soluble. Hence, medicinal products that are taken orally and are well-absorbed will pass the placental membranes. Drugs cross the placenta by passive diffusion, and a non-ionized drug of low molecular weight will cross the placenta more rapidly than a more polar drug. Given time, however, most drugs will achieve roughly equal concentrations on both sides of the placenta. Thus, the practical view to take when prescribing drugs during pregnancy is that the transfer of drugs to the fetus is inevitable. Most drugs have a lower molecular weight than 600–800, and will therefore be able to cross the placenta. The notable exceptions to this rule are the conjugated steroid and peptide hormones such as insulin and growth hormone. However, larger molecules (e.g. vitamin B_{12} and immunoglobulins) do cross the placenta via specific receptor-mediated processes. It should be noted that modified immunoglobulins used therapeutically, e.g. *abciximab*, do not cross the placenta but are metabolized by the placenta because they are only Fab fragments and do not have Fc terminals (see also Chapter 2.12; Miller 2003).

In the third month of pregnancy, the fetal liver is already capable of activating or inactivating chemical substances through oxidation (Juchau 1989). In the fetal compartment the detoxification of drugs and their metabolites takes place at a low level, certainly in the first half of pregnancy. This aspect, among others – such as excretion in the amniotic fluid – makes it understandable that accumulation of biological active substances might take place in the fetal compartment. The (at that time not yet existing) blood–brain barrier in the fetus is another characteristic that might be important for the possible fetotoxic effects of chemicals.

Although fetal treatment is still an exception, it is of interest that in the case of prevention of vertical infections, such as HIV-1, at the time of a functioning circulation and kidney excretion, antibiotics (*penicillins, cephalosporins*) and *antiretrovirals* concentrate in the fetal compartment. Such depot effects are also enhanced by recirculation of the medicinal product through swallowing of the excreted antibiotics in the amniotic fluid, thus contributing to a great extent to the therapeutic effect. Obviously, this effect is lost when an early amniorrhexis (rupture of the membranes) occurs (Gonser 1995).

1.9   Causes of developmental disorders

Wilson (1977), during a presentation in Vienna in 1973, presented an estimate of the causes of developmental disorders (Table 1.3). His most important observation, that about two-thirds of the causes are of unknown etiology, is still of current importance. This lack of clear causal connections explains the problems faced in primary prevention of developmental disorders.

Table 1.3 presents the estimates from different sources (Nelson 1989, Kalter 1983, Wilson 1977). In addition data are added from Saxony-Anhalt derived from a study of the late human geneticist Christine Rösch (2003) who meticulously analyzed the etiology of 4146 children born with major malformations from her birth

Table 1.3. Estimates of causes of developmental disorders (percentages)

	Wilson 1977	Kalter 1983	Nelson 1989	Rösch 2003
Monogenetic conditions	20	7.5	17.6	8.3
Chromosomal disorders	3–5	6.0	10.1	7.3
Environmental	8.5	5.0	6.1	2.0
Maternal infections		2.0		1.1
Maternal diabetes		1.4		0.1
Medicinal products		1.3		0.2
Other maternal conditions		0.3	2.9	0.6
Multifactorial and interactions	?	20	23	48.8
Unknown	65–70	61.5	43.2	33.6

registry (1987–2000) with 143,335 births in the registration area. The registration was limited to live births up to the completion of the first week.

Medicinal products and other chemical substances are estimated to account for only some percentage of developmental disorders, but they may play a more important role in the causation of defects through interaction with other (genetic) factors and maternal metabolic diseases. Table 1.4 presents an overview of the drugs and chemicals proven to be developmental toxicants in humans.

1.10 Embryo/fetotoxic risk assessment

There are different methods for assessing the embryo/fetotoxicity of medicinal products. The risk assessment process for new drugs is limited to experimental studies on laboratory animals. For drugs on the market, large epidemiological studies are of great value. In the case of thalidomide, more than 2 years passed before, in Germany, Dr Lenz's early suspicions about the phocomelia tragedy were accepted (Lenz 1988). It is generally accepted that the predictive value of animal teratogenicity and reproductive toxicity tests is in extrapolating results of chemicals into terms of human safety; however, such predictions are still not adequate. Hence, it can be understood that not all developmental toxic substances have been discovered by laboratory screening methods before they were used in humans. With the exception of androgens, several antimitotic drugs, sodium valproate and vitamin-A derivatives, all human teratogens were discovered earlier in man than in animals. Most of these discoveries were made from case studies by

Table 1.4. Medicinal products, chemicals and drugs of abuse with proven embryo/fetotoxic potential in humans

Agent	Indicating signs
ACE inhibitors and AT-II-receptor antagonists	Anuria
Alcohol	Fetal alcohol syndrome/effects
Androgens	Masculinization
Antimetabolites	Multiple malformations
Benzodiazepines	Floppy infant syndrome
Carbamazepine	Spina bifida, multiple malformations
Cocaine	CNS, intestinal and kidney damage
Coumarin anticoagulants	Coumarin syndrome
Diethylstilbestrol	Vaginal dysplasia and neoplasms
Ionizing radiation	Microcephaly, leukemia
Iodine overdose	Reversible hypothyroidism
Lead	Cognitive developmental retardation
Lithium	Ebstein-anomaly
Methyl mercury	Cerebral palsy, mental retardation
Misoprostol	Moebius-sequence, reduction defects of extremities
Penicillamine	Cutis laxa
Phenobarbital/primidone (anticonvulsive dose)	Multiple malformations
Phenytoin	Multiple malformations
Polychlorinated biphenyls	Mental retardation, immunological disorders, skin discoloration
Retinoids	Ear, CNS, cardiovascular, and skeletal disorders
Tetracycline (after week 15)	Discoloration of teeth
Thalidomide	Malformations of extremities, autism
Trimethadione	Multiple malformations
Valproic acid	Spina bifida, multiple malformations
Vitamin A (>25 000 IU/day)[1]	See retinoids

[1]Biologically, doses > 5000 IU/day are not required. The threshold for teratogenesis is much greater than 25 000 IU/day. Provitamin A = β-carotene harmless.
Note: Individual risk is dose- and time-dependent. The risk increases only two- to threefold at maximum with monotherapy or single administration of most substances in the list (see text). Never use this list for individual risk characterization or risk management! Drugs not mentioned in the list are not proven to be safe.

"alert" clinicians, and not primarily from epidemiological studies. Prospective cohort or retrospective case-control studies (see below) might provide the final evidence for such hypotheses (postmarketing surveillance).

In this respect, it is worth mentioning that in the 1970s collaboration was started among birth defects registries around the world. At present this International Clearinghouse for Birth Defects Monitoring Systems with its International Centre for Birth Defects Surveillance and Research in Rome (www.icbdsr.org) consists of programs monitoring several million newborns each year. Cooperative research is performed, but the main activity is the exchange of information collected within each program. The scope of this Clearinghouse includes fetal and childhood conditions of prenatal cause. A primary goal of the Clearinghouse is to detect changes in the incidence of specific malformations or patterns of malformations that may indicate the presence of chemicals (including medicinal hazards), to identify such hazards, and, if possible, eliminate them. Today, the FDA is requiring new drugs or suspicious medications to have pregnancy registries developed to monitor prospectively the incidence of birth defects in such drug-exposed pregnant women.

The process of assessing a reproductive or embryo/fetoxic effect of a drug includes the establishment of a biological plausibility and epidemiological evidence with the following criteria (according to Shepard 1994 and Wilson 1977):

- A sudden increase in the prevalence of a specific malformation is observed.
- An association is established between the introduction or an increased usage of a drug and an increased incidence of a specific malformation in a certain region and during a given time.
- Drug use must have taken place in the sensitive period for the induction of that specific malformation.
- It must be established that the drug and not the condition for which the drug is prescribed causes the specific malformation.
- The drug or its metabolite suspected of causing the malformation has to be proved capable of reaching the embryo or fetus.
- The findings have to be confirmed by another independent study.
- The results of specific laboratory animal studies might support the epidemiological findings.

In reproductive epidemiology, the principle of causal analytical studies of birth defects is simple: compare the observed number of exposed pregnancies with an adverse outcome with the expected number. However, this implies that the rate of adverse outcomes of pregnancy in the population and the rate of exposure must be known.

The easiest possible technique is to study all pregnancies, prospectively. This demands large numbers, producing many problems (such as mistakes in data entry and dealing with confounders that co-vary both with the exposure and the outcome), and a known ascertainment rate (Källén 1988).

The second type of causal analytical studies is the cohort approach (either historical or prospective), when adverse reproductive outcome is studied in a group of women defined by a specific exposure situation. The outcome in the exposed group is compared either with the total population or with an unexposed control cohort. The observed number of adverse outcomes is then compared with the expected number under the assumption that exposure does not affect outcome. Such cohort studies make it possible to examine many different outcomes after a specific exposure – e.g. spontaneous abortion, low birth weight, perinatal mortality, and different types of malformations. The big problem with cohort studies is often defining the cohort and identifying a sufficient number of women who have been exposed to the factor under study (Källén 1988).

Both types of analytical studies can be combined into a more powerful methodology: case-control studies within cohorts. These epidemiological studies lead to identification of a possible statistical association between the outcome and exposure. Källén (1988) elaborates clear examples of the meanings of such associations, and, among others, emphasizes the importance of not forgetting random variation as an explanation of the association. The latter is especially important when handling clusters (space–time aggregated occurrences) of adverse reproductive outcomes, often loosely suggested to be caused by an environmental agent or medicinal product.

The prolonged use of medicines during pregnancy occurs in cases of chronic (metabolic) diseases such as epilepsy, psychiatric illnesses, diabetes, and thyroid dysfunction. There are clear indications of developmental toxicity among these groups of medicines, and thus epidemiological investigations deserve a high priority. Greater uniformity in prescribing habits would enhance the likelihood of detecting causal factors of developmental disorders. The registration of new drugs developed for conditions requiring treatment during pregnancy should be based on comparative clinical trials in which not only the therapeutic but also the teratogenic properties are examined.

As mentioned earlier, developmental disorders are not only manifested as structural malformations – other embryo/fetotoxic effects include:

- spontaneous abortions
- intrauterine growth retardation

■ reversible functional postnatal effects, such as sedation, hypoglycemia, bradycardia, and withdrawal effects
■ central nervous system disorders, from motility disturbances to learning disabilities; immunological and fertility and reproductive disorders. Most of these are not apparent at birth but will be manifested much later, which explains why the prevalence of developmental disorders is about 3 percent at birth and about 8 percent or more at the age of 5 years.

1.11 Classification of drugs used in pregnancy

About 80 percent of pregnant women use prescribed or over-the-counter drugs. There is no doubt that even during pregnancy, drugs are often unjustifiably used. Healthcare professionals and pregnant women need to develop a more critical attitude to the use of drugs during pregnancy, or, more importantly, to the use of drugs during the fertile period, as well as exposures to occupational and environmental agents. These drugs and chemicals should only be taken or used when essential, thereby avoiding many unnecessary and unknown risks. The same obviously applies for social drugs like tobacco, alcohol, and addictive drugs.

Since 1984, classification systems have been introduced in the USA, Sweden and Australia. Classification is general, and of a "ready-made" fashion. These systems allow only for a general estimation of the safety of drugs during pregnancy and reproduction. The FDA classification as published in the Federal Register (2000) is not much different from the earlier one indicated in the previous edition of this book as being under "reconstruction". In the EU, a specification of the medicinal products to be used in pregnancy has to be given on the summary of product characteristics, including:

■ facts regarding human experience and conclusions from preclinical toxicity studies which are of relevance for the assessment of risks associated with exposure during pregnancy
■ recommendations on the use of the medicinal product at different times during pregnancy in respect of gestation
■ recommendations on the management of the situation of an inadvertent exposure, where relevant.

However, there are intrinsic problems with these categorization systems. It is doubtful whether the texts in the drug inserts will be updated frequently enough, and the use of the wording "contraindication in pregnancy" might result in unnecessary terminations of pregnancy (Briggs 2003). Moreover, labeling for pregnancy generally does not include specific advice regarding when the drug is used inadvertently during pregnancy (see also later).

1

Pregnancy

1 General commentary on drug therapy and drug risks in pregnancy

1.12   Paternal use of medicinal products

Husbands or partners are rarely, if ever, warned to avoid known embryo/fetotoxic medicinal products. Nevertheless, awareness is increasing that if males are exposed to reproductive toxic agents, these might damage their offspring. To date, no one is certain regarding the safety of substances that, after administration to males or via their occupational exposure, can cause birth defects.

Theoretically, there are three possible causes:

1. Substances such as cytostatics could damage the sperm itself genetically, or impair spermatogenesis or the maturation of sperm; it is also possible that the substance may become attached to sperm and transported during fertilization in the oocyte.
2. Agents might act through the semen. Many substances are excreted in semen and are present along with the sperm before, during and also (long) after the moment of conception, and undergo resorption through the vaginal mucosa, reaching the maternal circulation.
3. Toxic agents produced indirectly as a result of the action of, for example, drugs in the male may have an effect.

There have been case studies regarding immunosuppressants (review Weber-Schöndorfer 2005) and cytostatics that might indicate causality. No one believes at this moment that drugs taken by males are major contributors to developmental disorders, but many (experimental) investigators have concluded that these medicinal products *could* cause such disorders. Certainly, fertility disturbances are to be expected and have been reported with, for example, radiotherapy, cyclophosphamide, dibromochlorpropane, and lead (Friedman 2003, Sallmén 2003). Environmental agents with anti-androgenic or estrogenic activities, such as PCBs, dioxins and phthalates, are also incriminated in this respect (see review by Storgaard 2006). Casuistic cases have been mentioned with *mesalazine* in colitis ulcerosa (Chermesh 2004, Fisher 2004). Male occupational exposure to pesticides, heavy metals, organic solvents, radiation, and smoking (see Chapter 2.23) have also been associated with an increased risk of spontaneous abortions, developmental abnormalities and even childhood cancers (Aitken 2003). Acknowledging this possible cause of developmental toxicity should be considered when stimulating primary prevention of congenital disorders. The best (and indeed hygienic) way to take precautions is by the use of condoms when the man is taking medicinal products that are suspected to be harmful when ejaculated.

At present there are no data that justify elective termination of pregnancy (ETOP) because of paternal teratogenicity. The question of whether it is necessary to perform a chromosome analysis after using cytoxic or other mutagenic medicinal products has not yet been resolved. In practice, it is advisable to wait two spermatogenic cycles (about 6 months) after such treatment before conception is planned.

1.13 Communicating the risk of drug use in pregnancy

It is estimated that a pregnant woman takes about three to eight different drugs, partly as self-medication and partly prescribed. This average is not much different from the average drug use by non-pregnant women. There are, however, more questions about the safety of medicinal products used in pregnancy regarding the unborn – particularly in cases of unplanned pregnancies. In teratology counseling, a distinction must be made between the following two situations:

1. Risk communication before a pharmacotherapeutic choice has been made or before a pregnancy is initiated
2. Risk communication regarding the safety (or otherwise) of drugs used in pregnancy when drug exposure has already taken place, including risk communication in the case where a child is born with a developmental disorder following drug use during pregnancy.

In the latter situation, during pregnancy the question is whether or not fetal development is at risk, leading to discussion of whether additional (invasive) diagnostic procedures or even pregnancy termination are indicated. If there is the possibility that a child may be born with disorders, feelings of guilt might be the motivation for asking about risk; however, this situation is also frequently of importance when medical geneticists ask for specific details of genetic or environmental causations. Moreover, these issues are the subject of much debate in cases of legal procedures.

In our experience, these two risk communication situations require different approaches, which are dealt with separately below.

The safety warnings provided on package inserts or other sources such as the *Physician's Desk Reference* are so general, outdated and, in some cases, even misleading that the prescribing physician cannot make a "tailor-made" choice for the patient on such a basis. In some cases, these texts are written primarily to protect the drug producers and registration authorities from potential liability. The phrase "contraindicated in pregnancy" is in some cases correctly applied to an embryo/fetotoxic product, but it may also mean that experience with this drug in pregnancy has not been sufficiently documented.

Registration authorities and drug producers view drug risks differently from the clinician who is treating an individual patient. When, for example, a particular drug involves a relative risk (risk ratio) value of only 1.2 (which is indeed a very low risk), it is not essential that the clinician communicates the risk to an individual patient. To the drug producer, however, the same risk value implies an additional 400 malformed children per 100 000 exposed pregnancies, considering a spontaneous malformation rate of 2 percent.

1.14   Risk communication prior to pharmacotherapeutic choice

Drug administration during pregnancy means that both the mother and unborn child are exposed. The drug or metabolite concentration may be even higher in the embryonic or fetal compartment than it is in the mother. The fetus as an "additional" patient therefore demands a strict pharmacotherapeutic approach, as it is imperative to try to restore maternal health without endangering the development of the child. In severe conditions, such as bronchial asthma, diabetes mellitus, epilepsy or particular communicable diseases, treatment is obligatory regardless of pregnancy. In contrast, inessential products such as antitussive preparations, "pregnancy-supporting" substances, and high doses of vitamins and minerals should not be prescribed or used, as their potential risks outweigh their unproven benefits.

The following rules of thumb are applicable when prescribing drugs:

- Women of reproductive age must be asked, prior to drug prescription, whether an as-yet undetected pregnancy is possible, or whether they are planning a pregnancy. By the time a woman learns that she is pregnant, organogenesis has already progressed substantially.
- In chronic treatment of women of reproductive age, the possibility of pregnancy must be considered. In the case of drugs with teratogenic potential, effective contraceptive measures must be discussed and implemented. Products proven to be safe in pregnancy are the drugs of first choice for long-term treatment during the reproductive years.
- Some medicinal products (e.g. anticonvulsants) reduce the effectiveness of hormonal contraception.
- In general, drugs that have already been in use for several years should be the preferred choice during pregnancy, provided that they have not been substantially suspected of carrying risk. These products usually involve greater safety in their therapeutic efficacy in the mother and tolerability by the fetus. On the contrary,

recently introduced agents must be considered to be an unappraised risk; in many instances these products are also "pseudo-innovations" without any proven therapeutic advantage.

- If possible, monotherapy is preferred.
- The lowest effective dose should be prescribed.
- Non-drug treatment should be considered.
- The disease itself may be a greater fetotoxic risk than the appropriate drug therapy, as in diabetes mellitus. The same applies to severe psychic stress. An individual risk evaluation related to condition and treatment is necessary in these cases.

1.15   Risk communication regarding the safety (or otherwise) of drugs already used in pregnancy

A pregnant woman who uses a medicinal product must be given an individual risk assessment, and advice should be sought from a specialized institution when the assessment is difficult (see Appendix A for a list of such centers). A potential at-risk exposure should be handled in the same manner as a genetic or chromosomal disorder in a family. In the latter case, a special consultation will take place. A well-grounded individual risk assessment can help to allay unnecessary fears and avoid unnecessary diagnostic intervention, or the termination of a wanted and healthy pregnancy. A detailed maternal medical (obstetric) history, including all (drug) exposures with precise description of treatment intervals during embryogenesis, is an obligatory prerequisite.

When drug exposure has already taken place during pregnancy, a different approach is required from that used in cases of planning future pharmacotherapy. The latter allows the calm and fully confident selection of a safe drug. However, when the treatment has already begun, the pregnant patient will mainly be concerned about any possible disorder of the unborn. These different cases therefore require different communication strategies. When drug exposure has already taken place, the consultant should avoid vague comments that increase anxiety. Experimentally derived results or unconfirmed hypotheses based on individual case reports should not be referred to, as these could alarm the already anxious patient and perhaps lead to a drastic decision – for example, the termination of a wanted pregnancy based on a misinterpreted product warning such as "inadequately studied", "experimentally suspected" or "contraindicated in pregnancy". If no exposure-associated risk is known or strongly suspected, the woman should be given a straightforward answer: that there is no reason to worry about her pregnancy. In counseling her physician, it is advisable to use standard terminology such as: "it is unlikely that your patient has an increased risk for a developmental disorder as compared with the prevalence in the population". In the case of a developmental toxicant he should be provided with the relative risk, organ specificity, and recommended diagnostics.

For certain exposures, additional prenatal diagnostic procedures should be recommended. However, the intake of potentially embryo/fetotoxic substances does not require invasive diagnostic measures, such as intrauterine umbilical puncture, amniocentesis or chorion villous sampling with chromosomal analysis. It is important to add that teratology information services frequently intervene to prevent the unjustified termination of wanted pregnancies.

1.16   Teratology information centers

In 1990, two networks of teratology information services were established – one in Europe (ENTIS, or the European Network of Teratology Information Services, www.entisorg.com) and another in the Americas (OTIS, or the Organization of Teratology Information Specialists, www.otispregnancy.org). A teratology information service provides health professionals and patients with "tailor-made" information relating to the pertinent situation, illness and chemical exposure of the individual involved (Schaefer 2005). These services also conduct follow-up studies (case-registry studies and prospective cohort–control studies) to learn about what occurred during the course of pregnancy and the health of the newborn. Pregnancy outcomes of counseled patients are essential to identify more precisely the risk of medicinal products. This research relies on a detailed protocol of all chemical and medicinal exposures, maternal and paternal diseases and occupational conditions, the obstetric history, the course of the current pregnancy and the state of the newborn.

The institutions listed in Appendix A provide risk assessments of drug use in pregnancy (and during lactation). They belong to either the European Network of Teratology Information Services or the Organization of Teratology Information Specialists.

References

Aitken RJ, Sawyer D. The human spermatozoon – not waving but drowning. Adv Exp Med Biol 2003; 518: 85–98.

Barker DJP. Mothers, Babies and Health in Later Life, 2nd edn. Edinburgh: Churchill Livingstone, 1998.

Briggs GG, Freeman RK, Yaffe SJ. Classification of drugs for teratogenic risk: an anachronistic way of counseling: a reply to Merlob and Stahl. Birth Defects Res A 2003; 67: 207–8.

Briggs GG, Freeman RK, Yaffe SJ. Drugs in Pregnancy and Lactation, 7th edn. Baltimore: Williams & Wilkins, 2005.

Carney EW, Scialli AR, Watson RE et al. Mechanisms regulating toxicant disposition to the embryo during early pregnancy: an interspecies comparison. Birth Defects Res C Embryo Today 2004; 72: 345–60.

Chamberlain G. Organisation of antenatal care. Br Med J 1991; 302: 647.

Chermesh I, Eliakim R. Mesalazine-induced reversible infertility in a young male. Dig Liver Dis 2004; 36: 551–2.

Committee on Developmental Toxicology NAS/NRC. Scientific Frontiers in Developmental Toxicology and Risk Assessment. Washington, DC: National Research Council, 2000, pp. 10–25.

Elias SG, van Noord PA, Peeters PH et al. Childhood exposure to the 1944–1945 Dutch famine and subsequent female reproductive function. Hum Reprod 2005; 20: 2483–8.

Fisher JS. Environmental anti-androgens and male reproductive health: focus on phthalates and testicular dysgenesis syndrome. Reproduction 2004; 127: 305–15.

Friedman JM. Implications of research in male-mediated developmental toxicity to clinical counsellors, regulators, and occupational safety officers. Adv Exp Med Biol 2003; 518: 219–26.

Garbis-Berkvens JM, Peters PWJ. Comparative morphology and physiology of embryonic and fetal membranes. In: H Nau, WJ Scott (eds), Pharmacokinetics in teratogenesis, Vol. I. Boca Raton: CRC Press, 1987, pp. 13–44.

Gonser M, Stoll P, Kahle P. Clearance prediction and drug dosage in pregnancy. A clinical study on metildigoxin, and application to other drugs with predominant renal elimination. Clin Drug Invest 1995; 9: 197–205.

Gregg NM. Congenital cataract following German measles in mother. Trans Ophthalmol Soc Aust 1941; 3: 35–46.

Hale F. Pigs born without eyeballs. J Hered 1933; 24: 105–6.

Juchau MR. Bioactivation in chemical teratogenesis. Ann Rev Pharmacol Toxicol 1989; 29: 165–87.

Källén, B. Epidemiology of Human Reproduction. Boca Raton: CRC Press, 1988.

Kalter H, Warkany J. Congenital malformations. N Eng J Med 1983; 308: 424–31, 491–7.

Lander CM, Smith MT, Chalk JB et al. Bioavailability in pharmacokinetics of phenytoin during pregnancy. Eur J Clin Pharmacol 1984; 27: 105–10.

Lenz W. Kindliche Fehlbildungen nach Medikament während der Gravidität? Dtsch Med Wochenschr 1961; 86: 2555–6.

Lenz W. A Short History of Thalidomide Embryopathy. Teratology 1988; 38: 203–15.

Loebstein R, Lalkin A, Koren G. Pharmacokinetic changes during pregnancy and their clinical relevance. Clin Pharmacokinet 1997; 33: 328–43.

McBride WG. Thalidomide and congenital abnormalities. Lancet 1961; ii: 1358.

Miller RK, Mace K, Polliotti B et al. Marginal Transfer of ReoPro™ (abciximab) compared with immunoglobulin G (F105), insulin and water in the perfused human placenta in vitro. Placenta 2003; 24: 727–38.

Miller RK. Does the placenta protect against insult or is it the target? In Teratology Primer, Reston, VA: Teratology Society, 2005, pp. 22–26.

Nelson K, Holmes LB. Malformations due to presumed spontaneous mutations in newborn infants. N Engl J Med 1989; 320: 19–23.

Painter RC, Roseboom TJ, Bleker OP. Prenatal exposure to the Dutch famine and disease in later life: an overview. Reprod Toxicol 2005; 20: 345–52.

Rösch Chr. Aufgaben, Funktionen und Entwicklungperspektiven eines populations-
bezogenen Fehlbildungsregisters in Deutschland (Habilitationsschrift – PhD thesis). Magdeburg, 2003.

Sallmén M, Liesivuori J, Taskinen H et al. Time to pregnancy among the wives of
Finnish greenhouse workers. Scand J Work Environ Health 2003; 29: 85–93.

Schaefer C, Hannemann D, Meister R. Post-marketing surveillance system for drugs
in pregnancy – 15 years experience of ENTIS. Reprod Toxicol 2005; 20: 331–43.

Schardein JL. Chemically Induced Birth Defects, 4th edn. New York: Marcel Dekker,
2000.

Shepard TH. Letter: "proof" of teratogenicity. Teratology 1994; 50: 97.

St Clair D, Xu M, Wang P et al. Rates of adult schizophrenia following prenatal exposure to the Chinese famine of 1959–1961. J Am Med Assoc 2005; 294: 557–62.

Storgaard L, Bonde JP, Olsen J. Male reproductive disorders in humans and prenatal
indicators of estrogen exposure; a review of published epidemiological studies.
Reprod Toxicol 2006; 21: 4–15.

Weber-Schöndorfer C. Missbildungsrisiko bei Kindern unter Azathioprin-
Behandlung des Vaters. Arzneimittelbrief 2005; 39: 7–8.

Wilson JD. Embryotoxicity of drugs to man. In: JD Wilson, FC Frazer (eds),
Handbook of Teratology, Vol. 1. New York: Plenum Press, 1977, pp. 309–55.

Electronic databases offering an overview on published studies:

Reprotox: Information database on environmental hazards to human reproduction and
development. Reproductive Toxicology Center (RTC), 7831 Woodmont Ave, #375,
Bethesda, MD 20814; telephone: +1 301/514-3081; Internet: http://reprotox.org

Teris: Teratogen Information System and the on-line version of Shepard's Catalog of
Teratogenic Agents. University of Washington, TERIS Project, CHDD, Rm. 207 S.
Bldg., Box 357920, Seattle WA 98195-7920. Fax +1-206/543-7921, Email: ter-
isweb@u.washington.edu; Internet: http://depts.washington.edu/terisweb/teris/

Specific drug therapies during pregnancy

2

by authors listed below

Please note that in the following chapters drugs are discussed under their generic names. For trade names, please refer to the *Physician's Desk Reference* or comparable pharmacopoeias of your country.

Analgesics and anti-inflammatory drugs

2.1

Minke Reuvers and Christof Schaefer

2.1.1   Paracetamol (acetaminophen)

Pharmacology and toxicology

Paracetamol (*acetaminophen*) has both analgesic and antipyretic properties, and is well tolerated. In therapeutic doses, it does not inhibit prostaglandin synthesis. Its action is transmitted via a central point in the region of the hypothalamus. Paracetamol crosses the placenta easily. Indications that the chromatid breaks observed in lymphocytes (Hongslo 1991) might be clinically relevant have not been confirmed.

Earlier, as a result of individual case reports, a teratogenic potential in humans was suspected. Also recently, an association of gastroschisis and maternal treatment with paracetamol plus *pseudoephedrine* during the first trimester was observed in a retrospective study of 206 affected infants (Werler 2002). In one study, a significant reduction in the proportion of preterm birth was noted (Czeizel 2005). Another recent study discussed paracetamol use in late pregnancy as a causative factor for asthma and elevated IgE levels in later childhood (Shaheen 2002, 2005). However, other investigations (e.g. Cleves 2004) do not indicate a developmental risk with paracetamol. This also applies to suicide attempts with paracetamol (McElhatton 1997). Only when antidote treatment with *acetylcysteine* (which is also indicated in pregnancy) was for some reason unsuccessful and the mother suffered massive liver damage, was there also fetal liver damage (Wang 1997) (see also Chapter 2.22).

> **Recommendation.** Paracetamol/acetaminophen is the analgesic and antipyretic of choice. It can be used at usual dosages and at any stage of pregnancy.

2.1.2   Aspirin (acetylsalicylic acid)

Pharmacology

Depending on the dosage, *aspirin* (*acetylsalicylic acid*) (*ASA*) inhibits the synthesis of both prostaglandins and thromboxane. This gives rise to different treatment indications: with a low dosage of approximately 100 mg a day, thromboxane synthesis is inhibited with a reduction in the thrombocyte aggregation. This mechanism of action is used for thrombosis prophylaxis. The analgesic, antipyretic and antiphlogistic effects occur as a result of the inhibition of prostaglandin synthesis with individual doses from 500 mg. As a result of the limited therapeutic range in the antiphlogistic area (daily dosage of 3000 mg and more), acetylsalicylic acid has been largely supplanted as an antirheumatic by the newer, non-steroidal anti-inflammatory drugs (NSAIDs). Both low-dose and analgesia-dose usage is noted.

Salicylates are lipophilic; they are quickly absorbed after oral administration, they cross the placenta and distribute readily to the fetus. Metabolism and elimination via glucuronidation by the liver occurs only slowly in the fetus and newborn because of the still limited enzyme activity and the limited glomerular filtration rate.

Low-dose therapy

Low-dosage treatment with 75–300 mg daily is prescribed for thrombosis prophylaxis and for the prevention of pre-eclampsia. This therapy also seems effective in preventing abortions and other pregnancy complications in women with anticardiolipine or phospholipid antibodies as in systemic lupus erythematosus (Backos 1999; see also Chapter 2.9).

Many studies have examined the use of low-dose treatment to prevent high blood pressure in pregnancy and its consequences, such as intrauterine growth restriction. The Collaborative Low-dose Aspirin in Pregnancy Study (CLASP 1994), which studied 9000 women, provides a comprehensive look at this topic. The findings of the CLASP study did indicate that low-dose aspirin reduced fetal morbidity in a select population of women with early-onset pre-eclampsia. Several other single- and multicenter trials (nearly 30 000 pregnancies in total) were published. The ability of low-dose aspirin to prevent pre-eclampsia remains controversial, and this regards maternal as well as fetal outcome. Small benefits have been observed in specific groups (high-risk primigravidae, women with poor obstetric outcome). In one meta-analysis, aspirin treatment seemed to have, for women at moderate and high risk, a small but significant effect on reducing the rate of preterm birth, but did not reduce the rate of perinatal death (Kozer 2003). The small effect on altering preterm birth in women with moderate and high risk of pre-eclampsia currently does not justify the routine use of low-dose aspirin for prevention of pre-eclampsia in all patients (Kozer 2003, Heyborne 2000, Knight 2000, Caritis 1998, Sibai 1998).

Toxicology

Although salicylates in high doses can cause birth defects in some animal species, such effects in humans have not been identified until recently, in a retrospective investigation. A large prospective study of over 50 000 pregnancies did not uncover any evidence of teratogenicity, altered birth weight rates or perinatal deaths (Slone 1976). A retrospective study of 206 affected children, evaluating the relation between maternal use of cough/cold/analgesic medication and gastroschisis, found an elevated risk for the use of aspirin. Possible confounding with underlying illness cannot be ruled out, and definite conclusions cannot be drawn (Werler 2002). A meta-analysis of studies on ASA treatment in the first trimester showed a slightly increased risk for gastroschisis. The overall rate of birth defects was not increased (Kozer 2002). In a study on renal anomalies, more mothers of affected children reported ASA use in the first trimester compared to the control group (Abe 2003). However, considering the low number of exposed children, the result should be interpreted with caution. A study based on data of the Swedish medical birth registry could not find an association between ASA and cardiovascular defects (Källén 2003). Another study of over 19 000 pregnant women who had taken acetylsalicylic acid in the first or second trimester showed that intellectual development in early childhood, up to the age of 4 years, was not affected (Klebanoff 1988).

A study on prostaglandin inhibitors in very early pregnancy observed an increased risk for spontaneous abortion after ASA use around conception (Li 2003). Considering the low figures (5 of 22 exposed pregnancies) and other methodological limitations (no dosage specification), the results should be interpreted with caution.

Salicylate poisoning during pregnancy has been associated with intrauterine deaths. When an overdose has been taken, metabolic acidosis, as caused by salicylic acid, can occur more rapidly in the fetus with its already low arterial pH than in the mother, with serious consequences. Because fetal death in these cases is possible, maternal treatment or, in case of a potentially viable child, premature delivery should not be postponed (Palatnick 1998; see also Chapter 2.22).

Late pregnancy

The major pharmacologic action of aspirin (and the other NSAIDs) on the fetus is mediated through inhibition of prostaglandin synthesis. Like other prostaglandin synthesis inhibitors (see section 2.1.12), acetylsalicylic acid may decrease uterine contractions and prolong pregnancy and labor. For this reason, salicylates were once used for tocolysis. Inhibition of prostaglandin synthesis can, from about the twenty-eighth week to the end of pregnancy, lead to premature closing of the ductus arteriosus (botalli) and pulmonary hypertension (this was first documented with indomethacin therapy, but is also possible with acetylsalicylic acid – although not with low-dose therapy – and other NSAIDs; see section 2.1.12).

Aspirin also decreases platelet adhesiveness and aggregation, and among premature infants intracranial bleeding has been described many times when the mother took acetylsalicylic acid in the last week of her pregnancy. By contrast, in healthy full-term newborns analgesic doses seem only to have an effect on the laboratory parameters relevant to coagulation. There was no intracranial bleeding observed with these children.

When low-dose aspirin has been used, there is no risk of premature closure of the ductus arteriosus; maternal, fetal and neonatal hemostasis will not be affected (CLASP 1994, di Sessa 1994, Sibai 1993). There is only one case report where moderate cerebral bleeding in a term neonate is discussed in association with low-dose ASA; here, the prothrombin time and INR were elevated in the child's blood. There were no neurological symptoms reported (Sasisdharan 2001).

Recommendation. Aspirin is the analgesic and antipyretic of second choice in pregnancy. Paracetamol/acetaminophen is preferable. In the third trimester, salicylates should not be taken regularly and not at all in antiphlogistic doses. However, individual analgesic doses do not seem to represent an increased risk. For antiphlogistic indications, NSAIDs such as ibuprofen are preferable (with its restrictions; see section 2.1.12). When the mother is treated regularly with higher doses of acetylsalicylic acid from week 28 onward, the fetal ductus arteriosus must be observed with Doppler ultrasound. Consider also the fact that even a single analgesic dose of 500 mg can increase the risk of hemorrhage during delivery, especially in premature infants. Low-dose treatment with acetylsalicylic acid can be used unrestrictedly for appropriate indications (see also Chapter 2.9).

2.1.3   Pyrazolone derivatives

Pharmacology and toxicology

Metamizol (dipyrone), *phenazone (antipyrine)* and *propyphenazone* have become less important as analgesics and antipyretics because of undesirable effects on hematopoiesis. Other analgesics have superseded them. There are no indications of embryotoxic properties in humans. In a prospective study of 108 pregnant women with first-trimester exposure to metamizol, there were no indications for an increased risk of malformations or spontaneous abortion (Bar-Oz 2005). Findings from two other studies that discussed Wilms' tumor (Sharpe 1996) and leukemia (Alexander 2001) in association with prenatal metamizol exposure have not yet been confirmed by other authors, and should be interpreted with caution. Being a prostaglandin antagonist, the drug is considered to have the same effects as other NSAIDs when used in late pregnancy (see section 2.1.12).

Recommendation. The use of metamizol (dipyrone), phenazone (antipyrine) and propyphenazone should be abandoned. The analgesics of choice are paracetamol – in certain cases in combination with codeine or ibuprofen (until week 30). However, treatment with pyrazolone derivatives does not justify a termination of pregnancy.

2.1.4   Combination analgesic preparations

Recommendation. Combination preparations are not recommended, with the exception of paracetamol plus codeine. Although there are no concrete indications of any embryotoxic action in human beings, the imponderability of toxic risk increases with the number of ingredients. Furthermore, there are many combination products, which do not conform to good therapeutic practice. Inadvertent use of a combination of analgesic preparations does not justify either a termination of the pregnancy or invasive diagnostic procedures.

2.1.5   Opioid analgesics in general

Opioids are strong, centrally acting analgesics, which are similar in their action to morphine (the primary alkaloid in opium) and can lead to dependency. The opioids are divided into:

- Pure agonists: *morphine, codeine, hydromorphone* and *nicomorphine*; and synthetic agonists like *methadone* and its derivatives, *dextromoramide* and *dextropropoxyphene*, and *alfentanil, fentanyl, pethidine, piritramide, remifentanil, sufentanil* and *tramadol*.
- Partial agonists/antagonists: substances that have both properties, such as *buprenorphine, nalbuphine* and *pentazocine*.
- Pure antagonists: *naloxone* has its use as antidote.

With respect to their toxicity in pregnancy, the short-term therapeutic use of opiates (e.g. in the perinatal phase) should be evaluated differently from that of opiate abuse or substitution therapy for opiate abuse.

2.1.6   Morphine

Pharmacology and toxicology

Morphine is an opium alkaloid, derived from the seed capsule of the poppy plant. It has strong analgesic and sedative properties, and a high risk of dependency. Teratogenic effects have been observed in animal studies, but to date there are no indications that morphine, *hydromorphone* or *nicomorphine* increase the incidence of birth defects in humans. Administration of morphine or others during labor is associated with neonatal respiratory depression and also, in the case of abuse or long-term use, with withdrawal symptoms including tremors, irritability, sneezing, diarrhea, vomiting, and occasionally seizures (Kopecky 2000, Levy 1993; see also Chapter 2.21); these effects may be seen after administration of any opioid, but are believed to be more severe after morphine. Later-developing behavioral abnormalities in the offspring prenatally or perinatally exposed to opioids have been discussed in the literature. Experience with women who were on morphine (or methadone or buprenorphine) for treatment of addiction gives no indication of severe (lasting) adverse effects (Wunsch 2003).

2

Pregnancy

2.1 Analgesics and anti-inflammatory drugs

> **Recommendation.** If compellingly indicated, morphine may be used during pregnancy. Use near to term may cause neonatal respiratory depression, and long-term use may lead to withdrawal symptoms. For an evaluation of morphine abuse during pregnancy, see Chapter 2.21.

2.1.7   Codeine

Pharmacology and toxicology

Codeine is a morphine derivative with a more restricted analgesic and sedative effect than morphine. Codeine is available alone, primarily as an antitussive, or in an analgesic combination preparation with paracetamol and acetylsalicylic acid. Because codeine can cause dependency there are pregnant women who abuse it, taking 300–600 mg (sometimes even as much as 2000 mg) daily, or receive it as a heroin substitute.

Suspicions of a higher incidence of birth defects (Shaw 1992), as discussed in the literature earlier, have not been substantiated until now. Findings from a small retrospective study that discussed neuroblastoma in association with prenatal codeine exposure (Cook 2004) has not yet been confirmed by other authors and should be interpreted with caution.

There was no indication for teratogenicity in a study of approximately 100 pregnancies exposed to *oxycodone* during the first trimester (Schick 1996).

As with all opiate derivatives, therapy with codeine-containing medications up until birth can lead to postpartum respiratory depression in the infant, and also, mostly (but not exclusively) in the case of abuse, to withdrawal symptoms, characterized by tremor, jitteriness, diarrhea, and poor feeding (Khan 1997; see also Chapter 2.21).

> **Recommendation.** Codeine may be used as an analgesic for pregnant women if paracetamol is not sufficiently effective. When indicated, it may be used as an antitussive. The potential for dependency must be kept in mind. Use near to term may cause neonatal respiratory depression, and long-term use may lead to withdrawal symptoms.

2.1.8   Pethidine (meperidine)

Pharmacology

Because of its unparalleled spasmoanalgesic action during labor, *pethidine* is the analgesic of choice for this indication. When it is used during labor, the labor is not lengthened and the strength of the contractions is not diminished. Pethidine does not appear to influence either the severity of bleeding or the involution of the uterus postpartum.

During pregnancy, pethidine passes unimpeded to the fetus and can reach higher concentrations there than in the maternal serum. Because of the limited metabolic capacity in newborns, pethidine is decomposed only slowly and has a considerably lengthened half-life (18 hours as compared to 3–4 hours in adults; Caldwell 1978).

Toxicology

Pethidine is one of the most thoroughly studied spasmoanalgesics used in labor. The metabolic acidosis described after parenteral application (De Boer 1987, Kariniemi 1986) can probably be explained by individual overdose and the resultant hypotonic circulatory reaction in the mother. Epidemiologic studies have not uncovered an association between the use of pethidine during the first trimester and congenital malformations (Heinonen 1977). In newborns, pethidine can induce respiratory depression. Behavioral (for instance sucking behavior) and EEG disturbances, which may continue beyond the first few days of life, have been observed. The magnitude of these effects will vary with timing and dosing (Ransjö-Arvidson 2001, Hafström 2000, Nissen 1997). Because of the pharmacokinetics, observable effects are to be expected when maternal administration occurs between 1 and 4 hours before delivery. Multiple doses to the mother over a longer period of time result in accumulation of pethidine and its metabolite (Nissen 1997, Kuhnert 1985). Premature infants are at greater risk. Clinical studies have not uncovered lasting impairments of neonatal function.

The safety and efficacy of the different strategies for labor analgesia have been discussed extensively in the literature during the last decade. There are reports claiming that systemically administered pethidine (and other opioids) lack analgesic effectiveness for labor pain, but serve primarily to sedate the mother and, inadvertently, the neonate (Reynolds 1997, Olofsson 1996). Other strategies discussed include paracervical block, spinal blockade and epidural analgesia with local anesthetics or opioids. Combinations of epidural with parenteral analgesia and of epidural with spinal analgesia are also used (Eberle 1996). Epidural analgesia seems to be very effective in reducing pain during labor, but may also have some adverse effects.

> **Recommendation.** The spasmoanalgesic, pethidine, can be used during labor when there are critical indications for it; with premature births, however, it is relatively contraindicated. Use as an analgesic during pregnancy is not recommended; inadvertent use does not require either a termination of the pregnancy or additional diagnostic procedures.

2 Pregnancy

2.1 Analgesics and anti-inflammatory drugs

2.1.9   Fentanyl, alfentanil, remifentanil, and sufentanil

Pharmacology and toxicology

Fentanyl is used very commonly in obstetrics today. It is generally given intravenously and by epidural, but it is also available in oral, oromucosal and transdermal forms for analgesia. Placental transfer of fentanyl in early pregnancy has been demonstrated (Cooper 1999). There are no reports of teratogenic effects, but use during the first trimester or prolonged use during pregnancy is scarcely documented. A mild withdrawal syndrome without apparent long-term effects was observed after long-term, high-dose maternal treatment with a transdermal fentanyl patch (Regan 2000).

When used during labor, similar concentrations were found in both maternal and cord blood (Fernando 1997). Also, fentanyl was less frequently associated with maternal nausea, vomiting or prolonged sedation than was pethidine (Rayburn 1989). The risk that the neonate's breathing will be depressed seems slight. In most studies of women treated with this drug, there were no differences in respiratory depression, Apgar scores, the need for naloxone, and various other neurological parameters. There seems to be no difference in tolerability for the newborn, when used intravenously or as an epidural (Nikkola 1997).

Many publications describe the intravenous and epidural use of *alfentanil* in obstetrics. The tolerance for this drug among newborns seems similar to that for fentanyl, even though one researcher reported small neuromuscular irregularities in the first 30 minutes postpartum. The concentration in the cord was about 30% of the maternal value.

Fewer clinical investigations for *remifentanil* and *sufentanil* have been reported (Loftus 1995). In comparison to other analgesics, a lower rate of hypotonia was reported in women receiving *sufentanil* during delivery according to a study of 351 women (van der Velde 2001). However, there were more alterations in fetal heart rate, including bradycardias.

To date, there are no reports linking these drugs to teratogenicity when used during the first trimester.

Recommendation. Fentanyl and, when there are urgent indications, the other preparations can be used in every phase of pregnancy. When used shortly before the delivery, respiratory depression is possible as with all opiate analgesics.

2.1.10 Other narco-analgesics and centrally acting analgesics

Pharmacology and toxicology

Pentazocine is an opioid analgesic with weak antagonistic activity. It crosses the placenta readily at term. In combination with the antihistamine *tripelenamine*, pentazocine has been abused under the name "T's and Blues" as an intravenously injectable drug. In rats, this combination was associated with intrauterine growth restriction, and behavior abnormalities have been observed; similar effects have also been seen in humans after prenatal exposure (von Almen 1986). Gross malformations have not been observed.

Intravenous pentazocine and *methylphenidate* abuse during pregnancy have also been reported. Human reports on pentazocine-exposed pregnancies have not to date linked it with an increased risk of birth defects in the offspring (DeBooy 1993). If pentazocine has been used regularly until the end of pregnancy, typical opiate withdrawal symptoms such as restlessness, jitteriness, hypertonia, diarrhea, and vomiting must be reckoned with. Pentazocine can enhance uterine contractility.

Pentazocine, like *tilidine*, has been unable to establish itself as a substitute for pethidine in obstetrics. There is as yet no indication that tilidine has a teratogenic potential in humans.

Tramadol has been used with relative frequency in German-speaking areas without, as yet, any reports of specific embryotoxic effects. It is misused increasingly by drug-dependent patients. When used during labor, tramadol appears to produce less fetal respiratory depression, in comparison to older opioids (Viegas 1993). In recent reports, however, these findings were not confirmed (Keskin 2003). There are no documented studies on the use of tramadol in early pregnancy.

The same applies to *buprenorphine*, *dextro propoxyphene*, *flupirtin*, *meptazinol*, *nalbuphine*, *nefopam*, and *piritramide*.

All opiates similar to morphine can, depending on the treatment interval, the duration of use (long-term use as substitution for substance abuse) and dosage, lead to respiratory depression and withdrawal symptoms in the newborn.

Recommendation. In individual cases, treatment with the more established drugs (such as tramadol) can be considered during pregnancy. Depending on the indication, however, standard therapeutics such as paracetamol (possibly with codeine), ibuprofen (with restrictions; see section 2.1.12), or pethidine are preferable. If another drug mentioned in this section has been used during the first trimester, it does not require a termination of the pregnancy or invasive diagnostic procedures. Use of narco-analgesics near term may cause neonatal respiratory depression, and withdrawal symptoms when used long term.

2.1.11   Naloxone

Pharmacology and toxicology

Naloxone can reverse the respiratory depressive effect of opiates. In children whose mothers abused opiates during pregnancy, naloxone can cause withdrawal symptoms. No teratogenic potential has been described.

Recommendation. Naloxone may be used for appropriate indications.

2.1.12   Nonsteroidal anti-inflammatory drugs (NSAIDs)

Pharmacology

NSAIDs are the mainstay of antirheumatic therapy. Pregnancy-related conditions such as premature labor, polyhydramnios, and pregnancy induced hypertension have also been indications for treatment with NSAIDs.

This group of medications includes many drugs, and the number is still growing, so it is impossible to review them all. The most commonly used are *acemetacin, azapropazon, diclofenac, etofenamat, fenbufen, flufenamic acid, flurbiprofen, ibuprofen, indomethacin, indoprofen, ketoprofen, ketorolac, lonazolac, lornoxicam, mefenamic acid, meloxicam, nabumetone, naproxen, niflumic acid, nimesulide, piroxicam, proglumetacine, sulindac, suprofen, tenoxicam,* and *tiaprofenic acid.* Many of these can be obtained over the counter. The principal mode of action of this comprehensive group of drugs rests on inhibition of the synthesis of the prostaglandins; most of the currently available compounds are non-selective inhibitors of cyclooxygenase (COX), with an effect on the housekeeping COX-1 (inhibiting gastric, platelet and renal prostaglandin production), and COX-2, which is induced by inflammation. Meloxicam and nimesulide inhibit principally (but not selectively) COX-2. Most of these agents are reported to cross the placenta readily. Diclofenac has been shown in fetal tissues during the first trimester in concentrations similar to maternal blood levels. In contrast, only 10% of maternal naproxen values were found in the fetus (Siu 2002, 2000).

Toxicology

The ability of NSAIDs to compromise reproductive function by inhibition of ovulation (Stone 2002) and as causative agents for miscarriage (Nielsen 2004, 2001, Li 2003) is still under debate (Østensen 2004). Discontinuation of treatment with an NSAID is sometimes recommended in women who have been trying to conceive, without result, for a long period.

Until recently, first-trimester exposure to NSAIDs was not associated with an increased risk of birth defects. Results from two registry-based studies (Ofori 2006, Ericson 2001) indicate an increased risk of cardiac (septal) defects, which, however, could not be confirmed in other studies (Cleves 2004, Nielsen 2001). In another evaluation of the above-mentioned group (Källén 2003), using the same database, the association seemed to disappear. More studies are necessary to verify or reject earlier associations (Källén 2003).

The major pharmacologic action of NSAIDs on the fetus is mediated through the inhibition of prostaglandin synthesis. During the last trimester of pregnancy, NSAIDs can decrease uterine contractility and prolong pregnancy and labor. Indomethacin is the best-studied agent in this respect; it has been extensively used as a tocolytic agent in several prospective trials (Loe 2005).

Adverse effects, observed with indomethacin, have also been described for most of the non-selective COX-inhibitors. *Indomethacin* (and other NSAIDs) increases the risk of constriction of the ductus arteriosus, and affects renal function. Constriction is related to gestational age, being rare before week 27 but increasing with advancing gestational age to 50–70% at 32 weeks, rising as high as 100% when exposed from week 34 onwards. These effects appear not to be dose-dependent. Constriction resolved within 48 hours of stopping indomethacin. Exposure to indomethacin close to delivery may result in neonatal pulmonary hypertension (fatal in several patients) (Østensen 2001, Vermillion 1997, Moise 1993).

A persistent patent ductus arteriosus (PDA), unresponsive to indomethacin treatment and often needing surgical closure, has been observed. An apparently paradoxical effect, but as postulated by some of the authors, is that indomethacin may have damaged the intima of the ductus, thereby preventing spontaneous closure (Hammerman 1998, Norton 1993).

NSAIDs also affect fetal renal function, causing decreased urine output. For this effect, indomethacin has been used in the treatment of polyhydramnios. After maternal treatment with indomethacin (or with diclofenac, ibuprofen or naproxen), ultrasonography has demonstrated a reduction in the amount of amniotic fluid. These effects can be attributed to reduced kidney perfusion and an increase in the circulating vasopressins. Decreased urine output was reversible in most cases, and a study addressing the long-term effects on renal growth, structure or function in 2- to 4-year-old children did not find a correlation with perinatal indomethacin use (Ojala 2001). However, irreversible morphologic and functional renal damage with fetal oligohydramnios and persistent anuria was also reported following prolonged exposure (weeks), sometimes with fatal outcome. These effects are probably dose-related and have been observed following exposure during the last part of the second trimester and later (Cuzzolin 2001, Kaplan 1994, Van Der Heijden 1994).

Many case reports and retrospective studies have reported several adverse fetal effects when very preterm and very low birth weight (VLBW) infants have been exposed to NSAIDs – for example, an increased incidence of necrotizing enterocolitis (NEC) and intraventricular hemorrhages (IVH) in newborns (Ojala 2000, Major 1994, Norton 1993). In a retrospective study where indomethacin was used as first-line tocolytic, antenatal exposure to this drug was significantly associated with an increased incidence of IVH, but not with NEC or neonatal death (Doyle 2005).

The magnitude of the risks of indomethacin (NSAID) therapy during pregnancy is still a subject of debate in the literature. Serious sequelae, as mentioned above, seem to be related to longer duration (>72 hours) and/or a short time-lapse (<48 hours) between exposure and delivery. A recent meta-analysis, assessing neonatal safety of indomethacin tocolysis, did not identify a significantly increased risk of adverse effects, but the limited statistical power did not allow exclusion of any increased risk of adverse neonatal outcomes (Loe 2005). For further details on tocolysis, see Chapter 2.14.

It has not yet been demonstrated that the adverse effects observed with indomethacin are less marked when other NSAIDs are used. However, although experience is limited, because they share the same prostaglandin-inhibiting properties it must be suspected that all NSAIDs can have adverse effects during pregnancy.

There have been reports of persistent pulmonary hypertension after (probably prolonged) ductus constriction in fetuses antenatally exposed to *diclofenac* for analgesic or anti-inflammatory indications (Mas 1999, Zenker 1998). An additive constrictive effect of corticosteroids (betamethasone) on fetal ductus arteriosus was observed in a study where tocolysis with and without antenatal betamethasone was compared (Levy 1999).

Sulindac was thought, because of the limited ability of its active (sulfid)metabolites to cross the placenta, not to cause changes in fetal circulation (Carlan 1995, Kramer 1995, Rasanen 1995). However, further experience does not confirm this advantage (Kramer 1999).

There is no evidence that the agents with a stronger effect on COX-2 (meloxicam, *nimesulide*) have lesser fetal effects (Østensen 2001, Brent 1997). Neonatal *renal* insufficiency (even dialysis-dependent) has been reported after maternal use of nimesulide near term (Balasubramaniam 2000, Landau 1999, Peruzzi 1999), as has ductal constriction (Simbi 2002).

Phenylbutazone and the related compounds *famprofazone, kebuzone, mofebutazone,* and *oxyphenbutazon* have weak analgesic and antipyretic properties. However, they have strong anti-inflammatory properties based on their prostaglandin antagonism. Phenylbutazone derivatives can damage blood production; they lead to fluid retention and are strongly cumulative (elimination half-life 30–170 hours). These are undesirable qualities during pregnancy. Although teratogenicity has been observed in animal studies, until now there has been no indication of significant teratogenic potential in humans, but experience with its use during pregnancy is limited.

> **Recommendation.** Use of the more established NSAIDs like ibuprofen and diclofenac can be considered in the first two trimesters for anti-inflammatory therapy. From week 28 onward, (repeated) use of these agents for anti-inflammatory – or analgesic – indications is relatively contraindicated. If treatment is unavoidable, fetal circulation should be monitored regularly (once or twice a week) with (Doppler) sonography, and medication should be stopped as soon as signs of ductal constriction appear. Oligohydramnios should be ruled out. Tocolysis should be reckoned with. However, the use of prostaglandin antagonists for tocolysis is controversial, and should be reserved for special indications (see Chapter 2.14). If a drug, other than those mentioned above, of this group has been used in early pregnancy, it does not require a termination of pregnancy or additional invasive diagnostic procedures.

2.1.13   Selective cyclooxygenase-2 (COX-2) inhibitors

Pharmacology and toxicology

Because of their selective inhibition of COX-2, which is released in inflammatory processes, these newer agents are thought to have significantly fewer gastrointestinal side effects than the classic NSAIDs, and not to exert any antiplatelet effect. *Celecoxib, etoricoxib, lumiracoxib, parecoxib, rofecoxib,* and *valdecoxib* are among them. There are few case reports on their use in pregnancy (such as those collected by the producer of rofecoxib), and these do not to date indicate a teratogenic effect in humans. Data from animal studies did not demonstrate an embryotoxic risk; effects due to prostglandin-synthesis inhibition (constriction of ductus arteriosus) were observed, though.

In animal studies, COX-2 regulates the tone of the fetal ductus arteriosus and was present in the fetal kidney. As with classic NSAIDs, exposure during the third trimester may result in adverse cardiovascular and renal effects (Cuzzolin 2001, Østensen 2001) and treatment around the time of conception may lead to fertility problems (Pall 2001). A recent study comparing valdecoxib and placebo could not demonstrate an advantage with respect to total analgesic consumption when used during cesarean section. The authors concluded that adding *valdecoxib* after cesarean delivery under spinal anesthesia with intrathecal morphine is not supported at this time (Carvalho 2006).

> **Recommendation.** Selective COX-2 inhibitors are not recommended during pregnancy because of the lack of data. Inadvertent use during the first trimester does not require termination of pregnancy or invasive diagnostic procedures. Detailed fetal ultrasound may be considered.

2.1.14   Migraine medications

Migraine is an episodic headache disorder, sometimes preceded by a prodrome or an aura. The relationship between migraine and sex hormones (particularly estrogen) is well accepted, and prevalence of migraine is highest among women of childbearing age. When pregnant, migraine attacks most commonly occur during the first trimester. During pregnancy, 60–70% of the women improve. However, attacks often recur in the postpartum period (Silberstein 2004).

In migraine attacks there are three different phases:

1. The prodromal stage, with vasoconstriction of the vessels in the part of the brain affected
2. The painful stage, with vasodilatation
3. The edema stage, which involves increased vessel permeability and can last a long time.

There are different starting points for drug therapy. The drugs mentioned in the following section may be discussed in detail in other parts of this volume.

Ergot alkaloids

Ergot alkaloids, such as *ergotamine-tartrate* and *dihydroergotamine* (DHE), are helpful in many cases, but are contraindicated during pregnancy because of their ability to disrupt fetal blood supply, which can lead to fetal damage or death. They also can produce uterine contractions and perfusion disturbances in the placenta (Fox 2005, Silberstein 2004). Individual cases of birth defects due to vascular disruption and stillbirths have been observed (Hughes 1988, Schaefer unpublished observations). Epidemiological studies have not, as yet, documented a clear increase in the rate of birth defects (Raymond 1995). The other ergotamine derivatives, which are available in oral form, *lisuride* and *methysergide*, are not well studied for their tolerability during pregnancy, and should also be avoided (Fox 2005, Silberstein 2004).

Triptan-serotonin agonists

For severe acute attacks, *sumatriptan* (intranasal, s.c., oral or rectal application) is offered to patients who are unresponsive to other medications. Sumatriptan is a selective serotonin-receptor agonist, the receptors being present mainly in cranial vessels. More than 700 pregnancies have been studied prospectively by the producer in a registry and in some other prospective studies (GlaxoSmithKline 2005, Reiff-Eldridge 2000, O'Quinn 1999, Shuhaiber 1998, Eldridge 1997), and some 700 have been studied in retrospective studies (Källén 2001, Olesen 2000), the majority of them being exposed in the first trimester. These data do not indicate a teratogenic potential in human beings.

The manufacturer recorded 38 pregnancies exposed to *naratriptan* during the first trimester (GlaxoSmithKline 2005) without indication of teratogenicity. Animal experiments have shown skeletal and vascular anomalies associated with plasma concentrations only 2.5 times greater than the human therapeutic level.

There are almost 100 prospective and retrospective case reports on *rizatriptan* collected by the Swedish medical birth registry and the producer, and these do not indicate teratogenicity (Fiore 2005).

Among 28 pregnancies exposed to *zolmitriptan* during the first trimester, there were two major birth defects (microphthalmia plus cataract, ventricular septal defect). These data are insufficient for risk assessment.

There are insufficient data on *almotriptan*, *eletriptan*, and *frovatriptan*.

Other migraine medications

In the edema stage of a migraine, diuretics such as *furosemide* have proven useful for many (non-pregnant) patients. Diuretic-induced maternal hypovolemia, however, may impair placental perfusion, with possible adverse effects on fetal well-being (see Chapter 2.8).

For *clonidine*, *flunarizine*, *ketanserin*, and *pizotifen* there are insufficient data on the use during pregnancy.

> **Recommendation.** Migraine suffering is frequently positively influenced by pregnancy. Non-drug processes such as muscle relaxation therapy, biofeedback, acupuncture and acupressure, as well as changes in lifestyle and nutrition, are preferable in the prodromal stage and in the intervals that are free from pain. The analgesic of choice is paracetamol, perhaps combined with caffeine or codeine (see Chapter 2.1.7). Ibuprofen or aspirin can also be considered, but these should not be used from the early third trimester onwards. If necessary, antiemetics like *meclozine* or *metoclopramide* should be given prior to analgesics. To prevent dehydration, intravenous (i.v.) fluids should be given. To control nausea and pain, phenothiazines (*prochlorperazine*) can be administered intravenously, supplemented if necessary by i.v. narcotics (like codeine) or i.v. corticosteroids. Severe attacks can be treated with sumatriptan (preferably intranasal, s.c. or rectal); other "triptanes" should be used only when compellingly indicated.
> For prophylactic interval therapy, proven β-receptor blockers such as *propranolol* or *metoprolol* can be used, and when compellingly indicated tricyclic antidepressants can be considered.
> If one of the medications not recommended is taken, termination of pregnancy is not justified. Following an accidental injection of ergotamine derivatives in the last trimester, effects on contractions and fetal well-being can be determined by cardiotocography and ultrasound.

2.1.15   Additional analgesics

Gabapentine, *pregabalin*, *topiramate*, and *valproic acid* are antiepileptic drugs that are sometimes used in the treatment of (chronical) pain. During pregnancy, their use as an analgesic is not recommended and may even be contraindicated (see Chapter 2.10).

2.1.16   Additional antiphlogistics and antirheumatics

Disease-modifying antirheumatic drugs (DMARDs) are the pharmacological basis for the treatment of rheumatic diseases. DMARDs include *chloroquine* and *hydroxychloroquine*, *gold compounds*, *leflunomide*, *methotrexate*, and *cyclophosphamide* (see Chapter 2.12), *D-penicillamine*, *sulfasalazine* (see Chapter 2.6), *azathioprine* and *cyclosporine* (see Chapter 2.12). In case of necessity, NSAIDs, COX-2 inhibitors and glucocorticoids may be added to the DMARD therapy. Biologicals like the monoclonal antibodies *adalimumab*, *etanercept*, and *infliximab* (see Chapter 2.12) are only indicated if two DMARDs prove insufficient. The same applies to *anakinra*, which is prescribed in conjunction with methotrexate in case that methotrexate alone does not work. *Abatacept* is another new drug for rheumatic diseases.

Pharmacology and toxicology

Chloroquine and hydroxychloroquine, antimalarial drugs from the 4-aminochinoline group, are frequently used to treat rheumatoid arthritis and systemic lupus erythematosus (SLE), particularly when associated with antiphospholipid antibodies. In animal studies, the presence of chloroquine has been demonstrated in the fetal retina and in the central nervous system. Many studies investigating reproductive toxicology were in women receiving low-dose antimalarials for malaria prophylaxis. Chloroquine is neither embryo- nor fetotoxic when used in the usual dosage for malaria prophylaxis, or when used for the treatment of malarial infection in a 3-day course (Philips-Howard 1996; see also Chapter 2.6).

Damage to the fetal retina and inner ear has been linked to chloroquine therapy in human pregnancy; in these cases, chloroquine was used daily in high doses on a long-term basis (Hart 1964). Other studies covering more than 300 pregnancies with chloroquine or hydroxychloroquine treatment for SLE or rheumatic diseases do not demonstrate an increased risk of congenital malformations or other adverse effects (Costedoat-Chalumeau 2003, Parke 1996, Philips-Howard 1996). Ophthalmic and/or auditory evaluation, without detection of abnormalities, was performed in several studies (Motta 2005, Borba 2004, Klinger 2001, Levy 2001). The latter also addressed the maternal disease activity in a small, double-blind and placebo-controlled study with hydroxychloroquine: patients scored lower on disease-activity scales and had less need for *prednisone*. Following discontinuation of therapy in pregnant SLE, patients may precipitate a flare with harmful consequences for mother and child; it is thus considered to be reasonable to continue with antimalarials in SLE during pregnancy when there is no therapeutic alternative. Furthermore, stopping treatment at recognition of pregnancy will not prevent first-trimester exposure of the fetus, in view of the long half-life (Costedoat-Chalumeau 2005, Østensen 2001, Borden 2001, Janssen 2000). Due to lack of published associations with fetal toxicity, and in view of the greater tissue disposition of chloroquine, hydroxychloroquine is preferable to chloroquine (Borden 2001, Østensen 2001, Brent 1997).

Intramuscular (*aurothioglucose* and *aurothiomalate*) and oral (*auranofin*) gold salts are used for long-term therapy of chronic inflammatory conditions, such as rheumatoid arthritis, psoriatic arthritis and chronic juvenile arthritis (Østensen 2001). Unlike the results in animal studies, in humans no noteworthy teratogenic potential has been discovered to date. The placental transfer of gold compounds has, however, been proven, and gold has been detected in the fetal liver and kidneys. Cord serum levels have been reported to equal maternal serum concentrations. Case reports and case series, among them one in which 119 pregnant women were treated with gold for bronchial asthma in the first trimester, have not, however, shown any specific developmental disorders. As these data are insufficient to rule out a developmental risk, treatment with gold compounds should be discontinued as soon as pregnancy is recognized (Østensen 2001).

Leflunomide is a pyrimidine synthesis inhibitor, used more and more in the treatment of active rheumatoid arthritis. In studies in rats and rabbits with doses equivalent to human doses, leflunomide induced maternal toxicity, was embryotoxic (causing growth retardation and embryolethality) and induced birth defects (skeletal malformations, anophthalmia, microphthalmia, and hydrocephaly). About 50 case reports (Chambers 2004, Chakravarty 2003, observations by the authors, reports to the pharmaceutical company) on its use during human pregnancy do not yet indicate teratogenicity. However, data are insufficient to rule out developmental risks.

D-penicillamine works as a result of its structure as a chelating agent, and is therefore used as an antidote for metal poisoning and also as therapy for the copper storage illness, Wilson's disease. In addition, penicillamine has an antiphlogistic effect. In connection with prenatal exposure in the case of maternal cystinuria, chronic polyarthritis and Wilson's disease, five cases of inborn cutis laxa – some with inguinal hernia and with further very different and serious birth defects – have been described in the literature (Pinter 2004, Rosa 1986). In contrast, there are more than 100 cases with no noteworthy effects (Sinha 2004, Tarnacka 2000, Messner 1998, Dupont 1991, as well as unpublished experience). There is no clear-cut answer to whether penicillamine is responsible for the sometimes reversible disturbances in the development of the connective tissue. If there is a teratogenic risk at all, it is very slight.

A copper deficiency induced by the chelating agent, penicillamine, is unlikely to be the cause of teratogenic effects, since the neonatal copper concentration is not lowered by treatment for Wilson's disease. In addition, a chelating agent-induced zinc deficiency was discussed in association with the observed connective tissue defects.

Where penicillamine in the treatment for rheumatic diseases has been largely replaced by other antirheumatic drugs, it is one of the few available drugs for patients with Wilson's disease. In these patients, the benefit of continued treatment may outweigh the probably small (if any) teratogenic risk (Østensen 2001, Janssen 2000, Brent 1997). As penicillamine antagonizes *pyridoxine*, 25 mg vitamin B_6 (pyridoxin) should be supplemented during treatment.

Trientine is also used for the treatment of Wilson's disease. No adverse pregnancy outcomes were observed in a total of 13 women who were treated throughout their whole pregnancy with trientine (Devesa 1995). As trientine may cause anemia due to iron deficiency, iron should be supplemented during treatment.

For methotrexate and cyclophosphamide, see Chapter 2.13.

Recommendation. Sulfasalazine is the DMARD of first choice during pregnancy. Azathioprine, cyclosporine, hydroxychloroquine/chloroquine, as well as gold compounds and D-penicillamine are reserve treatment options.

If penicillamine is used for an illness outside the group of rheumatic conditions (e.g. Wilson's disease), the lowest possible dosage should be selected. Giving copper along with it as a preventive is not recommended, since the effectiveness of the penicillamine is diminished.

Women of childbearing potential should be started on leflunomide only when pregnancy tests are negative and safe contraception is in use. Leflunomide should be discontinued when pregnancy is planned. Due to the long half-life of up to more than 2 weeks, and the protracted elimination from the plasma, it is recommended that, before conception is attempted, a drug elimination procedure be performed (cholestyramine 8 g t.i.d. for 11 days). Plasma levels should be less than 0.02 mg/l. This level (extrapolated from animal studies) is considered not to cause an increased teratogenic or reproductive risk. To minimize exposure to the fetus in the case of an unplanned pregnancy, the same procedure is recommended (Brent 2001).

Cyclophosphamide, methotrexate (see Chapter 2.13), and biologicals are contraindicated during pregnancy. NSAIDs may be given until week 30, and prednisone/prednisolone throughout pregnancy (see section 2.1.12 and Chapter 2.15).

Treatment with the drugs not recommended in this section does not necessitate a termination of pregnancy or any invasive diagnostic procedures, even when low-dose methotrexate has been used. However, a detailed fetal ultrasound should be considered after treatment with any of these drugs.

2.1.17   Myotonolytics

Pharmacology and toxicology

Baclofen, carisoprodol, chlormezanone, clostridium botulinum toxin, dantrolene, fenyramidol, mephenesin, methocarbamol, orphenadrine, pridinol, quinine ethylcarbonate, tetrazepam, tizanidine, and *tolperisone* are available for treating muscle tension. There are anecdotal reports of normal pregnancy outcomes, but also of withdrawal syndromes (especially convulsions) after bacolofen treatment during pregnancy. There are five case reports on intrathecal *baclofen* therapy; three patients were treated throughout the whole pregnancy. All five newborns were healthy and did not show withdrawal symptoms (Roberts 2003, Munoz 2000). In two cases, 20–80 mg was taken orally throughout the whole pregnancy. Again there were no malformations, but both children suffered from withdrawal – one with seizures on day 7 (Ratnayaka 2001). The other newborn showed hyperirritability and respiratory problems (Moran 2004).

Following the use of *chlormezanone* during pregnancy, a fulminating hepatitis with a liver transplant and the birth of a healthy child has been reported (Bourliere 1992).

The available experience with the use of the other older and outdated treatments in pregnancy is not sufficient for a risk assessment.

> **Recommendation.** Myotonolytics are relatively contraindicated during pregnancy, and should be reserved for very special indications – e.g. dantrolene for malignant hyperthermia. Physiotherapeutic measures and anti-inflammatory agents or antirheumatics are preferable. In certain cases, the tension-releasing action of the better-studied diazepam can be used. Exposure to the myotonolytics mentioned does not require either a termination of the pregnancy or invasive diagnostic procedures.

2.1.18   Gout interval therapy

Pharmacology and toxicology

Gout seldom occurs before menopause. For women of childbearing age, therefore, gout therapy is only a minimal issue. Gout is caused by an elevated level of uric acid in the blood and in the tissue. Uric acid is the end product of purine metabolism. Interval treatment between gout attacks with uricosurics and *allopurinol* aims to lower uric acid levels.

Uricosurics, like *benzbromaron* and *probenecid*, promote the excretion of uric acid by inhibiting renal absorption.

Allopurinol causes a decrease of uric acid levels in blood by inhibiting the enzyme xanthine-oxidase. Since allopurinol is structurally similar to xanthines, there is the theoretic possibility that the drug or its metabolites will be incorporated into the nucleic acids of the embryo. In animal studies, allopurinol did not prove to be teratogenic in rats; in mice there was an increase in cleft palate. Experience in humans is limited to a few case reports. Due to additional confounding risk factors, like the maternal disease and other medications, these case observations do not permit assessment of the prenatal tolerability of allopurinol. Treatment during the third trimester has not been found to induce neonatal symproms (Gulmezoglu 1997).

There are no data on the use of benzbromaron during pregnancy.

Probenecid is transmitted to the embryo, but has proved itself to be well tolerated by both mother and baby.

> **Recommendation.** During pregnancy, probenecid is the drug of choice to achieve elimination of uric acid. Allopurinol is relatively contraindicated during pregnancy, since probenecid, a medication that has been proved to be safe, is available as an alternative. However, the use of allopurinol and benzbromaron do not justify a termination of pregnancy, but treatment should be switched to probenecid. After allopurinol use in the first trimester, a detailed fetal ultrasound should be considered.

2.1.19   Gout attack therapy

Pharmacology and toxicology

Apart from the nonsteroidal anti-inflammatory drugs (NSAIDs) such as ibuprofen, *colchicine* is the classic medication for gout attacks. Colchicine is a mitotic spindle poison, and is by this action capable of blocking cell division. It has mutagenic and genotoxic properties and, in various animal studies, an embryotoxic action. Mutagenic effects on lymphocytes have been described in patients who are treated with colchicine. Colchicine is the only effective therapy to prevent attacks of Familial Mediterranean Fever (FMF) and to treat the renal amyloidosis that often accompanies FMF and which may itself cause several maternal and fetal complications (Ben-Chetrit 2003, Mordel 1993). However, to date, teratogenic damage or other adverse pregnancy outcomes in women with long-term colchicine treatment for FMF have not been observed in several reports. In one study, evaluating the outcome of 225 completed pregnancies in mothers with FMF, the authors also did not find an unusual frequency of fetal abnormalities in the 131 prenatally (first trimester) exposed children (Rabinovitch 1992). This was confirmed in a retrospective study of 1124 infants born to mothers with FMF, where results indicated that the use of colchicine before or during pregnancy was not associated with adverse pregnancy outcomes (Barkai 2000). Two cases of aneuploidy (one trisomy 21, one Klinefelter) were found in a more recent group of 444 colchicine-treated women (viewed as a significantly increased rate by the same authors). Performing amniocentesis, in view of the possible chromosomal abnormalities and insufficient clinical data, is advocated by some (Berkenstadt 2005, Ben-Chetrit 2003, Barkai 2000) but not all (Mijatovic 2003) authors.

> **Recommendation.** Ibuprofen is the medication of choice in those rare cases of gout attacks during pregnancy, with the same restrictions as discussed in section 2.1.12. Colchicine is a drug of second choice. Inadvertent use does not justify a termination of the pregnancy or invasive diagnostic procedures. In case of FMF in pregnant women, long-term treatment with colchicine may be indicated to improve maternal and fetal outcome. After colchicine use in the first trimester, a detailed fetal ultrasound should be recommended.

References

Abe K, Honein MA, Moore CA. Maternal febrile illness, medication use, and risk of congenital renal anomalies. Birth Defects Res A 2003; 67: 911–18.

Alexander FE, Patheal SL, Biondi A et al. Transplacental chemical exposure and risk of infant leukemia with MLL gene fusion. Cancer Res 2001; 61: 2542–6.

Backos M. Pregnancy complications in women with recurrent miscarriage associated with antiphospholipid antibodies treated with low dose aspirin and heparin. Br J Obstet Gynaecol 1999; 106: 102–7.

Balasubramaniam J. Nimesulide and neonatal renal failure. Lancet 2000; 355: 575.

Barkai G, Meital Y, Chetrit A et al. Clinical and chromosomal outcome following colchicine exposure before and during pregnancy. Presentation at the 11th Annual Meeting of the European Network of Teratology Information Services, Jerusalem, March, 2000.

Bar-Oz B, Clementi M, Di Giantonio E. Metamizol (dipyrone, optalgin) in pregnancy, is it safe? A prospective comparative study. Eur J Obstet Gyn Reprod Biol 2005; 119: 176–9.

Ben Chetrit E, Levy M. Reproductive system in familial Mediterranean fever: an overview. Ann Rheum Dis 2003; 62(10): 916–19.

Berkenstadt M, Weisz B, Cuckle H et al. Chromosomal abnormalities and birth. defects among couples with colchicine treated familial Mediterranean fever. Am J Obstet Gynecol 2005; 193: 1513–16.

Borba EF, Turrini JR, Kuruma K et al. Chloroquine gestational use in systemic lupus erythematosus: assessing the risk of child ototoxicity by pure tone audiometry. Lupus 2004; 13: 223–7.

Borden MB, Parke AL. Antimalarial drugs in systemic lupus erythematosus – use in pregnancy. Drug Saf 2001; 24: 1055–63.

Bourliere M, LeTreut YP, Manelli JC et al. Chlormezanone-induced fulminant hepatitis in a pregnant woman: successful delivery and liver transplantation. J Gastroenterol Hepatol 1992; 7: 339–41.

Brent LH, Beckman DA, Brent RL. The effects of antirheumatic drugs on reproductive function. Reprod Toxicol 1997; 11: 561–77.

2

Pregnancy

Brent RL. Reproductive risks of Leflunomide (Arava™); a pyrimidine synthesis inhibitor: counseling women taking leflunomide before or during pregnancy and men taking leflunomide who are contemplating fathering a child. Teratology 2001; 63: 106–12.

Caldwell J, Notarianni LJ. Disposition of pethidine in childbirth. Br J Anaesth 1978; 50: 307–8.

Caritis S, Sibai B, Hauth J et al. Low-dose aspirin to prevent pre-eclampsia in women at high risk. N Engl J Med 1998; 338: 701–8.

Carlan SJ, O'Brien WF, Jones MH et al. Outpatient oral sulindac to prevent recurrence of preterm labor. Obstet Gynecol 1995; 85: 769–74.

Carvalho B, Chu L, Fuller A et al. Valdecoxib for postoperative pain management after cesarean delivery: a randomized, double-blind, placebo-controlled study. Anesth Analg 2006; 103: 664–70.

Chakravarty EF, Sanchez-Yamamoto D, Bush TM. The use of disease modifying antirheumatic drugs in women with rheumatoid arthritis of childbearing age: a survey of practice patterns and pregnancy outcomes. J Rheumatol 2003; 30: 241–6.

Chambers CD, Johnson DL, Macaraeg GR et al. Pregnancy outcome following early gestational exposure to leflunomide: The OTIS rheumatoid arthritis in pregnancy study (Abstract). Pharmacoepidemiol Drug Saf 2004; 14: S126–7.

CLASP Collaborative Group. CLASP: a randomized trial of low-dose aspirin for the prevention and treatment of preeclampsia among 9364 pregnant women. Lancet 1994; 343: 619–29.

Cleves MA, Savell VH, Raj S et al. Maternal use of acetaminophen and nonsteroidal anti-inflammatory drugs (NSAIDs), and muscular ventricular septal defects. Birth Defects Res A 2004; 70: 107–13.

Cook MN, Olshan AF, Guess HA et al. Maternal medication use and neuroblastoma in offspring. Am J Epidemiol 2004; 159: 721–31.

Cooper J, Jauniaux E, Gulbis B et al. Placental transfer of fentanyl in early human pregnancy and its detection in fetal brain. Br J Anaesth 1999; 82: 929–31.

Costedoat-Chalumeau N, Amoura Z, Duhaut P et al. Safety of hydroxychloroquine in pregnant patients with connective tissue diseases: a study of one hundred thirty-three cases compared with a control group. Arthritis Rheum 2003; 48: 3207–11.

Costedoat-Chalumeau N, Amoura Z, Duhaut P et al. Safety of hydroxychloroquine in pregnant patients with connective tissue diseases. Review of the literature. Autoimmunity Rev 2005; 4: 111–15.

Cuzzolin L, Dal Cere M, Fanos V. NSAID-induced nephrotoxicity from the fetus to the child. Drug Saf 2001; 24: 9–18.

Czeizel AE, Dudas I, Puho E. Short-term paracetamol therapy during pregnancy and a lower rate of preterm birth. Paediatr Perinat Epidemiol 2005; 19: 106–11.

De Boer FC, Shortland D, Simpson RL et al. A comparison of the effects of maternally administered meptazinol and pethidine on neonatal acid-base status. Br J Obstet Gynaecol 1987; 94: 256–61.

DeBooy VD, Seshia MM, Tenenbein M et al.: Intravenous pentazocine and methylphenidate abuse during pregnancy. Maternal lifestyle and infant outcome. Am J Dis Child 1993; 147: 1062–5.

Devesa R, Alvarez A, De las Heras G et al. Wilson's disease treated with trientine during pregnancy. J Pediatr Gastroenterol Nutr 1995; 20: 102–3.

di Sessa TG, Moretti ML, Khoury A et al. Cardiac function in fetuses and newborn exposed to low-dose aspirin during pregnancy. Am J Obstet Gynecol 1994; 171: 892–900.

2.1 Analgesics and anti-inflammatory drugs

Doyle NM, Gardner MO, Wells L et al. Outcome of very low birth weight infants exposed to antenatal indomethacin for tocolysis. J Perinatol 2005; 25(5): 336–40.

Dupont P, Irion O, Beguin F. Pregnancy and Wilson's disease. Am J Obstet Gynecol 1991; 165: 488–9.

Eberle RL, Norris MC. Labour analgesia. A risk–benefit analysis. Drug Saf 1996; 14: 239–51.

Eldridge RE, Ephross SA, and the Sumatriptan Registry Advisory Committee. Monitoring birth outcomes in the sumatriptan pregnancy registry. Teratology 1997; 55: 48.

Ericson A, Källén BA. Nonsteroidal anti-inflammatory drugs in early pregnancy. Reprod Toxicol 2001; 15: 371–5.

Fernando R, Bonello E, Gill P et al. Neonatal welfare and placental transfer of fentanyl and bupivacaine during ambulatory combined spinal epidural analgesia for labour. Anaesthesia 1997; 52: 517–24.

Fiore M, Shields KE, Santanello N et al. Exposure to rizatriptan during pregnancy: post-marketing experience up to 30 June 2004. Cephalgia 2005; 25: 685–8.

Fox AW, Diamond ML, Spierings EL. Migraine during pregnancy: options for therapy. CNS Drugs 2005; 19: 465–81.

GlaxoSmithKline. Sumatriptan and Naratriptan Pregnancy Registry. International Interim Report: 1 January 1996 through 30 April 2005. Wilmington, NC: GlaxoSmithKline, August 2005.

Gulmezoglu AM, Hofmeyr GJ, Oosthuisen MMJ. Antioxidants in the treatment of severe pre-eclampsia: An explanatory randomised controlled trial. Br J Obstet Gynaecol 1997; 104: 689–96.

Hafström M, Kjellmer I. Non-nutritive sucking by infants exposed to pethidine in utero. Acta Paediatr 2000; 89: 1196–200.

Hammerman C, Glaser J, Kaplan M et al. Indomethacin tocolysis increases postnatal patent ductus arteriosus severity. Pediatrics 1998; 102: E56.

Hart C, Naunton WRF. The ototoxicity of chloroquine phosphate. Arch Otolaryngol 1964; 80: 407–12.

Heinonen OP, Slone D, Shapiro S. Birth Defects and Drugs in Pregnancy. Littleton/USA: Publishing Sciences Group, 1977.

Heyborne KD. Preeclampsia prevention, lessons from the low-dose-aspirin therapy trials. Am J Obstet Gynecol 2000; 183: 523–8.

Hongslo JK, Brogger A, Bjorge C et al. Increased frequency of sister-chromatid exchange and chromatid breaks in lymphocytes after treatment of human volunteers with therapeutic doses of paracetamol. Mut Res 261; 1991: 1–8.

Hughes HE, Goldstein DA. Birth defects following maternal exposure to ergotamine, beta-blockers and coffeine. J Med Genetics 1988; 25: 3396–9.

Janssen NM, Genta MS. The effects of immunosuppressive and anti-inflammatory medications on fertility, pregnancy, and lactation. Arch Intern Med 2000; 160: 610–19.

Källén B, Lygner PE. Delivery outcome in women who used drugs for migraine during pregnancy with special reference to sumatriptan. Headache 2001; 41: 351–6.

Källén BAJ, Olausson PO. Maternal drug use in early pregnancy and infant cardiovascular defect. Reprod Toxicol 2003; 17: 255–61.

Kaplan BS, Restaino I, Raval DS et al. Renal failure in the neonate associated with in utero exposure to non-steroidal anti-inflammatory agents. Pediatr Nephrol 1994; 8: 700–704.

Kariniemi V, Rost J. Intramuscular pethidine (meperidine) during labor associated with metabolic acidosis in the newborn. J Perinat Med 1986; 14: 131–5.

Keskin HL, Keskin EA, Avsar AF et al. Pethidine versus tramadol for pain relief during labor. Intl J Gynaecol Obstet 2003; 82: 11–16.

Khan K, Chang J. Neonatal abstinence syndrome due to codeine. Arch Dis Child Fetal Neonatal Ed 1997; 76: 59–60.

Klebanoff MA, Betendes HW. Aspirin exposure during the first 20 weeks of gestation and IQ at four years of age. Teratology 1988; 37: 249–55.

Klinger G, Morad Y, Westall CA et al. Ocular toxicity and antenatal exposure to chloroquine or hydroxychloroquine for rheumatic diseases. Lancet 2001; 358: 813–14.

Knight M, Duley L, Henderson-Smart DJ et al. Antiplatelet agents for preventing and treating pre-eclampsia. Cochrane Database Syst Rev 2000; 2: CD000492.

Kopecky EA, Ryan ML, Barrett JF et al. Fetal response to maternally administered morphine. Am J Obstet Gynecol 2000; 183: 424–30.

Kozer E , Nikfar S, Costei A et al. Aspirin consumption during the first trimester of pregnancy and congenital anomalies: a meta-analysis. Am J Obstet Gynecol 2002; 187: 1623–30.

Kozer E, Costei AM, Boskovic R et al. Effects of aspirin consumption during pregnancy on pregnancy outcomes: meta-analysis. Birth Defects Res B, Dev Reprod Toxicol 2003; 68: 70–84.

Kramer WB, Saade G, Ou C et al. Placental transfer of sulindac and its active sulfide metabolite in humans. Am J Obstet Gynecol 1995; 172: 886–90.

Kramer W, Saade G, Belfort M et al. A randomized double-blind study comparing the fetal effects of sulindac to terbutaline during the management of preterm labor. Am J Obstet Gynecol 1999; 180: 396–401.

Kuhnert BR. Disposition of meperidine and normeperidine following multiple doses during labor. II. Fetus and neonate. Am J Obstet Gynecol 1985; 151: 410–15.

Landau D, Shelef I, Polacheck H et al. Perinatal vasoconstrictive renal insufficiency associated with maternal nimesulide use. Am J Perinatol 1999; 16: 441–4.

Levy M, Spino M. Neonatal withdrawal syndrome: associated drugs and pharmacologic management. Pharmacotherapy 1993; 13: 202–11.

Levy R, Matitiau A, Ben Arie A et al. Indomethacin and corticosteroids: an additive constrictive effect on the fetal ductus arteriosus. Am J Perinatol 1999; 16: 379–83.

Levy RA, Vilela VS, Cataldo MJ et al. Hydroxychloroquine (HCQ) in lupus pregnancy: double-blind and placebo-controlled study. Lupus 2001; 10: 401–4.

Li DK, Liu L, Odouli R. Exposure to non-steroidal anti-inflammatory drugs during pregnancy and risk of miscarriage: population based cohort study. Br Med J 2003; 327: 368.

Loe SM, Sanchez-Ramos L, Kaunitz AM. Assessing the neonatal safety of indomethacin tocolysis. A systemic review with meta-analysis. Obstet Gynecol 2005; 106: 173–9.

Loftus JR, Hill H, Cohen SE. Placental transfer and neonatal effects of epidural sufentanil and fentanyl administered with bupivacaine during labor. Anesthesiology 1995; 83: 300–308.

Major CA, Lewis DF, Harding J et al. Tocolysis with indomethacin increases the incidence of necrotizing enterocolitis in the low-birth-weight neonate. Am J Obstet Gynecol 1994; 170: 102–6.

Mas C, Menahem S. Premature in utero closure of the ductus arteriosus following maternal ingestion of sodium diclofenac. Aust NZ J Obstet Gynaecol 1999; 39: 106–7.

McElhatton P, Sullivan F, Volans G. Paracetamol overdose in pregnancy: analysis of the outcomes of 300 cases referred to the Teratology Information Service of the National Poisons Information Service. Reprod Toxicol 1997; 11: 85–94.

2

Pregnancy

2.1 Analgesics and anti-inflammatory drugs

Messner U, Gunter HH, Niesert S. Wilson disease and pregnancy. Review of the literature and case report {in German}. Z Geburtshilfe Neonatol 1998; 202: 77–9.

Mijatovic V, Hompes PGA, Wouters MGAJ. Familial Mediterranean fever and its implications for fertility and pregnancy. Eur J Obstet Gyn Reprod Biol 2003; 108: 171–6.

Moise KJ Jr. Effect of advancing gestational age on the frequency of fetal ductal constriction in association with maternal indomethacin use. Am J Obstet Gynecol 1993; 168: 1350–53.

Moran LR, Almeida PG, Worden S et al. Intrauterine baclofen exposure: a multidisciplinary approach. Pediatrics 2004; 114: E267–9.

Mordel N, Birkenfeld A, Rubinger D et al. Successful full-term pregnancy in familial Mediterranean fever complicated with amyloidosis: case report and review of the literature. Fetal Diagn Ther 1993; 8: 129–34.

Motta M, Tincani A, Faden D et al. Follow-up of infants exposed to hydroxychloroquine given to mothers during pregnancy and lactation. J Perinatol 2005; 25: 86–9.

Munoz FC, Marco DG, Perez AV et al. Pregnancy outcome in a woman exposed to continuous intrathecal baclofen infusion. Am Pharmacother 2000; 34: 956.

Nielsen GL, Sorensen HT, Larsen H et al. Risk of adverse birth outcome and miscarriage in pregnant users of non-steroidal anti-inflammatory drugs: population based observational study and case-control study. Br Med J 2001; 322: 266–70.

Nielsen GL, Skriver MV, Pedersen L et al. Danish group reanalyses miscarriage in NSAID users. Br Med J 2004; 328: 109.

Nikkola EM, Ekblad UU, Kero PO et al. Intravenous fentanyl PCA during labour. Can J Anaesth 1997; 44: 1248–55.

Nissen E, Widstrom A, Lilja G et al. Effects of routinely given pethidine during labour on infants' developing breastfeeding behaviour. Effects of dose-delivering interval and various concentrations of pethidine/norpethidine in cord plasma. Acta Paediatr 1997; 86: 201–8.

Norton ME, Merrill J, Cooper BAB et al. Neonatal complications after the administration of indomethacin for preterm labor. N Engl J Med 1993; 329: 1602–7.

Ofori B, Oraichi D, Blais L et al. Risk of congenital anomalies in pregnant users of non-steroidal anti-inflammatory drugs: A nested case-control study. Birth Defects Res B 2006; 77: 268–79.

Ojala R, Ikonen S, Tammela O. Perinatal indomethacin treatment and neonatal complications in preterm infants. Eur J Pediatr 2000; 159: 153–5.

Ojala R, Ala-Houhala M, Ahonen S et al. Renal follow up of premature infants with and without perinatal indomethacin exposure. Arch Dis Child Neonatal Ed 2001; 84: F28–33.

Olesen C, Steffensen FH, Sorensen HT et al. Pregnancy outcome following prescription for sumatriptan. Headache 2000; 40: 20–24.

Olofsson CH, Ekblom A, Ekman-Ordeberg G et al. Lack of analgesic effect in systematically administered morphine or pethidine on labour pain. Br J Obstet Gynaecol 1996; 103: 968–72.

O'Quinn S, Ephross SA, Williams V et al. Pregnancy and perinatal outcomes in migraineurs using sumatriptan: a prospective study. Arch Gynecol Obstet 1999; 263: 7–12.

Østensen M. Rheumatological disorders. Best Pract Res Clin Obstet Gynaecol 2001; 15(6): 953–69.

Østensen ME, Skomsvoll JF. Anti-inflammatory pharmacotherapy during pregnancy. Expert Opin Pharmacother 2004; 5: 571–80.

Palatnick W, Tenenbein M. Aspirin poisoning during pregnancy: increased fetal sensitivity. Am J Perinatol 1998; 15: 39–41.

Pall M, Fridén BE, Brännström M. Induction of delayed follicular rupture in the human by the selective COX-2 inhibitor rofecoxib: a randomized double-blind study. Hum Reprod 2001; 16: 1323–8.

Parke A, West B. Hydroxychloroquine in pregnant patients with systemic lupus erythematosus. J Rheumatol 1996; 23: 1715–18.

Peruzzi L, Gianoglio B, Porcellini MG et al. Neonatal end-stage renal failure associated with maternal ingestion of cyclooxygenase-type I selective inhibitor nimesulide as tocolytic. Lancet 1999; 354: 1615.

Phillips-Howard PA, Wood D. The safety of anti-malarial drugs in pregnancy. Drug Saf 1996; 14: 131–45.

Pinter R, Hogge WA, McPherson E. Infant with severe penicillamine embryopathy born to a women with Wilson's disease. Am J Med Genet 2004 A; 128: 294–8.

Rabinovitch O, Zemer D, Kukia E et al. Colchicine treatment in conception and pregnancy: two hundred thirty-one pregnancies in patients with familial Mediterranean fever. Am J Reprod Immunol 1992; 28: 245–6.

Ransjö-Arvidson AB, Matthiesen AS, Lilja G et al. Maternal analgesia during labor disturbs newborn behavior: effects on breastfeeding, temperature, and crying. Birth 2001; 28: 5–12.

Rasanen J, Jouppila P. Fetal cardiac function and ductus arteriosus during indomethacin and sulindac therapy for threatened preterm labor: a randomized study. Am J Obstet Gynecol 1995; 173: 20–25.

Ratnayaka BDM, Dhaliwal H, Watkin S. Neonatal convulsions after withdrawal of baclofen. Br Med J 2001; 323: 85.

Rayburn WF, Smith CV, Parriott, JE et al. Randomized comparison of meperidine and fentanyl during labor. Obstet Gynecol 1989; 74: 604–6.

Raymond GV. Teratogen update – ergot and ergotamine. Teratology 1995; 51: 344–7.

Regan J, Chambers F, Gorman W et al. Neonatal abstinence syndrome due to prolonged administration of fentanyl in pregnancy. Br J Obstet Gynaecol 2000; 107: 570–72.

Reiff-Eldridge R, Heffner C, Ephross S et al. Monitoring pregnancy outcomes after prenatal drug exposure through prospective pregnancy registries: a pharmaceutical company commitment. Am J Obstet Gynecol 2000; 182: 159–63.

Reynolds F, Crowhurst JA. Opioids in labour – no analgesic effect. Lancet 1997; 349: 4–5.

Roberts AG, Graves CR, Konrad PE et al. Intrathecal baclofen pump implantation during pregnancy. Neurology 2003; 61: 1156–7.

Rosa FW. Teratogen update: penicillamine. Teratology 1986; 33: 127–31.

Sasidharan CK, Kutty PM, Ajithkumar et al. Fetal intracranial hemorrhage due to antenatal low dose aspirin intake. Indian J Ped 2001; 68: 1071–2.

Schick B, Hom M, Tolosa J et al. Preliminary analysis of first trimester exposure to oxycodone and hydrocodone. Reprod Toxicol 1996; 10: 162.

Shaheen SO, Newson RB, Sherriff A et al. Paracetamol use in pregnancy and wheezing in early childhood. Thorax 2002; 57: 958–63.

Shaheen SO, Newson RB, Henderson AJ et al. Prenatal paracetamol exposure and risk of asthma and elevated immunoglobulin E in childhood. Clin Exp Allergy 2005; 35: 18–25.

Sharpe CR, Franco EL. Use of dipyrone during pregnancy and risk of Wilms' tumor. Brazilian Wilms' Tumor Study Group. Epidemiology 1996; 7: 533–5.

2

Pregnancy

2.1 Analgesics and anti-inflammatory drugs

Shaw GM, Malcoe LH, Swan SH et al. Congenital cardiac anomalies relative to selected maternal exposures and conditions during early pregnancy. Eur J Epidemiol 1992; 8: 757–60.

Shuhaiber S, Pastuszak A, Schick B et al. Pregnancy outcome following first trimester exposure to sumatriptan. Neurology 1998; 51: 581–3.

Sibai BM, Caritis SN, Thorn E et al. Prevention of preeclampsia with low-dose aspirin in healthy, nulliparous pregnant women. N Engl J Med 1993; 329: 1213–18.

Sibai BM. Prevention of preeclampsia: a big disappointment. Am J Obstet Gynecol 1998; 179: 1275–8.

Silberstein SD. Headaches in pregnancy. Neurologic Clin 2004; 22: 727–56.

Simbi KA, Secchieri S, Rinaldo M et al. In utero ductal closure following near-term maternal self-medication with nimesulide and acetaminophen. J Obstet Gynaecol 2002; 22(4): 440–41.

Sinha S, Taly AB, Prashanth LK et al. Successful pregnancies and abortions in symptomatic and asymptomatic Wilson's disease. J Neurol Sci 2004; 217: 37–40.

Siu SSN, Yeung JHK, Lau TK. A study on placental transfer of diclofenac in first trimester of human pregnancy. Hum Reprod 2000; 15: 2423–5.

Siu SSN, Yeung JHK, Lau TK. An in-vivo study on placental transfer of naproxen in early human pregnancy. Hum Reprod 2002; 17: 1056–9.

Slone D, Siskind V, Heinonen OP. Aspirin and congenital malformations. Lancet 1976; 1: 1373–5.

Stone S, Khamashta MA, Nelson-Piercy C. Nonsteroidal anti-inflammatory drugs and reversible female infertility: is there a link? Drug Saf 2002; 25: 545–51.

Tarnacka B, Rodo M, Cichy S et al. Procreation ability in Wilson's disease. Acta Neurol Scand 2000; 101(6): 395–8.

Van Der Heijden BJ, Carlus C, Narcy F et al. Persistent anuria, neonatal death, and renal microcystic lesions after prenatal exposure to indomethacin. Am J Obstet Gynecol 1994; 171: 617–23.

Van Der Velde M, Vercauteren M, Vandermeersch E. Fetal heart rate abnormalities after regional analgesia for labor pain: the effect of intrathecal opioids. Reg Anaesth Pain Med 2001; 26: 257–62.

Vermillion ST, Scardo JA, Lashus AG et al. The effect of indomethacin tocolysis on fetal ductus arteriosus constriction with advancing gestational age {see comments}. Am J Obstet Gynecol 1997; 177: 256–9.

Viegas OA, Khaw B, Ratnam SS. Tramadol in labour pain in primiparous patients. A prospective comparative clinical trial. Eur J Obstet Gynecol Reprod Biol 1993; 49: 131–5.

Von Almen WF, Miller JM. Ts and Blues in pregnancy. J Reprod Med 1986; 31: 236–9.

Wang PH, Yang MJ, Lee WL et al. Acetaminophen poisoning in late pregnancy. J Reprod Med 1997; 42: 367–71.

Werler MM, Sheehan JE, Mitchell AA. Association of vasoconstrictive exposures with risks of gastroschisis and small intestinal atresia. Epidemiology 2002; 14: 349–54.

Wunsch MJ, Stanard V, Schnoll SH. Treatment of pain in pregnancy. Clin J Pain 2003; 19: 148–55.

Zenker M, Klinge J, Kruger C et al. Severe pulmonary hypertension in a neonate caused by premature closure of the ductus arteriosus following maternal treatment with diclofenac: a case report. J Perinat Med 1998; 26: 231–4.

Antiallergic drugs and desensitization

2.2

Margreet Rost van Tonningen

To date, the treatment of allergic symptoms in pregnancy with anti-histamines has not been incriminated as being embryo- or fetotoxic. Some antihistamines are used for the treatment of hyperemesis gravidarum (see Chapter 2.4) and also as hypnotic drugs (see Chapter 2.11). The treatment of allergy with corticosteroids is described in Chapters 2.3 and 2.15, and with sodium cromoglycate in Chapter 2.3.

2.2.1   Antihistamines (H_1-blocker)

Pharmacology

Antihistamines are substances that competitively block the action of histamine on the histamine receptors. Histamine release results in the stimulation of H_1-receptors located on the smooth muscles of many organs, or H_2-receptors located in the mucosa of the stomach, producing an increase in acid secretion. Only the blocking of the H_1-receptors is essential in antiallergy therapy.

H_1-antihistamines are mostly used in antiallergy therapy; some are used as antiemetics and some as sedatives. The less sedating antihistamines are preferred for antiallergy therapy.

Of the first-generation antihistamines, *alimemazine, bamipine, brompheniramine, carbinoxamine, chlorpheniramine, chlorphenox-amine, clemastine, cyproheptadine, dexchlorpheniramine, dimetin-dene, diphenhydramine, hydroxyzine, mebhydroline, oxatomide, pheniramine, triprolidine,* and *tripelenamine* among others, have been or are still used as antiallergic drugs.

Second- and third-generation antihistamines such as *acrivastin, astemizole, azelastine, cetirizine, desloratadine, ebastin, fexofenadin, levocabastine, levocetirizine, loratadine, mequitazine, mizolastine, oxatomide, terfenadine,* and *tritoqualin* are less sedating than the first-generation agents. The half-lives for astemizole and for terfenadine are very long (20–26 hours, astemizole metabolites 9 days!). Serious cardiovascular events and potentially serious drug interactions have been reported with respect to terfenadine and astemizol. In many countries, astemizole and terfenadine have been removed from the market. Some of the above-mentioned drugs are only available for local use. For azelastine and oxatomide, see also Chapter 2.3.

Toxicology

First-generation antihistamines

A large number of pregnancies exposed to first-generation anti-histamines such as *chlorpheniramine, clemastine, dexchlorpheni-ramine, dimetindene, diphenhydramine, hydroxyzine, mebhydroline,* and *pheniramine* have been studied to date. No increased terato-genic risk has been detected (Gilbert 2005, Källén 2002, 2003, Schatz 1997, Lione 1996).

Only a limited number of pregnancies exposed to *brompheni-ramine, cyproheptadine, triprolidine,* and *tripelenamine* have been studied, but no increased risk of congenital malformations was noted (Mazzotta 1999). In animal experiments, cyproheptadine was toxic to fetal pancreatic cells. The comparable effects in humans have not been reported, but experience with the use of cyproheptadine in pregnancy is very limited.

One study uncovered an association between the use of antihist-amines during the 2 weeks preceding delivery and an increased risk of retrolental fibroplasia (Zierler 1986). Other investigators have not confirmed this association.

Diphenhydramine and *dimenhydrinate*, when used parenterally in late pregnancy, may stimulate uterine contractions, leading to concern about fetal hypoxia (Broussard 1998; see also Chapter 2.4).

Withdrawal symptoms (e.g. generalized tremulousness and diar-rhea) have been reported after the use of the antihistamines diphen-hydramine and hydroxyzine throughout pregnancy (Lione 1996). A recent publication reports on a term newborn with tonic–clonic seizures starting 4 hours after birth, whose mother had received 150 mg hydroxyzine per day for anxiolysis. The newborn's plasma levels paralleled those of its mother 6 hours after birth. The authors interpreted the seizures as withdrawal symptoms. The neurological development was uneventful at the age of 6 months (Serreau 2005).

Second- and third-generation antihistamines
Among 66 pregnant women exposed to *acrivastin* during early pregnancy, no indication for teratogenicity was observed (Källén 2002, Wilton 1998).

In prospective studies on *astemizole* use in 187 pregnancies, no association was found between astemizole exposure in the first trimester and the occurrence of congenital malformations or other adverse effects (Diav-Citrin 2003, Pastuszak 1998). However, like terfenadine, astemizole has been withdrawn in many countries because of cardiotoxicity.

There is a fair amount of experience with the use of *cetirizine* – an active metabolite of *hydroxyzine* – during pregnancy. In a very small prospective study (39 pregnancies), cetirizine use during the first trimester was not associated with a teratogenic risk (Einarson 1997). Two recent prospective controlled studies by members of the European Network of Teratology Information Services (ENTIS) demonstrated no increased risk of congenital malformations or other adverse effects after exposure to cetirizine during pregnancy, of which 292 were first-trimester exposures (Weber-Schöndorfer 2005, Paulus 2004). Data from the Swedish Medical Birth Registry on cetirizine exposure during pregnancy ($n = 917$) confirm these findings (Källén 2002).

Among 39 first-trimester exposures, there were no indications for teratogenicity of *ebastin* (Källén 2002).

Post-marketing prescription-event monitoring found no drug-related adverse outcome in 47 pregnancies exposed to *fexofenadine*, the active metabolite of terfenadine (Craig-McFeely 2001).

The best-studied second-generation antihistamine is *loratadine*. Data on more than 4000 exposed pregnancies are documented. The Swedish Medical Birth Registry reported finding a prevalence of hypospadias in male offspring that was twice that of the general population among approximately 3000 women who had taken loratadine in pregnancy (Källén 2001). This report had a number of design limitations. The finding of an increased risk of hypospadias was not confirmed in various subsequent studies and reports. Two prospective controlled studies found no increased risk of congenital malformations and no cases of hypospadias after exposure to loratadine in approximately 370 pregnancies, of which 336 were exposed at least during the first trimester (Diav-Citrin 2003, Moretti 2003). Unpublished data of the European Network of Teratology Information

Services (ENTIS) on loratadine exposure during pregnancy did not yield any case of hypospadias to date. Investigators at the Centers for Disease Control analyzed data from the National Birth Defects Prevention Study. The use of loratadine was identified in only 1.7% of the entire study population, and no statistical association with the use of loratadine (or other antihistamines) and hypospadias was detected in these data (Werler 2004). An examination of Danish birth registries, reported in abstract, identified cases of hypospadias and investigated prescription records for each case and a matched control group. This study did not find a significant association between maternal exposure to loratadine and an increased risk of hypospadias (Pedersen 2004). To date, continuous post-marketing surveillance has found no further evidence of an increased risk of hypospadias.

In prospective studies covering almost 300 pregnancies, and one record linkage study on *terfenadine* use during pregnancy, no increased risk of malformations could be detected after the first-trimester use (Diav-Citrin 2003, Loebstein 1999, Schick 1994). Data from the Swedish Medical Birth Registry on terfenadine exposure during pregnancy confirm these findings (Källén 2002). However, terfenadine has been withdrawn in many countries because of cardiotoxicity.

There are absent or few human data on the use of the following antihistamines: *bamipine, carbinoxamine, desloratadine, levocabastine, levocetirizine, mequitazin, mizolastine,* and *tritoqualin* (Gilbert 2005, Källén 2002).

Recommendation. First-generation H_1-blockers like chlorpheniramine, dexchlorpheniramine, mebhydroline, clemastine, and dimetindene can be used during pregnancy for the treatment of allergic conditions. As the best-studied second-generation antihistamine, loratadine can be used during pregnancy for the treatment of allergic conditions. Cetirizine could be an acceptable second choice. It should be noted that neonatal respiratory depression has been reported after perinatal use of some first-generation antihistamines. To date, the inadvertent use of the new and/or less well-documented antihistamines does not require termination of pregnancy or invasive diagnostic procedures. When feasible, local treatment with intranasal sodium cromoglycate, beclomethason or budesonide is preferred in conditions like allergic rhinitis etc. (see Chapter 2.3).

2.2.2   Glucocorticosteroids

See Chapters 2.3 and 2.15.

2.2.3   Mast cell stabilizers

See Chapter 2.3.

2.2.4   Immunotherapy

Pharmacology and toxicology

Allergen immunotherapy (*allergy shots*) is an antiallergy therapy in which continuously increasing doses of an allergen are injected subcutaneously. This therapy stimulates the production of immunoglobulins that bind the allergen before it can react with the mast cells. After immunotherapy, the allergic reaction on exposure to the allergen will be diminished because less histamine will be released by the mast cells. Immunotherapy is often effective for those allergic patients in whom the symptoms persist despite optimal environmental control and drug therapy. No specific embryo- or fetotoxic effects are to be expected after immunotherapy in pregnancy (Gilbert 2005, Shaikh 1993). However, a maternal anaphylactic reaction can cause hypotension and decreased uterine perfusion, which may result in fetal damage induced by fetal hypoxia (Luciano 1997).

> **Recommendation.** Allergen immunotherapy can be carefully continued during pregnancy in patients who benefit and are not experiencing adverse reactions. Due to the greater risk of anaphylaxis with increasing doses of immunotherapy, and a delay of several months before immunotherapy becomes effective, it is generally recommended that this therapy is not started during pregnancy. For the same reason, doses should not be increased. There is no indication for the termination of pregnancy or additional diagnostic procedures after immunotherapy during pregnancy.

References

Broussard CN, Richter JE. Nausea and vomiting of pregnancy. Gastroenterol Clin North Am 1998; 27: 123–51.

Craig-McFeely PM, Acharya NV, Shakir SA. Evaluation of the safety of fexofenadine from experience gained in general practice use in England in 1997. Eur J Clin Pharmacol 2001; 57: 313–20.

Diav-Citrin O, Shechtman S, Aharonovich A et al. Pregnancy outcome after gestational exposure to loratadine or antihistamines: a prospective controlled cohort study. J Allerg Clin Immunol 2003; 111: 1239–43.

Einarson A, Bailey B, Jung G et al. Prospective controlled study of hydroxyzine and cetirizine in pregnancy. Ann Allergy Asthma Immunol 1997; 78: 183–6.

2

Pregnancy

2.2 Antiallergic drugs and desensitization

Gilbert C, Mazzotta P, Loebstein R et al. Fetal safety of drugs used in the treatment of allergic rhinitis – a critical review. Drug Saf 2005; 28: 707–19.

Källén B, Olausson PO. Monitoring of maternal drug use and infant congenital malformations. Does loratadine cause hypospadias? Intl J Risk Saf Med 2001; 14: 115–19.

Källén B. Use of antihistamine drugs in early pregnancy and delivery outcome. J Matern Fetal Neonatal Med 2002; 11: 146–52.

Källén B, Mottet I. Delivery outcome after the use of meclozine in early pregnancy. Eur J Epidemiol 2003; 18: 665–9.

Lione A, Scialli A. The developmental toxicity of the H1 histamine antagonists. Reprod Toxicol 1996; 10; 247–55.

Loebstein R, Lalkin A, Addis A et al. Pregnancy outcome after gestational exposure to terfenadine: a multicenter, prospective controlled study. J Allerg Clin Immunol 1999; 104: 953–6.

Luciano R, Zuppa AA, Maragliano G et al. Fetal encephalopathy after maternal anaphylaxis. Case report. Biol Neonate 1997; 71: 190–93.

Mazzotta P, Loebstein R, Koren G. Treating allergic rhinitis in pregnancy. Safety considerations. Drug Saf 1999; 20: 361–75.

Moretti ME, Caprara D, Coutinho CJ et al. Fetal safety of loratadine use in the first trimester of pregnancy: a multicenter study. J Allerg Clin Immunol 2003;111: 479–83.

Pastuszak A, Schick B, D'Alimonte D et al. The safety of astemizole in pregnancy. J Allergy Clin Immunol 1996; 98: 748–50.

Paulus W, Schloemp S, Sterzik K et al. Pregnancy outcome after exposure to cetirizine/levocetirizine in the first trimester – a prospective controlled study {Abstract}. Reprod Toxicol 2004; 19: 258.

Pedersen L, Skriver MV, Soslashrensen HT. Maternal use of loratadine during pregnancy and risk of hypospadias in offspring: a Danish nested case control design. Pharmacoepidemiology Drug Saf 2004; 13(Suppl 1): S207.

Schatz M, Petitti D. Antihistamines and pregnancy. Ann Allergy Asthma Immunol 1997; 78(2): 157–9.

Schick B, Holm M, Librizzi R et al. Terfenadine (teldane) exposure in early pregnancy. Teratology 1994; 49: 417.

Serreau R, Komiha M, Blanc F et al. Neonatal seizures with maternal hydroxyzine hydrochloride in late pregnancy. Reprod Toxicol 2005; 20: 573–4.

Shaikh WA. A retrospective study on the safety of immunotherapy in pregnancy. Clin Exp Allergy 1993; 23: 857–60.

Weber-Schöndorfer C, Hannemann D, Schaefer C. The safety of cetirizine in pregnancy. a prospective controlled study of the Berlin TIS. Presentation at the 16th Annual Conference of the European Network of Teratology Information Services (ENTIS) 2005, Haarlem, The Netherlands.

Werler M, McCloskey C, Edmonds LD et al. Evaluation of an association between loratadine and hypospadias – United States, 1997–2001. J Am Med Assoc 2004; 291: 1828–30.

Wilton LV, Pearce GL, Martin RM et al. The outcomes of pregnancy in women exposed to newly marketed drugs in general practice in England. Br J Obstet Gynaecol 1998; 105: 882–9.

Zierler S, Purohit D. Prenatal antihistamine exposure and retrolental fibroplasia. Am J Epidemiol 1986; 123: 192–6.

Antiasthmatic and cough medication

2.3

Hanneke Garbis

2.3.1   Asthma and pregnancy

An increasing number of pregnancies (5–8%) are complicated by asthma. The course and severity of asthma can change during pregnancy, and may improve, remain unchanged or worsen.

Asthmatic women have an increased risk of pregnancy complications and adverse outcome, such as hypertensive disorders, preterm labor and delivery, intrauterine growth restriction, placenta praevia, cesarean delivery and low birth weight, especially when asthma is inadequately or poorly controlled (Beckmann 2003, Bracken 2003, Mihrshahi 2003, Wen 2001, Källén 2000, Alexander 1998, Demissie 1998). However, when asthma is aggressively controlled and well-managed, there has been no reported association with adverse infant and maternal outcomes or asthma complicating pregnancies (Olesen 2001, Jana 1995, Schatz 1995).

Stenius-Aarniala and colleagues report that there is no serious effect on pregnancy outcome if an acute asthma attack is adequately treated (Stenius-Aarniala 1996). The risk of suffering an acute attack is higher in patients using inadequate anti-inflammatory treatment.

Pregnant women with asthma should receive optimal treatment and be closely monitored (Cousins 1999). The commonly used drugs for the treatment of asthma do not pose a risk to pregnant women. These drugs are:

- inhaled selective β_2-adrenergic agonists
- inhaled corticosteroids
- inhaled anticholinergics
- systemic theophylline
- inhaled cromoglycic acid (sodium cromoglycate) for prevention of allergic asthma.

The drugs of first choice during pregnancy are inhaled short-acting β_2-adrenergic agonists and inhaled corticosteroids.

A number of reviews on the pathophysiology and management of asthma during pregnancy have been published (Murphy 2005, NAEPP Expert Panel Report 2005, Joint Committee of ACOG and ACAAI 2000, Schatz 1999, Liccardi 1998).

2.3.2   Selective β_2-adrenergic agonists

Pharmacology and toxicology

β_2-adrenergic drugs specifically act at β_2-receptors. The intermediate-acting β_2-adrenergic agonists *bitolterol, fenoterol, metaproterenol, pirbuterol, reproterol, salbutamol (albuterol), terbutaline*, and *tulobuterol*, and the long-acting β_2-adrenergic agonists *formoterol* and *salmeterol*, belong to this group and are used for the treatment of asthma.

β_2-agonists cause bronchodilation. They also inhibit uterine contractions in the second and third trimesters, and therefore are effective in the treatment of premature labor. They can be given orally, by inhalation, or by subcutaneous or intravenous injection. Inhalation is as effective as the other routes, and is preferred since the side effects are minimal.

β_2-agonists are well-absorbed when given orally, but have a low systemic availability. Plasma protein binding is low, elimination is by the kidneys, and the half-life (3–6 hours) is short in the intermediate-acting agonists but much longer (over 12 hours) in the long-acting agonists formoterol and salmeterol. β_2-agonists rapidly cross the placenta. Lyrenäs and colleagues found an increase in the clearance of terbutaline during pregnancy resulting in lower plasma concentrations (Lyrenäs 1986).

Therapy with inhaled β_2-adrenergic agonists appears to be safe during pregnancy. No increase in the rate of congenital malformations or other adverse pregnancy outcome has been reported (Schatz 2004, 1997, 1988). Most data are available for metaproterenol, salbutamol (albuterol) and terbutaline. There is insufficient experience with *bambuterol, clenbuterol, pirbuterol,* and tulobuterol during the first trimester; however, there is no indication yet for teratogenicity.

The experience with the use of the newer long-acting β_2-agonists formoterol and salmeterol during pregnancy is limited. High serum concentrations can occur with the use of these substances. In animal experiments, malformations have been found after prenatal exposure to salmeterol.

Adverse reactions in the fetus and the newborn (tremors, tachycardia, hypoglycemia, and hypokalemia) have been reported, especially when high doses of β_2-agonists are used. The effects are less common when used by inhalation, and they are reversible. Baker and Flanagan reported a case of maternal and fetal tachycardia after inadvertant inhalation of high doses of albuterol for 24 hours in week 33 (Baker 1997). The heart rate became normal after the discontinuation of albuterol.

High doses at the end of pregnancy can cause an inhibition of labor. Large intravenous doses of salbutamol as given for premature labor can produce hyperglycemic ketoacidosis in diabetic women.

> **Recommendation.** β_2-adrenergic agonists can be safely used during pregnancy. The short-acting salbutamol (albuterol), metaproterenol and terbutaline are first-choice drugs in the treatment of pregnant women. According to therapy guidelines, their use by inhalation is preferred. The dose may need to be adjusted. The long-acting β_2-agonists formoterol and salmeterol should only be used if they are essential to an optimal treatment. A tocolytic potential and betamimetic effects in the fetus have to be considered in case of a treatment at the end of pregnancy.

2.3.3   Corticosteroids

See also Chapter 2.15.

Pharmacology and toxicology

Inhaled corticosteroids are effective in the treatment of asthma and are first choice drugs. Stenius-Aarniala and colleagues reported that treatment with inhaled corticosteroids clearly reduces the risk of having an acute attack of asthma during pregnancy (Stenius-Aarniala 1996).

Inhaled corticosteroids have anti-inflammatory properties and increase the sensitivity of the bronchial system for β-adrenergic drugs. *Beclomethasone dipropionate, budesonide, flunisolide, fluticasone propionate, mometasone,* and *triamcinolone acetonide* are available for this purpose.

Topically active corticosteroids have minimal or no systemic side effects when used at the recommended doses. It is only high doses of inhaled corticosteroids that have been associated with systemic side effects, especially adrenal suppression (e.g. beclomethasone at a daily dose of 1500 µg or more).

All inhaled corticosteroids except for beclomethasone dipropionate pass into the systemic circulation as unchanged active drug. Beclomethasone dipropionate undergoes first-pass activation in the lungs and nose. They all are rapidly cleared after absorption.

Corticosteroids have been found to induce cleft palate in the mouse. There is no strong evidence that they are teratogenic in the human.

Beclomethasone has been used for many years in pregnant women without evidence of adverse effects on pregnancy or fetal development (Dombrowski 2004, 1997, Schatz 2004, 1997, Greenberger 1983).

In several large studies covering more than 6000 pregnancies, no increased incidence of congenital malformations or other adverse pregnancy outcome could be found after maternal exposure to inhaled budesonide (Gluck 2005, Norjavaara 2003, Källén 1999) and other inhaled cortisteroids (Rahimi 2006).

Maternal use of inhaled corticosteroids does not impair fetal growth (Rahimi 2006, Bakhireva 2005, Namazy 2005).

High doses of systemic corticosteroids for longer periods may cause intrauterine growth restriction, and are best avoided (Bakhireva 2005). In cases where higher doses are required, fetal growth should be monitored during treatment.

Several authors have found that pregnant women who used oral corticosteroids had an increased risk of hypertensive disorders. As oral corticosteroids were used mainly by women with severe asthma, it was difficult to separate the effects of the drug from those associated with the asthma. The authors concluded that, when indicated, there is no reason to withhold oral corticosteroids from pregnant women (Schatz 2004, 1997, Alexander 1998, Stenius-Aarniala

1988). Rahimi and colleagues could not confirm an increased risk of inhaled corticosteroids for hypertensive disorders (Rahimi 2006).

Intranasal corticosteroids are effective in the treatment of allergic rhinitis. They are safe, and there is no evidence of systemic effects. Bioavailability is higher than after inhalation, but the recommended dose for allergic rhinitis is lower than the dose given by inhalation. For this indication, beclomethasone has also been shown to be safe during pregnancy (Gilbert 2005). Data on pregnancy outcome after maternal exposure to intranasal budesonide are limited, but as pharmacological studies did show a much lower systemic exposure after intranasal administration, their safety is comparable to orally inhaled budesonide (Gluck 2005).

> **Recommendation.** Inhaled corticosteroids are the first drugs of choice for the treatment of asthma in pregnant women. The use of beclomethasone or budesonide is preferred, because these have been widely used in pregnancy and have a good safety record. Systemic use of the corticosteroids, prednisone, and its metabolite, prednisolone, is indicated in case of acute exacerbations of asthma or severe asthma during pregnancy. In the case of long-term treatment (for months), it is recommended that fetal growth and neonatal adrenal function be monitored, especially if higher doses are used. For allergic rhinitis, intranasal corticoids may be used. The use of inhaled or systemic corticosteroids in the first trimester is not an indication for the termination of pregnancy or for invasive diagnostics.

2.3.4   Anticholinergic drugs

Pharmacology and toxicology

Bronchodilating effects can also be achieved by drugs that act on the vagus nerve, such as anticholinergic drugs.

Inhaled *ipratropium bromide* is the drug of choice for the long-term treatment of chronic bronchitis. Its bronchodilating activity is about two-thirds of that of β_2-adrenergic drugs, and it may augment the bronchodilator responsiveness to β_2-agonists. Ipratropium is available as a single drug or in combination with a β_2-agonist (fenoterol and salbutamol). Side effects are minimal.

Data on the use of inhaled ipratropium during pregnancy are limited, but the drug has not been related to an increased risk of congenital malformations or other adverse pregnancy outcomes.

There is no or very limited experience with the treatment of *oxitropium bromide* and *tiotropium bromide* during pregnancy.

> **Recommendation.** Inhaled ipratropium bromide can be used during pregnancy if needed. Inadvertent use of oxitropium bromide or tiotropium bromide is not an indication for the termination of pregnancy or for specific diagnostics.

2.3.5   Theophylline

Pharmacology and toxicology

Theophylline is a methylxanthine and has been used for many years as a bronchodilator in the treatment and the prophylaxis of chronic asthma; it also has anti-inflammatory and immunomodulatory properties. Theophylline is also useful in the treatment of apnea in premature infants as it increases the sensitivity of the respiratory center in the brain, resulting in an increased respiratory frequency.

Theophylline acts by inhibiting phosphodiesterase enzymes which cause an increase in the intracellular concentration of *c*-AMP, and a subsequent relaxation of the smooth muscles in the airways and the pulmonary artery.

Since the availability of newer pharmacological agents, and because of concern about its toxicity, theophylline is no longer a first-line treatment. It may be added when severe symptoms do not respond rapidly to routine treatment with inhaled β_2-agonists and corticosteroids.

Theophylline has a narrow therapeutic index; therapeutic concentrations are between 10 and 20 μg/ml. It is demethylated and hydroxylated in the liver, and eliminated by the kidneys. The half-life in adults is about 5 hours.

During pregnancy the plasma protein binding of theophylline is reduced, resulting in an increase in the free drug. Moreover, the elimination of theophylline is decreased by about 25% in the third trimester (Connelly 1990, Gardner 1987). Therefore, serum concentrations should be monitored and the dose adjusted if necessary. It is recommended that theophylline plasma levels be kept between 8 and 12 μg/ml in pregnant asthmatics (NAEPP Expert Panel Report 2005, Connelly 1990).

Theophylline readily crosses the placenta, and is metabolized to caffeine in the fetal liver. Therapeutic levels of theophylline have been found in the newborn. The half-life in the newborn is 10–16 hours, but is even longer (up to 30 hours) in premature infants. As a result of the longer half-life, toxic concentrations may be reached in the neonate. Therefore, it is recommended that newborns be monitored for signs of toxicity, especially when premature.

There are conflicting data as to whether or not theophylline is associated with malformations. Park and colleagues reported three cases of severe cardiovascular malformations after prenatal exposure to theophylline (Park 1990), but other studies demonstrate no association with congenital malformations (Dombrowski 2004, Schatz 2004, 1997, Stenius-Aarniala 1995, Heinonen 1977). There is disagreement concerning data on the possible association between the use of theophylline and an increased risk of pre-eclampsia. The development of pre-eclampsia is most probably due to factors other than theophylline.

Theophylline causes changes in fetal breathing movements (Ishikawa 1996). Adverse effects such as vomiting, irritability, jitteriness, bradycardia or tachycardia, and cyanosis have been reported in the newborn. Due to the prolonged half-life of theophylline in the newborn, the effects disappear only slowly. Therefore, high doses of theophylline are best avoided during pregnancy, especially near term. Neonatal jaundice has been reported after the oral use of theophylline.

Gastrointestinal dysfunction in premature newborns has also been reported. Prenatal theophylline is used to enhance organ maturation and to avoid risks related to premature birth when the maternal disease does not allow the use of steroids. Gastric irritability and inhibition of the gut motility were seen in the newborn during the first days of life, but the risk of necrotizing enterocolitis was not increased (Zanardo 1996).

> **Recommendation.** Theophylline may be used for cases where the inhaled β_2-agonists and corticosteroids are insufficient to control the asthmatic diseases. Steady-state serum concentrations should be closely monitored, and maintained at 8–12 µg/ml. High doses should be avoided, especially near term, in order to avoid toxic concentrations in the newborn. Newborns, especially when preterm, should be monitored for adverse effects.

2.3.6   Cromoglycate, nedocromil, and Iodoxamide

Pharmacology and toxicology

Sodium cromoglycate is widely used in the prophylactic treatment of allergic diseases, especially bronchial asthma and allergic rhinitis. It inhibits histamine release from mast cells by a stabilizing effect on the cell membrane. It is usually given by inhalation or intranasally. The bioavailability following inhalation is low (<10%), and side effects are few.

Sodium cromoglycate can be safely used during pregnancy (Gilbert 2005). Schatz (1997) and Wilson (1982) report on the pregnancy outcome of asthmatic women who were treated throughout pregnancy with sodium cromoglycate. The incidence of congenital malformations in the offspring was not increased, and there were no adverse effects on the course of pregnancy.

Nedocromil sodium is not chemically related to sodium cromoglycate, but has similar pharmacological and pharmacokinetic properties; and it suppresses the influx of eosinophils into allergic lesions. There is insufficient experience with the use of nedocromil and *lodoxamide* during pregnancy.

> **Recommendation.** Sodium cromoglycate can be safely used in pregnant women for the prophylactic treatment of allergic diseases such as asthma and allergic rhinitis. Lodoxamide and nedocromil should be avoided until data on their safety during pregnancy are available. Inadvertent use does not require any intervention.

2.3.7   Other mast cell inhibitors

Pharmacology and toxicology

Ketotifen and *oxatomide* are second-generation H_1-receptor antagonists. They not only inhibit mast cell degranulation, but also have antihistaminic and antianaphylactic effects by blocking histamine receptors. There is no primary role for these agents in the management of asthmatic disease, but they can be used when oral therapy is preferred.

Azelastine has a similar activity, and also protects against leukotriene-induced bronchospasms. There are no data on the safety of ketotifen, oxatomide and azelastine for pregnant women.

> **Recommendation.** The use of ketotifen, oxatomide, and azelastine should be avoided during pregnancy. Inadvertent use does not require any intervention.

2.3.8   Antileukotrienes

Pharmacology and toxicology

Leukotrienes are involved in the pathogenesis of both acute and chronic asthma. They cause increased bronchoconstriction, mucous secretion, and vascular permeability. The action of leukotrienes can be blocked via inhibition of their production, e.g. with *zileuton*, or by blocking the leukotriene receptors with a new pharmacological class of drugs, e.g. *montelukast* and *zafirlukast*. Antileukotrienes are well tolerated, but data on their use during pregnancy are scarce.

There are limited data on pregnancy outcomes after maternal use of montelukast. In two prospective studies with small numbers, no increased rates of congenital malformations, preterm births, or low birth weights were found (Bakhireva 2006, Sarkar 2005). Several prospective and retrospective cases of limb reduction defects have been reported to the manufacturer and in international reports, but a causative relationship between montelukast and limb defects has not yet been established. It should be used only in patients with recalcitrant asthma with known favorable response before pregnancy.

> **Recommendation.** Apart from selected cases, antileukotrienes should be avoided in pregnant women. The use of montelukast and zafirlukast may be considered in patients with recalcitrant asthma who have shown a uniquely favorable response prior to pregnancy. The use of zileuton should be avoided, because of non-reassuring animal data (Namazy 2004). In the case of first-trimester use of antileukotrienes, a detailed fetal scan should be offered. It is not an indication for the termination of pregnancy.

2.3.9   Monoclonal antibodies and other asthma medications

Pharmacology and toxicology

A new approach in asthma therapy is the use of monoclonal antibodies against IgE. *Omalizumab* was introduced in 2005. There is no experience with its use in pregnancy yet.

The so-called PDEH-type-4 agent *roflumilast* has not yet been licensed. It has anti-inflammatory but no bronchodilating properties, is orally available, and may be effective in chronic obstructive lung diseases. There is no experience in pregnancy with roflumilast or with *cilomilast*.

> **Recommendation.** The use of these new agents should be avoided in pregnancy. In the case of first-trimester exposure, a detailed fetal scan should be offered. It is not an indication for the termination of pregnancy.

2.3.10   Expectorants and mucolytic agents

Pharmacology and toxicology

Expectorants and mucolytic agents enhance or facilitate the clearance of mucus in the respiratory tract.

Ambroxol is a metabolite of *bromhexine*, and has been used in the prevention of neonatal respiratory distress syndrome with no reported maternal or fetal/neonatal side effects.

N-acetylcysteine is a derivative of the amino acid L-cysteine, and is used as a mucolytic agent and an antidote in paracetamol (acetaminophen) poisoning. Although the documented data on its use as a mucolytic during pregnancy are scarce, it seems to be safe when used in low doses.

Carbocysteine is a mucus regulator rather than a mucolytic agent.

Guaifenesin and *guaiacol* stimulate the clearance of viscous mucus via stimulation of the gastropulmonary vagal reflex, but they have no effect on the thickness of the mucus. There is no evidence of an increased risk of congenital malformations or other adverse effects on pregnancy outcome.

Mesna is an expectorant that breaks the disulfide bonds in mucopolysaccharides present in the mucus. Data on human pregnancy outcome are not available.

Potassium iodide also has mucolytic properties. However, it may suppress fetal thyroid function.

> **Recommendation.** N-acetylcysteine, ambroxol and bromhexine are first-choice mucolytics during pregnancy, if (oral) fluid therapy, and other non-medical treatment is not effective. Iodine-containing mucolytics are contraindicated, especially after the first trimester. Inadvertent short-term use of the other expectorants and mucolytics does not require any intervention.

2.3.11   Antitussives

Pharmacology and toxicology

Codeine is the most widely used antitussive. It is a derivative of morphine, and has strong antitussive and analgesic properties. Because of its analgesic action, it is also used in compound antitussive preparations. An association between the prenatal use of codeine and congenital malformations has not been shown. When codeine is used in high doses for longer periods, or near term, respiratory depression and withdrawal symptoms can occur in the neonate (see also Chapter 2.1).

Dextromethorphan has no analgesic properties, but its antitussive effect is similar to that of codeine. Its use is considered safe during pregnancy. Einarson and associates reported pregnancy outcomes of women who had used dextromethorphan during pregnancy, most of them in the first trimester. No increased incidence of congenital malformations or other adverse pregnancy outcomes was found (Einarson 2001). In another recent study, an association between congenital malformations and prenatal exposure to dextromethorphan could not be established (Martínez-Frias 2001).

There is no experience in the use of other antitussives, such as *benproperine, clobutinol, dropropizine, eprazinone, noscapin, pentoxyverin*, and *pipacetate*, during pregnancy.

> **Recommendation.** In the case of persistent dry cough, codeine and dextromethorphan can be given in all trimesters of pregnancy. Higher doses given for longer periods, or use near delivery, can cause neonatal withdrawal symptoms and respiratory depression. Inadvertent use of other antitussives does not require any intervention.

2.3.12   Non-selective β-adrenergic agonists

Non-selective β-adrenergic agonists are not recommended for asthma treatment. Some of these drugs are used in oral OTC drugs for the common cold. These combinations do not follow good therapeutic practices, and are not recommended during pregnancy.

Hexoprenaline, isoprenaline, and orciprenaline

Pharmacology and toxicology

Hexoprenaline, isoprenaline (isoproterenol), and *orciprenaline* have a stimulating effect on β-receptors. They are non-selective β-adrenergic agents that act on both β_1- and β_2-receptors, and therefore have unwanted side effects on cardiac and metabolic functions, central nervous system, and motility of the gastrointestinal tract.

There is no experience in the use of orciprenaline and hexoprenaline during pregnancy. Limited experience with isoprenaline does not show adverse effects on embryonal and fetal development.

> **Recommendation.** *Hexoprenaline, isoprenaline*, and *orciprenaline* should not be given to pregnant women. Only specific β_2-adrenergic drugs are recommended during pregnancy. Inadvertent use is not an indication for the termination of pregnancy.

▶ Adrenalin (epinephrine)

Pharmacology and toxicology

Adrenalin (*epinephrine*) is a catecholamine, which is normally present in the body. It has both α- and β-adrenergic properties, and causes a slight vasoconstriction in the bronchi. Adverse effects on the cardiovascular system are so severe that it is not indicated for the treatment of bronchial asthma. $β_2$-adrenergic agents are preferred. In the case of acute spastic airway obstruction, adrenalin may be effective when given subcutaneously or as an aerosol. Due to α-adrenergic effects, systemic application can impair uterine blood flow resulting in fetal hypoxia. Catecholamines cross the placenta where they are inactivated. There is no clear evidence of an increased risk of congenital malformations when using adrenalin in human pregnancy (Heinonen 1977).

Adrenalin is also available in combination with local anesthetics. Adverse effects during pregnancy have not been reported following the use of such preparations.

> **Recommendation.** The systemic use of adrenaline during pregnancy is restricted to emergency cases. Inadvertent use is not an indication for the termination of pregnancy. Local anesthetics with adrenaline may be used during pregnancy.

▶ Ephedrine and other sympathomimetics

Pharmacology and toxicology

Ephedrine, pseudoephedrine, phenylephrine, and related compounds are α-adrenergic receptor agonists, which cause blood-vessel constriction. It has been demonstrated that α-adrenergic receptor agonists slow uterine blood flow, but their effects have not been sufficiently studied in relation to most reproductive outcomes in animals or humans. Ephedrine is one of the first drugs that was used for the treatment of asthma. It causes an increased release of catecholamines, and has both α- and β-adrenergic properties. It has a short duration of action. Ephedrine is no longer in use for the treatment of asthma because of the unwanted side effects, especially on the cardiovascular system. Pseudoephedrine, phenylephrine, and *phenylpropanolamine* are sometimes used in combination with dextromethorphan, doxylamine, etc., for treating the common cold.

Pseudoephedrine is often used to reduce airflow resistance in the nasal cavity. Ephedrine, and phenylephrine, have been associated with hemorrhages and cardiovascular and limb malformations in animal models. Risk of ventricular septal defects was associated with decongestant use in pregnant women in one recent study (review in Werler 2006). The vasoconstrictive effects of these drugs raise the hypothesis that their use in early pregnancy might increase the risk of vascular disruption defects. Decongestant use in the first trimester has been discussed in association with small increases in risks of gastroschisis, small intestinal atresia, and hemifacial microsomia (review in Werler 2006). The majority of decongestant use is in oral form, and the question of whether intranasal formulations carry risk has not been adequately addressed.

Recommendation. The systemic use of ephedrine and other sympathomimetics should be avoided during pregnancy. Inadvertent use is not an indication for the termination of pregnancy.

References

Alexander S, Dodds L, Armson BA. Perinatal outcomes in women with asthma during pregnancy. Obstet Gynecol 1998; 92: 435–40.

Baker ER, Flanagan MR Fetal atrial flutter associated with maternal beta-sympathomimetic drug exposure. Obstet Gynecol 1997; 89: 861.

Bakhireva LN, Jones KL, Schatz M et al. Asthma medication use in pregnancy and fetal growth. J Allergy Clin Immunol 2005; 116: 503–9.

Bakhireva LN, Jones KL, Chambers CD. Safety of leukotriene receptor agonists in pregnancy. Birth Def Res A 2006; 76: 314.

Beckmann CA. The effects of asthma on pregnancy and perinatal outcomes. J Asthma 2003; 40: 181–7.

Bracken MB, Triche EW, Belanger K et al. Asthma symptoms, severity and drug therapy: a prospective study of effects on 2205 pregnancies. Obstet Gynecol 2003; 102: 739–52.

Briggs GG, Freeman RK, Yaffe SJ. Drugs in Pregnancy and Lactation, 7th edn. Philadelphia, PA: Lippincott Williams & Wilkins, 2005.

Connelly TJ, Ruo TI, Frederiksen MC et al. Characterization of theophylline binding to serum proteins in pregnant and nonpregnant women. Clin Pharmacol Ther 1990; 47: 68–72.

Cousins L. Fetal oxygenation, assessment of fetal well-being and obstetric management of the pregnant patient with asthma. J Allergy Clin Immunol 1999; 103: S343–9.

Demissie K, Breckenridge MB, Rhoads GG. Infant and maternal outcomes in the pregnancies of asthmatic women. Am J Respir Crit Care Med 1998; 158: 1091–5.

Dombrowski MP. Pharmacologic therapy of asthma during pregnancy. Obstet Gynecol Clin North Am 1997; 24: 559–74.

Dombrowski MP, Schatz M, Wise R et al. Randomized trial of inhaled beclomethasone dipropionate versus theophylline for moderate asthma during pregnancy. Am J Obstet Gynecol 2004; 190: 737–44.

Einarson A, Lyszkiewicz D, Koren G. The safety of dextromethorphan in pregnancy: results of a controlled study. Chest 2001; 119: 466–9.

Gardner MJ, Schatz M, Cousins L et al. Longitudinal effects of pregnancy on the pharmacokinetics of theophylline. Eur J Clin Pharmacol 1987; 31: 289–95.

Gilbert C, Mazzotta P, Loebstein R et al. Fetal safety of drugs used in the treatment of allergic rhinitis. A critical review. Drug Saf 2005; 28: 707–19.

Gluck PA, Gluck JC. A review of pregnancy outcomes after exposure to orally inhaled or intranasal budesonide. Curr Med Res Opin 2005; 21: 1075–84.

Greenberger PA, Patterson R. Beclomethasone dipropionate for severe asthma during pregnancy. Ann Intern Med 1983; 98: 478–80.

Heinonen OP, Slone D, Shapiro S. Birth Defects and Drugs in Pregnancy. Littleton, NH: Publishing Sciences Group, 1977.

Ishikawa M, Yoneyama Y, Power GG et al. Maternal theophylline administration and breathing movements in late-gestation human fetuses. Obstet Gynecol 1996; 88: 973–8.

Jana N, Vasishta K, Saha SC et al. Effect of bronchial asthma on the course of pregnancy, labour and perinatal outcome. J Obstet Gynaecol 1995; 21: 227–32.

Joint Committee of the American College of Obstetricians and Gynecologists (ACOG) and the American College of Allergy, Asthma and Immunology (ACAAI). Position statement. The use of newer asthma and allergy medications during pregnancy. Ann Allergy Asthma Immunol 2000; 84: 475–80.

Källén B, Rydhstroem H, Åberg A. Congenital malformations after the use of inhaled budesonide in early pregnancy. Obstet Gynecol 1999; 93: 392–5.

Källén B, Rydhstroem H, Åberg A. Asthma during pregnancy – a population based study. Eur J Epidemiol 2000; 16: 167–71.

Liccardi G, D'Amato M, D'Amato G. Asthma in pregnant patients: pathophysiology and management. Monaldi Arch Chest Dis 1998; 53: 151–9.

Lyrenäs S, Grahnén A, Lindberg B et al. Pharmacokinetics of terbutaline during pregnancy. Eur J Clin Pharmacol 1986; 29: 619–23.

Martínez-Frias ML, Rodriguez-Pinilla E. Epidemiologic analysis of prenatal exposure to cough medicines containing dextromethorphan: no evidence of human teratogenicity. Teratology 2001; 63: 38–41.

Mihrshahi S, Belousova E, Marks GB et al. Pregnancy and birth outcomes in families with asthma. J Asthma 2003; 40: 181–7.

Murphy VE, Gibson PG, Smith R et al. Asthma during pregnancy: mechanisms and treatment implications. Eur Respir J 2005; 25: 731–50.

NAEPP Expert Panel Report. Managing asthma during pregnancy: recommendations for pharmacologic treatment – 2004 update. J Allergy Clin Immunol 2005; 115: 34–46.

Namazy JA, Schatz M. Update in the treatment of asthma during pregnancy. Clin Rev Allergy Immunol 2004; 26: 139–48.

Namazy JA, Schatz M, Long L et al. Use of inhaled steroids by pregnant asthmatic women does not reduce intrauterine growth. J Allergy Clin Immunol 2005; 113: 427–32.

Norjavaara E, Gerhardsson de Verdier M. Normal pregnancy outcomes in a population-based study including 2968 pregnant women exposed to budesonide. J Allergy Clin Immunol 2003; 111: 736–42.

Olesen C, Thrane N, Nielsen GL et al for the EUROMAP group. A population-based prescription study of asthma drugs during pregnancy: changing the intensity of asthma therapy and perinatal outcomes. Respiration 2001; 68: 256–61.

Park JM, Schmer V, Myers TL. Cardiovascular anomalies associated with prenatal exposure to theophylline. Southern Med J 1990; 83: 1487–8.

Rahimi R, Nikfar S, Abdollahi M. Meta-analysis finds use of inhaled corticosteroids during pregnancy safe: a systematic meta-analysis review. Hum Exper Toxicol 2006; 25: 447–52.

Sarkar M, Koren G. Pregnancy outcome following gestational exposure to montelukast: a prospective controlled study: PI-83. Clin Pharmacol Therapeutics 2005; 77: 30.

Schatz M, Zeiger RS, Harden KM et al. The safety of inhaled β-agonist bronchodilators during pregnancy. J Allergy Clin Immunol 1988; 82: 686–95.

Schatz M, Zeiger RS, Hoffman CP et al. Perinatal outcomes in the pregnancies of asthmatic women: a prospective controlled analysis. Am J Respir Crit Care Med 1995; 151: 1170–74.

Schatz M, Zeiger RS, Harden K et al. The safety of asthma and allergy medications during pregnancy. J Allergy Clin Immunol 1997; 100: 301–6.

Schatz M. Interrelationship between asthma and pregnancy. A literature review. J Allergy Clin Immunol 1999; 103: S330–36.

Schatz M, Dombrowski MP, Wise R et al. The relationship of asthma medication use to perinatal outcomes. J Allergy Clin Immunol 2004; 113: 1040–45.

Stenius-Aarniala B, Piirilä P, Teramo K. Asthma and pregnancy: a prospective study of 198 pregnancies. Thorax 1988; 43: 12–18.

Stenius-Aarniala B, Ritkonen S, Teramo K. Slow-release theophylline in pregnant asthmatics. Chest 1995; 107: 642–7.

Stenius-Aarniala B, Hedman J, Teramo KA. Acute asthma during pregnancy. Thorax 1996; 51: 411–14.

Wen SW, Demissie K, Liu S. Adverse outcomes in pregnancies of asthmatic women: results from a Canadian population. Ann Epidemiol 2001; 11: 7–12.

Werler MM. Teratogen update: pseudoephedrine. Birth Def Res A 2006; 76: 445–52.

Wilson J. Utilisation du cromoglycate de sodium au cours de la grossesse. Acta Therapeutica 1982; 8(Suppl): 45–51.

Zanardo V, Trevisanuto D, Cagdas S et al. Prenatal theophylline and necrotizing enterocolitis in premature newborn infants. Ped Med Chir 1996; 18: 153–6.

2

Pregnancy

2.3 Antiasthmatic and cough medication

Antiemetics

2.4

Lee H. Goldstein and Matitiahu Berkovitch

2.4.1 Nausea and vomiting in pregnancy

Of all pregnant women, 50–80% suffer from nausea and vomiting of pregnancy (NVP), also known as morning sickness – although symptoms may persist throughout the whole day. Usually limited to the first trimester, NVP may continue for the entire pregnancy.

NVP may range from mild discomfort to severe vomiting and nausea, weight loss, dehydration and metabolic compromise. In severe cases, NVP can be fatal. The death of the famous Charlotte Brontë, author of *Jane Eyre* (1855), reflects the potential severity of NVP and the fact that at that time (the turn of the twentieth century) no therapy was considered necessary, as NVP was attributed solely to psychological factors and as such was not treated medically. NVP may pose a serious socioeconomic burden, as 25% of women suffering from NVP miss work as a result of their symptoms (Vellacott 1988).

The pathogenesis of NVP has been attributed to multiple factors such as elevated levels of β-hCG, prostaglandin levels (by relaxing the gastroesophageal sphincter), gastric dysrhythmia, vitamin B_6 deficiency, and hyperolfaction. Psychological factors (depression, anxiety, eating disorders), once considered the only etiology of NVP, might in fact be a result of the NVP. A genetic predisposition has been suggested based on the concordance in monozygotic twins, variation within ethnic groups, and the fact that siblings and mothers of patients with NVP are likely to have experienced NVP themselves (Goodwin 2002).

NVP has been postulated to protect the embryo by encouraging the mother to avoid potentially harmful or teratogenic foods and beverages (Furneaux 2001, Profet 1992, Hook 1976). For women suffering NVP, it may be reassuring to know that NVP is associated with less chance of spontaneous abortions and a reduced risk of congenital heart defects (Boneva 1999).

Women with past pregnancies complicated by severe forms of NVP or hyperemesis gravidarum may benefit by pre-emptive therapy, initiated as soon as the patient becomes aware of her pregnancy and before the symptoms of NVP appear. Twenty-five women with severe NVP in previous pregnancies were administered antiemetic therapy before symptoms of NVP became evident, and gradually increased the dosage of the antiemetic therapy as the NVP emerged. The severity of the NVP was significantly reduced in comparison to a group of women with the same maternity history of severe NVP in previous pregnancies who initiated antiemetic treatment only when the nausea and vomiting appeared (Koren 2004).

2.4.2   Diet manipulations and treatment

Nausea and vomiting is a common predicament in early pregnancy. Patients can be reassured of the benign nature of their condition and should be encouraged to use the various treatment options that have been proven efficacious with little risk to the fetus.

The treatment options for NVP range from conservative measures such as reassurance and diet manipulations in the mildly symptomatic women to drug therapy and, if necessary, in severe and intractable cases, intravenous rehydration and total parenteral nutrition (Koren 2000, Broussard 1998). Therapeutic pregnancy termination might be considered in severe intractable cases; however, this option is seldom utilized.

Dietary measures are often suggested for the mildly symptomatic women, although little evidence supports these measures. Women may benefit from frequent and small meals, with high carbohydrate and low fat content. Salty foods may be tolerated better in the morning, and sour or tart beverages may be tolerated better than water (Quinlan 2003).

An algorithm of treatment would depend on the women's preferences and the availability of the different modes of therapy. It would seem sensible to start treatment with dietary measures, lifestyle modifications and vitamin B_6. If symptoms persist, treatment with metoclopramide or diclectine (if available) should be started. The first- and some of the second-generation antihistamines are a good option, and if they fail then ondansetron would be the next choice. Intractable cases are best treated with intravenous antiemetics and steroids, and rehydration therapy; in severe cases, parenteral nutrition should be considered. Vitamin B1 should be administered in severe protracted cases in order to prevent thiamine deficiency. Alternative or complementary therapy such as acustimulation, hypnosis, and ginger can be considered at any stage. Hypnosis has proved efficient in a small number of trials, and the evidence for acustimulation as treatment of NVP is mixed. Ginger is safe and efficient when applied in the correct quantities and to women with certain yin-yang characteristics. These modes of therapy may be beneficial and are probably harmless to the pregnancy, and so may be worth a try if the woman is willing.

2.4.3   Complementary treatment options

Complementary therapy has become very popular in Western countries. Many people prefer complementary or "natural" therapy to medical therapy, believing that "natural" treatment is less harmful. Pregnant women and their doctors have been reluctant to use medical therapy during pregnancy, especially during the first trimester, when symptoms of NVP are worse, and so may prefer alternative therapy. See also Chapter 2.19.

The following section presents a review on the various alternative therapies available for NVP, and the evidence, if any, of efficacy and safety.

2.4.4   Acupuncture and acupressure

Acupuncture is a popular form of Chinese medicine, based on the notion that vital life energy (*qi*) flows through dozens of paths (meridians) throughout the human body. Illness is thought to be the result of obstructed or misdirected energy flow, and stimulating of acupoints within the meridian system is believed to restore health by correcting this flow. By inserting very thin needles 5 mm deep under the skin, different organs can be influenced via the meridians. Many acupoints influence the upper gastrointestinal tract, but the acupoint studied most by Western scientists is the P6 (*Nei Guan*), located on the anteromedial aspect of the forearm at a three-finger distance from the wrist crease, between the palmaris longus and flexor carpi radialis tendons. This point can be activated using needles (acupuncture) or by pressure (acupressure) applied by an acupressure band.

Numerous explanations have been proposed to explain the antiemetic influence of acupuncture and acupressure. The acupuncture needle presumably affects the diffuse noxious inhibitory controls of the spinal cord, causing secretion of β-endorphins (analgesic effect) and ACTH from the hypothalamus. The surge of ACTH causes an elevation of blood cortisol levels, influencing the brain stem emetic center (Streitberger 1998, Foster 1987, Malizia 1979). The acupuncture directly affects the upper GI tract by enhancing gastric myoelectrical activity and vagal tone (Li 1992).

Recently, acupuncture has been reported to have a relatively low incidence of complications, mostly temporary, in large population studies (total of 65 000 patients) (MacPherson 2001, Vincent 2001, White 2001). A trial comparing 4 weeks of traditional acupuncture, P6 acupuncture and placebo on NVP of approximately 600 pregnant women concluded that acupuncture in early pregnancy reduced or resolved nausea and dry retching earlier than if women waited for their symptoms to resolve spontaneously, but did not influence vomiting (Smith 2002A). There was no difference between the groups with regard to the incidence of spontaneous abortion, stillbirth or neonatal death. The incidence of major malformations was no larger than the incidence in the general population (3% total), and the overall risk of pregnancy complications did not differ between groups (antepartum hemorrhage, pregnancy-induced hypertension, pre-eclampsia and preterm birth). There were no differences in any birth outcomes, such as gestational age, weight, length, and head circumference (Smith 2002B). Also, P6 acupressure was useful in reducing nausea, vomiting, and dry retching (Markose 2004, Dundee 1988). Meta-analysis of the studies in 1306 patients summarized in the Cochrane database demonstrated mixed evidence, and did not clearly prove acupressure or acupuncture to be more effective than standard dietary and lifestyle advice

(Jewell 2003). Acustimulation, which is electrical stimulation of the P6 acupoint, does seem to be effective, but further trials are warranted (Rosen 2003).

Recommendation, see 2.4.6.

2.4.5   Hypnosis

Hypnotherapy may be used as an adjunct to medical therapy in patients with NVP, or hyperemesis gravidarum. In a study of 138 patients hospitalized with refractory hyperemesis gravidarum, 88% stopped vomiting after one to three sessions of medical hypnosis (Simon 1999, Fuchs 1994). The hypnotic state induces a deep state of psychological relaxation, with a corresponding decrease in sympathetic tone. Symptoms associated with hypersympathetic arousal tend to remit. Patients might be given suggestions during the hypnotic state to relax their stomach and throat muscles, causing their nausea, gagging, and vomiting to subside.

Recommendation, see 2.4.6.

2.4.6   Ginger

Ginger is used in Asian and Indian medicine to treat nausea, indigestion, diarrhea, stomachache, and flatulence, and is used with caution for treating NVP. It has been found to be effective in treatment of motion sickness and postoperative nausea (Bone 1990, Mowry 1982).

Concern has been expressed regarding the safety of ginger's use by pregnant women due to the mutagenic activity of 6-gingerol, one of the constituents of ginger (Nakamura 1982). The whole rhizome, however, is not mutagenic due to the substance zingerone, which suppresses the mutagenic activity of 6-gingerol (Nakamura 1982). Ginger has been claimed to inhibit platelet aggregation, and theoretically could affect testosterone receptor binding and sex steroid differentiation of the fetus; however, no clinical evidence has suggested that this is the case (Guh 1995, Backon 1991, Murphy 1988). In a large prospective trial following women who took various types of ginger during the first trimester, there was no evidence of an increased rate of major malformations (Portnoi 2003).

A number of trials have shown the efficacy of ginger in NVP. The first trial involved 27 women hospitalized with hyperemesis gravidarum who were randomized to receive ginger capsules four times daily (total 1 g daily) versus placebo in a double-blind, crossover designed study. The ginger significantly reduced the symptoms of hyperemesis, reducing both the degree of nausea and the number of attacks of vomiting (Fischer-Rasmussen 1990). Two additional trials proved the efficacy of ginger in reducing symptoms of NVP in women without hyperemesis gravidarum. Ginger treatment was associated with reduced nausea and vomiting in one trial (70 participants), and nausea and retching only in the other trial (120 participants). Participants in both trials were treated with 1–1.25 g of ginger daily in four doses. The side effects were minor – mostly mild gastrointestinal discomfort – and no adverse effects were noted for the pregnancy or for the fetus (Willetts 2003, Vutyavanich 2001).

These trials employed dry capsules of ginger rhizome. Ginger biscuits, however, might worsen the symptoms of NVP due to their sugar content, which could cause surges of blood glucose levels, associated with worsening of symptoms (Tiran 2002). Exacerbation of the symptoms of NVP after taking ginger might also be associated with the yin-yang principle of the traditional Chinese medicine; ginger is considered a yang (or hot) remedy, and would help women with deficient yang energy or *qi*. The NVP of *qi*-deficient women is characteristically worse in the morning, and improves after eating and resting. Women with excess yang energy characteristically report nausea at other times of the day that worsens after meals. These women would benefit, according to the Chinese traditional medicine, from a yin or "cool" remedy such as peppermint (Tiran 2002).

In summary, ginger is efficient for NVP and has not been associated with malformations; however, larger trials are required, see also Chapter 2.19.

> **Recommendation.** Complementary therapies for treating NVP, such as acustimulation, hypnosis, and ginger, have proved in some cases to be efficient, although more large-scale studies are needed. Acustimulation and hypnosis are often expensive and difficult to obtain reliably, but may be a good solution for women who are reluctant to use pharmacological therapy for NVP.

2.4.7   Antihistamines (H$_1$-blockers)

Pharmacology and toxicology

The first- and some of the second-generation antihistamines are effective and safe treatment for nausea and vomiting of pregnancy. The antihistamines that are indicated for nausea and vomiting are *buclizine, cyclizine, dimenhydranate, diphenhydramine, doxylamine, hydroxyzine*, and *meclizine*. The drawback of the first-generation antihistamines is their sedative effect; however, the fact that they have been on the market for so long, with no evidence of adverse effects on the newborn, is very reassuring. The newer antihistamines,

such as meclizine, are also safe and less sedating. A large meta-analysis of 24 studies with more than 200 000 participating women
showed no increased risk for major malformations; on the contrary,
it seemed that the use of antihistamines for NVP might even be protective (Seto 1997). Another large prospective study on antihistamine use in the first trimester, involving more than 18 000 infants,
failed to demonstrate any adverse effect on the birth outcome. The
outcome of the pregnancies was more favorable than the controls
with respect to preterm births, low birth weight, and perinatal death
(Källén 2002).

Buclizine is a piperazine-derivative antihistamine; it acts centrally and via the labyrinthine apparatus to suppress nausea and
vomiting. There is very little evidence supporting use during pregnancy, although it is probably safe – as are the other related antihistamines, such as cyclizine and meclizine.

Cyclizine is a piperazine-derivative antihistamine with anticholinergic properties that exerts its antiemetic effect via direct effects on
the labyrinthine apparatus, the chemoreceptor trigger zone, and possibly by increasing the muscular tone of the lower esophagus. The
antihistaminic effect lasts for 4–6 hours only.

Dimenhydrinate is the chlorotheophylline salt of diphenhydramine,
and inhibits labyrinthine stimulation and the vestibular system. As
with diphenhydramine, dimenhydrinate is safe during early pregnancy
(Mazzota 2000), but should be avoided during the third trimester due
to its potential to stimulate uterine contractions (Brost 1996).

Diphenhydramine is an ethanolamine antihistamine that acts by
competitively antagonizing histamine at the H$_1$ histamine receptor.
Diphenhydramine is a first-generation antihistamine that is mainly
used as a sedative, although it is safe and effective as an antiemetic
during pregnancy (Mazzota 2000). Diphenhydramine has oxyctocin-
like effects, especially when given intravenously or in an overdose,
and may cause uterine contractions (Brost 1996); therefore, it should
not be given during the third trimester.

Doxylamine is an antihistamine, marketed with *pyridoxine* alone
or together with *dicyclomine* (an antispasmodic), that has been used
worldwide by millions of pregnant women as an effective treatment
for NVP. In the mid-1970s, limb and various gastrointestinal malformations were suspected to be associated with the combination.
Numerous studies, retrospective and prospective, failed to prove an
association; nevertheless, *Bendectin* (Lenotan in Germany and
Debendox in the UK) was withdrawn from the market in most
European countries and in the USA (Einarson 1988, Barash 1986,
Sheffield 1985). Following withdrawal from the market, an impres-
sive surge in rates of hospitalization rates due to NVP was observed,
and no difference in the rate of malformations (Neutel 1995). To
date, *Diclectin*, a generic version of doxylamine combined with

pyridoxine, is marketed in Canada (only). Outside of Canada, this combination may be used by combining the two medications.

Meclizine (meclozine) is a piperazine antihistamine with anticholinergic and antiemetic activity. The antiemetic effects appear to be related to inhibition of the emetic center in the brain stem, vestibular nucleus, and labyrinth. The onset of effect takes 1 hour, but the effect is prolonged – usually 24 hours – so once-daily dosing is appropriate.

Meclizine is the antiemetic antihistamine of choice when doxylamine is unavailable. It has a long-lasting effect in approximately 90% of patients, and there is no evidence of adverse consequences to the child (Broussard 1998).

> **Recommendation.** First- and second-generation antihistamines are a safe and effective treatment for NVP. Doxylamine should be the first choice, preferably combined with vitamin B6 (Diclectin, if available); otherwise, second-generation antihistamines such as meclizine should be used because of the sedative effects of the first-generation antihistamines.

2.4.8   Dopamine antagonists

Pharmacology and toxicology

The dopamine antagonists used to treat NVP are *metoclopramide, phenothiazines, domperidone, droperidol,* and *trimethobenzamide*.

Metoclopramide is an effective antiemetic that acts both centrally (causing dopamine blockade in the chemoreceptor trigger zone and decreasing sensitivity of the visceral nerves that transmit GI impulses to the central emetic center) and peripherally by stimulating motility of the upper gastrointestinal tract and increasing the lower esophageal sphincter basal tone. Metoclopramide counteracts some of the physiological changes during pregnancy that may lead to nausea or vomiting, such as decreased lower esophageal sphincter tone (van Thiel 1977), and decreased propulsive motility time and increased transit time of the small intestine.

Metoclopramide is effective as antiemetic therapy for all stages of NVP, including hyperemesis gravidarum, and has been used to manage NVP successfully at home using a continuous subcutaneous pump (Buttino 2000).

No adverse fetal effects were reported in a number of studies when metoclopramide was administered during the first and second trimesters, with no significant risk of major malformations (Berkovitch 2002, 2000, Magee 2002, Sørensen 2000). A prospective follow-up of 175 women exposed to metoclopramide during the first trimester established that the rates of major malformations, spontaneous abortions, and birth weight were comparable with controls, although the metoclopramide group had a significantly higher rate of premature births (8.1% vs 2.4%) (Berkovitch 2002). No adverse birth outcomes (birth weight, major malformations, preterm delivery) were found in a study of 309 women, identified from the Danish Medical Birth Registry, exposed to metoclopramide during the first trimester of pregnancy (Sørensen 2000).

Phenothiazines like *chlorpromazine, perphenazine, prochlorperazine, promethazine*, and *trifluoperazine* significantly decrease NVP (Fitzgerald 1955, Lask 1953), and a meta-analysis of 2948 patients demonstrated no evidence of teratogenicity (Magee 2002; see also Chapter 2.11).

Domperidone shows no teratogenicity in animals (Shepard 1992), but there are insufficient data regarding use in humans.

One trial combined *droperidol* with diphenhydramine for treatment of 80 women with hyperemesis gravidarum. This is the only published trial of exposure to droperidol in the first trimester. In comparison to another group exposed to various antiemetics, the combination of intravenous droperidol (1–1.25 mg/h) and diphenhydramine shortened the length of hospitalization and reduced readmissions (Nageotte 1996).

Pooling the results of three studies on *trimethobenzamide* (two cohort and one case control), there was no increased risk for malformations. In comparison to placebo alone or in combination with pyridoxine, trimethobenzamide significantly improved symptoms of NVP (Magee 2002).

> **Recommendation.** Dopamine antagonists are widely used for treatment of NVP, especially in countries where Benedectin is unavailable. Metoclopramide seems safe and efficacious, and has less of the sedating properties of the phenothiazines; it should probably be first choice among the dopamine antagonists.

2.4.9   Pyridoxine (vitamin B$_6$)

Pharmacology and toxicology

Pyridoxine has been empirically recommended for NVP for more than 40 years, although no association has ever been found between vitamin B$_6$ levels and NVP (Schuster 1985). Pyridoxine requirements increase during pregnancy, although low serum concentrations are usually normal until the second or third trimester.

Proof of efficacy has been obtained in two large trials showing a significant reduction of nausea and the number of vomiting episodes (Vutyavanich 1995, Sahakian 1991). The first trial demonstrated efficacy in severe NVP only, but the second trial, larger and more adequately powered, showed efficacy in moderate and mild NVP as well. Pyridoxine was administered for 3–5 days, but the maximum benefit was during the first 3 days of treatment, and the beneficial effect appeared to diminish with time (Vutyavanich 1995). There is no indication for teratogenicity, even with higher than standard doses (Atanackovic 2001). Another study found that 50 mg pyridoxine i.m. along with 10 mg metoclopramide orally (on request every 6 hours) was more efficient in treating hyperemesis during the first trimester than prochlorperazine or promethazin as monotherapy. Again, there was no increased malformation rate in either group (Bsat 2003).

It is important to note that the large doses of pyridoxine are neurologically detrimental in non-pregnant patients, and therefore maximum doses of 80 mg per day are warranted (Schaumburg 1983).

> **Recommendation.** For NVP, 40 mg/d should be used initially and the maximum 80 mg/d can be tried. If vitamin B_6 alone is not successful, then combining with the antihistamine doxylamine (10 mg), a combination similar to Diclectin (available in Canada), may improve the efficacy.

2.4.10   Thiamine (vitamin B_1)

Pharmacology and toxicology

Vitamin B_1 has no antiemetic properties, although it should be kept in mind especially for those cases of hyperemesis gravidarum with vomiting for more than 3 weeks. Thiamine deficiency has been described in 20 cases, causing memory loss, ataxia, nystagmus, visual disturbances, permanent neurological symptoms, and even maternal death (Gardian 1999).

> **Recommendation.** Consider treatment with vitamin B_1 as an adjunctive to other antiemetic therapy for prolonged hyperemesis gravidarum: 100–500 mg thiamine intravenously for 3 days, and then maintenance of 2–3 mg daily. Intravenous dextrose should not be given without prior administration of thiamine, as the metabolism of the dextrose consumes the remaining B_1 and may worsen symptoms.

2.4.11   Serotonin antagonists

Pharmacology and toxicology

Ondansetron is a selective serotonin-(5-HT3)-antagonist, used for treating chemotherapy-induced nausea and vomiting. Ondansetron binds to the serotonin receptors located on the vagal neurons lining the gastrointestinal tract and blocks signaling to the vomiting center in the brain, thus preventing nausea and vomiting.

Although widely used for severe cases of NVP, there is scarce information regarding fetal safety. In the largest study published to date, the outcome of 176 pregnancies exposed to ondansetron between the fifth and ninth weeks of gestation was no different from a control group with regard to fetal outcome and major malformations. There was a slight but insignificant increase in the rate of hypospadias (three cases); although the sample size lacked power to show the apparent six-fold increase in this anomaly (Einarson 2004). There is insufficient information on the other serotonin-antagonists *dolasetron*, *granisetron*, *palonosetron*, and *tropisetron* during pregnancy.

> **Recommendation.** Ondansetron should be used only if other antiemetics fail, due to the lack of safety studies. The use of a serotonin antagonist is not, in itself, an indication either for invasive diagnostic procedures or for termination of pregnancy. After use in the first trimester, a detailed fetal ultrasound should be considered.

2.4.12   Glucocorticoids

Pharmacology and toxicology

Corticosteroids have been proposed to modify the chemoreceptor trigger zone in the brain, and are used to control nausea and emesis associated with chemotherapy (Italian Group for Antiemetic Research 2000, Safari 1998).

Corticosteroids are currently used to treat intractable hyperemesis gravidarum, the most extreme form of NVP. These patients have severe nausea and vomiting, causing weight loss and dehydration and occasionally requiring hospitalization. In the first randomized trial examining intramuscular ACTH versus placebo, 32 women with hyperemesis gravidarum were studied. There was no difference in response between the two groups (Ylikorkal 1979). A number of randomized controlled studies have since been published: 25 patients were randomized to receive 40 mg *prednisolone* daily versus placebo. The only difference among the groups was that the sense of well-being improved in the prednisolone group (Nelson-Piercy 2001). In a randomized, double-blind trial that compared parenteral followed by oral corticosteroids versus placebo for treatment of intractable hyperemesis gravidarum, the corticosteroids had no effect on the hyperemesis gravidarum and did not reduce recurrent hospitalizations. In addition, all patients were treated with promethazine and metoclopramide (Yost 2003). When compared with promethazine, however, a short course of *methylprednisolone* was more effective than promethazine (Safari 1998). Treatment with oral prednisolone promptly resolved symptoms if given specifically to the subset of patients with the more severe hyperemesis, defined as weight loss of greater than 5% (Moran 2002). For safety of glucocorticoids in pregnancy, see Chapter 2.15.

> **Recommendation.** Corticosteroids may be effective therapy for severe intractable hyperemesis gravidarum associated with dehydration. Their use is not, in itself, an indication either for invasive diagnostic procedures or for termination of pregnancy.

2.4.13   Other agents with antiemetic properties

Pharmacology and toxicology

With respect to the antiemetics such as *alizapride* and *aprepitant*, used primarily in oncology, there is insufficient experience to estimate prenatal risk.

Betahistine, a histamine analog, and the antihistamines *cinnarizine* and *flunarizin* have long been in use, and no increase in birth defects after clinical use has been shown. However, the absence of controlled studies on the use of these agents during pregnancy argues against their routine use. Betahistine and cinnarizine are both effective for treatment of vestibulair vertigo, as in Menière's syndrome.

Scopolamine is a parasympatholytic used transdermally in patch form as antiemetic treatment. Among 309 pregnant women exposed to scopolamine in the first trimester, no increase in the rate of birth defects was seen (Heinonen 1977). Other studies have also given no indication of an increase in birth defects after clinical use. Scopolamine crosses the placenta, and can cause anticholinergic symptoms such as tachycardia and decreased heart rate variability in the fetus. This effect could, at least theoretically, interfere with the detection of hypoxia-induced fetal bradycardia.

> **Recommendation.** Betahistine, cinnarizine, flunarizin, scopolamine, and, most particularly, alizapride and aprepitant should only be used when those substances recommended in the previous sections have failed. The use of any other antihistamine or antiemetic is not, in itself, an indication either for invasive diagnostic procedures or for termination of pregnancy.

References

Atanackovic G, Navioz Y, Moretti ME et al. The safety of higher than standard dose of doxylamine-pyridoxine (Diclectin) for nausea and vomiting of pregnancy. J Clin Pharmacol 2001; 41: 842–5.

Backon J. Ginger in preventing nausea and vomiting of pregnancy: a caveat due to its thromboxane synthetase activity and effect on testesterone binding. Eur J Obstet Gynecol Reprod Biol 1991; 42: 163–4.

Barash CI, Lasagna L. The Benedectin saga: voluntary discontinuation. J Clin Res Drug Dev 1986; 1: 277–92.

Berkovitch M, Elbirt D, Addis A et al. Fetal effects of metoclopramide therapy for nausea and vomiting of pregnancy. N Engl J Med 2000; 343: 445–6.

Berkovitch M, Mazzota P, Greenberg R et al. Metaclopramide for nausea and vomiting of pregnancy: a prospective multicenter international study. Am J Perinatology 2002; 19: 311–16.

Bone ME, Wilkinson DJ, Young JR et al. Ginger root – a new antiemetic. The effect of ginger root on postoperative nausea and vomiting after major gynecological surgery. Anaesthesia 1990; 45: 669–71.

Boneva RS, Moore CA, Botto L et al. Nausea during pregnancy and congenital heart defects: a population-based case-control study. Am J Epidemiol 1999; 149(8): 717–25.

Brost BC, Scardo JA, Newman RB. Diphenhydramine overdose during pregnancy: lessons from the past. Am J Obstet Gynecol 1996; 175(5): 1376–7.

Broussard CN, Richter JE. Nausea and vomiting of pregnancy. Gastroenterol Clin North Am 1998; 78: 1–3.

Bsat FA, Hoffman DE, Seubert DE. Comparison of three outpatient regimens in the management of nausea and vomiting in pregnancy. J Perinatol 2003; 23: 531–5.

Buttino L Jr, Coleman SK, Bergauer NK et al. Home subcutaneous metoclopramide therapy for hyperemesis gravidarum. J Perinatol 2000; 20: 359–62.

Dundee JW, Sourial FB, Ghaly RG et al. P6 acupressure reduces morning sickness. J R Soc Med 1988; 81: 456–7.

Einarson A, Meltepe C, Navioz Y et al. The safety of ondansetron for nausea and vomiting of pregnancy: a prospective comparative study. Br J Obstet Gynecol 2004; 111: 940–43.

Einarson TR, Leeder JS, Koren G. A method for meta-analysis of epidemiological studies. Drug Intell Clin Pharm 1988; 22: 813–24.

Fischer-Rasmussen W, Kjaer SK, Dahl C et al. Ginger treatment of hyperemesis gravidarum. Eur J Obstet Gynecol Reprod Biol 1990; 38: 19–24.

Fitzgerald JPB. The effect of promethazine in nausea and vomiting of pregnancy. NZ Med J 1955; 54: 215–18.

Foster JM, Sweeney BP. The mechanisms of acupuncture analgesia. Br J Hosp Med, 1987; 38: 303–12.

Fuchs K, Paldi E, Abramovici H et al. Treatment of hyperemesis gravidarum. Am J Clin Hypn 1994; 37: 1–11.

Furneaux EC, Langley–Evans AJ, Langley-Evans SC. Nausea and vomiting of pregnancy: an endocrine basis and contribution to pregnancy outcome. Obstet Gynecol Survey 2001; 56: 775–82.

Gardian G, Voros E, Jardanhazy T et al. Wernicke's encephalopathy induced by hyperemesis gravidarum. Acta Neurol Scand 1999; 99: 196–8.

Goodwin TM. Nausea and vomiting of pregnancy: an obstetric syndrome. Am J Obstet Gynecol 2002; 186: S184–9.

2

Pregnancy

Guh JH, Ko FN, Jong TT et al. Antiplatelet effect of gingerol isolated from *Zingiber officinale*. J Pharmacy Pharmacol 1995; 47: 329–32.

Hook EB. Changes in tobacco smoking and ingestion of alcohol and caffeinated beverages during early pregnancy: are these consequences, in part, of feto-protective mechanisms diminishing maternal exposure to embryotoxins? In: S Kelly, EB Hook, DT Janrich et al (eds), Birth Defects: Risks and Consequences. New York: Academic Press, 1976, 173–83.

Italian Group for Antiemetic Research. Dexamethasone alone or in combination with ondansetron for the prevention of delayed nausea and vomiting induced by chemotherapy. N Engl J Med 2000; 342: 1554–9.

Jewell D, Young G. Interventions for nausea and vomiting in early pregnancy. Cochrane Database Systematic Reviews 2003, Issue 4. Art No.: CD000145.DOI: 10.1002/14651858.CD000145.

Källén B. Use of antihistamine drugs in early pregnancy and delivery outcome. J Matern Fetal Neonatal Med 2002; 11: 146–52.

Koren G, Bishai R. Nausea and Vomiting of Pregnancy: State of the Art. Toronto: Motherisk, 2000.

Koren G, Maltepe C. Pre-emptive therapy for severe nausea and vomiting of pregnancy and hyperemesis gravidarum. J Obstet Gynecol 2004; 24: 530–33.

Lask S. Treatment of nausea and vomiting of pregnancy with anti-histamines. Br Med J 1953; 1: 652–3.

Li Y, Tougas G, Chiverton SG et al. The effect of acupuncture on gastrointestinal function and disorders. Am J Gastroenterol 1992; 87: 1372–81.

MacPherson H, Thomas K, Walters S et al. The York Acupuncture Safety Study: prospective survey of 34,000 treatments by traditional acupuncturists. Br Med J 2001; 323: 486–7.

Magee LA, Mazzotta P, Koren G. Evidence-based view of safety and effectiveness of pharmacology therapy for nausea and vomiting of pregnancy (NVP). Am J Obstet Gynecol. 2002; 186(Suppl 5): S256–61.

Malizia E, Andreucci G, Paolucci D et al. Electroacupuncture and peripheral beta-endorphin and ACTH levels. Lancet 1979; 2: 535–6.

Markose MT, Ramanathan K, Vijayakumar J. Reduction of nausea, vomiting and dry retches with P6 acupressure during pregnancy. Intl J Gynecol and Obstet, 2004; 85: 168–9.

Mazzota P, Magee LA. A risk–benefit assessment of pharmacological and non-pharmacological treatment for nausea and vomiting of pregnancy. Drugs 2000; 59: 781–800.

Moran P, Taylor R. Management of hyperemesis gravidarum: the importance of weight loss as a criterion for steroid therapy. Q J Med 2002; 95: 153–8.

Mowry DB, Clayson DE. Motion sickness ginger and psychophysics. Lancet 1982; 1: 655–7.

Murphy PA. Alternative therapies for nausea and vomiting of pregnancy. Obstet Gynecol 1988; 91: 149–55.

Nageotte MP, Briggs GC, Towers CV et al. Droperidol and diphenhydramine in the management of hyperemesis gravidarum. Am J Obstet Gynecol 1996; 174: 1801–6.

Nakamura H, Yamatoto T. Mutagen and antimutagen in ginger, *Zingiber officinale*. Mut Res 1982; 103: 119–26.

Nelson-Piercy C, Fayers P, De Sweit M. Randomized, double blind, placebo-controlled trial of corticosteroids for the treatment of hyperemesis gravidarum. Br J Obstet Gynecol 2001; 108: 9–15.

2.4 Antiemetics

Neutel CI, Johansen HL. Measuring drug effectiveness by default: the case of Bendectin. Can J Public Health 1995; 86: 66–70.

Portnoi G, Chng LA, Karimi-Tabesh L et al. Prospective comparative study of the safety and effectiveness of ginger for the treatment of nausea and vomiting in pregnancy. Am J Obstet Gynecol 2003; 189: 1374–7.

Profet M. Pregnancy sickness as adaptation: a deterrent to maternal ingestion of teratogens. In: JH Barlow, L Cosmides, J Tooby (eds), The Adapted Mind: Evolutionary Psychology and the Generation of Culture. New York: Oxford University Press, 1992, pp. 327–65.

Quinlan JD, Hill DA. Nausea and vomiting of pregnancy. Am Fam Physician 2003; 68: 121–8.

Rosen T, de Vaciana M, Miller HS et al. A randomized controlled trial of nerve stimulation for relief of nausea and vomiting in pregnancy. Obstet Gynecol 2003; 102: 129–35.

Safari HR, Fassett MJ, Souter IC et al. The efficacy of methylprednisolone in the treatment of hyperemesis gravidarum: A randomized, double blind, controlled study. Am J Obstet Gynecol 1998; 179: 921–4.

Sahakian V, Rouse D, Sipes S et al. Vitamin B6 is effective therapy for nausea and vomiting of pregnancy: a randomized, double blind, placebo-controlled trial. Obstet Gynecol 1991; 78: 33–6.

Schaumburg H, Kaplan J, Windebank A et al. Sensory neuropathy from pyridoxine abuse: a new megavitamin syndrome. N Engl J Med 1983; 309: 445–8.

Schuster K, Baily LB, Dimperio D et al. Morning sickness and vitamin B6 status of pregnant women. Hum Nutr Clin Nutr 1985; 39: 75–9.

Seto A, Einarson T, Koren G. Pregnancy outcome following first trimester exposure to antihistamines: meta-analysis. Am J Perinatol 1997; 14: 119–24.

Sheffield LJ, Batagol R. The creation of therapeutic orphans – or, what have we learned from the Debendox fiasco? Med J Aust 1985; 143: 143–7.

Shepard TH. Catalog of Teratogenic Agents, 7th edn. Baltimore, MD: Johns Hopkins University Press, 1992.

Simon E. Hypnosis in the treatment of hyperemesis gravidarum {Letter}. Am Fam Physician 1999; 60: 56, 61.

Smith CA (A), Crowther CA, Beilby J. Acupuncture to treat nausea and vomiting in early pregnancy: randomized controlled trial. Birth 2002; 29: 6–14.

Smith CA (B), Crowther CA, Beilby J. Pregnancy outcome following women's participation in a randomized controlled trial of acupuncture to treat nausea and vomiting in early pregnancy. Comp Ther Med 2002; 10: 78–83.

Sørensen HT, Nielsen GL, Christensen K et al. Br J Clin Pharmacol 2000; 49: 264–8.

Streitberger K, Kleinhenz J. Introducing a placebo needle into acupuncture research. Lancet 1998; 352: 364–5.

Tiran D. Nausea and vomiting in pregnancy: safety and efficacy of self-administered complimentary therapies. Complementary Ther Nursing Midwif 2002; 8: 191–6.

Van Thiel DH, Gavaler JS, Joshi SN et al. Heartburn of pregnancy. Gastroenterology 1977; 72: 666–8.

Vellacott ID, Cooke EJ, James CE. Nausea and vomiting in early pregnancy. Intl J Obstet Gynecol 1988; 27: 57–62.

Vincent C. The safety of acupuncture. Br Med J 2001; 323: 467–8.

Vutyavanich T, Wontrangan S, Ruangsri R. Pyridoxine for nausea and vomiting of pregnancy: a randomized, double blind, placebo-controlled trial. Am J Obstet Gynecol 1995; 173: 881–4.

Vutyavanich T, Kraisarin T, Ruangsri RA. Ginger for nausea and vomiting in pregnancy: randomized, double masked, placebo-controlled trial. Obstet Gynecol 2001; 97: 577–82.

White A, Hayhoe S, Hart A et al. Adverse events following acupuncture: prospective survey of 32,000 consultations with doctors and psychotherapists. Br Med J 2001; 323: 485–6.

Willetts KE, Ekangaki A, Eden JA. Effect of ginger extract on pregnancy induced nausea: a randomized controlled trial. Aust NZ J Obstet Gynaecol 2003; 43: 139–44.

Ylikorkala O, Kauppila A, Ollanket ML. Intramuscular ACTH or placebo in the treatment of hyperemesis gravidarum. Acta Obstet Gynecol Scand 1979; 58: 453–5.

Yost NP, McIntire DD, Wians FH et al. A randomized, placebo-controlled trial of corticosteroids for hyperemesis due to pregnancy. Obstet Gynecol 2003; 102: 1250–54.

2

Pregnancy

Gastrointestinal and antilipidemic agents and spasmolytics

2.5

Margreet Rost van Tonningen

2.5.1 Gastritis and peptic ulcer during pregnancy

During pregnancy, motility changes occur throughout the gastrointestinal tract. These changes are largely attributed to increased levels of progesterone and estrogen. The mechanisms promoting gastroesophageal reflux during gestation primarily involve decreased lower esophageal sphincter (LES) pressure and a decrease in the sphincter's adaptive responses, but mechanical factors may also be important.

Gastroesophageal reflux and heartburn are common during pregnancy. In mild cases, lifestyle and dietary modifications alone may be all that is required to improve the symptomatic relief. If drug treatment is indicated, first-line therapy includes antacids or sucralfate. H_2-blockers or proton-pump inhibitors should be reserved for patients with more severe symptoms, refractory to antacid or sucralfate therapy (Katz 1998).

Interestingly, in contrast, the frequency, symptoms and complication rate of peptic ulcer disease appear to decrease during pregnancy (Cappell 1998).

2.5.2   Antacids and sucralfate

Pharmacology

Antacids are basic compounds which neutralize hydrochloric acid in the gastric secretions. For this purpose, the following are used:

- *sodium hydrogen carbonate, aluminum hydroxide, aluminum phosphate, algeldrate, calcium carbonate, magnesium(hydr)oxide, magnesium carbonate*, and *magnesium trisilicate*
- combination preparations of *aluminum, magnesium*, and *carbonate*
- the structurally newer aluminum–magnesium complexes *almasilate, hydrotalcite*, and *magaldrate*; and the aluminum saccharide combination, *sucralfate*.

Regarding *aluminum-containing antacids*, the bioavailability of ingested aluminum is reported to be 0.01–1% (Greger 1993). Priest reports, referring to studies employing ^{26}Al as a tracer, that approximately 0.01% of ingested aluminum, as aluminum hydroxide, may be absorbed. Co-administration of citrate may enhance the uptake a tenth-fold, up to 0.14%. Excretion occurs primarily through the kidneys; about 2% of aluminum entering the blood is retained within the body for years (Priest 2004). Renal failure may reduce renal excretion of aluminum. Because of its molecular structure, the aluminum bound in the newer complex preparations like magaldrate may be more poorly absorbed in comparison to aluminum in classical antacids. It has been shown in animal studies that the absorbed aluminum salts can also reach the fetus (Domingo 2000). Aluminum-containing antacids can be constipating.

Regarding *calcium-containing antacids*, about 15–30% of oral calcium carbonate intake is absorbed. In patients with normal kidney function, there is no danger of hypercalcemia with normal therapeutic use. High intake of calcium carbonate antacids has been associated with (life-threatening) milk-alkali syndrome during pregnancy (Gordon 2005).

2

Pregnancy

2.5 Gastrointestinal and antilipidemic agents and spasmolytics

Regarding *magnesium-containing antacids*, about 5–10% of oral magnesium intake may be absorbed. Magnesium-containing antacids have a laxative effect.

Chronic consumption of high doses of antacids can cause alterations in mineral metabolism.

Sucralfate, a water-soluble aluminum salt of a sulfated polysaccharide, attaches to the surface of an ulcer and thus protects the mucosa from further injury by acid and pepsin. The systemic absorption of sucralfate is negligible.

Toxicology

Antacids are generally considered safe in pregnancy. The available data do not suggest teratogenic effects or other developmental toxicity associated with normal therapeutic use of antacids during pregnancy.

It has been proposed that the aluminum absorbed from aluminum-containing antacids could lead to functional disturbances in potentially sensitive organs in the fetus, such as the central nervous system and the kidneys. A 1998 case report has described a 9-year-old with a fatal neurodegenerative disorder, whose mother had taken an excessive amount of aluminum hydroxide (an average of 15 000 mg daily) throughout the entire pregnancy. The authors postulate that the high levels of aluminum ingested by this mother during pregnancy resulted in neurologic impairment in this infant (Gilbert-Barness 1998). However, with normal therapeutic use there have been no clinical indications of teratogenic effects or other developmental toxicity.

In a case reported by Robertson (2002), it is suggested that maternal ingestion of high doses of calcium carbonate-containing antacid may have temporarily suppressed neonatal parathormone production, causing neonatal seizures secondary to late neonatal hypocalcemia. However, there have been no clinical indications of teratogenic effects or other developmental toxicity with normal therapeutic use.

Antacids containing sodium bicarbonate can induce maternal and fetal metabolic alkalosis and fluid overload (review by Richter 2003, Cappell 1998, Katz 1998).

Compounds containing magnesium trisilicate, when used long term and in high doses, can lead to nephrolithiasis, hypotonia, respiratory distress and cardiovascular impairment in the fetus (review by Richter 2003, Cappell 1998, Katz 1998).

Generally speaking, magnesium salts can inhibit contractions (see Chapters 2.8 and 2.14), but after oral ingestion as an antacid, with its limited systemic absorption, such an effect is unlikely to occur.

Antacids may interfere with iron absorption (review by Richter 2003, Cappell 1998, Katz 1998).

> **Recommendation.** Antacids and sucralfate may be used during all phases of pregnancy. The unrestricted/long-term use of antacids during pregnancy should be avoided. Among the aluminum-containing antacids, magaldrate and sucralfate may be considered the drugs of choice because of their apparently limited aluminum absorption.

2.5.3   H$_2$-receptor antagonists

Pharmacology and toxicology

Cimetidine, famotidine, nizatidine, ranitidine, and *roxatidine* promote the healing of stomach and duodenal ulcers by blocking the H$_2$-receptors in the gastric mucosa. In this way, the stimulation by histamine, which induces the secretion of hydrochloric acid, is prevented. Pepsin production is reduced as well. H$_2$-receptor antagonists are used to treat gastroesophageal reflux and peptic ulcer disease. These agents are all well-absorbed and cross the placenta.

Cimetidine showed weak anti-androgenic effects in some animal experiments. However, there are no reports of human sexual developmental disorders in infants exposed to cimetidine *in utero* (review by Richter 2003).

The best-studied agent is *ranitidine*, with documented experience on approximately 1500 exposed pregnancies altogether, followed by cimetidine, with documentation for approximately 800 exposed pregnancies. In one prospective controlled study on H$_2$-blockers (mostly ranitidine), no increased risk of major malformations was found after first-trimester exposure (Magee 1996). Other studies on H$_2$-blockers (mostly ranitidine and cimetidine), based on linkage of record/prescription databases with birth registers, also argue against a teratogenic potential in humans (Ruigomez 1999, Källén 1998). A large prospective study by the European Network of Teratology Information Services (ENTIS) on 553 pregnancies exposed to H$_2$-blockers – 335 to ranitidine, 113 to cimetidine, 75 to famotidine, 15 to nizatidine and 15 to roxatidine – confirms earlier data that the use of ranitidine and cimetidine during pregnancy does not significantly increase the risk of major malformations or other pregnancy complications (Garbis-Berkvens 2005).

One case report noted a possible association between transient neonatal liver impairment with hyperbilirubinemia and cimetidine exposure during the last month of gestation (Glade 1980), but this finding has not been confirmed in other studies. There is considerable experience in the use of cimetidine and ranitidine in late pregnancy; no adverse neonatal effects were attributed to their use. When cimetidine

2

Pregnancy

2.5 Gastrointestinal and antilipidemic agents and spasmolytics

or ranitidine is given to reduce the risk of aspiration during a cesarean section, it is well tolerated by the mother and the fetus (Broussard 1998, Cappell 1998).

There is very limited experience in the use of *famotidine, nizatidine*, and *roxatidine* in pregnancy (see the aforementioned ENTIS study); data are insufficient for a well-grounded risk assessment, but there are no indications of a teratogenic risk in humans as yet.

Recommendation. During pregnancy, H_2-receptor antagonists may be prescribed when antacids or sucralfate have failed. Ranitidine – the best-studied agent – may be preferable to cimetidine because of a theoretical concern about the anti-androgenic properties of cimetidine. The use of one of the other H_2-receptor antagonists is not grounds for either the termination of pregnancy or invasive diagnostic procedures.

2.5.4   Proton-pump inhibitors

Pharmacology and toxicology

Proton-pump inhibitors such as *omeprazole, esomeprazole, lansoprazole, pantoprazole*, and *rabeprazole* suppress gastric acid secretion by inhibiting the H^+/K^+-ATPase enzyme system on the surface of the parietal cell. Proton-pump inhibitors are used to treat gastroesophageal reflux and peptic ulcers. *Omeprazole* has been shown to be well-absorbed and to cross the placenta.

The best-studied agent is *omeprazole*, with documented experience on approximately 1300 exposed pregnancies altogether. In one prospective controlled study on omeprazole use in 113 pregnancies, the authors found no association between exposure during the first trimester and an increased risk for major malformations (Lalkin 1998). Other studies on omeprazole, based on linkage of record/prescription databases with birth registers, yielded similar results (Källén 2001, Ruigomez 1999). The aforementioned studies were all included in a meta-analysis (Nikfar 2002). A recently published prospective controlled study by the ENTIS on 410 pregnancies exposed to proton-pump inhibitors – 295 to omeprazole, 62 to lanzoprazole and 53 to pantoprazole – suggests that proton-pump inhibitors do not represent a major teratogenic risk in humans (Diav-Citrin 2005).

In multiple human studies, oral administration of omeprazole during labor and delivery to prevent aspiration of gastric acid was well tolerated by mother and fetus (Cappell 1998).

Experience in the use of *lansoprazole, rabeprazole*, and *pantoprazole* in pregnancy is very limited (see the pertinent ENTIS study) and insufficient for a well-grounded risk assessment, but there are, to date, no indications of a teratogenic potential in humans.

> **Recommendation.** Omeprazole is a drug of choice for reflux esophagitis in pregnancy. For other treatment indications, proton-pump inhibitors are second-choice drugs during pregnancy when antacids, sucralfate, and ranitidine are not effective. In such a case, omeprazole, the proton-pump inhibitor with the largest experience, should again be chosen. Treatment with other proton-pump inhibitors is not grounds for the termination of the pregnancy. Detailed fetal ultrasonography during the second trimester can be considered.

2.5.5   Bismuth salts

Pharmacology and toxicology

With the discovery of the relationship between the occurrence of gastric and duodenal ulcers and infection with the bacterium *Helicobacter pylori*, bismuth salts, which were formerly used as a nonspecific antidiarrheal and antiulcer drug, have experienced a renaissance in recent years. Bismuth combinations have antimicrobial effects against *Helicobacter pylori*. *Bismuth subcitrate, bismuth subsalicylate, bismuth subcarbonate, bismuth subnitrate, dibismuthtris (-tetraoxodialuminate)*, and *bismuth III-citrate hydroxide complex* are available. Salicylate is released from bismuth subsalicylate and rapidly absorbed (see Chapter 2.1 for acetylsalicylic acid). Bismuth nitrate can form nitrite.

The data available for bismuth exposure in pregnancy are not sufficient for a well-grounded risk assessment (Friedman 1990). There have been no indications of a specific teratogenic effect in humans as yet.

> **Recommendation.** Bismuth salts are relatively contraindicated during pregnancy. When antimicrobial treatment for *H. pylori* is necessary, the use of macrolides is preferred (see Chapter 2.6).

2.5.6   Additional ulcer therapeutics

Pharmacology and toxicology

Carbenoxolone appears to act by stimulating the synthesis of protective mucus, and has no direct effect on the production of hydrochloric

2 — Pregnancy

2.5 Gastrointestinal and antilipidemic agents and spasmolytics

acid. It has mineral corticoid-like effects, and may produce sodium and water retention and hypokalemia.

Methantheline, an anticholinergic drug, is used for the treatment of peptic ulcer disease (see also spasmolytics).

Pirenzepine is an anticholinergic drug (so-called M_1-receptor blocker), which apparently works selectively in the stomach, reducing the secretion of gastric acid; up to 25% is absorbed.

Proglumide is a cholecystokinine antagonist with an inhibitory effect on gastric secretion.

Because of a lack of human studies for carbenoxolone, methantheline, pirenzepine, and proglumide, a well-grounded risk assessment is not possible.

Misoprostol is a synthetic prostaglandin E_1 analog with antisecretory and mucosal protective properties, used to treat or prevent NSAID-induced gastric ulcers. Oral use of misoprostol induces uterine contractions that can result in uterine bleeding or abortion. There is a report of fetal death in the thirty-first week of pregnancy as a result of tonic uterine contractions after the ingestion of a high dosage with the intention of committing suicide (Bond 1994).

In Brazil and Central America, misoprostol is used as an illegal abortifacient. In Brazil, cases of Moebius sequence were observed in children whose mothers had tried to induce abortion with misoprostol (see Chapter 2.14 for details).

Few data are available on the inadvertent therapeutic (gastric ulcers) use of misoprostol during pregnancy. In a French collaborative study of 125 pregnancies exposed to misoprostol, 61 patients used misoprostol for prevention of NSAID-induced gastrointestinal lesions. Although the study was too small to draw conclusions, no increased risk for major malformations was noted and no consistent pattern of malformations was seen. In particular, Moebius sequence and limb-reduction defects were not observed (Bellemin 1999). However, the timing of exposures for all of these cases may not be during the most sensitive periods for inducing Moebius sequence and limb-reduction defects.

Recommendation. Carbenoxolone, misoprostol, pirenzepine, and proglumide should not be used during pregnancy. Their inadvertent use does not necessitate the termination of the pregnancy or invasive diagnostic procedures. In the case of inadvertent misoprostol use during the first trimester, a detailed fetal ultrasound examination during the second trimester should be offered to evaluate morphologic development; however, the features of Moebius sequence may not be identifiable using this technique (see Chapter 2.14 for details).

2.5.7 *Helicobacter pylori* therapy

In recent years, antibiotic treatment of *H. pylori* has fundamentally altered the therapy of gastric and duodenal ulcers. It is recommended that treatment should consist of triple therapy, namely a proton-pump inhibitor and two of the following antibiotics: clarithromycin, metronidazole, and amoxicillin. Several different regimens are used; the choice depends on local patterns of bacterial resistance and regional preference. An example of an effective regimen is: *omeprazole* 20 mg, *amoxicillin* 1000 mg and *clarithromycin* 500 mg, all given twice daily for 1 week. Generally these triple therapy regimens achieve an eradication rate of about 90%. However, in case of bacterial resistance to clarithromycin or metronidazole, effectiveness decreases to less than 50%.

Quadruple therapy with *omeprazole*, *bismuth*, *tetracycline*, and *metronidazole* is used when triple therapy fails or may be ineffective because of local bacterial resistance.

In a publication of several cases, it is discussed that when the symptoms of hyperemesis gravidarum are persistent into the second trimester, active peptic ulcer disease from *H. pylori* could be the cause (Jacoby 1999). The results of several studies do not support an involvement of *H. pylori* infection in the generation of gastrointestinal symptoms during pregnancy, although a possible relationship with severe forms of emesis is suggested by Larraz (Weyermann 2003, McKenna 2003, Larraz 2002).

Recommendation. Eradication of *H. pylori* with triple therapy can be undertaken during pregnancy when clearly indicated. As mentioned in Chapter 2.6, amoxicillin can be safely used during pregnancy in the usual doses. There are as yet no clear indications of embryo- or fetotoxic effects due to the use of macrolides such as, for instance, clarithromycin, during human pregnancy, although data on clarithromycin are still limited (see Chapter 2.6). Based on experimental results, metronidazole may be evaluated more cautiously; however, human data do not indicate an increased risk (see Chapter 2.6). At least during the first trimester, application of metronidazole should be carefully considered. This applies as well to the proton-pump inhibitors, among which the oldest medication, omeprazole, should have preference. Quadruple therapy is not recommended during pregnancy, because tetracyclines are contraindicated after the fifteenth week of gestation (see Chapter 2.6), and bismuth salts are relatively contraindicated because of lack of human studies (see section 2.5.5).

Pregnancy

2.5 Gastrointestinal and antilipidemic agents and spasmolytics

2.5.8   Acids

Pharmacology and toxicology

For digestive problems caused by too little production of stomach acid, *glutamic acid* and *citric acid* with *pepsin proteinase* are available. There are no detailed studies in animals or humans concerning the use of these agents during pregnancy. No embryotoxic damage has been observed as yet, and it is unlikely, based upon the mode of action, that these agents would be teratogenic.

> **Recommendation.** For appropriate indications, these therapies may be taken during pregnancy.

2.5.9   Atropine and other anticholinergic spasmolytics

Pharmacology and toxicology

Atropine, a belladonna-alkaloid, is a classic parasympatholytic, which inhibits the action of acetylcholine by competitively blocking muscarine receptors. With local application (in the eye), systemic availability is negligible when applied properly. l-Atropine is the biologically active enantiomer, and is sometimes encountered under the name *hyoscyamine*.

Atropine reaches concentrations in the fetus equivalent to those in the mother within a few minutes. Although atropine may alter fetal heart rate or inhibit fetal breathing after systemic application, exposure to this drug during pregnancy has not been associated with adverse developmental effects or significant fetotoxicity at recommended therapeutic dosages.

Atropine-like belladonna-alkaloids and their derivatives are parasympathicolytic agents, used in the relief of visceral spasms of the gastrointestinal tract and of colic of the biliary and genitourinary systems; some of these agents are used in the treatment of peptic ulcer. Mydriasis (for diagnostical purpose), respiratory tract disorders, urinary incontinence and Parkinsonism are other indications.

Atropine-like belladonna alkaloids such as *scopolamine* and *homatropine*, and the tertiary amine derivatives of these belladonna alkaloids such as *flavoxate, oxybutynin, tolterodine, cyclopentolate*, and *tropicamide*, have central (CNS) and peripheral effects similar to those of atropine. With systemic use, effects similar to those of atropine cannot be ruled out. *Scopolamine* has an hypnotic action.

It is also available as a mydriatic, and as a patch for prevention of motion sickness (see Chapter 2.4). *Homatropine*, *cyclopentolate*, and *tropicamide* are available as a mydriatic.

Flavoxate, *oxybutynin*, and *tolterodine* are smooth-muscle relaxants for the urinary tract or bladder.

The quaternary ammonium derivatives of atropine-like belladonna alkaloids have peripheral effects similar to those of atropine; central (CNS) effects are negligible. With systemic application, peripheral effects similar to those of atropine cannot be ruled out. The quaternary ammonium derivatives are mostly used as spasmolytics and for gastrointestinal disorders. Among them, *butylscopolamine* is the most widely used spasmolytic. Butylscopolamine is poorly absorbed after oral administration. Two cases of eclamptic seizures after the intravenous administration of butylscopolamine in patients with severe pre-eclampsia were reported (Kobayashi 2002).

Others are *clidinium*, *glycopyrronium*, *methantheline*, *methylscopolamine*, *pipenzolate*, *pipoxolan*, *propantheline*, and *trospium chloride*. There are no detailed studies in humans concerning the use of these anticholinergic drugs during pregnancy. The same applies to the antispasmodics *denaverin*, *hymecromon*, *mebeverine*, *papaverine*, *phenamazide*, *pinaverium*, and *tiropramide*.

Specific embryotoxic effects in humans have not thus far been observed with the use of the belladonna alkaloids and derivatives mentioned, but documented experience is very limited.

Diclofenac, a nonsteroidal anti-inflammatory drug (NSAID), and as such a prostaglandin synthetase inhibitor, is used as a spasmolytic in the relief of kidney and biliary colic (see Chapter 2.1).

Recommendation. Anticholinergics, including atropine, can be used throughout pregnancy when strongly indicated. Functional effects, i.e. on the fetal heart rate, must be considered with systemic use. Butylscopolamine is the spasmolytic of choice in this group of medications. Diagnostic application of anticholinergics in the eye can be undertaken during pregnancy. Diarrhea should not be treated routinely with anticholinergics.

2.5.10   Cholinergics

Pharmacology and toxicology

In the past 30 years, numerous publications have appeared on use of *pyridostigmine* and *neostigmine* during pregnancy for the treatment of the autoimmune illness myasthenia gravis. According to these experiences, the use of these cholinergics has not been associated with congenital malformations or other adverse effects (review by Tellez-Zenteno 2004, Batocchi 1999). In 10–15% of babies born to mothers with myasthenia gravis, transient signs of neonatal myasthenia are noted, which are apparently caused by the placental transfer of receptor-blocking antibodies and not associated with the cholinergic therapy. In a few cases, placental transfer of receptor-blocking antibodies results in fetal/neonatal arthrogryposis multiplex congenita (AMC) (Polizzi 2000).

There is insufficient published information concerning the use during pregnancy for other cholinergics, *ambenonium, aneth-oltrithion, bethanechol, carbachol, ceruletide, edrophonium, distigmine,* and *physostigmine.*

> **Recommendation.** For appropriate indications, such as glaucoma, myasthenia, or intestinal or bladder atonia, the cholinergics (e.g. neostigmine, pyridostigmine, carbachol, distigmine and physostigmine) may be used during pregnancy. If another medication in this group is used accidentally, this does not require termination of pregnancy or invasive diagnostic procedures.

2.5.11   Other prokinetic agents

Pharmacology and toxicology

Metoclopramide, bromopride, cisapride, and *domperidon* are licensed for treating motility disturbances in the upper intestinal tract. *Dexpanthenol* is used for intestinal atonia.

Metoclopramide is discussed in Chapter 2.4.

In a prospective, controlled multicenter study, the authors concluded that exposure to *cisapride* during pregnancy was not associated with an increased risk of malformations or other adverse effects, although the sample size (88 first-trimester exposures) is too small to draw conclusions as yet (Bailey 1997). Cisapride has been withdrawn from the market in some countries because of serious side effects such as fatal cardiac arrhythmias.

Experience in the use of *bromopride* and *domperidon* during pregnancy is insufficient for a well-grounded risk assessment.

> **Recommendation.** Metoclopramide is the drug of choice for motility disturbances (with nausea) in the upper gastrointestinal tract. An (accidental) use of the other agents does not require termination of pregnancy or invasive diagnostic procedures.

2.5.12   Constipation during pregnancy

Constipation is common during pregnancy, occurring in up to one-third of women. Constipation during pregnancy is probably caused by progesterone-related changes in both small bowel and colon motility, and by the increased absorption of water and electrolytes during pregnancy. The subjective experience of the pregnant woman (a feeling of fullness due to the growing uterus) certainly also plays a role. Therefore, before prescribing laxatives it must be determined whether there is, in fact, any constipation (hard, dry stool, painful, less than three times a week).

Therapeutically, an improvement should first be attempted with dietary changes, including increased fluid and fiber intake, training of the defecation reflex, and increased physical activity. When these measures are not successful, it may be necessary to use a laxative to enhance the effectiveness of defecation.

Habituation to these medications, resulting in the abuse of excessively high doses, should be counteracted because water loss, electrolyte imbalance and, in advanced pregnancy, uterine contractions, can endanger the fetus.

Laxatives should only be used in pregnancy when dietary and physical measures have been unsuccessful. In this case, stool-bulking agents are the drugs of choice (Bonapace 1998).

2.5.13   Stool-bulking agents

Pharmacology and toxicology

Stool-bulking agents are non-absorbed substances that increase in volume when absorbing water; they promote intestinal peristalsis. Foods with high cellulose content, such as wheat bran, linseed, psyllium, and wheat germ, as well as agar-agar, carboxymethyl-cellulose, guar gum, ispaghula, methylcellulose, and sterculia, belong to this group of laxatives.

> **Recommendation.** All stool-bulking and absorbent substances are seen as safe in pregnancy, and should be used preferentially.

2.5.14   Hyperosmotic and saline laxatives

Pharmacology and toxicology

Lactulose, a poorly absorbed disaccharide, and its analog, *lactitol*, increase osmolar tension, creating an increase in water collection, distension, peristalsis, and evacuation. Lactulose is widely used, and in moderate use it is well tolerated. Poorly absorbed alcohols such as *mannitol* and *sorbitol* are used with the same effect. *Macrogol* works similarly; macrogols with a molecular weight of more than 3000 are not absorbed.

Saline laxatives are poorly absorbed as well; they work in a similar way to lactulose, but use saline to create an increase in fluid accumulation. Isotonic solutions are recommended because hypertonic solutions have the disadvantage that they remove significant quantities of fluid from the body. The salts, which are most appropriate as saline laxatives, are *sodium sulfate* and *magnesium sulfate*; *potassium–sodium tartrate, magnesium citrate, potassium bitartrate*, and *potassium citrate* are also used. Generally speaking, magnesium salts can inhibit contractions (see Chapters 2.8 and 2.14), but after oral ingestion as a laxative, with its limited systemic absorption, this effect is unlikely to occur.

> **Recommendation.** After stool-bulking agents, lactulose is the first-choice laxative in pregnancy. Lactitol, mannitol, and sorbitol, as well as the saline laxative sodium sulfate, can also be used as laxatives during pregnancy. However, sodium sulfate in higher doses and magnesium sulfate are contraindicated in pregnant women with cardiac or renal insufficiency, because absorption of sodium or magnesium can mean an additional burden for them. Other salts are not recommended.

2.5.15 Diphenylmethanes

Pharmacology and toxicology

The diphenylmethane *phenolphthalein* and its derivatives *bisacodyl* and *sodium picosulfate* have a laxative effect by stimulating the colon peristalsis; hence they are stimulant laxatives. Up to 15% of phenolphthalein is absorbed, and after glucuronidation is excreted in the urine (reddish coloring). Only about 5% of bisacodyl is absorbed.

Neither teratogenic nor fetotoxic effects have been observed with diphenylmethanes (Bonapace 1998).

> **Recommendation.** When constipation needs to be treated with medication and neither bulk nor osmotic laxatives like lactulose work effectively enough, bisacodyl is the drug of choice throughout the entire pregnancy.

2.5.16   Anthraquinone derivatives

Pharmacology and toxicology

Anthraquinone derivatives with a laxative action occur in a number of plants: *folia sennae, rhizoma rhei, cortex frangulae,* and *aloe.* They have a laxative effect by directly stimulating colonic smooth muscles. Anthraquinone derivatives occur as glycosides. After the sugar portion is cleaved in the intestine, these agents are partially absorbed and excreted in the urine (colored!). Anthraquinone derivatives do not appear to be teratogenic. Reported experience is the most extensive with *senna* laxatives. No stimulating effect on uterine contractions or other side effects relevant to pregnancy were noted when senna laxatives were used in pregnancy (Anonymous 1992).

A stimulating effect on uterine muscles as well as the risk of meconium passage *in utero* as a result of the direct action of the aloe ingredient *aloin* have been discussed.

> **Recommendation.** Anthraquinone derivatives should be avoided during pregnancy because some of them have a stimulating effect on uterine contractions. However, treatment with them does not necessitate either termination of the pregnancy or invasive diagnostic procedures.

2.5.17   Castor oil

Pharmacology and toxicology

Castor oil (*oleum ricini*) is a triglyceride that is hydrolyzed in the small intestine to release glycerol and ricinoleic acid. This causes a laxative effect by irritating the intestinal mucosa. Castor oil is a laxative with a harsh action; it is not appropriate for long-term therapy. In addition, it has a very unpleasant taste. No specific embryotoxic effects have been observed in human beings; however, studies during early pregnancy have to our knowledge not been reported. Many authors warn against a possible uterine contraction-stimulating effect. Steingrub (1988) reported a single case of amniotic fluid embolism associated with ingestion of castor oil, which was taken in an effort to induce labor.

> **Recommendation.** Castor oil should not be used during pregnancy because it may stimulate uterine contraction. Nevertheless, exposure does not require any action other than changing medication.

2.5.18   Lubricants and emollient laxatives

Pharmacology and toxicology

Paraffinum subliquidum (mineral oil) interferes with the intestinal absorption of fat-soluble substances, including fat-soluble vitamins such as vitamin K, and can therefore affect fetal development; neonatal hypoprothrombinemia and hemorrhage have been reported (Bonapace 1998). The fact that limited amounts are absorbed and can lead to granulomatous reactions, as well as the risk of lipoid pneumonia if aspirated, generally limit the therapeutic value of paraffinum subliquidum (Gatusso 1994).

Docusate is an emollient laxative which also has some stimulant activity in the colon. It affects the function of the intestinal mucosa, and may enhance the uptake of other drugs and thus increase their potential toxicity. No increased risk of malformations has been observed after use of docusate during pregnancy (Bonapace 1998). There is a single case report of clinically manifest neonatal hypomagnesemia after maternal overuse of oral docusate sodium (Schindler 1984).

> **Recommendation.** Paraffinum subliquidum is contraindicated during pregnancy. Nevertheless, exposure does not require any action other than changing medication. Docusate can be used in low doses when indicated. Stool-bulking agents, lactulose or bisacodyl are preferred.

2.5.19   Antidiarrheals

For acute diarrhea, symptomatic therapy with fluid replacement and maintenance of electrolyte balance is the mainstay of treatment during pregnancy. If infectious enteritis has an invasive course (bloody stools, high fever), antibiotic treatment may be necessary.

Pharmacology and toxicology

Diphenoxylate is available for inhibiting intestinal motility. It is a pethidine derivative, which reacts with opiate receptors, but it does not have analgesic properties.

Loperamide is related to diphenoxylate with respect to structure and action. Its systemic bioavailability is less than 1%. Experience indicates that its central action is less opiate-like than that of diphenoxylate, because very little loperamide enters the CNS. In a prospective controlled study on 105 pregnant women, of whom 89 had used loperamide in the first trimester, no increased risk of malformations was noted. However, women who took loperamide throughout pregnancy had babies that tended to be 200 g smaller (Einarson 2000).

There are no indications of specific teratogenic effects for either of these drugs; however, documented experience is not large (Bonapace 1998).

The same applies to *tannin albumate*.

Recommendation. Only rarely does acute diarrhea require treatment that goes beyond dietary measures. In cases where a drug-induced inhibition of intestinal motility is indicated, loperamide can be chosen.

2.5.20   Drugs for chronic inflammatory bowel disease

Inflammatory bowel disease (IBD) often affects young adults, and young women with IBD may become pregnant. Several earlier retrospective studies suggest that the rates of prematurity, fetal loss, and congenital malformations in IBD approximate the incidence of these findings in the normal population (review by Katz 2001). Recent population-based studies, however, have demonstrated an increased risk of preterm delivery and have documented neonates born to mothers with IBD to have lower birth weight and to be small for gestational age (Dominitz 2002, Nørgård 2000, Fonager 1998, Kornfeld 1997). Two studies also reported an increased risk of malformations, contradicting earlier findings (Nørgård 2003, Dominitz 2002). Disease symptoms and activity play a dominant role in determining pregnancy outcome. Active inflammatory bowel disease in pregnancy has been associated with low birth weight, higher rates of spontaneous abortion, prematurity, and perinatal complications. Therefore, optimal treatment of (active) IBD is important in improving pregnancy outcome (review by Friedman 2002, Katz 2001). The severity of the disease and the potential for drug toxicity determine the choice of treatment.

Pharmacology

Choices for treatment of ulcerative colitis and Crohn's disease include sulfonamides, 5-amino-salicylic acids, glucocorticoids, immunosuppressives like azathioprine and also methotrexate, 6-mercaptopurine, thioguanine, and monoclonal antibodies like infliximab are being used. Heparin has been used to treat refractory ulcerative colitis.

Sulfasalazine, a combination of a sulfonamide part and 5-amino-salicylic acid (5-ASA), was for a long time the drug of choice for

IBD. A significant clinical obstacle to the use of sulfasalazine in inflammatory bowel disease is the frequency of side effects due to the sulfonamide moiety. In most cases, the antiphlogistically active part of sulfasalazine – 5-ASA – is just as effective by itself for treating chronic inflammatory bowel disease, without the side effects. 5-ASA has been available for some years as a single substance – *mesalazine* (*mesalamine*), and is currently a first-line drug in the treatment of IBD.

Mesalazine-delivering drugs differ in the systemic bioavailability of mesalazine. Up to 50% of mesalazine is absorbed when taken orally. 5-amino-salicylic acid transits the placenta, and fetal plasma concentrations of the drug are lower than in maternal plasma (Christensen 1994).

Olsalazine, used as treatment and as prophylaxis against recurrence of chronic inflammatory bowel disease, is a double molecule consisting of two mesalazine parts.

For *balsalazide*, mesalazine is coupled to an inert molecule.

For *glucorticosteroids*, see Chapter 2.15; for *immunomodulating agents*, see Chapter 2.12; and for *cytostatic drugs*, see Chapter 2.13.

Toxicology

Substantial experience with use of *sulfasalazine* in human beings demonstrates that sulfasalazine therapy is not teratogenic (overview by Connell 1999). Concerns that the sulfonamide moiety might potentiate kernicterus in the prenatally exposed newborn are more of a theoretical nature. In a case report, reversible neonatal neutropenia was associated with maternal sulfasalazine therapy of 3 g daily (Levi 1988).

Mesalazine has been prescribed frequently in pregnancy without indications as yet that there may be a teratogenic activity or other adverse potential, when used at recommended doses (overview by Connell 1999, Marteau 1998). Renal insufficiency was reported in a newborn whose mother took 2–4 g of oral mesalazine daily from the third to the fifth months of pregnancy (Colombel 1994); a prostaglandin antagonism of the 5-ASA was suggested as the cause by the authors. To date, no prostaglandin antagonism-like effects of 5-ASA on the fetal ductus arteriosus have been reported.

A prospective controlled study on 165 women exposed to mesalazine during pregnancy confirms earlier results that the use of mesalazine during pregnancy does not significantly increase the risk of major malformations or other pregnancy complications. It was suggested by the authors that the increase in the rate of preterm deliveries and decrease in the mean birth weight, which were reported in this study, could be attributed to the disease (Diav-Citrin 1998). A recently published small, controlled cohort study on 5-ASA exposure during pregnancies complicated by IBD – based on data from a prescription registry – reported an increased risk of stillbirth and preterm birth only in patients with ulcerative colitis; no increased risk of malformations was noted. However, it was difficult to distinguish the specific effects of disease activity and the 5-ASA drugs (Nørgård 2003). In an as yet unpublished study of the ENTIS, data on 318 prospectively followed pregnancies exposed to mesalazine do not suggest a teratogenic risk or other drug-related adverse effects, even when used in high doses. An increase in the rate of preterm deliveries, a higher rate of neonates with low birth weight, and a lower mean birth weight were reported in the exposed group; however, in quiescent disease no statistically significant differences in pregnancy outcome were found comparing exposed cases with controls, except for a lower mean birth weight with Crohn's disease (Rost van Tonningen 2004, unpublished data).

There is limited or no experience with use of *olsalazine* and *balsalazide* in pregnancy.

For *glucorticosteroids*, see Chapter 2.15.

Documented experience – principally involving renal transplant recipients – with the use of *azathioprine* during pregnancy does not demonstrate an increased risk of malformations. Some small studies report the use of azathioprine during pregnancy for the treatment of inflammatory bowel disease as well, with similar results (review by Alstead 2003). See Chapter 2.12 for details.

Documented experience with the use of *6-mercaptopurine* during pregnancy is still insufficient for a definitive risk assessment. See Chapter 2.13 for details.

A case report describes the use of low-dose *6-thioguanine* during two pregnancies for the treatment of Crohn's disease refractory to other therapy. The pregnancies resulted in two healthy infants (De Boer 2005). See Chapter 2.13 for details.

In the post-marketing surveillance of *infliximab*, used in the treatment of Crohn's disease and rheumatoid arthritis, a number of pregnancies have been reported with no increase in adverse events (Katz 2004). However, experience is too limited for a definitive risk assessment. See Chapter 2.12 for details.

Successful treatment of an acute flare of steroid-resistant Crohn's disease during pregnancy with unfractioned *heparin* has been reported (Prajapati 2002).

Recommendation. Mesalazine is the drug of choice for treatment of chronic inflammatory bowel disease during pregnancy. Dosage should be as required for optimal treatment of the inflammatory bowel disease, as undertreatment may have adverse effects on pregnancy and the fetus due to active disease. Sulfasalazine and olsalazine may also be used if necessary. Corticosteroids may also be used, locally as well as systemically, when indicated (see Chapter 2.15 for details). Immunosuppressive agents such as azathioprine should only be used when compellingly indicated (see Chapter 2.12). 6-mercaptopurine, 6-thioguanine and infliximab should be avoided if possible, and only be used when the aforementioned agents have failed (see Chapters 2.12 and 2.13). Methotrexate should not be prescribed (see Chapter 2.13).

2.5.21   Dimeticon and plant-based carminatives

Pharmacology and toxicology

Substances that relieve meteorism are collectively referred to as *carminatives*. Among these are caraway, anise, and peppermint with their active essential oils. They are viewed as safe in pregnancy (see also Chapter 2.19).

Dimeticon/simethicone is a silicone product that is used as an antiflatulent. It defoams and disperses gas bubbles that accumulate in the gastrointestinal tract, causing meteorism. In this way, it makes transport of the intestinal contents easier. It is not absorbed, and is well-tolerated during pregnancy.

Recommendation. Dimeticon/simethicone and the plant-based substances, which contain anise, caraway, or peppermint, may be used throughout the pregnancy as carminatives.

2.5.22   Chenodeoxycholic acid and ursodeoxycholic acid

Pharmacology and toxicology

Ursodeoxycholic acid (UDCA) is a naturally occurring bile acid that has been used to change the composition of bile in an effort to dissolve gallstones, and in the management of chronic cholestatic disorders. It also has been used as a therapy for intrahepatic cholestasis of pregnancy. Intrahepatic cholestasis of pregnancy is characterized by maternal pruritis with elevated serum bile acids and liver-function test abnormalities, and associated with an increased rate of fetal distress, stillbirth, premature deliveries, and perinatal morbidity. One study reported that only high levels of serum bile acids ($= 40\,\mu$mol/l) were associated with increased fetal risks (Glantz 2004). Ursodeoxycholic acid improves pruritis and biochemical abnormalities in patients with intrahepatic cholestasis of pregnancy (Roncaglia 2004, Reyes 2000, McDonald 1999). It is too early to say whether the use of UDCA improves fetal outcome in pregnancies affected by intrahepatic cholestasis of pregnancy, but several studies suggest better perinatal outcome (Zapata 2005, Palma 1997, Diaferia 1996). In a randomized study on 84 pregnant women with intrahepatic cholestasis of pregnancy who received either ursodeoxycholic acid or cholestyramine, pruritus was more effectively reduced by ursodeoxycholic acid than by cholestyramine, as were the biochemical abnormalities; babies were delivered significantly closer to term by patients treated with ursodeoxycholic acid than those treated with cholestyramine (Kondrackiene 2005).

As yet, there are no definitive studies on the use of ursodeoxycholic acid in early pregnancy, only for the second and third trimesters. There have not been reports of fetal damage following the treatment of a pregnant woman with intrahepatic cholestasis (Zapata 2005, Roncaglia 2004, Reyes 2000, McDonald 1999, Palma 1997, Diaferia 1996).

There is no documented experience with the use of *chenodeoxycholic acid* in pregnancy. In experimental animal studies, fetal liver damage has been noted after large maternal doses of this agent. This effect has not been described in humans as yet.

> **Recommendation.** Ursodeoxycholic acid should be avoided during the first 3 months of pregnancy. If a patient becomes pregnant during treatment, the medication should be stopped, except when chronic use is necessary for primary biliary cirrhosis. Ursodeoxycholic acid can be used in the second and third trimesters for the treatment of intrahepatic cholestasis of pregnancy when indicated. Chenodeoxycholic acid should not be used during pregnancy. Treatment in the first trimester with bile acids does not require termination of the pregnancy or invasive diagnostic procedures.

2.5.23 Clofibrine acid derivatives and analogs

Pharmacology and toxicology

Clofibrate is a lipid reducer that acts on the triglycerides and, to a limited extent, on cholesterol. It is used for primary hyperlipidemia. Clofibrate has been withdrawn from the market in some countries because of serious side effects. In animal studies, clofibrate was identified in fetal tissue and was capable of inducing fetal hepatic enzymes. Because of the reduced glucuronide conjugation of clofibrate in the fetus, it is possible that fetal accumulation of the drug could occur with treatment towards the end of pregnancy.

The analog products *bezafibrate, etofibrate, fenofibrate, ciprofi-brate*, and *gemfibrozil* can be evaluated pharmacologically and tox-icologically in the similar manner as clofibrate.

Experience with clofibrate – and primarily with the other ingredients – is very limited and insufficient for risk assessment, but no reports linking the use of clofibrate with congenital defects have been located.

> **Recommendation.** Clofibrate, like bezafibrate, etofibrate, fenofibrate, and gemfibrozil, should not be prescribed during pregnancy. Inadvertent treat-ment with these lipid reducers during pregnancy does not necessitate either termination of pregnancy or invasive diagnostic procedures.

2.5.24   Cholesterol synthesis-enzyme inhibitors

Pharmacology and toxicology

The lipophylic statins *atorvastatin, fluvastatin, lovastatin (mevinolinic acid), pitavastatin, simvastatin*, and hydrophilic statins *pravastatin* and *rosuvastatin*, are used to treat hyperlipidemia and hypercholes-terolemia. These agents reduce the biosynthesis of cholesterol through a competitive inhibition of the rate-limiting enzyme, 3-hydroxy-3-methylglutaryl coenzyme A (HMG CoA) reductase.

The proliferation-inhibiting properties of some of these agents ('-statin'-induced apoptosis) with respect to tumors/malignant dis-eases are an ongoing topic of discussion.

A case study (Ghidin 1992) described a newborn with birth defects (VATER-association) following maternal treatment with *lovastatin* in the first trimester; the mother had taken dexampheta-mine at the same time. Another case report described the occur-rence of a neural tube defect in a fetus exposed to lovastatin (Hayes 1995).

A collection of human malformations – including the aforemen-tioned cases, holoprocencephaly, other CNS malformations, and limb anomalies – involving first-trimester exposure to the lipophylic HMG-CoA reductase inhibitors *atorvastatin, cerivastatin, lovastatin*, and *simvastatin* has been published. The authors suggest a possible link to abnormal Sonic Hedgehog signaling. Cholesterol binding to Sonic Hedgehog protein is required for this protein to play a signal-ing role in embryonic development. The same authors hypothesized that statins may affect fetal development by lowering *in utero* cho-lesterol biosynthesis. No malformations were reported after expo-sure to hydrophilic statins (Edison 2005A, 2004). In this collection, a cardiac malformation was misclassified as holoprosencephaly (Edison 2005B). These cases were based upon spontaneous uncontrolled reports, and are not proof of a causal association.

On the other hand, experience of the manufacturers involving prospectively collected data on pregnancy exposure to simvastatine (191 cases) and lovastatin (34 cases), and retrospectively collected cases, did not demonstrate an increase in adverse pregnancy outcome compared to general population rates obtained from the US CDC. No specific pattern of anomalies was identified in either the prospective or the retrospective reports. The authors report that a case with hydrocephalus was misclassified as holoprosencephaly in their earlier study by Manson (Pollack 2005, Manson 1996). However, data are still insufficient to exclude a teratogenic risk.

There are no published studies on use of atorvastatin, cerivastatin, fluvastatin, pitavastatin, pravastatin, and rosuvastatin in human pregnancy. To date, the only case of holoprosencephaly in a fetus, involving exposure to statins during pregnancy, was exposed to cerivastatin (withdrawn from clinical use in 2001).

Experimental animal studies with these agents do not indicate a substantial teratogenic risk; only very high-dose lovastatin exposure of pregnant rats resulted in abnormalities of the skeleton and gastroschisis in the offspring. Holoprosencephaly as a marker of Sonic Hedgehog dysfunction due to impaired cholesterol biosynthesis has been supported by rat studies; however, the exact relation remains to be clarified. It is clear, however, that the role of cholesterol in embryonic development must be taken into account (Roux 2000).

> **Recommendation.** Atorvastatin, fluvastatin, lovastatin, pitavastatin, pravastatin, rosuvastatin, and simvastatin should not be prescribed during pregnancy; discontinuing this medication would not significantly impair the long-term treatment of hyperlipidemia, and their safety has not been proven. In addition, theoretical considerations concerning the role of cholesterol in embryo development argue against the intentional use of statins during pregnancy. Nevertheless, inadvertent treatment with these drugs does not require termination of the pregnancy, but a detailed fetal ultrasound to confirm normal morphologic development may be considered.

2.5.25   Cholestyramine and other lipid reducers

Pharmacology and toxicology

Cholestyramine is an anion-exchange resin which is not absorbed systemically. It binds bile acids, producing an insoluble complex which is excreted in the stool. This leads to a reduction of cholesterol and the low-density (LD) lipoproteins in the serum. Cholestyramine is used in pregnancy for the treatment of obstetric cholestasis to relieve the itching. Ursodeoxycholic acid is, however, more effective than cholestyramine in intrahepatic cholestasis of pregnancy (see ursodeoxycholic acid; Kondrackiene 2005). There is at least a theoretical risk for the fetus because, in addition to bile acids, cholestyramine also binds other lipophile substances – such as fat-soluble vitamins and medications. One case report concerning the gestational use of cholestyramine has described severe intracranial hemorrhage in a fetus; vitamin K deficiency was suspected (Sadler 1995).

Individual case studies argue against teratogenic properties (Landon 1987).

Other lipid reducers, such as *acipimox, colestipol, β-sitosterin, ezetimibe xantinol and inositol nicotinate*, and *probucol*, have not been sufficiently studied for pregnancy effects. Little systemic absorption of colestipol is believed to occur. As with the related agent *cholestyramine*, colestipol can bind and impede the absorption of a variety of nutrients, including the fat-soluble vitamins.

For these medications, too, there have not, as yet, been indications of specific teratogenic effects.

> **Recommendation.** Cholestyramine – and, as a second choice, colestipol – may be used for intrahepatic cholestasis of pregnancy or when the use of a lipid reducer is strongly indicated. If used, sufficient supplementation of fat-soluble vitamins should be considered. These vitamins must be taken at a different time than the medication. Acipimox, β-sitosterin, ezetimibe, xantinol and inositol nicotinate, and probucol should not be used in pregnancy. However, their (inadvertent) use does not require either an interruption of the pregnancy or invasive diagnostic procedures.

2.5.26   Appetite suppressants, obesity and weight loss

Pharmacology and toxicology

Amfepramone (synonym *diethylpropion*), *clobenzorex*, *dexfenfluramine*, *fenfluramine*, *fenproporex*, *mazindol*, *mefenorex*, *norpseudoephedrine*, *phentermine*, and *sibutramine* are used as appetite suppressants. Amfepramone, clobenzorex, fenproporex, mefenorex, and phentermine share the pharmacological properties of amphetamines; dexfenfluramine, fenfluramine, and sibutramine stimulate the release of serotonin and block its reuptake; norpseudoephedrine is a sympathomimetic amine; mazindol is a tricyclic drug structurally unrelated to amphetamine, but with the same actions as amphetamine.

Orlistat inhibits intestinal lipase and reduces fat absorption, which results in weight reduction.

Concerns about these medications have been repeatedly mentioned because of results in animal experiments and in connection with individual case studies. Because some of these drugs are vasoactive substances, it has been suggested that the perfusion-reducing effect could theoretically lead to vascular disruption-related birth defects.

A French collaborative study by Teratology Information Services, which evaluated 168 pregnancies primarily exposed to dexfenfluramine, did not provide any indication of teratogenic properties in this appetite suppressant (Vial 1992).

Pregnancy outcome in 98 prospectively ascertained pregnancies, exposed to the combination of fenfluramine and phentermine in early pregnancy, has been reported. No increased risk of malformations or other adverse effects was noted in this controlled study, although data are still insufficient for definitive conclusions (Jones 2002).

In two small case series, 11 live births (normal healthy babies) were reported after first-trimester exposure to sibutramine (Kadioglu 2004, Einarson 2004).

There is no or very limited experience with the use of mazindol or orlistat in pregnancy.

Obesity and weight loss

It has been hypothesized by other authors that disturbances in temperature regulation or ketoacidosis connected with weight loss could be responsible for embryotoxic damage such as, for instance, neural tube defects (Robert 1995, 1994).

Several publications discuss the association of maternal obesity and pregnancy complications, including birth defects (Scialli 2006). A preconceptionally existing maternal obesity is, according to a retrospective case-control study on 277 neural tube defect cases and controls, associated with at least a two-fold increased risk for neural tube defects, independent of periconceptional intake of folic acid and vitamins (Shaw 2000A). A prospective study evaluating 1451 children of obese mothers (Body mass index (BMI) $\geq 30\,\mathrm{kg/m^2}$) found an increased malformation rate (11.1%) with more than expected cases of encephalopathy, truncus arteriosus communis, and Potter sequence (Wiesel 2001). It is controversially discussed whether cardiovascular defects are more frequent among infants of obese mothers (Correa-Villasesor 2004). Another retrospective study observed significantly more obstructive renal anomalies in children of mothers with decreased fertility and a BMI $\geq 25\,\mathrm{kg/m^2}$ (Honein 2003). Cedergen and co-workers (2005) report an increase of cleft lip/palate if maternal BMI is $\geq 29 \, \text{kg/m}^2$. An impaired glucose metabolism or undiagnosed diabetes mellitus may be responsible for the observed increase of birth defects.

In another retrospective case-control study on 538 neural tube defect cases and 539 non-malformed controls, maternal lowered weight gain during pregnancy was associated with an increased risk of neural tube defects among offspring, especially when weight gain was less than 5 kg. The effect was independent of folic acid intake. According to Shaw and associates (2000B), it is not clear whether the lowered weight gain is cause of or caused by the neural tube defect. The same cases and controls were studied on dieting behaviors; the data suggest that restricted food intake during the first trimester may be associated with increased neural tube defect risk (Carmichael 2003).

> **Recommendation.** Appetite suppressants are contraindicated during pregnancy. Accidental ingestion does not necessitate a termination of the pregnancy. In the case of abuse or long-term use during pregnancy, as well as after a considerable loss of weight in early pregnancy, a detailed fetal ultrasound is recommended to evaluate morphologic development; screening for neural tube defects using maternal serum or amniotic fluid α-fetoprotein can be considered.

References

Anonymous. Risk assessment for senna during pregnancy. Pharmacology 1992; 44(Suppl 1): 20–22.

Alstead EM, Nelson PC. Inflammatory bowel disease in pregnancy. Gut 2003; 52: 159–61.

Bailey B, Addis A, Lee A et al. Cisapride use during human pregnancy: a prospective, controlled multicenter study. Dig Dis Sci 1997; 42: 1848–52.

Batocchi AP, Majolini L, Evoli A et al. Course and treatment of myasthenia gravis during pregnancy. Neurology 1999; 52: 447–52.

Bellemin B, Carlier P, Vial T et al. Misoprostol exposure during pregnancy: a French collaborative study. Presentation at the 10th Annual Conference of the European Network of Teratology Information Services (ENTIS), Madrid, 1999.

Bonapace ES Jr, Fisher RS. Constipation and diarrhea in pregnancy. Gastroenterol Clin North Am 1998; 27: 197–211.

Bond GR, van Zee A. Overdosage of misoprostol in pregnancy. Am J Obstet Gynecol 1994; 71: 561–2.

Broussard CN, Richter JE. Treating gastroesophageal reflux disease during pregnancy and lactation: what are the safest therapy options? Drug Saf 1998; 19: 325–37.

Cappell MS, Garcia A. Gastric and duodenal ulcers during pregnancy. Gastroenterol Clin North Am 1998; 27: 169–95.

2

Pregnancy

Carmichael SL, Shaw GM, Schaffer DM et al. Dieting behaviors and risk of neural tube defects. Am J Epidemiol 2003; 158: 1127–31.

Cedergren M, Källén B. Maternal obesity and the risk for orofacial clefts in the offspring. Cleft Palate-Craniofacial J 2005; 42: 367–71.

Christensen LA, Rasmussen SN, Hansen SH et al. Disposition of 5-aminosalicylic acid and N-acetyl-5-aminosalicylic acid in fetal and maternal body fluids during treatment with different 5-aminosalicylic acid preparations. Acta Obstet Gynaecol Scand 1994; 73: 399–402.

Colombel JF, Brabant G, Gubler MC et al. Renal insufficiency in infant: side-effect of prenatal exposure to mesalazine? Lancet 1994; 344: 620–21.

Connell W, Miller A. Treating inflammatory bowel disease during pregnancy: risks and safety of drug therapy. Drug Saf 1999; 21: 311–23.

Correa-Villasenor A, Alverson CJ. Maternal obesity and cardiovaskular malformations. Birth Def Res A 2004; 70: 257.

De Boer NKH, van Elburg RM, Wilhelm AJ et al. 6-Thioguanine for Crohn's disease during pregnancy: thiopurine metabolite measurements in both mother and child. Scand J Gastroenterol 2005; 40: 1374–7.

Diaferia A, Nicastri PI, Tartagni N. Ursodeoxycholic acid therapy in pregnant women with cholestasis. Intl J Gynaecol Obstet 1996; 52: 133–40.

Diav-Citrin O, Park YH, Veerasuntharam G et al. The safety of mesalamine in human pregnancy: a prospective controlled cohort study. Gastroenterology 1998; 114: 23–8.

Diav-Citrin CO, Arnon J, Shechtman S et al. The safety of proton pump inhibitors in pregnancy: a multicentre prospective controlled study. Aliment Pharmacol Ther 2005; 21: 269–75.

Domingo JL, Gomez M, Colomina MT. Risks of aluminium exposure during pregnancy. Science 2000; 1: 479–87.

Dominitz JA, Young JCC, Boyko EJ. Outcomes of infants born to mothers with inflammatory bowel disease: a population-based cohort study. Am J Gastroenterol 2002; 97: 641–8.

Edison RJ, Muenke M. Mechanistic and epidemiologic considerations in the evaluation of adverse birth outcomes following gestational exposure to statins. Am J Med Genet A 2004; 131A: 287–98.

Edison RJ (A), Muenke M. Gestational exposure to lovastatin followed by cardiac malformation misclassified as holoprosencephaly. N Engl J Med 2005; 352: 2759.

Edison RJ (B), Schnur RE, Ennis S et al. Potential teratogenicity of statin drugs : an update. Birth Def Res A 2005; 73: 298.

Einarson A, Mastroiacovo P, Arnon J et al. Prospective, controlled, multicentre study of loperamide in pregnancy. Can J Gastroenterol 2000; 14: 185–7.

Einarson A, Bonari L, Sarkar M et al. Exposure to sibutramine during pregnancy: a case series. Eur J Obstet Gyn Reprod Biol 2004; 116: 112.

Fonager K, Sorensen HT, Olsen J et al. Pregnancy outcome for women with Crohn's disease: a follow-up study based on linkage between national registries. Am J Gastroenterol 1998; 93: 2426–30.

Friedman JM, Little BB, Brent RL et al. Potential human teratogenicity of frequently prescribed drugs. Obstet Gynecol 1990; 75: 594–9.

Friedman S, Regueiro MD. Pregnancy and nursing in inflammatory bowel disease. Gastroenterol Clin North Am 2002; 31: 265–73.

Garbis-Berkvens JM, Diav-Citrin O et al. Pregnancy outcome after exposure to ranitidine and other H2-blockers. A Collaborative Study of the European Network of Teratology Information Services. Reprod Toxicol 2005; 19: 453–8.

2.5 Gastrointestinal and antilipidemic agents and spasmolytics

Gatusso JM, Kamm MA. Adverse effects of drugs used in the management of constipation and diarrhoea. Drug Saf 1994; 10: 47–65.

Ghidin A, Sicherer S, Willner J. Congenital abnormalities (Vater) in baby born to mother using lovastatin. Lancet 1992; 339: 1416–17.

Gilbert-Barness E, Barness LA, Wolff et al. Aluminum toxicity. Arch Ped Adolescent Med 1998; 152: 511–12.

Glade G, Saccar GR, Pereira GR. Cimetidine. Transient liver impairment in the newborn. Case report. Am J Dis Child 1980; 134: 87–8.

Glantz A, Marschall HU, Mattsson LA. Intrahepatic cholestasis of pregnancy: relationships between bile acid levels and fetal complication rates. Hepatology Baltimore, MD 2004; 40: 467–74.

Gordon MV, McMahon LP, Hamblin PS. Life-threatening milk-alkali syndrome resulting from antacid ingestion during pregnancy. Med J Aust 2005; 182: 350–51.

Greger JL. Aluminum metabolism. Annu Rev Nutr 1993; 13: 43–63.

Hayes A, Gilbert A, Lopez, G et al. Mevacor – a new teratogen? Am J Hum Genet 1995; 57: A92.

Honein MA, Moore CA, Watkins ML. Subfertility and prepregnancy overweight/obesity: possible interaction between these risk factors in the etiology of congenital renal anomalies. Birth Def Res A 2003; 67: 572–7.

Jacoby EB, Porter KB. *Helicobacter pylori* infection and persistent hyperemesis gravidarum. Am J Perinatal 1999; 16: 85–8.

Jones KL, Johnson KA, Dick LM et al. Pregnancy outcomes after first trimester exposure to phentermine/fenfluramine. Teratology 2002; 65: 125–30.

Kadioglu M, Ulku C, Yaris F et al. Sibutramine use in pregnancy: report of two cases. Birth Def Res A 2004; 70: 545–6.

Källén BA. Delivery outcome after the use of acid-suppressing drugs in early pregnancy with special reference to omeprazole. Br J Obstet Gynaecol 1998; 105: 877–81.

Källén BA. Use of omeprazole during pregnancy – no hazard demonstrated in 955 infants exposed during pregnancy. Eur J Obstet Gynecol Reprod Biol 2001; 96: 63–8.

Katz JA, Pore G. Inflammatory bowel disease and pregnancy. Inflam Bowel Dis 2001; 7: 146–57.

Katz JA, Antoni C, Keenan GE et al. Outcome of pregnancy in women receiving infliximab for the treatment of Crohn's disease and rheumatoid arthritis. Am J Gastroenterol 2004; 99: 2385–92.

Katz PO, Castell DO. Gastroesophageal reflux disease during pregnancy. Gastroenterol Clin North Am 1998; 27: 153–67.

Kobayashi T, Sugimura M, Tokunaga N et al. Anticholinergics induce eclamptic seizures. Semin Thromb Hemost 2002; 28: 511–14.

Kondrackiene J, Beuers U, Kupcinskas L. Efficacy and safety of ursodeoxycholic acid versus cholestyramine in intrahepatic cholestasis of pregnancy. Gastroenterology 2005; 129: 894–901.

Kornfeld D, Cnattingius S, Ekbom A. Pregnancy outcomes in women with inflammatory bowel disease – a population-based cohort study. Am J Obstet Gynecol 1997; 177: 942–6.

Lalkin A, Loebstein R, Addis A et al. The safety of omeprazole during pregnancy: a multicenter prospective controlled study. Am J Obstet Gynecol 1998; 179(3 Pt 1): 727–30.

Landon MB, Soloway RD, Freedman LJ et al. Primary sclerosing cholangitis and pregnancy. Obstet Gynecol 1987; 69: 457.

Larraz J, Marin N, Pineiro L et al. Lack of relationship between infection by *Helicobacter pylori* and vomiting that usually occurs during pregnancy, although possible relationship with severe forms of emesis. Rev Esp Enferm Dig 2002; 94: 417–22.

Levi S, Liberman M, Levi AJ et al. Reversible congenital neutropenia associated with maternal sulphasalizine therapy {Letter}. Euro J Pediatr 1988; 48: 174–5.

Magee LA, Inocencion G, Kamboj L et al. Safety of first trimester exposure to histamine H_2-blockers. Dig Dis Sci 1996; 41: 1145–9.

Manson JM, Freyssinges C, Ducrocq MB et al. Postmarketing surveillance of lovastatin and simvastatin exposure during pregnancy. Reprod Toxicol 1996; 10: 439–46.

Marteau P, Tennenbaum R, Elefant E et al. Foetal outcome in women with inflammatory bowel disease treated during pregnancy with oral mesalazine microgranules. Aliment Pharmacol Ther 1998; 12: 1101–18.

McDonald JA. Cholestasis of pregnancy. J Gastroenterol Hepatol 1999; 14: 515–18.

McKenna D, Watson P, Dornan J. *Helicobacter pylori* infection and dyspepsia in pregnancy. Obstet Gynecol 2003; 102: 845–9.

Nikfar S, Abdollahi M, Moretti ME et al. Use of proton pump inhibitors during pregnancy and rates of major malformations: a meta-analysis. Dig Dis Sci 2002; 47: 1526–9.

Nørgård B, Fonager K, Sorensen HT et al. Birth outcomes of women with ulcerative colitis: a nationwide Danish cohort study. Am J Gastroenterol 2000; 95: 3165–70.

Nørgård B, Erzsebet P, Pedersen L et al. Risk of congenital abnormalities in children born to women with ulcerative colitis: a population-based, case-control study. Am J Gastroenterol 2003; 98: 2006–10.

Palma J, Reyes H, Ribalta J et al. Ursodeoxycholic acid in the treatment of cholestasis of pregnancy. A randomised double blind study controlled with placebo. J Hepatol 1997; 27: 1022–8.

Polizzi A, Huson SM, Vincent A. Teratogen update: maternal myasthenia gravis as a cause of congenital arthrogryposis. Teratology 2000; 62: 332–41.

Pollack PS, Shields KE, Burnett DM et al. Pregnancy outcomes after maternal exposure to simvastatin and lovastatin. Birth Def Res A 2005; 73: 888–96.

Prajapati DN, Newcomer JR, Emmons J et al. Successful treatment of an acute flare of steroid-resistant Crohn's colitis during pregnancy with unfractionated heparin. Inflam Bowel Dis 2002; 8: 192–5.

Priest ND. The biological behaviour and bioavailability of aluminium in man, with special reference to studies employing ^{26}Al as a tracer: review and study update. J Environ Monit 2004; 6: 375–403.

Reyes H, Sjovall J. Bile acids and progesterone metabolites in intrahepatic cholestasis of pregnancy. Ann Med 2000; 32: 94–106.

Richter JE. Gastroesophageal reflux disease during pregnancy. Gastroenterol Clin North Am 2003; 32: 235–61.

Robert E, Francannet CH, Shaw G. Neural tube defects and maternal weight reduction in early pregnancy. Reprod Toxicol 1994; 8: 448.

Robert E, Francannet CH, Shaw G et al. Neural tube defects and maternal weight reduction in early pregnancy. Reprod Toxicol 1995; 9: 57–9.

Robertson WC Jr. Calcium carbonate consumption during pregnancy: an unusual cause of neonatal hypocalcemia. J Child Neurol 2002; 17: 853–5.

Roncaglia N, Locatelli A, Arreghini et al. A randomised controlled trial of ursodeoxycholic acid and S-adenosyl-l-methionine in the treatment of gestational cholestasis. Br J Obstet Gynecol 2004; 111: 17–21.

Rost van Tonningen MM, Schaefer C, Elefant E et al. Pregnancy outcome after exposure to mesalazine. A Collaborative Study of the European Network of Teratology Information Services (ongoing).

Roux C, Wolf C, Mulliez N et al. Role of cholesterol in embryonic development. Am J Clin Nutr 2000; 71(5 Suppl): S1270–79.

Ruigomez A, Gargia-Rodriguez LA, Cattaruzzi C et al. Use of cimetidine, omeprazole, and ranitidine in pregnant women and pregnancy outcomes. Am J Epidemiol 1999; 150: 476–81.

Sadler LC, Lane M, North R. Severe fetal haemorrhage during treatment with cholestyramine for intrahepatic cholestasis of pregnancy. Br J Obstet Gynaecol 1995; 102: 169–70.

Scialli AR. Teratology Public Affairs Committee Position Paper: Maternal obesity and pregnancy. Birth Def Res A 2006; 76: 73–7.

Schindler AM. Isolated neonatal hypomagnesemia associated with maternal overuse of stool softener. Lancet 1984; 2: 822.

Shaw GM (A), Todoroff K, Finnell RH et al. Spina bifida phenotypes in infants or fetuses of obese mothers. Teratology 2000; 61: 376–81.

Shaw GM (B), Todoroff K, Carmichael SL et al. Lowered weight gain during pregnancy and risk of neural tube defects among offspring {Abstract}. Teratology 2000; 61: 451.

Steingrub JS, Lopez T, Teres D et al. Amniotic fluid embolism associated with castor oil ingestion. Crit Care Med 1988; 16: 642–3.

Tellez-Zenteno JF, Hernandez-Ronquillo L, Salinas V et al. Myasthenia gravis and pregnancy: clinical implications and neonatal outcome. BMC Musculoskel Dis 2004; 5: 42.

Vial T, Robert E, Carlier P et al. First-trimester in utero exposure to anorectics: a French collaborative study with special reference to dexfenfluramine. Intern J Risk Saf Med 1992; 3: 207–14.

Weyermann M, Brenner H, Adler G et al. *Helicobacter pylori* infection and the occurrence and severity of gastrointestinal symptoms during pregnancy. Am J Obstet Gynecol 2003; 189: 526–31.

Wiesel A, Stolz G, Schlaefer K et al. Does maternal obesity increase the risk of congenital anomalies? Reprod Toxicol 2001; 15: 561–85.

Zapata R, Sandoval L, Palma J et al. Ursodeoxycholic acid in the treatment of intrahepatic cholestasis of pregnancy. A 12-year experience. Liver Intl 2005; 25: 548–54.

Anti-infective agents

2.6

Hanneke Garbis, Margreet Rost van Tonningen, and Minke Reuvers

2.6.1   Penicillins

Pharmacology and toxicology

Penicillins belong to the β-lactam antibiotics. They inhibit cell-wall synthesis in bacteria and have bactericidal properties. Similar metabolic pathways do not exist in mammals, and therefore penicillins and related β-lactam antibiotics have a low toxicity profile for both the pregnant and non-pregnant patient when used in therapeutic doses. Only penicillin allergy may present a problem. In such cases, *erythromycin* is an alternative.

The group of penicillins includes *amoxicillin, ampicillin, azidocillin, azlocillin, bacampicillin, cloxacillin, dicloxacillin, flucloxacillin, mezlocillin, nafcillin, oxacillin, panamecillin, penicillin G and V, phenoxymethylpenicillin, piperacillin,* and *propicillin.* Penicillins are sometimes used in combination with β-lactamase inhibitors such as *clavulanic acid, sulbactam*, and *tazobactam*. Penicillins cross the placenta in low concentrations, and can be detected in amniotic fluid. Elimination of penicillins is more rapid in pregnant women, and therefore dosage or dosage intervals should be adjusted if necessary (Heikkilä 1994, Chamberlain 1993).

There is no evidence that penicillins have teratogenic or embryo/fetotoxic properties (Berkovitch 2004, Jepsen 2003, Dencker 2002, Larsen 2001, 2000, Czeizel 2000A, 1998). Czeizel (2001A) found a higher prevalence of cleft palate after prenatal exposure to ampicillin in the second and third months of pregnancy, but they state that the risk is probably not real but due to chance. Pregnant women who are treated with penicillin for syphilis may develop the Jarisch–Herxheimer reaction – a febrile reaction, often with headache and myalgia. Fetal monitoring is recommended in such cases, as uterine contractions may occur (Myles 1998). There are no differences between the various penicillins regarding their safety in pregnancy.

> **Recommendation.** Penicillins can be safely used during pregnancy in the usual doses; they are the antibiotics of choice in pregnancy.

2.6.2   Cephalosporins

Pharmacology and toxicology

Cephalosporins also belong to the β-lactam antibiotics, but their pharmacokinetic and antibacterial properties are different from those of penicillins. They may cause hypersensitivity reactions. Some patients with penicillin allergy also react with cephalosporins. Cephalosporins are classified according to their antimicrobial activity.

First-generation cephalosporins are *cefaclor, cefradin, cefadroxil, cefalexin, cefalotine,* and *cefazolin.*

Second-generation cephalosporins are *cefamandole, ceftnetazol, cefoxitin,* and *cefuroxime.*

Third-generation cephalosporins are *cefdinir, cefetamet, cefixime, cefodizim, cefoperazone, cefotaxime, cefotetan, cefpirome, cefpodoxime, cefprozil, cefsulodin, ceftazidime, ceftibuten, ceftizoxime, ceftriaxone,* and *latamoxef.*

Cefipime is a fourth-generation cephalosporin.

Second- and third-generation cephalosporins, especially cefotetan, are increasingly associated with severe immune hemolytic anemia (Garratty 1999).

Cephalosporins cross the placenta, and can reach therapeutic levels in amniotic fluid and fetal tissues (Mitchell 2001). Elimination in pregnant women is faster, and it may be necessary to adjust dosage (Heikkilä 1994).

There is no evidence of teratogenic or embryo/fetotoxic properties (Czeizel 2001B, Berkovitch 2000).

In a recent study, Manka (2000) reported that the physical and mental development was normal in children of women who had been treated with cefuroxim at any time during pregnancy.

> **Recommendation.** Cephalosporins can be used safely during pregnancy if needed. The older cephalosporins are preferred.

2.6.3   Other β-lactam antibiotics and β-lactamase inhibitors

Pharmacology and toxicology

Aztreonam, imipenem, loracarbef, and *meropenem* are synthetic β-lactam antibiotics, belonging to the groups of *carbapenems* or *carbacefems*. They have excellent antimicrobic activity against gram-negative bacteria, especially against enterobacteria. Their stability for bacterial β-lactamase is the same as for third-generation cephalosporins.

Sulbactam and *tazobactam* are β-lactamase inhibitors which are used in combination with β-lactam antibiotics such as ampicillin or cephalosporins.

Clavulanic acid is also a β-lactamase inhibitor, and is used in combination with amoxicillin or ticarcillin.

β-lactam antibiotics and β-lactamase inhibitors cross the placenta and can be found in high concentrations in the fetus. They are more rapidly eliminated during pregnancy (Heikkilä 1994).

There is no evidence for teratogenicity or other adverse effects on pregnancy outcome after maternal use of amoxicillin/clavulanic acid (Czeizel 2001C, Berkovitch 2004).

> **Recommendation.** β-lactam antibiotics from this group and β-lactamase inhibitors can be used during pregnancy when strongly indicated, such as in cases where penicillins or cephalosporins have been ineffective.

2.6.4   Macrolide antibiotics

Pharmacology and toxicology

Macrolides inhibit bacterial protein synthesis and have bacteriostatic properties. *Erythromycin* is the oldest of the macrolides. *Azithromycin, clarithromycin, dirithromycin, josamycin, midecamycin, oleandomycin,* and *roxithromycin* are newer macrolides. Azithromycin belongs to the azalides, a new class of macrolides which resemble erythromycin but have different pharmacokinetic profiles and antibacterial activity. The newer macrolides have a longer half-life and fewer gastrointestinal side effects.

Little is known about the pharmacokinetics in pregnant women. Maternal and fetal serum levels are low and may vary; fetal plasma concentrations are 5–20% of maternal plasma concentrations. In a study using *in vitro* perfusion of placentas at term, Heikkinen (2000) found that the transplacental transfer of the macrolides erythromycin, roxithromycin, and azithromycin was relatively low (<5%). In patients scheduled for elective cesarean section who were given azithromycin 6–168 hours before the procedure, high placental levels were found. Fetal serum levels of azithromycin, however, were low (Ramsey 2003). Data from a recent study suggest that in patients who are treated in the third trimester, gastrointestinal absorption of erythromycin may be delayed; severe adverse gastrointestinal events may forewarn of subtherapeutic plasma concentrations which could have consequences for the treatment outcome (Larsen 1998).

Erythromycin has always been considered a safe and effective antibiotic during pregnancy. Data on more than 7000 first-trimester exposures do not support an association between erythromycin and congenital malformations (Briggs 2005, Czeizel 1999). In a recent study, however, Källén (2005) reported an increased rate of cardiovascular malformations (1.8%), especially ventricular and atrial septal defects. They conclude that even if the association is causal, the individual risk for an infant is still low. The same authors also found an increased incidence of pyloric stenosis (0.2%). Louik (2002), on the contrary, did not find an increased risk of pyloris stenosis as did Cooper (2002), but the last publication reports a possible association with other macrolides. The association between prenatal exposure to erythromycin and other macrolides and infant pyloric stenosis is still uncertain.

Erythromycin estolate and *troleandomycin* may adversely influence maternal liver function; hepatotoxicity is especially seen in the second half of pregnancy, and is reversible. Fetal development is not impaired in such cases (Lewis 1991, McCormack 1977).

Available data on the newer macrolides are still limited. Several studies are available on the pregnancy outcome after *clarithromycin* exposure. Cardiovascular malformations have been reported in rat species after prenatal exposure to clarithromycin, but so far no evidence exists that prenatal exposure in the human does increase the rate of cardiovascular or other major malformations (Drinkard 2000, Einarson 1998, Schick 1996). Einarson (1998) found only a significantly higher rate of spontaneous abortions in the exposed group (122 first-trimester exposures), which might be due to confounding factors such as maternal diseases.

Spiramycin is recommended during pregnancy for the treatment of maternal toxoplasmosis to prevent congenital toxoplasmosis. Adverse effects have not been reported.

Recommendation. Erythromycin is still the drug of choice among the macrolides during pregnancy. Erythromycin estolate and troleandomycin should not be given in the second and third trimesters. Newer macrolides such

2

Pregnancy

2.6 Anti-infective agents

as azithromycin, clarithromycin, josamycin, and roxithromycin are second-choice macrolides. Spiramycin is the drug of choice for the treatment of toxoplasmosis during the first trimester.

2.6.5   Lincomycin and clindamycin

Pharmacology and toxicology

Lincomycin and its derivative *clindamycin* inhibit bacterial protein synthesis and have bacteriostatic and bacteriocidal activity.

No teratogenic or fetotoxic effects have been reported for lincomycin in 302 pregnancies (Czeizel 2000B).

Clindamycin may cause pseudomembranous colitis, which recently has also been reported after intravaginal application (Trexler 1997). The drug is best avoided during pregnancy.

Intravaginal clindamycin appears to be effective in the treatment of bacterial vaginosis, but is less effective in preventing the increased incidence of adverse pregnancy outcome caused by bacterial vaginosis (Joesoef 1999; see also Chapter 2.14).

Recommendation. Clindamycin and lincomycin are only indicated during pregnancy when penicillins, cephalosporins, erythromycin or the other macrolides are not effective. Inadvertent use of these agents is not an indication for termination of pregnancy or for additional prenatal diagnostic procedures.

2.6.6   Tetracyclines

Pharmacology and toxicology

Tetracyclines are among the first antibiotics which became available, and are still widely used. They are broad-spectrum antibiotics and have bacteriostatic activity by inhibiting protein synthesis. *Chlortetracycline, doxycycline, minocycline, oxytetracycline*, and *tetracycline* belong to this group.

Tetracyclines cross the placenta, and they bind strongly to calcium ions (especially tetracycline itself).

From the sixteenth week of pregnancy, tetracyclines are strongly bound in this way in developing tooth and bone structures, causing brown discoloration of deciduous teeth and inhibition of bone growth. In the 1950s, tetracyclines were also commonly used in late pregnancy. This resulted in many reports in the 1960s of brown discoloration of teeth in children who were prenatally exposed to tetracyclines. Since then, the use of tetracyclines has been contraindicated during pregnancy.

Inadvertent first-trimester use of tetracyclines occurs frequently, and has not been associated with an increased risk of other congenital malformations. The results of two population-based case-control studies suggested that oxytetracycline was associated with an increased incidence of congenital malformations when treatment occurred in the second month of pregnancy (Czeizel 1997, 2000C). The number of first-trimester exposures in controls and cases was, however, very small, and there are no other studies confirming this suspicion.

In the past, the use of tetracyclines, especially in high doses or via intravenous administration in the second half of pregnancy, has been associated with severe maternal hepatic toxicity. As tetracyclines are now contraindicated in this stage of pregnancy, this should no longer occur.

> **Recommendation.** Tetracyclines are contraindicated beyond the fifteenth week of gestation. In the first trimester, they are considered to be second-line therapy. Doxycycline should be preferred in such cases. Inadvertent use of tetracyclines, even after the fifteenth week, is not an indication for termination of pregnancy or for invasive prenatal diagnostic procedures.

2.6.7   Sulfonamides, trimethoprim, atovaquone, and pentamidine

Pharmacology and toxicology

Sulfonamides are among the oldest antibiotics. They inhibit the metabolism of bacteria and have bacteriostatic properties. They cross the placenta well; fetal concentrations are 50–90% of maternal plasma concentrations. Sulfonamides compete with bilirubin for binding sites on albumin.

Sulfonamides have not been associated with an increased incidence of congenital malformations. Due to their bilirubin-mobilizing capacity, they may increase the risk of hyperbilirubinemia in the neonate when used near to delivery.

Most sulfonamides are used in combination with other antibiotics. *Cotrimoxazole* is a combination of *sulfamethoxazole* and *trimethoprim* (see below).

2

Pregnancy

2.6 Anti-infective agents

Sulfasalazine is a combination of *sulfapyridine* and *5-amino salicylic acid*, which has been used for many decades as an antirheumatic drug and in the treatment of inflammatory bowel disease. The bilirubin-mobilizing capacity of sulfapyridine is low (see also Chapter 2.5).

Sulfadiazine in combination with *pyrimethamine* is used in the treatment of toxoplasmosis.

Sulfalene and *sulfadoxine* are used in combination with pyrimethamine in the treatment and prophylaxis of malaria (see section 2.6.28).

Sulfamethizole and *sulfafurazole* have been prescribed in the past to treat urinary tract infections, but are no longer in use.

Sulfadicramide is used in ocular preparations.

Trimethoprim antagonizes folic acid in bacteria, but does not affect the human enzyme system with similar potency. Measurable folate depression will occur only with high doses or in those patients who are already folate-depleted. At the usual doses, hematological side effects of trimethoprim or cotrimoxazole have been rare, even after long-term use (Kinzie 1984).

Trimethoprim alone or in combination with sulfamethoxazole attains high renal tissue levels, and is therefore effective in the treatment of urinary tract infections. Levels of trimethoprim and sulfamethoxazole are unchanged during pregnancy.

Very high doses of trimethoprim have produced teratogenic effects (cleft palate) in rats. However, there is no strong evidence to suggest that trimethoprim or cotrimoxazole cause a serious risk of teratogenicity in the human (Czeizel 1990, Brumfitt 1973). Trimethoprim has been used for many decades in non-pregnant subjects and also in pregnant women. At the moment, there is an ongoing discussion concerning the association between the use of folic-acid antagonists and an increased risk of congenital malformations (Shepard 2002, Hernandez-Dias 2001, 2000). Trimethoprim is not a drug of first choice, but is an alternative if penicillins or cephalosporins are ineffective. The risk of folic-acid depletion after low doses of trimethoprim is small. It is recommended that folic acid be supplied in the usual dosage for pregnant women (0.5 mg daily) if trimethoprim is needed in the first trimester.

Tetroxoprim is also a folic-acid antagonist and is used in combination with a sulfonamide, but there are insufficient data on use during pregnancy.

Atovaquone and *pentamidine* are used in the treatment of *Pneumocystis carinii* infections. Experience with the use of both drugs during pregnancy is limited. Pentamidine given to rats in doses similar to those recommended for human use had embryotoxic but no teratogenic effects. Pentamidine in aerosol form has a high affinity for lung tissue, but circulating amounts are small. The dose which a healthcare worker will receive is likely to be lower than the dose received by a patient.

> **Recommendation.** Sulfonamides, trimethoprim, and cotrimoxazole may be safe alternative drugs for antibiotic treatment of urinary tract infections when penicillins and cephalosporins are ineffective. When trimethoprim or cotrimoxazole are needed in the first trimester, folic-acid supplementation (0.5 mg daily) is recommended for theoretical reasons. Tetroxoprim should not be given during pregnancy because of a lack of safety data. Atovaquone and pentamidine should only be given in cases of life-threatening infections and when other antibiotics are ineffective. Although the risk for a pregnant healthcare worker is probably small after aerosol exposure, regular occupational exposure to pentamidine should be avoided until more data on its safety are available. Inadvertent use of tetroxoprim, atovaquone or pentamidine is not an indication for termination of pregnancy or for invasive prenatal diagnostic procedures.

2.6.8   Quinolones

Pharmacology and toxicology

Quinolones impair bacterial DNA metabolism by inhibiting DNA gyrase. They have bactericidal activity at normal doses; at higher doses they have also bacteriostatic properties by inhibiting bacterial RNA and protein synthesis. Quinolones have a high affinity for cartilage and bone tissue; this affinity is highest in immature cartilage.

Pipemidic acid, cinoxacin, and *nalidixic acid* belong to the group of older quinolones. They concentrate in the urinary tract. Few data on their safety during pregnancy are available.

The newer *fluoroquinolones* have more favorable efficacy and pharmacokinetic properties, and are therefore suitable for the treatment of systemic infections. *Ciprofloxacin, enoxacin, fleroxacin, gatifloxacin, grepafloxacin, levofloxacin, lomefloxacin, moxifloxacin, norfloxacin, ofloxacin, pefloxacin, rosoxacin*, and *sparfloxacin* belong to the fluoroquinolones group.

Quinolones cross the placenta and are found in the amniotic fluid at low concentrations. Umbilical cord concentrations of ciprofloxacin, pefloxacin, and ofloxacin have been found to be lower than maternal blood concentrations (Giamarellou 1989).

The use of fluoroquinolones in the first trimester of pregnancy has not been associated with an increased risk of major malformations or other adverse effects on pregnancy outcome (Larsen 2001,

Loebstein 1998, Schaefer 1996, Berkovitch 1994). Most data are available for norfloxacin and ciprofloxacin and, to a lesser extent, for ofloxacin and pefloxacin. There are no or few data for the other fluoroquinolones. Quinolones have not been found to be teratogenic in animals.

Animal experiments have shown that quinolones can cause damage to the cartilage of immature animals and the fetus, resulting in arthropathy. The sensitivity is highest in the dog. The effects are dependent on the dose and duration of treatment, and occur only in the sensitive period.

Musculoskeletal dysfunctions have so far not been found after prenatal exposure in humans (Loebstein 1998, Berkovitch 1994, Peled 1991). Wogelius (2005) expressed concern that prenatal use of fluoroquinolones may be associated with an increased risk of bone malformations. However, the study on 130 women who redeemed a prescription for fluoroquinolones during the first trimester or 30 days before conception did not find a significant increase of (such) birth defects (Wogelius 2005).

Recommendation. Quinolones should only be used in case of complicated infections resistant to the antibiotics of choice in pregnancy. Ciprofloxacin and norfloxacin should then be chosen, because of their relatively large documented experience. Even the first-trimester use of a quinolone antibiotic is not an indication for termination of pregnancy, but detailed fetal ultrasonography can be offered in such cases.

2.6.9   Nitrofurantoin and other drugs for urinary tract infections

Pharmacology and toxicology

Nitrofurantoin is an antiseptic drug which has been used for many decades as an effective agent for the treatment and prophylaxis of urinary tract infections and asymptomatic bacteriuria in pregnancy. High concentrations appear only in the urinary tract; maternal and fetal serum concentrations are low; marked placental transfer does not occur. Nitrofurantoin has not been associated with an increased risk of congenital malformations (Briggs 2005, Ben-David 1994).

Nitrofurantoin may cause hemolytic reactions, especially in patients with glucose-6-phosphatase dehydrogenase deficiency, but except for one case (Bruel 2000) hemolytic anemia in the newborn has never been reported after *in utero* exposure to nitrofurantoin (Gait 1990).

2

Fosfomycin is a broad-spectrum antibiotic which inhibits cell-wall synthesis and is indicated for the treatment of uncomplicated urinary tract infections, especially acute cystitis. A single dose produces therapeutic concentrations in the urine which may last for 1–3 days (Stein 1998). Fosfomycin appears to be safe for use during pregnancy (Reeves 1992).

Methenamine mandelate and *methenamine hippurate* are antiseptic agents for the treatment of urinary tract infections. In urine, formaldehyde is produced from methenamine. In general, they are controversially discussed drugs. Adverse effects on pregnancy outcome have not been reported, but documented experience is very limited.

> **Recommendation.** Nitrofurantoin and fosfomycin can be given during pregnancy to treat urinary tract infections when the antibiotics of choice have been ineffective. Methenamine is contraindicated during pregnancy. Inadvertent use is not an indication for termination of pregnancy or for invasive prenatal diagnostic procedures.

2.6.10   Aminoglycosides

Pharmacology and toxicology

The aminoglycosides *amikacin, gentamycin, kanamycin, neomycin, netilmycin, paromomycin, spectinomycin, streptomycin*, and *tobramycin* inhibit protein synthesis in gram-negative bacteria and have bactericidal activity. Aminoglycosides rapidly cross the placenta. After parenteral administration, fetal plasma concentrations vary between 20 and 40% of maternal plasma concentrations. Gastrointestinal absorption is minimal.

Administration of aminoglycosides to pregnant women may result in cumulation of the drug in fetal plasma, amniotic fluid, and the kidneys (Jin 1992, Bourget 1991, Bernard 1977).

Renal elimination of aminoglycosides is more rapid in pregnant women, and has been reported for gentamycin in obstetric patients by Zaske (1980). This may lead to subtherapeutic serum concentrations. Congenital hearing loss has been documented in association with prenatal exposure to *streptomycin* and *kanamycin*, but not with the use of *gentamycin* and *tobramycin*. However, a case of severe hearing loss after maternal use of gentamycin has been reported (Sanchez-Sainz-Trapaga 1998). The most sensitive period is the first 4 months of pregnancy.

In animal experiments, dose-dependent fetal nephrotoxicity has been reported after prenatal exposure to aminoglycosides (Mantovani 1992, Mallie 1988). Although fetal nephrotoxicity has not been reported in human pregnancy, a theoretical risk exists because aminoglycosides concentrate in the fetal kidneys. There has been one case of renal dysplasia after prenatal exposure to gentamycin and corticosteroids for which a causal relationship could not be excluded (Hulton 1995). Another case of renal anomaly has been reported after first-trimester exposure to gentamycin and ciprofloxacin by Yaris (2004).

> **Recommendation.** Aminoglycosides are not recommended for parenteral use during pregnancy. They should only be administered in case of life-threatening infections. In those cases, maternal serum levels should be carefully monitored and dose should be adjusted if necessary. Treatment with aminoglycosides in pregnancy is not an indication for termination of pregnancy or for invasive prenatal diagnostic procedures. When higher doses have been used, renal function should be monitored in the neonate and an auditory test should be performed. If local or oral application of aminoglycosides is indicated they can be given because systemic absorption is minimal by these routes.

2.6.11 Chloramphenicol

Pharmacology and toxicology

Chloramphenicol and *thiamphenicol* inhibit bacterial protein synthesis and have bacteriostatic activity.

Chloramphenicol is relatively toxic, and can cause severe agranulocytosis. It crosses the placenta well and can reach therapeutic concentrations in the fetus.

Sufficient experience with the use of chloramphenicol is available. There is no evidence that chloramphenicol increases the incidence of congenital malformations.

Chloramphenicol should not be used in the last weeks of pregnancy as, owing to inadequate metabolism in the neonate, toxic concentrations can be reached which may cause the "gray baby syndrome" (feeding problems, vomiting, ash-gray skin, respiratory distress, and cardiovascular collapse), which may be fatal in the neonate.

Recommendation. Chloramphenicol and thiamphenicol are contraindicated during pregnancy unless there is a serious indication. Treatment during the first trimester is not an indication for termination of pregnancy or for invasive prenatal diagnostic procedures.

2.6.12   Metronidazole and other nitroimidazole antibiotics

Pharmacology and toxicology

The nitroimidazole antibiotic *metronidazole* is an antibacterial and antiprotozoal agent used in trichomonas infections, amebiasis, giardiasis, bacterial vaginosis, and anaerobic infections. It acts as an electron acceptor in the metabolism of the bacteria, and causes growth disturbances in the susceptible microorganism. Active metabolites that interact with and disrupt the DNA-synthesis are responsible for the effect. After oral and intravenous administration, concentrations as high as those in the mother are reached in the embryo/fetus. Significant systemic absorption occurs after vaginal application, exposing the fetus as well.

Because metronidazole is mutagenic in bacterial tests and carcinogenic in some animals (review by Dobias 1994), it was feared that it could also be mutagenic and carcinogenic in humans. Such effects have not been reported. A 20-year ongoing study gave no indication of an elevated risk for malignancies after metronidazole therapy (Beard 1988). In a retrospective study, no increased risk of childhood cancer associated with *in utero* exposure to metronidazole was found; only a non-significant association with neuroblastoma was observed (Thapa 1998). Metronidazole does not appear to have teratogenic effects in the human, according to considerable experience (Caro-Paton 1997, Burtin 1995, Piper 1993). A recent prospective controlled study on 228 women exposed to metronidazole in pregnancy, 86% of whom with first-trimester exposure, confirmed these findings (Diav-Citrin 2001).

Metronidazole is now being recommended by some investigators for the treatment of bacterial vaginosis in pregnancies at high risk for preterm delivery, as a strategy to decrease this risk. For this purpose, oral therapy against possible subclinical genital upper tract infection seems to be more effective than intravaginal therapy (Donders 2000, review by Joesoef 1999). A review by Yudin confirms that vaginal treatment regimens of bacterial vaginosis are ineffective in preventing preterm birth (Yudin 2005; see also Chapter 2.14).

Nimorazole and *tinidazole*, both registered for the treatment of trichomonas infections, amebiasis, and bacterial vaginosis, cannot be evaluated sufficiently because of lack of human data. The same applies to *ornidazole*.

> **Recommendation.** If strongly indicated, metronidazole can be used in pregnancy. For treatment of trichomoniasis, a single oral dose of 2 g should be used. Parenteral administration is only indicated for life-threatening anaerobic infections. Protracted vaginal treatment of vaginosis should be avoided because it is not considered effective enough; moreover, it exposes the fetus for longer. Metronidazole is preferred over nimorazole and tinidazole. Treatment with nimorazole, ornidazole or tinidazole during pregnancy does not require termination of pregnancy or invasive diagnostic procedures. However, a detailed fetal ultrasound may be considered after first-trimester exposure to these compounds.

2.6.13 Polypeptide antibiotics

Pharmacology and toxicology

Vancomycin, colistin, polymyxin B, and *teicoplanine* belong to the polypeptide antibiotics. Polypeptide antibiotics increase the permeability of the cytoplasma membrane of sensitive bacteria. They work against gram-positive bacteria.

For example, *vancomycin* is used against multiresistant staphylococcus. Experience with treatment in human pregnancy is limited; neither malformations nor nephrotoxicity or auditory impairment were seen in neonates (Reyes 1989). There is a case report of a woman who became hypotensive when vancomycin was infused too rapidly during labor; the fetus exhibited a bradycardia during the hypotensive episode (Hill 1985).

Colistin and *polymyxin B* have as yet not shown teratogenic properties in humans, although documented experience is very limited (Kazy 2005). Experience with *teicoplanine* is insufficient for a risk assessment.

> **Recommendation.** Vancomycin should only be used in case of life-threatening bacterial infections. Also, colistin, polymyxin B and (especially) the little-tested teicoplanine should only be used if compellingly indicated. The use of these substances is not in itself an indication either for termination of pregnancy or for invasive diagnostic procedures.

2.6.14 Antimycotics in general

For the treatment of mycosis, topical therapy with the older agents is to be considered safe in pregnancy.

There is less experience and fewer data with systemic agents. If systemic therapy is actually necessary, then there should be a careful choice from this group of questionable drugs.

Lately it has become "fashionable" to use antimycotics for treatment of aspecific symptoms supposedly associated with the harmless presence of fungus in the stool; in pregnancy, at least, this should be omitted.

The treatment of asymptomatic colonization of the vagina is unnecessary (Sobel 2000).

2.6.15   Nystatin

Pharmacology and toxicology

Nystatin is an antimycotic that is effective against candida infections of the skin and mucosa, and is not absorbed. It is bound to ergosterol in the cell membrane of the fungi, and causes a disturbance in the permeability of the cell membrane. Extensive data on intravaginal application of nystatin during pregnancy do not give any indication of embryo/fetotoxic effects (King 1998). Nystatin use is limited by lower efficacy rates and by the need for longer duration of treatment required with this agent.

> **Recommendation.** Nystatin can be used throughout pregnancy without restriction. It is a drug of choice for the treatment of superficial candida infections of the mucous membranes of mouth, intestine, and vagina, but may be less effective than newer agents.

2.6.16   Clotrimazole and miconazole for topical use

Pharmacology and toxicology

Clotrimazole and *miconazole* are antimycotics belonging to the group of imidazole derivatives. These agents inhibit the ergosterol biosynthesis, thereby causing disturbances in the permeability and function of the cell membrane. Systemic absorption of these agents is minimal. Clotrimazole is only used for the local treatment of mycosis of the skin and mucosa. In studies comparing intravaginal use of imidazoles to nystatin, imidazoles have superior cure rates and lower relapse rates. In a population-based study it was found that vulvovaginal clotrimoxazole treatment during pregnancy reduces the prevalence of preterm birth significantly (Czeizel 2004A).

Considerable experience with clotrimazole and miconazole for the local therapy of vaginal mycosis in pregnancy did not show any embryotoxic potential of these topical antifungal agents (King 1998). For miconazole these findings were confirmed in a population-based case control study (Czeizel 2004B).

> **Recommendation.** Clotrimazole and miconazole are topical antimycotics of choice in pregnancy.

2.6.17   Other local "conazole" antimycotics

Pharmacology and toxicology

Bifonazole, croconazole, econazole, fenticonazole, isoconazole, ketoconazole, omoconazole, oxiconazole, sertaconazole, sulconazole, and *tioconazole* are imidazole derivatives, and structurally and functionally related to clotrimazole. No teratogenic effects have been observed as a result of local treatment with these antimycotics. For econazole, these findings were confirmed in a population-based case control study (Czeizel 2003A). They are, however, less tried than clotrimazole and miconazole (King 1998).

> **Recommendation.** Bifonazole, croconazole, econazole, fenticonazole, isoconazole, ketoconazole, omoconazole, oxiconazole, sertaconazole, sulconazole, and tioconazole are second-choice antimycotics for local therapy. Nystatin, clotrimazole, and miconazole are preferred.

2.6.18   Other local antimycotics

Pharmacology and toxicology

Amorolfin, ciclopiroxolamine, nafiifin, terbinafine, tolciclate, and *tolnaftate* have been insufficiently studied with regard to their prenatal toxicity. As yet, there is no substantial indication for an increased risk of malformations after local use.

A population-based case-control study on vaginal *natamycin* treatment during pregnancy did not show an increased teratogenic risk (Czeizel 2003B).

> **Recommendation.** Amorolfin, ciclopiroxolamine, naftifin, terbinafine, tolciclate, and tolnaftate are to be avoided during pregnancy. The use of these substances is not, in itself, an indication either for a termination of pregnancy or for invasive diagnostic procedures. Natamycin is a second-choice antimycotic for local therapy. Nystatin, clotrimazole, and miconazole are preferred.

2.6.19   "Conazole" antimycotics for systemic use

Pharmacology and toxicology

Itraconazole and *miconazole* are systemically used antimycotics belonging to the group of imidazole derivatives. These agents inhibit the ergosterol biosynthesis, thereby causing disturbances in the permeability and functions of the fungal cell membrane. In animal experiments, they cross the fetal–placental barrier easily.

Fluconazole and *ketoconazole* are triazole derivates. Their activity matches that of the structurally related imidazole derivatives.

In animal experiments, teratogenic effects have been observed after administration of very high doses of these antimycotics.

Concerning the use of *fluconazole* in pregnancy, there was a report of three children with craniofacial, skeletal, and cardiac malformations, similar to those seen in animal studies. Because of meningitis, their mother had used high doses of fluconazole (400–800 mg daily) through or beyond the first trimester on a long-term basis (Pursley 1996). A fourth case was reported of a child with similar malformations, whose mother was also treated, with high doses of fluconazole on a long-term basis for meningitis. They all shared some characteristics with the Antley–Bixler syndrome (Aleck 1997). Another malformed baby with encephalocele and an aorta emerging from the right ventricle was published. The mother had been taken a single fluconazole dose for vaginal candidiasis around conception, which makes a causal relation unprobable (Sanchez 1998). Recently, another case with craniofacial and skeletal abnormalities was reported after prenatal exposure to high doses of fluconazole on a long-term basis (Lopez-Rangel 2004).

In a prospectively studied controlled cohort of 226 women, first-trimester exposure to low-dosage regimens (150 mg/d) of fluconazole for vaginal candidiasis did not appear to cause an increased risk of malformations (Mastroiacovo 1996). In an unpublished (to date) ongoing prospective study by the European Network of Teratology Information Services (ENTIS) concerning the new systemic "conazole" antimycotics, preliminary data on 191 fluconazole-exposed pregnancies give no indication of an increased risk of malformations. Fluconazole was mostly used very early in pregnancy on a short-term basis and in low doses (Vial 2001). In several other studies, based on linkage of prescription databases with birth registries, first-trimester exposure to low-dosage regimens of fluconazole for vaginal candidiasis did not appear to cause an increased risk of malformations. These studies included more than 400 first-trimester exposures (Jick 1999, Sørensen 1999, Inman 1994).

Experience with use of *itraconazole* in pregnancy is still fairly limited. In the aforementioned prospective study by ENTIS, preliminary data on 182 itraconazole-exposed pregnancies show no increased teratogenic risk in humans after short-term use in the first trimester (Vial 2001). In a recent controlled prospective study, the first-trimester use of itraconazole in 198 pregnancies did not seem to be associated with an increased teratogenic risk either (Bar-Oz 2000). A small study, based on linkage of prescription databases with birth registries, yielded similar results (Jick 1999).

Ketoconazole is an inhibitor of steroid synthesis, and as such is also used for the treatment of Cushing's syndrome. Ketoconazole inhibits testosterone synthesis as well. Whether these properties have a possible effect on fetal corticosteroid synthesis and may cause abnormalities in the development of male fetuses exposed to ketoconazole prenatally is unknown. However, in two case reports treatment of Cushing's syndrome with ketoconazole during pregnancy resulted in healthy male and female infants. The male infant was prenatally exposed throughout pregnancy, except for the third to seventh weeks; the female infant was exposed during the late third trimester. No disturbed sexual differentiation or neonatal adrenal insufficiency were observed (Berwaerts 1999, Amado 1990). In the aforementioned prospective study by ENTIS concerning the new systemic "conazole" antimycotics, preliminary data on 280 ketoconazole-exposed pregnancies give no indication of an increased teratogenic risk in humans after short-term systemic use in the early first trimester (Vial 2001).

Experience with systemic use of *miconazole* in pregnancy is limited to a few cases, in which no adverse effects on pregnancy outcome were seen after first-trimester exposure (Vial 2001).

> **Recommendation.** In particular during the first trimester, systemic antimycotic therapy with fluconazole, ketoconazole, miconazole or itraconazole should be used only if compellingly indicated. For treatment of serious disseminated mycoses, amphotericin B is the preferred drug in early pregnancy. For treatment of vaginal candidiasis where local treatment has failed, low-dose fluconazole, as the best documented "conazole" compound for this indication, is preferred. Treatment during pregnancy is not an indication for termination of pregnancy, but a detailed ultrasound examination of fetal anatomy should be considered after first-trimester use.

2.6.20   Amphotericin B

Pharmacology and toxicology

Amphotericin B can be applied locally or can be used as a systemic therapy for mycosis – for instance, in systemic candida infection, cryptococcosis, and coccidiomycosis. Amphotericin B is bound to ergosterol in the fungal cell membrane, and causes a disturbance in the permeability of the cell membrane. This antimycotic can cause febrile reactions, electrolyte disorders, and nephrotoxicity, when administered parenterally. Amphotericin B crosses the placenta and may be retained in the placenta and other tissues, prolonging exposure for the fetus and neonate. This effect may have contributed to reported transient neonatal renal dysfunction (Dean 1994).

There are several case reports of small numbers of pregnant women being treated with amphotericin B without an apparent increased risk of malformations (Ely 1998, review by Dean 1994); however, the number of reported cases is too small for a definitive risk assessment. Experience with the newer lipid formulations of amphotericin B is still very limited. To date, there is only one report of the use of amphotericin B liposome for the treatment of visceral leishmaniasis in a pregnant patient during the second trimester; no adverse effects were reported (King 1998).

> **Recommendation.** Local application is considered safe. Parenteral use of amphotericin B in pregnancy should be restricted to dangerous disseminated mycoses.

2.6.21   Flucytosine

Pharmacology and toxicology

Flucytosine is effective against *Cryptococcus neoformans* and many candida species. It is used in systemic infections with these pathogens, and works through inhibition of DNA synthesis. There is concern about adverse developmental and reproductive effects of this agent because in the fungus cell flucytosine is metabolized to – among others – 5-fluorouracil, a cytostatic agent. To a lesser degree, this reaction is also to be expected in the human organism. In animal experiments, flucytosine has a teratogenic effect in doses that are lower than those used in human therapy. As yet, no malformations have been reported in humans; however, there is practically no published experience with the use of flucytosine in the first trimester. Limited experience in the second and third trimesters of pregnancy with flucytosine for treatment of life-threatening disseminated cryptococcosis has yielded no adverse fetal outcomes (Ely 1998).

> **Recommendation.** Flucytosine should only be used for life-threatening disseminated fungal infections. Such a treatment during the first trimester does not require termination of pregnancy, but detailed fetal ultrasonography should be considered.

2.6.22   Griseofulvin

Pharmacology and toxicology

Griseofulvin is an organically derived antifungal agent; it is used as an oral preparation for the treatment of dermatophytosis of skin, hair and nails. Because it is deposited in keratine, it is suitable for the therapy of nail mycoses. In animal experiments it has a teratogenic effect and, moreover, a carcinogenic effect in high doses.

Experience in human pregnancy is limited. In one report, two pairs of conjoined twins were observed after use of griseofulvin in pregnancy (Rosa 1987); however, in contrast to this report, data from two birth defect registries did not uncover an association between griseofulvin and conjoined twinning or other anomalies (Knudsen 1987, Metneki 1987). The birth rate of conjoined twins might be 1:100 000 births.

> **Recommendation.** Because it is not prescribed for life-threatening fungal infections, therapy with griseofulvin is contraindicated in pregnancy. However, if inadvertent exposure has occurred, neither termination of pregnancy nor invasive diagnostic procedures are required. A detailed ultrasound examination can be considered.

2.6.23   Terbinafine

Pharmacology and toxicology

Terbinafine is used for both oral and topical therapy of nail mycoses and various tineal skin infections. There is little experience with its use during human pregnancy. In an ongoing study, the Canadian Motherisk program reports on 54 pregnancies exposed to terbinafine; of these, 24 were exposed to systemic therapy and 23 to topical; 24 were exposed during the first trimester. Data collected thus far appear to suggest no increased risk for major malformations (Sarkar 2003).

> **Recommendation.** Terbinafine should not be used during pregnancy, because data on pregnancy outcome are lacking and nail mycosis is not a condition requiring urgent treatment. Inadvertent pregnancy exposure does not require termination of pregnancy. Detailed fetal ultrasonography can be considered after first-trimester exposure.

2.6.24   Malaria prophylaxis and therapy in pregnancy

Apart from pregnant women living in malaria areas, ever more often pregnant women are traveling in tropical countries and asking for appropriate malaria prophylaxis. As multidrug resistance of the parasite is emerging, a general recommendation is increasingly more difficult. Prophylaxis against and treatment for malaria tropica, caused by *Plasmodium falciparum*, is especially difficult. Pregnancy enhances the clinical severity of falciparum malaria, especially in the primiparous or non-immune woman. Pregnancy alters a woman's immunity to malaria, making her more susceptible to malaria infection and increasing the risk of illness, severe anemia, and death. Maternal malaria increases the risk of spontaneous abortion, stillbirth, prematurity, and low birth weight, and thus results in excess infant mortality (Shulman 2003). Therefore, mosquito-bite prevention, prophylaxis, and treatment of malaria should not be shortened or omitted in an ongoing pregnancy. Depending on the drug, the chemoprophylaxis must be continued for up to 4 weeks after leaving the malarial region. Traveling to areas with multidrug-resistant malaria should be avoided if possible.

For travelers to malaria-endemic areas, generally chloroquine is the drug of choice for malaria prophylaxis during pregnancy, in some situations in combination with proguanil. If resistance for these agents is likely, mefloquine is second choice. No antimalarial prophylactic regimen gives complete protection, but good chemoprophylaxis does reduce the risk of fatal disease (WHO 2005A).

For women living in falciparum-endemic areas, the WHO recommends insecticide-treated nets (ITNs) and intermittent preventive treatment (IPT) in areas with stable transmission, and ITNs and effective case management of malarial illness in areas with unstable transmission, as prevention and management of malaria during pregnancy (WHO 2005B).

For treatment of malarial infection in the first trimester, chloroquine (if the parasite is fully-sensitive!) and quinine are usually the drugs of choice; in the second and third trimesters, in addition to quinine and chloroquine, artesiminin derivatives, sulphadoxin/pyrimethamin (see also Chapter 2.18.7), and amodiaquine can be used. Mefloquine should only be used if no other drug is available.

The choice of drug for malaria prophylaxis and treatment during pregnancy depends on the local pattern of antimalarial drug resistance, the severity of the malaria, and the degree of pre-existing immunity. It is important to be well informed about the current recommendations for prophylaxis and treatment of malaria in the area to be visited (review by Shulman 2003).

2.6.25   Chloroquine

Pharmacology and toxicology

Chloroquine, an antimalarial drug from the 4-aminochinoline group, is a rapidly-acting blood schizonticide, destroying the asexual blood forms of all *Plasmodium* species. Chloroquine resistance is common in many malaria-endemic regions. This resistance mainly concerns the pathogenic parasite of the severe and often deadly progressing malaria tropica (pathogen: *Plasmodium falciparum*). However, resistance against chloroquine has also been observed in *Plasmodium vivax*, the pathogenic parasite of the less severely progressing malaria tertiana.

Chloroquine is neither embryo- nor fetotoxic when used in the usual dosage for malaria prophylaxis, and when used for the treatment of the malarial infection in a 3-day course (Philips-Howard 1996). A study on the use of chloroquine in a 3-day course for the treatment of *Plasmodium vivax* infection during the first trimester of pregnancy confirms these findings (McGready 2002).

Damage to the fetal retina and inner ear has been linked to chloroquine therapy in pregnancy; in these cases, chloroquine was used daily in high doses on a long-term basis (Hart 1964). Such long-term, high-dose therapy may be used for other indications – for instance, in chronic inflammatory diseases. However, small series of patients taking large doses of (hydroxy)chloroquine during pregnancy for treatment of systemic lupus erythematosus did not show an increased risk of congenital malformations or other adverse effects (Parke 1996; see also Chapter 2.1).

> **Recommendation.** Chloroquine is the drug of choice for prophylaxis and treatment of malaria during all phases of pregnancy if the parasite is sensitive, and if appropriate for the type and severity of the malarial infection. If chloroquine resistance of the parasite is likely or has been demonstrated, other drugs must be used for the prophylaxis and treatment of malaria. It is important to keep informed of current recommendations for the region in question.

2.6.26   Proguanil

Pharmacology and toxicology

Proguanil is an older agent for malaria prophylaxis. It is a folic-acid antagonist. Owing to the increasing appearance of chloroquine-resistant malaria species, proguanil has experienced a revival. In some tropical areas, it is the drug of choice for malaria prophylaxis. Proguanil is used alone or in combination with chloroquine for malaria prophylaxis and, more recently, in combination with *atovaquone* for malaria prophylaxis and treatment (see Chapter 2.6.33 regarding atovaquone). There is no indication of embryotoxic effects (Philips-Howard 1996).

> **Recommendation.** Proguanil can be prescribed in all phases of pregnancy. Proguanil alone or in combination with chloroquine is the malaria prophylaxis of choice in regions where chloroquine alone does not give adequate protection. If resistance of the parasite is likely or has been demonstrated, other drugs must be used for the prophylaxis of malaria. It is important to keep informed of current recommendations for the region in question.

2.6.27   Mefloquine

Pharmacology and toxicology

Mefloquine is a very effective antimalarial drug. It is a potent, long-acting blood schizonticide that destroys the erythrocytic forms of all *Plasmodium* species. It is still effective against most chloroquine-resistant pathogens, except for clearly defined regions of multidrug resistance.

As yet, experience with first-trimester use of mefloquine for prophylaxis in several hundred pregnancies gives no indication for a teratogenic potential in humans (Schlagenhauf 1999, Philips-Howard 1998, unpublished experience by the European Network of Teratology Information Services, ENTIS). More extensive experience with mefloquine prophylaxis in the second and third trimesters of pregnancy gave no clear indication for mefloquine-associated adverse effects (Schlagenhauf 1999, Philips-Howard 1996).

Cumulative evidence is reassuring, and has led the WHO and the US CDC&P to sanction the use of mefloquine in the second and third trimesters of pregnancy both for prophylaxis and treatment (Schlagenhauf 1999, WHO 1996A). However, one group of investigators reported that their data provided evidence that mefloquine treatment during pregnancy may be associated with stillbirth: women who were treated with mefloquine in pregnancy had a significant greater risk of stillbirth than did women treated with quinine alone (Nosten 1999).

> **Recommendation.** Mefloquine can be used for prophylaxis or treatment of malaria in cases with chloroquine/proguanil-resistant *P. falciparum*. It is important to keep informed of current recommendations for the region in question. Exposure to mefloquine in the first trimester does not require termination of pregnancy or invasive diagnostic procedures.

2.6.28   Pyrimethamine, sulfadoxine and dapsone

Pharmacology and toxicology

Pyrimethamine is an inhibitor of folic-acid synthesis and a well-tried malaria prophylactic agent in pregnancy. However, nowadays it is only used in combination with sulfonamides and sulfones such as *sulfadoxine, sulfalene*, and *dapsone*; these agents are also inhibitors of folic-acid synthesis.

Severe cutaneous reactions like erythema exsudativum multiforme and Stevens–Johnson syndrome were reported as unwanted side effects of the combination *sulfadoxin/pyrimethamine*. Therefore, use of the combination for malariaprophylaxis is not recommended, but the combination is used for treatment of acute chloroquine-resistant falciparum malaria and as intermittent preventive treatment (IPT) for prevention of malaria-associated adverse effects during pregnancy in women living in malaria-endemic areas. Pregnant women suffering from resistant malaria forms were successfully treated with the combination sulfadoxine/pyrimethamine (Philips-Howard 1996). Intermittent preventive treatment (ITP) with sulfadoxin/ pyrimethamine seems to be the most effective in preventing the adverse outcomes associated with malaria in pregnancy in countries where *Plasmodium falciparum* is sensitive, although the spread of resistance is affecting its efficacy (Newman 2003).

The combination *dapson/pyrimethamine* is used for prophylaxis of chloroquine-resistant malaria. Significant side effects like agranulocytosis have restricted its use (for dapsone, see also tuberculostatics). Data on pregnancy outcome after the use of this combination during pregnancy for malaria prophylaxis and treatment are limited and insufficient for a well-grounded risk assessment (review by Brabin 2004).

Pyrimethamine, in combination with a long-acting sulfonamide, is also used therapeutically for toxoplasmosis infection of the fetus, in particular after the first trimester. The effectiveness of the various schedules for prevention and treatment of toxoplasmosis is an ongoing topic of discussion (Wallon 1999).

Because of embryotoxic effects in animal experiments, there were initial objections against use of these folic acid antagonists in early pregnancy (see also trimethoprim). Currently, there is an ongoing discussion concerning the association between the use of folic-acid antagonists and an increased risk of congenital malformations (Shepard 2002, Hernandez-Diaz 2001, 2000).

Recommendation. If indicated, the combination sulfadoxine/pyrimethamine can be used during pregnancy for the treatment of acute chloroquine-resistant malaria tropica; the combination can also be used in intermittent preventive treatment (IPT) in the second and third trimesters although it is not recommended for prophylaxis. Significant side effects have restricted the use of dapsone/pyrimethamine for prophylaxis of chloroquine-resistant malaria tropica. This combination should be considered as second choice in pregnancy. It is important to keep informed of current recommendations for the region in question. Pyrimethamine, in combination with a long-acting sulfonamide, can be used for the prevention/treatment of *toxoplasmosis* infection of the fetus.

2.6.29   Quinine

Pharmacology and toxicology

Quinine is the oldest antimalarial agent. It has a good and rapid schizonticide activity against the erythrocytic forms of all *Plasmodium* species. In spite of relatively high toxicity and a narrow therapeutic range, it is used more often for the treatment of chloroquine-resistant malaria today. Concentrations in the fetus are just as high as in the mother, and are potentially toxic. There are some reports describing eye defects and hearing loss in children after use of quinine in pregnancy. However, in those cases considerably higher doses had generally been administered than are used nowadays for the treatment of acute malaria. There is no evidence of an increased risk of abortion or preterm delivery with the use of a standard dosage of quinine for treatment of acute malaria (Philips-Howard 1996). In a study on the use of quinine for the treatment of *Plasmodium falciparum* infection during the first trimester of pregnancy ($n = 165$) these findings were confirmed, as no increased rates of spontaneous abortion, congenital malformations, stillbirth or low birth weight were found (McGready 2002).

Pregnancy outcome has been compared between mefloquine-treated and quinine-treated pregnant women. Women who were treated with mefloquine in pregnancy had a significant greater risk of stillbirth than did women treated with quinine alone; there was no difference in risk of congenital malformations (Nosten 1999).

A trial comparing quinine-clindamycine ($n = 64$) with artesunate ($n = 65$) for the treatment of falciparum malaria during the second or third trimesters of pregnancy found no serious adverse effects, no increase in stillbirths or congenital malformations above expected rates, and no negative impact on child development for both regimens (McGready 2001A). A small trial comparing quinine with artesunate-atovaquone-proguanil ($n = 39$) for the treatment of falciparum-malaria during the second or third trimesters of pregnancy found no serious adverse effects and no significant differences in birth weight, gestational age, congenital malformation rates, or in growth and developmental parameters of infants (McGready 2005).

Especially in the last part of pregnancy, severe maternal hypoglycemia has been induced by quinine therapy.

Induction of contractions with high doses of quinine cannot be excluded. Quinine is a component of some analgesic compounds and of certain beverages, although in lower and apparently non-embryotoxic doses.

> **Recommendation.** In pregnancy, quinine can be used for therapy of acute chloroquine-resistant falciparum malaria. The potential risk for the fetus due to the therapy is much less than the hazards due to the severe maternal disease. Attention should be paid to possible maternal hypoglycemia. Even though embryotoxic effects due to quinine in analgesic compounds are not to be expected, these agents should be avoided because they do not conform to good therapeutical practice.

2.6.30   Halofantrine

Pharmacology and toxicology

Halofantrine is a malaria drug with a rapid schizonticide activity against the erythrocytic forms of those *Plasmodium* species that are resistant to chloroquine and other malaria drugs. Halofantrine lengthens the QT interval in the ECG. Halofantrine can provoke life-threatening arrhythmias in patients with cardiac disease, and in combination with other arrhythmogenic agents.

Experience with the use of halofantrine in human pregnancy is too limited for a defined risk assessment.

> **Recommendation.** Halofantrine should only be used in those cases of severe falciparum malaria which cannot be effectively treated with better-studied and less toxic agents (e.g. chloroquine, quinine, artemisinin derivatives, mefloquine). Halofantrine is not indicated in other malaria forms, like malaria tertiana. In cases of predisposition to cardiac rhythm disturbances, other malaria drugs should definitely be selected. Treatment with halofantrine does not require termination of pregnancy. To evaluate fetal morphologic development, a detailed ultrasound examination can be considered after first-trimester exposure.

2.6.31   Primaquine

Pharmacology and toxicology

Primaquine, an 8-aminochinoline derivative, acts against vivax and ovale malaria by destroying the exoerythrocytic forms of the malaria parasite. It is used after suppressive therapy with chloroquine to eliminate the pathogen completely to prevent a relapse of vivax and ovale malaria. Primaquine should not be used in pregnancy because of the potential risk of hemolytic effects in the fetus. As yet, there are no studies that permit a well-grounded risk assessment. However, there is no substantial evidence for a teratogenic potential in humans (Philips-Howard 1996).

> **Recommendation.** Primaquine should not be used in pregnancy. Instead, it is recommended that weekly prophylaxis be continued in these cases, with 300 mg chloroquine base, until delivery. After delivery, therapy with primaquine can be started. Inadvertent pregnancy exposure during the first trimester requires neither termination of pregnancy nor invasive diagnostic procedures.

2.6.32 Artemisinin derivatives

Pharmacology and toxicology

Artemisinin derivatives like *artesunate, artemether, artemether dihydroartemisinin*, and artemotil are the most potent antimalarials available. These compounds combine rapid blood schizonticide activity with a wide therapeutic index. Artemisinin derivatives are used nowadays as artimisin-based-combination therapy (ACT) or as monotherapy for the treatment of multidrug-resistant falciparum malaria. Recommended artimisin-based combinations are artemether plus lumefantrine, artesunate plus sulphadoxine/pyrimethamine, artesunate plus amodiaquine, and artesunate plus mefloquine.

Very limited experience with artemisinin use in the second and third trimesters did not demonstrate any adverse effects on the children (Philips-Howard 1996). In a prospective treatment study, artesunate ($n = 528$) or artemether ($n = 11$) was used to treat 539 episodes of acute *P. falciparum* malaria (44 episodes occurred during the first trimester). Birth outcomes were not significantly different from community rates for abortion, stillbirth, congenital abnormality, or mean duration of gestation. An earlier report from the same group on 83 women treated with artemisinin derivatives appears to be a subset of the more recent publication (McGready 2001B, 1998). In Gambia, a total of 287 pregnant women were exposed to artesunate plus sulphadoxine/pyrimethamine during a mass drug administration, and no increased risk of adverse pregnancy outcome was noted, comparing the exposed to the non-exposed pregnancies; 35 women were exposed in the first trimester (Deen 2001). In a small study ($n = 28$), no increased risk of adverse pregnancy outcome was found after the use of artemether for the treatment of falciparum malaria in the second or third trimester of pregnancy (Adam 2004A).

2 *Pregnancy*

2.6 Anti-infective agents

These reassuring data have led the WHO to sanction the use of artemisinin derivatives in the second and third trimesters of pregnancy for treatment of multidrug-resistant falciparum malaria (WHO 2002). However, first-trimester experience is still too limited for a well-grounded risk assessment.

> **Recommendation.** The artemisinin derivatives can be used as monotherapy or as ACT (e.g. artesunate plus sulphadoxine/pyrimethamine, artesunate plus mefloquine) in the second and third trimesters of pregnancy for treatment of multidrug-resistant falciparum malaria. During first trimester, artemisinin derivatives should only be used if there is no safe and effective alternative. Inadvertent use of these antimalarials during the first trimester does not require termination of pregnancy. To evaluate fetal morphologic development, a detailed ultrasound examination can be considered after first-trimester exposure to artemisinin derivatives.

2.6.33   Other malarial agents

Pharmacology and toxicology

As multidrug resistance of the parasite to the well-known medicines is emerging – especially for *Plasmodium falciparum* (malaria tropica) – more than 10 combinations of various antimalarial drugs are used. In some regions, the combination of *chloroquine* plus *pyrimethamine* or *doxycycline* has proven effective. *Clindamycin* combined with *quinine* is used to treat multidrug-resistant malaria in pregnancy in some areas (Alecrim 2000). A recent trial comparing quinine-clindamycine ($n = 64$) with artesunate ($n = 65$) for the treatment of falciparum malaria during the second or third trimester of pregnancy found no serious adverse effects, no increase in stillbirths or congenital malformations above expected rates, and no negative impact on child development (McGready 2001A).

Amodiaquine is a malarial agent related to chloroquine. To date, there is no indication for specific teratogenic effects (review by Thomas 2004). Severe side effects such as toxic hepatitis and fatal agranulocytosis were attributed to the use of amodiaquine as prophylaxis. This and increasing drug resistance precludes its use for prophylaxis, but it is used therapeutically (Alecrim 2000). In a recent study, 900 pregnant women with a gestational age of 16 weeks or more and *P. falciparum* asexual stage parasitaemia were randomly assigned chloroquine, sulphadoxine-pyrimethamine, amodiaquine, or amodiaquine plus sulphadoxine-pyrimethamine. No serious liver toxic effects or white blood cell dyscrasias were noted. The authors concluded that amodiaquine alone or in combination with sulphadoxine-pyrimethamine, although associated with minor side effects, is most effective when used to treat malaria in pregnancy (Tagbor 2006). There was no significant difference with respect to the rates of spontaneous abortion, prematurity, stillbirth, and birth defects. However, considering the methodological limitations of the study and the limited experience with first-trimester exposure, these results do not rule out embryotoxic effects.

Atovaquone is a new antimalarial agent. Used in combination with proguanil, it seems to be very effective against multidrug-resistant *Plasmodium falciparum* as prophylaxis and treatment. As yet, there is very little documented experience of the use of this combination in human pregnancy. A small trial comparing quinine with artesunate-atovaquone-proguanil ($n = 39$) for the treatment of falciparum malaria during the second or third trimester of pregnancy found no significant differences in birth weight or gestational age, the congenital malformations rates, or the growth and developmental parameters of infants (McGready 2005). In a small study, no increased risk of adverse pregnancy outcome was noted after the use of atovaquone-proguanil for the treatment of falciparum malaria in 22 third-trimester pregnant women; the pharmacokinetics of atovaquone appeared to be influenced by the pregnancy status (Na-Bangchang 2005).

Lumefantrine is used in combination with artemether in the treatment of malaria disease. There is no documented experience of its use in pregnancy.

Recommendation. The antimalarial agents in this section are reserve drugs for the treatment of malaria. When indicated, clindamycin can be used in pregnancy (see clindamycin). Doxycycline should not be used after the fifteenth week of pregnancy (see tetracyclines). Significant side effects have precluded the use of amodiaquine for prophylaxis. It should be considered as a second-choice drug in pregnancy; safer antimalarials are preferred. Atovaquone should only be used in pregnancy if there is no safe and effective alternative for the treatment of acute multidrug-resistant malaria. Inadvertent use of these antimalarials does not require termination of pregnancy. To evaluate fetal morphologic development, a detailed ultrasound examination can be considered after first trimester exposure to atovaquone.

2.6.34 Tuberculosis and pregnancy

The indications for treatment of active tuberculosis in pregnant women are no different from those for non-pregnant women. Transmission and infection are felt to be the same as in the non-pregnant individual, and pregnancy does not seem to influence the course of the disease (Laibl 2005, Tripathy 2002, Espinal 1996).

Untreated tuberculosis represents a greater hazard to the mother and her fetus than does the treatment of the disease (Bothamley 2001, Raju 1998, Brost 1997). There are slight differences in the recommendations of the different organizations in the world, such as the WHO, the International Union against Tuberculosis and Lung Disease (IUATLD), and several national organizations (Frieden 2003). Treatment considerations depend on disease status and drug resistance. Some treatment schedules recommend delaying preventive therapy until after delivery in pregnant women with only a positive tuberculin skin test (PPD) but a negative chest radiograph, unless they have a high risk of progressing to active disease (for example, HIV patients, diabetics, recent converters, and those who are close contacts of a person with an active disease). For the treatment of active tuberculosis, *isoniazide* (INH), *rifampicin*, and *ethambutol* are considered to be the first-line antituberculous drugs during pregnancy; a regimen including *pyrazinamide* for the first 2 months can be considered. A particular problem is the increasing incidence of single- and multidrug-resistant tuberculosis (MDR-TB). Therefore, treatment should always consist of at least two, but usually three or more, drugs. Pregnant women with MDR-TB may also require second-line antituberculous drugs; the necessity for treatment should be weighed against the risk for the fetus on an individual base (Laibl 2005, Frieden 2003, Shin 2003, Tripathy 2002, Bothamley 2001, Raju 1998, Brost 1997). A major cause of tuberculosis resistance and treatment failure is medication non-compliance. Because of the seriousness of tuberculosis in pregnancy, the importance of daily intake should be emphasized and this should be supervised if necessary.

2.6.35   Isoniazid (INH)

Pharmacology and toxicology

Isoniazid has proven to be a highly effective drug against many strains of mycobacterium, and can be used for tuberculous prophylaxis and for treatment of an active disease during pregnancy. Although INH can cross the placenta, it does not appear to be teratogenic. An increased rate of malformations, as mentioned in earlier publications, has not been confirmed. As isoniazid increases pyridoxine metabolism, which may be responsible for CNS toxicity, INH therapy in the pregnant woman should be combined with pyridoxine. As a possible increased risk of INH-induced hepatotoxicity in pregnant women has been reported in the literature, it is recommended that liver-function tests should be performed at least monthly in INH-treated pregnant women (Laibl 2005, Bothamley 2001, Raju 1998).

Recommendation. Isoniazid is the drug of choice for prophylaxis and treatment of tuberculosis in pregnancy. It should be combined with pyridoxine (vitamine B$_6$). Liver-function tests should be performed at least monthly.

2.6.36   Rifampicin

Pharmacology and toxicology

Rifampicin is indicated as part of a multidrug regimen for the treatment of active tuberculosis in pregnancy. Rifampicin can cross the placenta. Because rifampicin inhibits DNA-dependent RNA polymerase, there has been concern that it might interfere with fetal development. Until now, no reports in the literature have confirmed this fear; the risk of congenital malformations seems not to be increased. Several observations suggest that concomitant rifampicin administration may enhance the hepatotoxicity of INH. As rifampicin influences vitamin K synthesis and is associated with an increased risk of hemorrhagic complications in the mother as well as in the newborn, prophylactic administration of vitamin K to the mother and the neonate is advised.

Recommendation. Rifampicin is a drug of choice for the treatment of tuberculosis during pregnancy. When used near term, prophylactic vitamin K should be administered to the mother and neonate to prevent hemorrhagic complications (see vitamin K, Chapter 2.9). Rifampicin may also be given prophylactically to prevent meningococci infection.

2.6.37   Ethambutol

Pharmacology and toxicology

Ethambutol has bacteriostatic properties and is used in combination with either INH or rifampin, or both. Like INH and rifampin, it can cross the placenta, but the risk of congenital malformations when used during pregnancy appears to be low. There are no reports indicating that ethambutol can cause ocular toxicity in the fetus, as it does in adults when given in higher doses.

Recommendation. Ethambutol is a first-line drug for treatment of tuberculosis during pregnancy in combination with INH and rifampicin.

2.6.38   Pyrazinamide (PZA)

Pharmacology and toxicology

Pyrazinamide is a bactericidal antituberculous drug that (in non-pregnant patients) is routinely used as a first-line agent, having permitted the introduction of a short course (6-month) regimen. Use of PZA during pregnancy is not adequately documented, but adverse outcomes were not found in a small study (Davidson 1995). A small risk of birth defects cannot be excluded based upon current reports. Its use is limited to cases where susceptibility to PZA and resistance to first-line antituberculous drugs is suspected or documented (Laibl 2005, Bothamley 2001).

> **Recommendation.** Pyrazinamide (PZA) can be used during pregnancy in those cases where resistance of the other first-line drugs is suspected or documented.

2.6.39   Aminoglycosides in tuberculosis

Pharmacology and toxicology

Streptomycin, an aminoglycoside with bactericidal properties, is frequently used in combination with other antituberculous drugs in the non-pregnant patient. Fetal ototoxicity is documented, and use during pregnancy is contraindicated (see section 2.6.10).

Other aminoglycosides, used as second-line drugs in antituberculous treatment (*kanamycin, amikacin*, and the newer *capreomycin*), possibly share the same ototoxic potential, and they should be avoided during pregnancy (Shin 2003, Brost 1997).

> **Recommendation.** Streptomycin (a first-line drug in the non-pregnant patient) and kanamycin, amikacin, and capreomycin (second-line drugs) are contraindicated during pregnancy because of their ototoxic properties. Inadvertent use does not require termination of pregnancy or invasive diagnostic procedures, but hearing tests should be performed after birth.

2.6.40   Para-aminosalicylic acid (PAS)

Pharmacology and toxicology

Para-aminosalicylic acid (4-amino salicylic acid) is a folic acid-synthesis inhibitor. It was commonly used with INH in the 1950s and 1960s. Because of its (gastrointestinal) side effects, it is often not tolerated during pregnancy and is scarcely used anymore. There have been no indications for embryo- or fetotoxic potential.

> **Recommendation.** Para-aminosalicylic acid (PAS) is a second-line drug that is not recommended during pregnancy. Inadvertent use does not require termination of pregnancy or invasive diagnostic procedures.

2.6.41 Quinolones in tuberculosis

Pharmacology and toxicology

Quinolones (*ciprofloxacin, levofloxacin, ofloxacin*, and *sparfloxacin*) have become the mainstay of multidrug-resistant tuberculosis (MDR-TB) treatment regimens in the past few years (Frieden 2003, Raju 1998). Their use during pregnancy is discussed in section 2.6.8.

> **Recommendation.** Quinolones (ciprofloxacin, ofloxacin, levofloxacin, and sparfloxacin) are second-line drugs for the treatment of MDR-TB. As their safety has not been established, they should only be used in the pregnant patient when the benefit for the mother outweighs possible fetal risk. In such a case ciprofloxacine should be preferred, because of its relatively large documented experience.

2.6.42 Other second-line antituberculous drugs

Pharmacology and toxicology

Ethionamide and *protionamide* are effective in the treatment of many strains of mycobacterium. There are no adequate data regarding their use in pregnancy.

Cycloserine is a broad-spectrum antibiotic, used in combination with other medications after the failure of first-line antituberculosis agents. Information is lacking about its use during pregnancy.

Rifabutine (used also for *Myobacterium avium* infections in HIV-patients) and *rifapentine* are both semisynthetic rifamycin derivatives. A few case reports of normal pregnancy outcomes do not allow for a risk estimation of their use during pregnancy.

Terizidon has not been evaluated for its use during pregnancy.

> **Recommendation.** Ethionamide, protionamid, cycloserine, rifabutine, rifapentine, and terizidon are not recommended during pregnancy. Inadvertent use does not require termination of pregnancy or invasive diagnostic procedures. However, a detailed fetal ultrasound may be considered after first-trimester exposure.

2.6.43   Dapsone

Pharmacology and toxicology

Because of increasing multidrug resistance, it was expected that *dapsone*, used mainly in the treatment of leprosy, would become more important in the treatment of tuberculosis. However, it is scarcely used for the treatment of tuberculosis currently. From its use in leprosy patients, dapsone does not appear to have an increased teratogenic potential (Bhargava 1996). Case reports of hemolytic anemia in the mother and child have been published. However, the risk cannot be estimated due to a paucity of documented data.

> **Recommendation.** During pregnancy, dapsone should be reserved for specific indications.

2.6.44   Aciclovir and other herpes antivirals

Pharmacology and toxicology

Aciclovir (*acyclovir*) is an acyclic nucleoside analog, highly specific for HSV-infected cells. It inhibits viral ribonucleotide production in Herpes 1 and 2 and in varicella zoster infections. *Valaciclovir* is the prodrug of aciclovir, with the benefit of a greater bioavailability and a longer half-life (less frequent dosing). Aciclovir can cross the placenta, and fetal aciclovir levels are comparable to maternal levels once a steady state is reached. It is concentrated in the amniotic fluid, approximately four-fold, but does not concentrate in the fetus (Frenkel 1991). There is substantial experience with systemic use of aciclovir during pregnancy. The manufacturer initiated the Acyclovir Pregnancy Registry (June 1984–April 1999). In total, the outcomes of 1234 prospectively registered pregnancies were obtained; 756 infants were exposed during the first trimester and 291 in the third trimester. There was no evidence of an increased risk of congenital defects or adverse fetal or neonatal outcomes in this study (Stone 2004). The same applies to other publications. In total, more than 1800 infants are reported to have been prenatally exposed without any apparent drug-related adverse outcome (Scott 1999). Many studies have been conducted to evaluate the safety and efficacy of systemic aciclovir for the treatment of genital herpes in pregnancy, with the objective of preventing transmission of the virus and subsequent serious neonatal herpes. Of neonatal herpes, 85% results from viral transmission near delivery. To date, the conclusions and recommendations made are not definitive, but as maternal primary and nonprimary first-episode genital herpes seem to have the greatest risk for prolonged shedding and transmitting the virus, treatment of these conditions is generally viewed as justified. Treatment of recurrent episodes of genital herpes, when there is no or minimal risk of transmission, is not routinely recommended, but can be considered when maternal infection is severe (Brown 2005, Hill 2005, Scott 1999, RCOG 1998). To reduce the need for cesarean delivery in women with symptomatic genital herpes, antiviral suppressive therapy initiated at 36 weeks to all asymptomatic HSV-2 seropositive pregnant women is presently a focus of discussion (Brown 2005, Whitley 2004, Watts 2003). Intravenous administration is required in patients with life-threatening conditions like disseminated herpes infection or varicella pneumonia.

After topical use of aciclovir, there will be only minimal resorption through the skin.

Valaciclovir, the prodrug of aciclovir, has an increased bioavailability to the mother (and possibly to the fetus). Pregnancy outcomes were obtained from 111 prospectively registered pregnancies in the Valaciclovir Pregnancy Registry (same manufacturer), including 29 infants exposed in the first trimester and 50 in the third trimester. Although no apparent adverse outcomes were reported, these data, together with those from some other small studies, provide insufficient information for a risk evaluation.

There are a few case reports describing normal pregnancy outcome after first-trimester treatment with *ganciclovir* (Pescovitz 1999). However, these data are inadequate to evaluate the safety of ganciclovir in pregnancy. The same applies to the prodrug *valganciclovir*, and *penciclovir* or its prodrug *famciclovir*. In animal studies, embryotoxicity of ganciclovir was reported.

Recommendation. Topical use of aciclovir is, regarding the minimal systemic absorption, probably safe. Oral treatment should be considered when first-episode genital herpes is diagnosed in a pregnant woman, to prevent neonatal infection by vertical transmission of the virus. Intravenous administration is indicated for treatment of life-threatening maternal infections like varicella pneumonia or disseminated herpes simplex infection. It should not be routinely administered in case of uncomplicated herpes zoster. The use of famciclovir, ganciclovir, penciclovir or valaciclovir is not recommended during pregnancy because of insufficient data. Inadvertent use does not require termination of pregnancy or invasive diagnostic procedures.

2.6.45   Antiviral drugs for influenza

Pharmacology and toxicology

Amantadine, oseltamivir, and *zanamivir* are the available drugs for prophylaxis or treatment of influenza-virus infection. *Amantadine* (against influenza A) has been on the market for a long time now. It is a drug with dopaminergic activity, and is therefore also used in Parkinsonian-like disorders. In one animal study the drug was found to be teratogenic (no specific anomalies were mentioned), but no other reports of teratogenicity have been located. A few case reports describe malformations in the offspring, but none of these reports provide sufficient information for any conclusion about developmental toxicity. In a letter to the editor (Rosa 1994), 64 pregnancies were reported where first-trimester exposure to amantadine had occurred. There were five congenital defects (three statistically expected), one of which was a cardiovascular defect. The author concluded that no definite conclusion could be drawn from these numbers, but that if there is any risk with amantadine it is not high, based on the available data.

Experience during pregnancy with *oseltamivir* or *zanamivir* (against influenza A and B, the latter especially in HIV-infected patients) is insufficient for a risk assessment. Reports from animal studies have not clearly indicated the teratogenic potentials of these drugs.

Recommendation. Amantadine, oseltamivir, and zanamivir are not recommended during pregnancy, and should be reserved for vital indications. Inadvertent use does not require termination of pregnancy or invasive diagnostic procedures. However, a detailed fetal ultrasound may be considered after first-trimester exposure.

2.6.46   Ribavirin

Pharmacology and toxicology

Ribavirin is an antiviral with broad-spectrum activity. Severe viral infections, like hepatitis C (in combination with interferon then) and respiratory syncytial virus (RSV) infection in young infants, may be an indication. It was found to be teratogenic and/or embryo-lethal in several animal studies. The infants of nine women who were treated with ribavirin for severe measles during the second half of pregnancy did not have an increased incidence of anomalies (Atmar 1992). A woman treated at 7 weeks' gestation with ribavirin by injection at 200 mg/d for 3 days had a normal child (Rezvani 2006). Because of the potential absorption of this agent by hospital staff (when ribavirin aerosol is administered to the patient), concern has been expressed regarding the possible exposure of pregnant healthcare workers to this drug. There is insufficient information regarding exposure to this drug during pregnancy to make any conclusion about its safety. A Ribavirin Pregnancy Registry (www.ribavirinpregnancyregistry.com) has been established to follow women who have conceived while taking the medication, or whose spouse has taken the medication. This Registry also includes women who have concluded their therapy within the previous 6 months, because of the long half-life of Ribavirin.

> **Recommendation.** Ribavirin should be used in pregnancy only for life-threatening infections. Detailed ultrasound diagnosis can be considered after first-trimester exposure. Pregnant hospital staff should refrain from administering ribavirin aerosol to patients on a regular base.

2.6.47   Other antiviral drugs

Pharmacology and toxicology

Brivudine is being used in varicella zoster and HSV-I infections; *cidofovir* and *foscarnet* are indicated for severe cytomegaly (CMV) infections. No published data on their use during pregnancy are available.

> **Recommendation.** Use of brivudine, cidofovir, and foscarnet during pregnancy should be reserved for vital indications. When one of these drugs has been used during the first trimester, termination of pregnancy is not advocated; however, a detailed ultrasound diagnosis may be considered.

2.6.48   HIV prophylaxis and therapy

HIV therapy (ART, antiretroviral therapy) may be indicated for maternal as well as for fetal reasons. During the recent past the treatment guidelines for HIV-infected adults have been changing, and for pregnant women the treatment should focus both on the fetal protection and on the optimal antiretroviral therapy of the mother.

Treatment decisions for HIV-infected women should consider the present and future health of the mother, prevention of perinatal transmission, and toxicity limitation to the antiretroviral-exposed fetus (US Dept of Health Guidelines 2005, http://aidsinfo.nih.gov., US Public Health Service Task Force 2004, WHO).

Nucleoside reverse transcriptase inhibitors (NRTIs), non-nucleoside reverse transcriptase inhibitors (NNRTIs) and protease inhibitors (PIs) are used currently, mostly in combination, for the treatment of HIV infections. In the pregnant HIV patient, highly active antiretroviral therapy (HAART) is being used more frequently, especially in developed countries.

- The NRTIs used are *abacavir, didanosine, emtricitabine, lamivudine, stavudine, tenofovir, zalcitabine*, and *zidovudine*
- The NNRTIs used are *delavirdine, efavirenz*, and *nevirapine*
- The PIs are *amprenavir, atazanavir, fosamprenavir, indinavir, lopinavir, nelfinavir, ritonavir, saquinavir*, and *tipranavir*
- *Enfuvirtide* is a fusion inhibitor.

Pharmacology and toxicology

Zidovudine, also known as *azidothymidine* (*AZT*), is a pyrimidine analog used in the treatment of HIV-1 and HIV-2 infections. AZT is a nucleoside reverse transcriptase inhibitor (NRTI). Pharmacokinetic studies indicate that AZT crosses the placenta; fetal AZT levels are found to be similar to or higher than maternal levels. The administration of zidovudine monotherapy to the mother (and to the infant after birth) rapidly became standard practice once it had been shown to reduce mother-to-child transmission by two-thirds (AIDS Clinical Trial Group, protocol 076, 1994). In combination with other antiretroviral drugs such as *lamivudine* and, recently, with HAART, the risk of perinatal transmission has decreased even more and is presently around 1–2%.

Zidovudine is the best-studied compound; the manufacturer has recorded pregnancy outcomes of more than 1000 pregnant women exposed in the first trimester. The rate of adverse outcomes was not different from that expected (Watts 2004, Covington 2004A, Antiretroviral Pregnancy Registry 2004 (www.apregistr.com and www.pregnancyregistry.gsk.com/antiretroviral.html)). This is confirmed by the experience from several other trials (Fowler 2000, Mofenson 2000A), where again no adverse fetal effects of zidovudine were described, except for a small decrease in hemoglobin levels at birth which resolved by 12 weeks of age (review by Mofenson 2000B). No long-term sequelae regarding growth or neurological, immunologic or neurodevelopmental characteristics have been found in the 234 zidovudine-exposed children from the PACTG 076 study, who were followed for as long as 6 years, and no cancers have been detected (Culnane 1999, Hanson 1999). A study in monkeys prenatally exposed to zidovudine at comparable human levels revealed abnormalities in mitochondrial structure and function in heart and skeletal muscle. There has been concern about the possibility that this mitochondrial dysfunction might adversely affect development, particularly cardiac function. Although a group of French investigators has identified 12 children with possible mitochondrial dysfunction from a series of 2644 infants treated with zidovudine and other nucleoside-analog reverse-transcriptase inhibitors (Barrett 2003, Blanche 1999), evidence was not considered conclusive (Morris 1999) and other studies were reassuring (Arnold 2002, Lipshultz 2000, Culnane 1999, Hanson 1999). However, the risk is not considered large, compared to the major reduction in perinatal HIV-transmission that has been associated with the prenatal administration of this agent. After combination therapy of lamivudine/ zidovudine, some severe adverse outcomes (anemia, neutropenia, and mitochondrial dysfunction) occurred (Mandelbrot 2001). A recent report (Witt 2007) demonstrated the genotoxic potential for ZDV but not for other anti-HIV agents via the induction of micronucleated reticulocytes in cord blood and mother's blood. Based upon these investigations, it is recommended that long term monitoring of the ZDV exposed infants should continue.

Lamivudine is a cytidine analog used as a reverse transcriptase antagonist in the therapy of retroviral infection. Lamivudine appears to cross the human term placenta by simple diffusion, with cord blood levels at term similar to maternal blood levels. The manufacturer has again recorded pregnancy outcomes of more than 1000 pregnant women exposed in the first trimester, and the rate of adverse outcomes was not different from that expected (Watts 2004, Antiretroviral Pregnancy Registry 2004).

For *nelfinavir, stavudine, nevirapine*, and *abacavir*, pregnancy outcomes after first-trimester exposure were also monitored in the pregnancy registry of the manufacturer. The rate of adverse outcomes was not different from that expected. Although the numbers (between 250 and 450 exposures of each drug) are not sufficient for definite conclusions, the findings might be viewed as reassuring (Covington 2004B, Watts 2004, Antiretroviral Pregnancy Registry 2004). Increased maternal hepatotoxicity is observed in pregnant women treated with *nevirapine* (Hitti 2004).

Limited data are available regarding birth defects after prenatal exposure to *efavirenz*. There have been retrospective reports of neural tube defects, including three cases of meningomyelocele and one Dandy Walker syndrome, after first-trimester exposure to *efavirenz*-containing regimens (de Santis 2002). In monkeys, similar defects were observed. However, prospectively followed pregnancies in 206 women exposed to *efavirenz* in the first trimester resulted in 188 live births, of which 5 had a birth defect, none of them being a neural tube defect (Martin 2005).

In a series of 233 HIV-infected women treated with protease inhibitors (PIs), HAART including PIs was confirmed to be effective in preventing perinatal transmission. In this multicenter, retrospective study, prematurity and low birth weight were not significantly increased compared with other studies where HIV-infected pregnant women were not treated with PIs (Morris 2005).

Based on three cases of fatal lactic acidosis in pregnant women treated with a combination of stavudine and didanosine, the manufacturer issued a warning in 2001 to alert clinicians to an apparent increased risk of liver disease and pancreatitis in women treated with this drug combination.

Data on antiretroviral drugs not mentioned here are too limited for any conclusions about their safety during pregnancy.

A recent prospective controlled study of the neurodevelopment of 39 exposed children demonstrated that perinatal highly active antiretroviral therapy exposure is not associated with altered development and behavior at 18–36 months of age (Alimenti 2006).

> **Recommendation.** Treatment decisions for HIV-infected women should consider the present and future health of the mother, the prevention of perinatal transmission, and toxicity limitation to the antiretroviral-exposed fetus. In cases of compelling maternal or fetal (preventing transmission in zidovudine resistance) indications, combination ART or HAART with one or more of the abovementioned substances should be applied. Management must remain individually based, using HIV RNA levels throughout pregnancy and previous disease and obstetric history to plan optimal ART for the mother and child. After combination ART in the first trimester, a detailed ultrasound diagnosis should be considered. Treatment should be conducted in specialized centers and according to established regimen guidelines. Long term follow up of ZDV prenatally exposed infants should continue upon recent genotoxic results.

2.6.49   Mebendazole and flubendazole

Pharmacology and toxicology

Most infections of adults with common nematodes like ascaris and trichuris will be asymptomatic, and there is rarely an indication for treatment during pregnancy. Severe infections with hookworms may cause anemia, responsible, if during pregnancy, for increased perinatal mortality and morbidity worldwide. The WHO estimates that as many as 44 million pregnant women throughout the world are infected with hookworms (WHO 1996B).

Mebendazole is a highly effective and well-tolerated drug against nematodes in the gastrointestinal tract (such as enterobius, ascaris, trichuris, ankylostoma – pinworms, round-worms, whipworms, and hookworms). The drug is poorly absorbed from the gut. Mebendazole exerts its action through inhibition of glucose uptake by the parasite, causing its starvation and death. Mebendazole had teratogenic effects in some animal studies. Conflicting results of several case reports and (retrospective) studies in hundreds of human pregnancies (including many first-trimester exposures) do not allow a well-founded estimation of human risk. However, an increased risk of congenital malformations was not observed in a study of over 400 pregnant women exposed to mebendazole in the first trimester (de Silva 1999). This was confirmed in a controlled prospective study, where 192 pregnancy outcomes were evaluated and compared with a matched control group (Diav-Citrin 2003). There was no increase in the rate of major malformations. In another prospective study on anthelmintics during pregnancy, where 64 women were exposed to mebendazole in the first trimester (Reuvers-Lodewijks 1999), only one malformation (bilateral clubfoot) was observed, which is below the expected background rate. Although numbers are too small for any definite conclusion, mebendazole does not appear to represent a major teratogenic risk. Improvement of pregnancy outcomes (regarding stillbirths, perinatal deaths, and birth weight) was observed when mebendazole was used during the second and third trimesters in developing countries, where intestinal helminthiasis is endemic (de Silva 1999).

Flubendazole is structurally related to mebendazole. Teratogenicity has been reported in rats. No significant increase in major malformations was observed in a prospective study of 150 pregnancies after exposure to flubendazole in the first trimester (Reuvers-Lodewijks 1999), and a smaller prospective investigation covering 11 pregnancies (Choi 2005; see also section 2.6.50).

> **Recommendation.** Mebendazole may be used during pregnancy with helmintic infections that require treatment, but during the first trimester should only be used when strictly indicated and when treatment cannot be delayed. For the treatment of pinworms, pyrvinium, if available, is preferred. Inadvertent use during the first trimester does not require termination of pregnancy or additional diagnostic procedures. The same applies to flubendazole.

2.6.50   Pyrviniumembonate

Pharmacology and toxicology

Pyrviniumembonate, which is not available in all countries, is effective against enterobius (pinworms) and is very poorly absorbed from the gastrointestinal tract. Embryo- or fetotoxicity has not been observed.

> **Recommendation.** Pyrviniumembonate is the drug of choice for the treatment of enterobiasis/oxyuriasis.

2.6.51   Albendazole and thiabendazole

Pharmacology and toxicology

Albendazole is a highly effective broad-spectrum anthelmintic, structurally related to mebendazole. It also kills the parasite through inhibition of the glucose uptake. It is the first-line drug for the treatment of alveolar forms of echinococcosis (*Echinococcus multilocularis*), and also for the advanced cystic forms (*Echinococcus granulosus*). During a mass drug administration for lymphatic filiriasis in Ghana, 50 women were inadvertently (because their pregnancy was not recognized) treated with *ivermectin* and *albendazole*; their pregnancy outcomes were compared with those of 293 women with a recognized pregnancy who were not treated. Of the 39 children who were exposed during the first trimester, 1 congenital malformation (a hearing impairment), versus 5 of the untreated group, was reported. The authors concluded that there was no evidence of increased risk after exposure to ivermectin and albendazole (Gyapong 2003). One Down syndrome was observed in a small prospective study of albendazole ($n = 12$) and flubendazole ($n = 11$) (Choi 2005). No malformations were observed among 24 children born after first-trimester exposure to albendazole in a prospective study (Reuvers-Lodewijks 1999).

Thiabendazole is indicated for the treatment of strongyloidiasis, larva migrans cutanea, and trichinosis. There are no reports of thiabendazole use during human pregnancies.

> **Recommendation.** When there is a vital indication for the treatment of echinococcosis, albendazole may be used during all stages of pregnancy. However, a small risk of birth defects cannot be excluded. For all other indications, more established anthelmintics should be used. When used during the first trimester, a detailed ultrasound diagnosis is recommended.

2.6.52   Niclosamide

Pharmacology and toxicology

Niclosamide is an effective anthelmintic against most human cestodes. It appears to act by inhibiting respiration of the parasite, and is hardly absorbed in the gastrointestinal tract. The drug has been widely used for a long time, and is not suspected of causing an increased risk for birth defects to date; however, experience in humans is not well-documented. In a prospective follow-up study of 39 pregnant women exposed in the first trimester, one child was born with a minor malformation (Reuvers-Lodewijks 1999), which is below the expected background rate.

> **Recommendation.** Only when there is a clear need for treatment of a cestode infection should niclosamide be used during pregnancy; treatment during the first trimester should be restricted to vital indications. However, a small risk of birth defects cannot be excluded. When used during the first trimester, a detailed ultrasound diagnosis is recommended.

2.6.53   Praziquantel

Pharmacology and toxicology

Praziquantel is a highly effective broad-spectrum anthelmintic against many trematodes and cestodes, but is also the first-line drug against schistosomiasis (bilharziosis). No teratogenicity has been reported in animal studies. A case report of a normal child, born after treatment of the mother from weeks 8 to 11, has been published (Paparone 1996). In a retrospective study, during treatment of their mothers for schistosomiasis 88 children were exposed to praziquantel (47 during the first trimester); no increase in adverse outcomes was reported (Adam 2004B). The same research team also followed and evaluated prospectively 25 pregnancy outcomes after exposure (6 during the first trimester) to praziquantel. Apart from one spontaneous abortion, no adverse outcomes were observed (Adam 2005). In another prospective study on anthelmintics, four pregnant women treated in the first trimester delivered four normal children (Reuvers-Lodewijks 1999). The health benefits, for both mother and unborn child, that are gained from the treatment for schistosomiasis are viewed by many to outweigh by far the probably very small risk of adverse pregnancy outcome (Olds 2003, Savioli 2003, WHO 2002).

> **Recommendation.** Praziquantel is not recommended during pregnancy when other better-established anthelmintics are available. Treatment should be reserved for specific vital indications. Inadvertent use does not require termination of pregnancy or invasive diagnostic procedures. It is the first-line drug against bilharziosis.

2.6.54   Pyrantel

Pharmacology and toxicology

Pyrantel is a broad-spectrum anthelmintic that acts by inhibition of cholinesterase, causing spastic paralysis and subsequent death of the parasite. Published experience on its use during pregnancy is not sufficient to determine risk.

> **Recommendation.** Pyrantel is not recommended during pregnancy because better-established anthelmintics are available for all indications. Inadvertent use does not require termination of pregnancy or invasive diagnostic procedures. A detailed ultrasound diagnosis may be considered when pyrantel has been used during the first trimester of pregnancy.

2.6.55   Ivermectin and diethylcarbamazine

Pharmacology and toxicology

Ivermectin is a highly effective drug in the treatment of onchocerciasis (river blindness) and lymphatic filiriasis. Reports from animal studies do not indicate a teratogenic potential of this drug. In some cases inadvertent exposure during pregnancy has occurred without apparent adverse effects (Gyapong 2003), but data are not sufficient for risk estimation.

Diethylcarbamazine is used for the treatment of filiriasis and onchocercosis. No teratogenicity was reported in animal studies. No publications regarding use during human pregnancies have been located.

> **Recommendation.** Ivermectin treatment during pregnancy should be reserved for compelling indications. Inadvertent use does not require termination of pregnancy or invasive diagnostic procedures. The same applies to diethylcarbamazine.

2.6.56   Hyperthermia

Hyperthermia can be caused by fevers and by environmental exposure to heat sources. Maternal temperature increases are transmitted to the fetus. For several decades it has been demonstrated that elevated body temperature can cause malformations in animal studies. There is growing evidence that the same also applies to humans; mild exposure during the pre-implantation period and more severe exposure during embryonic and fetal development often result in prenatal death and abortion. Hyperthermia also causes a wide range of structural and functional defects. The central nervous system (CNS) is most at risk, probably because it cannot compensate for the loss of prospective neurons by additional divisions by the surviving neuroblasts, and it remains at risk at stages throughout pre- and postnatal life, although its possible effects at these stages have not been studied in detail (Edwards 2006). There are indications that some malformations, such as neural tube defects (Shaw 1998), but also heart defects, renal anomalies, and gastroschisis, were more frequently observed after prolonged periods of high fever in early pregnancy (e.g. Abe 2003, Chambers 1998). In this prospective study, 115 pregnant women with high fever (38.9° C for 24 hours or more) were compared with 147 women with moderate fever (<38.9° C, or <24 hours) and with women without fever. About 80% of these febrile periods occurred in the first trimester. The relative risk for congenital malformations calculated in this study, however, was not of statistical significance. In a cohort study of 24 040 pregnant women, where 1145 pregnancies resulted in a miscarriage or stillbirth, there was no evidence that fever in the first 16 weeks of pregnancy is associated with fetal death was found (Andersen 2002). In a commentary it was pointed out that the main limitation of this study was that the risk of fetal death before week 6 could not be assessed, and therefore no definite conclusions could be made (Chambers 2006). The question of whether elevated body temperature may be responsible for the so-called "vascular disruption disorders", where developing organs are deprived of sufficient blood supply, is still under discussion (Martínez-Frías 2001, Graham 1998). A rise in body temperature of $\approx$ 2° C for more than 24 hours is acknowledged nowadays to be associated with an increased risk of developmental defects.

An increased risk from sauna or hot-tub bathing has been discussed (Li 2003, Milunsky 1992), but data are not sufficient for definite conclusions (Chambers 2006, Herz-Picciotto 2003). However, in view of the relatively large volume of animal data and the association between high maternal fever and NTDs, a risk cannot be excluded. In a hot-tub (39–40° C), body temperature (studied in non-pregnant women) may reach 38.9° C after only 10–20 minutes (Harvey 1981). Women of reproductive age and who may be pregnant should limit exposure to hot-tubs to less than 15 minutes in 39° C water and less than 10 minutes in 40° C water (Chambers 2006). Time limits for hot-tubs are shorter than for saunas; the latter permit greater heat loss by evaporation and perspiration. In Finland, where sauna bathing is very common, even during pregnancy, no association with adverse pregnancy outcomes has been detected.

Use of electric blankets or heated waterbeds has not demonstrated any additional risk of congenital malformations to date. The use of birthing pools has raised some concern in a case report (Rosevaer 1993), where, after staying in water of 39° C for several hours, two mothers delivered infants in poor condition; both newborns died shortly afterwards.

> **Recommendation.** When high fever does arise in early pregnancy, paracetamol (acetaminophen) should be taken to lower the body temperature, together if necessary with other measurements such as cool wrappings and sufficient fluid intake. Saunas or hot-tubs should not exceed 10 minutes. In general, sources of possible overheating should be avoided. In cases of high fever episodes in early pregnancy, diagnostic measurements such as detailed fetal ultrasound should be considered.

2.6.57   Traveling

When pregnant patients are traveling long distances, or going abroad, several possible risks should be discussed:

- Prophylactic measurements to prevent infections (for malaria prophylaxis, see section 2.6.24; for vaccinations, see Chapter 2.7)
- The risk of other infections (fever, fluid loss), and required therapy
- In long-distance air travel, cosmic radiation, the increased risk of thrombotic events due to prolonged immobilization, decreased air (oxygen) pressure comparable with an altitude of approximately 2500 m, and physical and psychic stress.

No specific malformations have been associated with established vaccinations or with malaria prophylaxis. However, with some of them there is insufficient experience with use in pregnancy (see Chapter 2.7). It should be pointed out that the increased physical stress associated with long-distance travel in predisposed women might increase their risk for spontaneous abortion. Another risk is of "common" infections, due to altered hygienic standards in the destination country. The accompanying fever, dehydration or other complications may also endanger the fetus.

The quantity of ionizing radiation in air travel will vary according to several conditions, but as far as we know doses will not be high enough to incorporate an additional risk of malformations.

Staying at high altitudes carries the problem of decreased air pressure and the risk of high altitude sickness. Although a decreased birth weight in infants born to mothers who live at (moderate) high altitudes has been observed, a short-term stay in conditions with moderate decreased air pressure does not seem to carry a risk of fetal hypoxia. Fetal oxygen supply at very high altitudes (>3300 m or 11 000 ft) cannot be guaranteed, and the risk of maternal high altitude sickness may endanger the mother and child. Healthy pregnant women can probably stay at a moderately high altitude for a short period, but avoiding exercise, or maintaining hydration and waiting several days for acclimatization before starting moderate exercise, is recommended (Jean 2005, Rodway 2004, Niermeyer 1999). Heavy exercise with increasing body temperature must be avoided (Samuel 1998). During long-distance flights, air pressure and the oxygen partial pressure are kept to the same level as at an altitude of 2500 m, which carries no risk for healthy (pregnant) individuals.

2

Pregnancy

> **Recommendation.** The need for long journeys, especially to tropical destinations, by pregnant women should be critically evaluated. Women with a history of spontaneous abortion should preferably postpone their journey. Women with risk factors for spontaneous abortion, pre-eclampsia or placental abruption, or whose babies are at risk of intrauterine growth restriction (IUGR), should not go to (very) high altitudes. When a journey has been made during pregnancy without any complications, further diagnostic procedures are not warranted.

References

Abe K, Honein MA, Moore CA. Maternal febrile illnesses, medication use, and the risk of congenital renal anomalies. Birth Def Res A 2003; 67: 911–18.

ACOG Technical Bulletin. Pulmonary Disease in Pregnancy, No. 224. Intl J Gynaecol Obstet 1996; 54: 187–96.

Adam I (A), Elwasila E, Ali DAM et al. Artemether in the treatment of falciparum malaria during pregnancy in eastern Sudan. Trans R Soc Trop Med Hyg 2004; 98: 509–13.

Adam I (B), Elwasila ET, Homeida M. Is praziquantel therapy safe during pregnancy? Trans R Soc Trop Med Hyg 2004; 98: 540–43.

Adam I, Elwasila E, Homeida M. Praziquantel for the treatment of schistosomiasis mansoni during pregnancy. Ann Trop Med Parasitol 2005; 99: 37–40.

Aleck KA, Bartly DL. Multiple malformation syndrome following fluconazole use in pregnancy: report of an additional patient. Am J Med Genet 1997; 72: 253–6.

Alecrim WD, Espinosa FEM, Alecrim MGC. *Plasmodium falciparum* infection in the pregnant patient. Infect Dis Clin North Am 2000; 14: 83–95.

Alimenti A, Forbes JC, Oberlander TF et al. A prospective controlled study of neurodevelopment in HIV-uninfected children exposed to combination antiretroviral drugs in pregnancy. Pediatrics 2006; 118: 1139–45.

Amado JA, Pesquera C, Gonzalez EM et al. Successful treatment with ketoconazole of Cushing's syndrome in pregnancy. Postgrad Med J 1990; 66: 221–3.

Andersen AMN, Vastrup P, Wohlfahrt J et al. Fever in pregnancy and risk of fetal death: a cohort study. Lancet 2002; 360(9345): 1552–6.

Antiretroviral Pregnancy Registry Steering Committee. Antiretroviral Pregnancy Registry Interim Report for 1 January 1989 through 31 July 2004. Wilmington, NC: Registry Coordinating Center, 2004 (available at www.apregistr.com).

Arnold SR, Degani N, King SM: Retrospective study to characterize the effects of antiretroviral therapy in infants born to HIV-infected mothers. Pediatr Res 2002; 51(4 Pt 2): 282A.

Atmar RL, Englund JA, Hammill H. Complications of measles during pregnancy. Clin Infect Dis 1992; 14: 217–26.

2.6 Anti-infective agents

Bar-Oz B, Moretti ME, Bishai R et al. Pregnancy outcome after in utero exposure to itraconazole: a prospective cohort study. Am J Obstet Gynecol 2000; 183: 617–20.

Barret B, Tardieu M, Rustin P et al. Persistent mitochondrial dysfunction in HIV-1-exposed but uninfected infants: clinical screening in a large prospective cohort. AIDS 2003; 17: 1769–85.

Beard CM, Noller Kl, O'Fallon WM et al. Cancer after exposure to metronidazole. Mayo Clin Proc 1988; 63: 147–53.

Ben-David S, Einarson T, Ben-David Y et al. The safety of nitrofurantoin during the first trimester of pregnancy: meta–analysis. Fund Clin Pharmacol 1994; 28: 248–51.

Berkovitch M, Patuszak A, Gazarian M et al. Safety of the new quinolones in pregnancy. Obstet Gynecol 1994; 84: 535–8.

Berkovitch M, Segal-Socher I, Greenberg R et al. First trimester exposure to cefuroxim: a prospective cohort study. Br J Clin Pharmacol 2000; 50: 161–5.

Berkovitch M, Diav-Citrin O, Greenberg R et al. First-trimester exposure to amoxycillin/clavulanic acid: a prospective, controlled study. Br J Clin Pharmacol 2004; 58: 298–302.

Bernard B, Abate M, Thielen PF et al. Maternal–fetal pharmacological activity of amikacin. J Infect Dis 1977; 135: 925–32.

Berwaerts J, Verhelst J, Mahler C et al. Cushing's syndrome in pregnancy treated by ketoconazole: case report and review of the literature. Gynecol Endocrinol 1999; 13: 175–82.

Bhargava P, Kuldeep CM, Mathur NK: Antileprosy drugs, pregnancy and fetal outcome. Intl J Lepr Other Mycobact Dis 1996; 64: 457.

Blanche S, Tardieu M, Rustin P et al. Persistent mitochondrial dysfunction and perinatal exposure to antiretroviral nucleoside analogues. Lancet 1999; 354: 1084–9.

Bothamley G. Drug treatment for tuberculosis during pregnancy – safety considerations. Drug Saf 2001; 24: 553–65.

Bourget P, Fernandez H, Delouis C et al. Pharmacokinetics of tobramycin in pregnant women. Safety and efficacy of a once-daily dose regimen. J Clin Pharm Ther 1991; 16: 167–76.

Brabin BJ, Eggelte TA, Parise M et al. Dapsone therapy for malaria during pregnancy – maternal and fetal outcomes. Drug Saf 2004; 27: 633–48.

Briggs GG, Freeman RK, Yaffe SJ. Drugs in Pregnancy and Lactation, 7th edn. Philadelphia, PA: Lippincott Williams & Wilkins, 2005.

Brost BC, Newman RB. The maternal and fetal effects of tuberculosis therapy. Obstet Gynecol Clin North Am 1997; 24: 659–73.

Brown ZA, Gardella C, Wald A et al. Genital herpes complicating pregnancy. Obstet Gynecol 2005; 106(4): 845–56.

Bruel H, Guillemant V, Saladin TC et al. Anémie hémolytique chez un nouveau – né aprés prise maternelle de nitrofurantoine en fin de grossesse. Arch Pédiatr 2000; 7: 745–7.

Brumfitt W, Pursell R. Trimethoprim sulfamethoxazole in the treatment of bacteriuria in women. J Infect Dis 1973; 128: S657–63.

Burtin P, Taddio A, Ariburno O et al. Safety of metronidazole in pregnancy: a meta-analysis. Am J Obstet Gynecol 1995; 172: 525–9.

Caro-Paton T, Carvajal A, Martin de Diego I et al. Is metronidazole teratogenic? A meta-analysis. Br J Clin Pharmacol 1997; 44(2): 179–82.

Chamberlain A, White S, Bawdon R et al. Pharmacokinetics of ampicillin and sulbactam in pregnancy. Am J Obstet Gynecol 1993; 168: 667–73.

Chambers CD, Johnson KA, Dick LM et al. Maternal fever and birth outcome: a prospective study. Teratology 1998; 58: 251–7.

Chambers CD. Risks of hyperthermia associated with hot tub or spa use by pregnant women. Birth Def Res A 2006; 76: 569–73.

Choi JS, Han JY, Ahn HK. Fetal outcome after exposure to antihelminthics albendazole and flubendazole during early pregnancy. Birth Def Res A 2005; 73: 349.

Cooper WO, Ray WA, Griffin MR. Prenatal description of macrolide antibiotics and infantile hypertrophic pyloric stenosis. Obstet Gynecol 2002; 100: 101–6.

Covington DL (A), Tilson H, Elder J et al. Assessing teratogenicity of antiretroviral drugs: monitoring and analysis plan of the Antiretroviral Pregnancy Registry. Pharmacoepidemiol Drug Saf 2004; 13: 537–45.

Covington DL (B), Conner SD, Doi PA et al. Risk of birth defects associated with nelfinavir exposure during pregnancy. Obstet Gynecol 2004; 103: 1181–9.

Culnane M, Fowler MC, Lee SS et al. Lack of long-term effects of in utero exposure to zidovudine among uninfected children born to HIV-infected women. J Am Med Assoc 1999; 281: 151–7.

Czeizel AE. A case-control analysis of the teratogenic effects of co-trimoxazole. Reprod Toxicol 1990; 4: 305–13.

Czeizel AE, Rockenbauer M. Teratogenic study of doxycycline. Obstet Gynecol 1997; 89: 524–8.

Czeizel AE, Rockenbauer M, Olsen J. Use of antibiotics during pregnancy. Eur J Obstet Gynecol 1998; 81: 1–8.

Czeizel AE, Rockenbauer M, Sørensen HT et al. A population-based case-control teratologic study of oral erythromycin treatment during pregnancy. Reprod Toxicol 1999; 13: 531–6.

Czeizel AE (A), Rockenbauer M, Olsen J et al. Oral phenoxymethylpenicillin treatment during pregnancy. Results of a population-based Hungarian case-control study. Arch Gynecol Obstet 2000; 263: 178–81.

Czeizel AE (B), Rockenbauer M, Sorensen HT, Olsen J. A teratological study of lincosamides. Scand J Infect Dis 2000; 32: 579–80.

Czeizel AE (C), Rockenbauer M. A population-based case-control study of oral oxytetracycline treatment during pregnancy. Eur J Obstet Gynecol Reprod Biol 2000; 88: 27–33.

Czeizel AE (A), Rockenbauer M, Sørensen HT et al. A population-based case-control teratologic study of ampicillin treatment during pregnancy. Am J Obstet Gynecol 2001; 185: 140–7.

Czeizel AE (B), Rockenbauer M, Sørensen HT et al. Use of cephalosporins during pregnancy and in the presence of congenital malformations. A population-based case-control study. Am J Obstet Gynecol 2001; 184: 1289–96.

Czeizel AE (C), Rockenbauer M, Sørensen HT et al. Augmentin treatment during pregnancy and the prevalence of congenital malformations. A population-based case-control teratologic study. Eur J Obstet Gynecol 2001; 97: 188–92.

Czeizel AE (A), Kazy Z, Vargha P. A population-based case-control teratological study of vaginal econazole treatment during pregnancy. Eur J Obstet Gyn Reprod Biol 2003; 111: 135–40.

Czeizel AE (B), Kazy Z, Vargha P. A case-control teratological study of vaginal natamycin treatment during pregnancy. Reprod Toxicol 2003; 17: 387–91.

Czeizel AE (A), Fladung B, Vargha P. Preterm birth reduction after clotrimazole treatment during pregnancy. European J Obstet Gyn Reprod Biol 2004; 116: 157–63.

Czeizel AE (B), Kazy Z, Puho E. Population-based case-control teratologic study of topical miconazole. Congenital Anomalies 2004; 44: 41–5.

Davidson PT. Managing tuberculosis during pregnancy. Lancet 1995; 346: 199–200.

2

Pregnancy

2.6 Anti-infective agents

Dean JL, Wolf JE, Rancini AC et al. Use of amphotericin B during pregnancy: case report and review. Clin Infect Dis 1994; 18: 364–8.

Deen JL, von Seidlein L, Pinder M et al. The safety of the combination artesunate and pyrimethamine-sulfadoxine given during pregnancy. Trans R Soc Trop Med Hyg 2001; 95: 424–8.

Dencker BB, Larsen H, Jensen ES et al. Birth outcome of 1886 pregnancies after exposure to phenoxymethylpenicillin in utero. Clin Microbiol Infect 2002; 8: 196–201.

De Santis M, Carducci B, de Santis L et al. Periconceptional exposure to efavirenz and neural tube defects. Arch Intern Med 2002; 162(3): 355.

De Silva NR, Sirisena JLGJ, Gunasekera DPS et al. Effect of mebendazole therapy during pregnancy on birth outcome. Lancet 1999; 353: 1145–9.

Diav-Citrin O, Gotteiner T, Shechtman S et al. Pregnancy outcome following gestational exposure to metronidazole: a prospective controlled cohort study. Teratology 2001; 63: 186–92.

Diav-Citrin O, Shechtman S, Arnon J. Pregnancy outcome after gestational exposure to mebendazole: a prospective controlled cohort study. Am J Obstet Gynecol 2003; 188: 282–5.

Dobias L, Cerna M, Rössner P et al. Genotoxicity and carcinogenicity of metronidazole. Mutation Res 1994; 317: 177–94.

Donders GG. Treatment of sexually transmitted bacterial diseases in pregnant women. Drugs 2000; 59(3): 477–85.

Drinkard CR, Shatin D, Clouse J. Postmarketing surveillance of medications and pregnancy outcomes: clarithromycin and birth malformations. Pharmacoepidemiol Drug Saf 2000; 9: 549–56.

Edwards MJ, Shiota K, Smith MSR et al. Hyperthermia and birth defects. Reprod Toxicol 1995; 9: 411.

Edwards MJ. Review: Hyperthermia and fever during pregnancy. Birth Def Res Part A 2006; 76: 507–16.

Einarson A, Philips E, Mawji F et al. A prospective controlled multicentre study of clarithromycin in pregnancy. Am J Perinatal 1998; 9: 523–5.

Ely EW, Peacock JE Jr, Haponik EF et al. Cryptococcal pneumonia complicating pregnancy. Medicine Baltimore 1998; 77: 153–67.

Espinal MA, Reingold AL, Lavandera M. Effect of pregnancy on the risk of developing active tuberculosis {see comments}. J Infect Dis 1996; 173(2): 488–91.

Fowler MG. Follow-up of children exposed to perinatal antiretrovirals. Teratology 2000; 61: 395–6.

Frenkel LM, Brown ZA, Bryson YJ et al. Pharmacokinetics of acyclovir in the term human pregnancy and neonate. Am J Obstet Gynecol 1991; 164: 569–76.

Frieden TR, Sterling TR, Munsiff SS et al. Tuberculosis. Lancet 2003; 362: 887–99.

Gait JE. Hemolytic reactions to nitrofurantoin in patients with glucose-6-phosphate dehydrogenase deficiency: theory and practice. DICP 1990; 24: 1210–13.

Garratty G, Leger RM, Arndt PA. Severe immune hemolytic anemia associated with prophylactic use of cefotetan in obstetric and gynecologic procedures. Am J Obstet Gynecol 1999; 181: 103–4.

Giamarellou H, Kolokythas, Petrikkos G et al. Pharmacokinetics of three newer quinolones in pregnant and lactating women. Am J Med 1989; 87(Suppl 5A): S49–51.

Graham JM, Edwards MJ, Edwards MJ. Teratogen update: gestational effects of maternal hyperthermia due to febrile illnesses and resultant patterns of defects in humans. Teratology 1998; 58: 209–21.

Gyapong JO, Chinbuah MA, Gyapong M. Inadvertent exposure of pregnant women to ivermectin and albendazole during mass drug administration for lymphatic filariasis. Trop Med Intl Health 2003; 8: 1093–101.

Hanson IC, Antonelli TA, Sperling RS et al. Lack of tumors in infants with perinatal HIV-1 exposure and fetal/neonatal exposure to zidovudine. J Acq Immune Defic Syndr Hum Retrovirol 1999; 20: 463–7.

Hart CW, Naunton RF. The ototoxicity of chloroquine phosphate. Arch Otolaryngol 1964; 80: 407–12.

Harvey MAS, McRorie MM, Smith DW. Suggested limits to the use of hot tubs and sauna by pregnant women. Can Med Assoc J 1981; 125: 50–54.

Heikkilä A, Erkkola R. Review of beta-lactam antibiotics in pregnancy. The need for adjustment of dosage schedules. Clin Pharmacokin 1994; 27: 49–62.

Heikkinen T, Laine K, Neuvonen PJ et al. The transplacental transfer of the macrolide antibiotics erythromycin, roxithromycin and azithromycin. Br J Obstet Gynaecol 2000; 107: 770–75.

Hernandez-Diaz S, Werler MM, Walker AM et al. Folic acid antagonists during pregnancy and the risk of birth defects. N Engl J Med 2000; 343: 1608–14.

Hernandez-Diaz S, Werler MM, Walker AM et al. Neural tube defects in relation to use of folic acid antagonists during pregnancy. Am J Epidemiol 2001; 153: 961–8.

Herz-Picciotto I, Howards PP. Invited commentary: hot tubs and miscarriage – methodological and substantiveb reasons why the case is weak. Am J Epidemiol 2003; 158: 938–40.

Hill J, Roberts S. Herpes simplex virus in pregnancy: new concepts in prevention and management. Clin Perinatol 2005; 32(3): 657–70.

Hill LM. Fetal distress secondary to vancomycin-induced maternal hypotension. Am J Obstet Gynecol 1985; 153: 74–5.

Hitti J, Frenkel LM, Stek AM et al. Maternal toxicity with continuous nevirapine in pregnancy – results from PACTG 1022. JAIDs 2004; 36(3): 772–6.

Hulton S-A, Kaplan BS. Renal dysplasia associated with in utero exposure to gentamycin and corticosteroids. Am J Med Genet 1995; 58: 91–3.

Inman W, Pearce G, Wilton L. Safety of fluconazole in the treatment of vaginal candidiasis. A prescription-event monitoring study, with special reference to the outcome of pregnancy. Eur J Clin Pharmacol 1994; 46: 115–18.

Jensen P, Skriver MV, Floyd A et al. A population-based study of maternal use of amoxycillin and pregnancy outcome in Denmark. Br J Clin Pharmacol 2003; 55: 216–21.

Jick SS. Pregnancy outcomes after maternal exposure to fluconazole. Pharmacotherapy 1999; 19: 221–2.

Jin ZK. Effects of gentamycin on the fetal kidneys. Chinese J Obstet Gynecol 1992; 27: 157–8.

Joesoef MR, Schmid GP, Hillier SL. Bacterial vaginosis: a review of treatment options and potential clinical indications for therapy. Clin Infect Dis 1999; 28(Suppl 1): S57–65.

Källén B, Otterblad AJ, Olausson P, Danielsson BR. Is erythromycin therapy teratogenic in humans? Reprod Toxicol 2005; 20: 209–14.

Kazy Z, Puho E, Czeizel AE. Parenteral polymyxin B treatment during pregnancy. Reprod Toxicol 2005; 20: 181–2.

King CT, Rogers PD, Cleary JD et al. Antifungal therapy during pregnancy. Clin Infect Dis 1998; 27(5): 1151–60.

Kinzy BJ, Taylor JW. Trimethoprim and folinic acid. Ann Intern Med 1984; 101: 565.

Knudsen LB. No association between griseofulvin and conjoined twinning. Lancet 1987; 2: 1097.

Laibl VR, Sheffield JS. Tuberculosis in pregnancy. Clin Perinatol 2005; 32: 739–47.

Larsen B, Glover DD. Serum erythromycin levels in pregnancy. Clin Therapeut 1998; 20: 971–7.

2 Pregnancy

2.6 Anti-infective agents

Larsen H, Nielsen GL, Sørensen HT et al. A follow-up study of birth outcome in users of pivampicillin during pregnancy. Acta Obstet Gynecol Scand 2000; 79: 379–83.

Larsen H, Nielsen GL, Schønheyder HC et al. Birth outcome following maternal use of fluoroquinolones. Intl J Antimicrob Agents 2001; 18: 259–62.

Lewis JH. Drug hepatotoxicity in pregnancy. Eur J Gastroenterol Hepatol 1991; 3: 883–91.

Li DK, Janevic T, Odouli R et al. Hot tub use during pregnancy and the risk of miscarriage. Am J Epidemiol 2003; 158: 931–7.

Lipshultz SE, Easley KA, Orav J et al. Absence of cardiac toxicity of zidovudine in infants. N Engl J Med 2000; 343: 759–66.

Loebstein R, Addis A, Ho E et al. Pregnancy outcome following gestational exposure to fluoroquinolones: a multicenter prospective controlled study. Antimicrob Agents Chemother 1998; 42: 1336–9.

Lopez-Rangel E, Van Allen MI. Prenatal exposure to fluconazole: an identifiable dysmorphic phenotype. Birth Def Res A 2004; 70: 261.

Louik C, Werler MM, Mitchell AA. Erythromycin use during pregnancy in relation to pyloris stenosis. Am J Obstet Gynecol 2002; 186: 288–90.

Mallie JP, Coulon G, Billerey C et al. In utero aminoglycosides-induced nephrotoxicity in rat neonates. Kidney Intl 1988; 33: 36–44.

Mandelbrot L, Landreau-Mascaro A, Rekacewicz C et al. Lamivudine-zidovudine combination for prevention of maternal–infant transmission of HIV-1. J Am Med Assoc 2001; 285: 2083–93.

Manka W, Solowiow R, Okrzeja D. Assessment of infant development during an 18-month follow-up after treatment of infections in pregnant women with cefuroxime axetil. Drug Saf 2000; 22: 83–8.

Mantovani A, Macri C, Stazi AV et al. Tobramycin-induced changes in renal histology of fetal and newborn Sprague-Dawley rats. Teratog Carcinog Mutagen 1992; 12: 19–30.

Martin CL. Update on the teratogenicity of efavirenz. AIDS Rev 2005; 7: 246.

Martínez-Frías ML, Mazario MJG, Caldas CF et al. High maternal fever during gestation and severe congenital limb disruptions. Am J Med Genet 2001; 98: 201–3.

Mastroiacovo P, Mazzone T, Botto LD et al. Prospective assessment of pregnancy outcomes after first trimester exposure to fluconazole. Am J Obstet Gynaecol 1996; 175: 1645–50.

McCormack WM, George H, Donner A et al. Hepatotoxicity of erythromycin estolate during pregnancy. Antimicrob Agents Chemother 1977; 12: 630–35.

McGready R, Cho T, Cho JJ et al. Artemisinin derivates in the treatment of falciparum malaria in pregnancy. Trans R Soc Trop Med Hyg 1998; 92: 430–3.

McGready R (A), Cho T, Samuel L et al. Randomized comparison of quinine-clindamycin versus artesunate in the treatment of falciparum malaria in pregnancy. Trans R Soc Trop Med Hyg 2001; 95: 651–6.

McGready R (B), Cho T, Keo NK et al. Artemisinin antimalarials in pregnancy: a prospective treatment study of 539 episodes of multidrug-resistant *Plasmodium falciparum*. Clin Infect Dis 2001; 33: 2009–16.

McGready R, Thwai KL, Cho T et al. The effects of quinine and chloroquine antimalarial treatments in the first trimester of pregnancy. Trans R Soc Trop Med Hyg 2002; 96: 180–84.

McGready R, Ashley EA, Moo E et al. A randomized comparison of artesunate-atovaquone-proguanil versus quinine in treatment for uncomplicated falciparum malaria during pregnancy. J Infect Dis 2005; 192: 846–53.

Metneki J, Czeizel A. Griseofulvin teratology. Lancet 1987; 1: 1042.

Milunsky A, Ulcickas M, Rothman KJ et al. Maternal heat exposure and neural tube defects. J Am Med Assoc 1992; 268: 882–5.

Mitchell TF, Pearlman MD, Chapman RL et al. Maternal and transplacental pharmacokinetics of cefazolin. Obstet Gynecol 2001; 98: 1075–9.

Mofenson LM (A). Prenatal exposure to zidovudine – benefits and risks. N Engl J Med 2000; 343: 803–5.

Mofenson LM (B), McIntyre JA. Advances and researches in the prevention of mother-to-child HIV-1 transmission. Lancet 2000; 355: 2237–44.

Morris AAM, Carr A. HIV nucleoside analogues: new adverse effects on mitochondria? Lancet 1999; 354: 1046–7.

Morris AB, Dobles AR, Cu-Uvin S et al. Protease inhibitor use in 233 pregnancies. J Acq Immune Defic Synd 2005; 40: 30–33.

Myles TD, Elam G, Park-Hwang E et al. The Jarisch–Herxheimer reaction and fetal monitoring changes in pregnant women treated for syphilis. Obstet Gynecol 1998; 92: 859–64.

Na-Bangchang K, Manyando C, Ruengweerayut R et al. The pharmacokinetics and pharmacodynamics of atovaquone and proguanil for the treatment of uncomplicated falciparum malaria in third-trimester pregnant women. Eur J Clin Pharmacol 2005; 61: 573–82.

Newman RD, Parise ME, Slutsker L et al. Safety, efficacy and determinants of effectiveness of antimalarial drugs during pregnancy: implications for prevention programmes in *Plasmodium falciparum*-endemic sub-Saharan Africa. Trop Med Intl Health 2003; 8: 488–506.

Nosten F, Vincenti M, Simpson J et al. The effects of mefloquine treatment in pregnancy. Clin Infect Dis 1999; 28: 808–15.

Olds GR. Administration of Praziquantel to pregnant and lactating women. Acta Trop 2003; 86: 185–95.

Paparone PW, Menghetti RA. Case report: neuro-cysticercosis in pregnancy. NJ Med 1996; 93: 91–4.

Parke AL, Rothfield NF. Antimalarial drugs in pregnancy – the North American experience. Lupus 1996; 5(Suppl l): S67–9.

Peled Y, Friedman S, Hod M et al. Ofloxacin during the second trimester of pregnancy. DICP 1991; 25: 1181–2.

Pescovitz MD. Absence of teratogenicity of oral ganciclovir used during early pregnancy in a liver transplant recipient. Transplantation 1999; 67: 758–9.

Philips-Howard PA, Wood D. The safety of antimalarial drugs in pregnancy. Drug Saf 1996; 14: 131–45.

Philips-Howard PA, Steffen R, Kerr I et al. Safety of mefloquine and other antimalarial agents in the first trimester of pregnancy. J Travel Med 1998; 5: 121–6.

Piper JM, Mitchell EF, Ray WA. Prenatal use of metronidazole and birth defects. Obstet Gynecol 1993; 82: 348–52.

Pursley TJ, Blomquist IK, Abraham J et al. Fluconazole-induced congenital anomalies in three infants. CID 1996; 22: 336–40.

Raju B, Schluger NW. Tuberculosis and pregnancy. Sem Respir Crit Care Med 1998; 19: 295–306.

Ramsey PS, Vaules MB, Vasdev GM et al. Maternal and transplacental pharmacokinetics of azithromycin. Am J Obstet Gynecol 2003; 188: 714–18.

RCOG (Royal College of Obstetricians and Gynaecologists). Smith JR, Cowan FM, Munday P. The management of herpes simplex infection in pregnancy. Br J Obstet Gynaecol 1998; 105: 255–60.

2

Pregnancy

2.6 Anti-infective agents

Reeves DS. Treatment of bacteriuria in pregnancy with single dose fosfomycin trometamol: a review. Infection 1992; 20(Suppl 4): S313–16.

Reuvers-Lodewijks WE. ENTIS – study on anthelmintics during pregnancy. Presentation on the 10th Annual Meeting of the European Network of Teratology Information Services 1999, Madrid.

Reyes MP, Ostrea EM, Cabinian AE et al. Vancomycin during pregnancy: does it cause hearing loss or nephrotoxicity in the infant? Am J Obstet Gynecol 1989; 161: 977–81.

Rezvani M, Koren G. Pregnancy outcome after exposure to injectable ribavirin during embryogenesis. Reprod Toxicol 2006; 21: 113–15.

Rosa F, Hernandez C, Carlo WA. Griseofulvin teratology, including two thoracopagus conjoined twins. Lancet 1987; 1: 171.

Rosa F. Amantadine pregnancy experience. Reprod Toxicol 1994; 8: 531.

Rosevear SK, Fox R, Marlow N et al. Birthing pools and the fetus. Lancet 1993; 342: 1048–9.

Samuel BU, Barry M. The pregnant traveler. Infect Dis Clin North Am 1998; 12: 325–54.

Sanchez JM, Moya G. Fluconazole teratogenicity. Prenat Diagn 1998; 18: 862–9.

Sanchez-Sainz-Trapaga C, Gutierrez-Fonseca R, Ibanez-Ruiz C et al. Relationship between a case of severe hearing loss and use of gentamycin in the pregnant mother. An Esp Pediatr 1998; 49: 397–8.

Sarkar MS, Rowland K, Koren G. Pregnancy outcome following gestational exposure to terbinafine: a prospective comparative study. Birth Def Res A Clin Mol Teratol 2003; 67: 390.

Savioli L, Crompton DW, Neira M. Use of anthelminthic drugs during pregnancy. Am J Obstet Gynecol 2003; 188: 5–6.

Schaefer C, Amoura–Elefant E, Vial T et al. Pregnancy outcome after prenatal quinolone exposure. Evaluation of a Case Registry of the European Network of Teratology Information Services (ENTIS). Eur J Obstet Gynecol Reprod Biol 1996; 69: 83–9.

Schick B, Horn M, Librizzi R et al. Pregnancy outcome following exposure to clarithromycin. Reprod Toxicol 1996; 10: 162.

Schlagenhauf P. Mefloquine for malaria chemoprophylaxis 1992–1998: a review. J Travel Med 1999; 6(2): 22–33.

Scott LL. Prevention of perinatal herpes: prophylactic antiviral therapy? Clin Obstet Gynecol 1999; 42(1): 134–48.

Shaw GM, Todoroff, Velie EM et al. Maternal illness, including fever, and medication use as risk factors for neural tube defects. Teratology 1998; 57: 1–7.

Shephard TH, Brent RL, Friedman JM et al. Update on new developments in the study of human teratogens. Teratology 2002; 65: 153–61.

Shin S, Guerra D, Rich M et al. Treatment of multidrug-resistant tuberculosis during pregnancy: a report of 7 cases. Clin Infect Dis 2003; 36: 996–1003.

Shulman CE, Dorman EK. Reducing childhood mortality in poor countries; importance and prevention of malaria in pregnancy. Trans R Soc Trop Med Hyg 2003; 97: 30–35.

Sobel JD. Use of antifungal drugs in pregnancy – a focus on safety. Drug Saf 2000; 23: 77–85.

Sørensen HT, Nielsen Gl, Olesen et al. Risk of malformation and other outcomes in children exposed to fluconazole in utero. Br J Clin Pharmacol 1999; 48: 234–8.

Stein GE. Single-dose treatment of acute cystitis with fosfomycin tromethamine. Ann Pharmacother 1998; 32: 215–17.

Stone KM, Reiff ER, White AD et al. Pregnancy outcomes following systemic prenatal acyclovir exposure: Conclusions from the International Acyclovir Pregnancy Registry, 1984–1999. Birth Def Res A 2004; 70: 201–7.

Tagbor H, Bruce J, Browne E et al. Efficacy, safety, and tolerability of amodiaquine plus sulphadoxine-pyrimethamine used alone or in combination for malaria treatment in pregnancy: a randomised trial. Lancet 2006; 368: 1349–56.

Thapa PB, Whitlock JA, Brockman-Worrell KG et al. Prenatal exposure to metronidazole and risk of childhood cancer: a retrospective cohort study of children younger than 5 years. Cancer 1998; 83(7): 1461–8.

Thomas F, Erhart A, D'Alessandro U. Can amodiaquine be used safely during pregnancy? Lancet Infect Dis 2004; 4(4): 235–9.

Trexler MF, Fraser TG, Jones MP. Fulminant pseudomembranous colitis caused by clindamycin phosphate vaginal cream. Am J Gastroenterology 1997; 92: 2112–13.

Tripathy SN, Tripathy SN. Tuberculosis and pregnancy. Intl J Gynaecol Obstet 2003; 80: 247–53.

Vial T. ENTIS Study on Conazole Antimycotics During Pregnancy. Personal communication, 2001.

Wallon M, Liou C, Garner P et al. Congenital toxoplasmosis: systemic review of evidence of efficacy of treatment in pregnancy. Br Med J 1999; 318: 1511–14.

Watts DH, Brown ZA, Money D et al. A double-blind, randomized, placebo-controlled trial of acyclovir in late pregnancy for the reduction of herpes simplex virus shedding and cesarean delivery. Am J Obstet Gynecol 2003; 188: 836–43.

Whitley R. Neonatal herpes simplex virus infection. Curr Opin Infect Dis 2004; 17: 243–6.

WHO (A). Drug Information. Mefloquine: an update on safety issues. Reports on individual drugs 1996; 10: 58–60.

WHO (B). World Health Report 1996: Fighting Disease, Fostering Development. WHO 1996; 43.

WHO. Assessment of the Safety of Artemisinin Compounds in Pregnancy. Report of two informal consultations convened by WHO in 2002. WHO/CDS/MAL/2003.1094 and WHO/RBM/TDR/Artemisinin/03.1.

WHO (A). International Travel and Health Publication 2005; Malaria (http://whqlib doc.who.int/publications/2005/9241580364_chap7.pdf).

WHO (B). Malaria Control Today. Current WHO Recommendations. Working document, March 2005 (http://www.who.int/malaria/docs/MCT_workingpaper.pdf).

Witt KL, Cunningham CK, Patterson KB et al. Elevated frequencies of micronucleated erthroyctes in infants exposed to zidovudine in utero and postpartum to prevent mother-to-child transmission of HIV. Environ Mol Mutagen 2007; 48: 322-9.

Wogelius P, Nørgaard M, Gislum M et al. Further analysis of the risk of adverse birth outcome after maternal use of fluoroquinolones. Intl J Antimicrobial Agents 2005; 26: 323–6.

Yaris F, Kesim M, Kadioglu M et al. Gentamicin use in pregnancy. A renal anomaly. Saudi Med J 2004; 25: 958–9.

Yudin MH. Bacterial vaginosis in pregnancy: diagnosis, screening, and management. Clin Perinatol 2005; 32: 617–27.

Zaske DE, Cipolle RJ, Strate RG et al. Rapid gentamycin elimination in obstetric patients. Obstet Gynecol 1980; 56: 559–64.

2

Pregnancy

2.6 Anti-infective agents

Vaccines and immunoglobulins

2.7

Paul Peters

2.7.1 Vaccination and pregnancy

Protective and booster immunizations should be carried out before pregnancy. Even though no embryotoxic or teratogenic effects have been proven for any vaccine, the indications for immunization, especially in the first trimester, should be limited strictly to rare situations. With live vaccines, the risk of a fetal infection from the vaccine is more of a theoretical nature, but routine immunization should be avoided during pregnancy. Another reason for avoiding vaccinations in early pregnancy is the possible risk of maternal hyperthermia (see Chapter 2.6) as a reaction to the vaccine. This risk is moderate, but common to almost all types of vaccines. If fever occurs, it should be treated with paracetamol (acetaminophen) as soon as it occurs. A third reason for avoiding vaccinations, especially in later stages of pregnancy, would be that postnatally the developing child might not recognize the antigen and since the immune system has become tolerant no seroconversion would be the result.

When there is a high infection risk without protection from prior immunization, a vaccination should be pursued in the interest of both mother and child, even during pregnancy. Candidate vaccines should be immunogenic, safe, and cause minimal reactions. The potential effect on the incidence of communicable diseases in the newborn and young infant will increase as more candidate vaccines that could be administered during pregnancy become available. In the future, infections such as herpes simplex virus infection, cytomegalovirus, and human immunodeficiency virus infection could be prevented with this intervention (Munoz 2001). Details of different compounds are discussed below.

The use of *thiomersal* (*ethyl mercury*) as a preservative in vaccines has been debated (Bigham 2005), since ethyl mercury might be a risk for the brain of the unborn or developing child. However, the blood–brain barrier passage of ethyl mercury is much more difficult than for the known fetotoxicant methyl mercury. There are as yet no data indicating embryotoxicity for the unborn related to ethyl mercury in vaccines (about 5 µg). According to the WHO, thiomersal will stay in the vaccines where necessary for developing countries (Bigham 2005). In these countries, the so-called "cold-chain" might not be optimal to prevent vaccines to be contaminated.

In general, and this holds for all successful vaccines and vaccinations, the advantages of protection and prevention of the population from the pertinent diseases outweigh by far the individual adverse reactions that vaccines might cause.

Pregnancy

2.7 Vaccines and immunoglobulins

2.7.2   Cholera vaccine

The cholera vaccine contains inactivated vibrios of the serotypes Inaba and Ogawa. There are no studies on the use of this vaccine during pregnancy. Protection is incomplete and only short-term. Antibiotic treatment of a cholera infection is obviously the choice during pregnancy. It should, however, be considered that there is already a high antibiotic resistance among vibrios. Thus, no universally valid recommendations for infection prophylaxis in pregnancy can be made, because the appropriate procedure depends on the situation of the individual case (e.g. length of the trip, destination, housing conditions). Pregnant women who must travel in epidemic areas should, in any case, strictly adhere to the basic hygienic measures: "boil it, cook it, peel it or forget it."

Recommendation. If compellingly indicated, assuming that travel to an endemic area cannot be postponed, vaccination should also be performed during pregnancy.

2.7.3   Hemophilus influenza b (HIB) vaccine

Hemophilus b conjugate vaccine is a combination of the capsular polysaccharides or oligosaccharides purified from HIB type b bound with various proteins. Two reports and a review have described the maternal immunization with the capsular polysaccharide vaccine of HIB during the third trimester of pregnancy to achieve passive immunity in the fetus and newborn. No adverse effects were observed in the newborns (review in Briggs 2005).

Recommendation. Vaccination results in pregnancy are lacking; discussion about the innocuity and effectivity are still ongoing.

2.7.4   Hepatitis A vaccine

Hepatitis A infection is usually not more severe during pregnancy than at other times, and does not affect the outcome of pregnancy. There have been reports, however, of acute fulminate conditions in pregnant women during the third trimester, when there is also an increased risk of premature labor and fetal death. These events have occurred in women from developing countries, and may have been related to underlying malnutrition. The hepatitis A virus is rarely transmitted to the fetus, but this can occur during viremia or from fecal contamination at delivery (Tanaka 1995).

Hepatitis A vaccine contains inactivated hepatitis A viruses that are cultivated from human cell cultures. Its use in pregnancy has not been systematically investigated. However, there is no indication of developmental toxicity.

2

Pregnancy

> **Recommendation.** Pregnant women without immunity to hepatitis A need protection before traveling to developing countries. Based on the experience with other inactivated viral vaccines, hepatitis A vaccine can be given to the pregnant woman at high risk of infection. Immune globulin is safe and effective in preventing hepatitis A, but immunization with one of the hepatitis A vaccines gives a more complete and prolonged protection.

2.7.5   Hepatitis B vaccine

A biotechnologically produced non-reproducible surface antigen is used as hepatitis B vaccine (HBV). It is therefore a non-infectious vaccine, and no risks to the fetus have been reported following vaccination of their mothers in pregnancy (ACOG 1993). Immunization of groups at risk is recommended; if possible, it should be given after the twelfth week of pregnancy. Ayoola (1987) described a series of 72 pregnant Nigerians who were seronegative for hepatitis B and were given two intramuscular doses of vaccine in the third trimester. One month after the second dose, 84% were anti-HBs positive. No significant adverse effects were observed in the mothers or their newborns. Passive transfer of anti-HBs occurred in 59% of the newborns. The antibodies disappeared rapidly in these infants, and by 3 months only 23% had detectable antibodies (Ingardia 1999, Reddy 1994). No HBsAg carrier status developed in this group. In contrast, the infants born to HBsAg-positive mothers had a cumulative rate of HBV events of 20%. The authors concluded that HBV vaccine is safe and immunogenic in pregnant women. The passive immunity conferred on the infants is of short duration (Lee 2006). Therefore, in, for example, The Netherlands, newborns from HBsAg-positive mothers will be vaccinated immediately or otherwise within 48 hours after birth, preferably following the administration of hepatitis-B immunoglobulin with booster vaccinations at the ages of 3, 4 and 11 months, according to the Dutch Health Council advice (Geelen 2006).

2.7 Vaccines and immunoglobulins

Recommendation. Vaccination of pregnant mothers in hepatitis B high-risk populations may provide adequate protection before the child is vaccinated. There are no negative adverse effects to be expected.

2.7.6   Human Papilloma Virus (HPV) vaccine

In June 2006 the US FDA licensed the first vaccine developed to prevent cervical cancer and other diseases in females caused by certain types of genital human papillomavirus (HPV) types (6, 11, 16 and 18), responsible for 70% of cervical cancers and 90% of genital warts. The duration of the protection is unclear. Current studies (with 5-year follow-up) indicate that the vaccine is effective for at least 5 years (Anonymous 2006). The vaccine has not been causally associated with adverse outcomes of pregnancy or adverse reactions to the developing fetus. However, data on vaccination in pregnancy are limited.

Recommendation. The HPV vaccine is not recommended in pregnancy. Inadvertent exposure during pregnancy is not a reason for invasive diagnostics or for interruption of pregnancy.

2.7.7   Influenza vaccine

Pregnant women are supposed to have an increased risk of influenza infection and complications. Evaluation of more than 2000 pregnancies exposed to influenza vaccine could not demonstrate an increased risk of maternal complications or adverse fetal outcomes associated with the vaccine (Naleway 2006, Munoz 2005). The selected vaccine should be the vaccine advised for that influenza season. The American College of Obstetricians and Gynecologists (ACOG) (1991) recommended that the vaccine should be given only to pregnant women with serious underlying diseases (chronic diseases or pulmonary problems). In contrast, the Advisory Committee on Immunization Practices recommends standing orders, programs or reminders for patients and providers as strategies to improve vaccination rates during pregnancy, which are estimated to be less than 10%. The Joint Committee on Vaccination and Immunisations (JCVI 2006) in the UK agreed in June 2006 that pregnant women were at an increased risk of morbidity and mortality from seasonal influenza, and recommended that women in the second and third trimesters should be routinely offered vaccination. A study (Hartert 2003) on respiratory hospitalizations among pregnant women during influenza seasons revealed that the further advanced the pregnancy, the more vulnerable the women appeared. At 37–42 weeks of pregnancy, they were nearly five times more likely to end up in hospital with influenza than were women who were up to 6 months' pregnant. There have been only a few and small studies of the effect of the influenza vaccination on the fetus, but they have shown no ill effects.

> **Recommendation.** Influenza vaccination in the influenza season before planning a pregnancy is preferred, but there are no indications of an adverse effect of vaccination during pregnancy for the mother, or on the fetal outcome.

2.7.8   Measles and mumps vaccines

There is insufficient documented experience with the use of these vaccines during pregnancy.

Measles (rubeola) vaccine is a live attenuated virus vaccine. Although transplacental passage of this vaccine has never been demonstrated, the vaccine should not be used during pregnancy because fetal infection with the attenuated virus cannot be excluded. Because this vaccine is normally administered together with the rubella vaccine, its contraindications are similar. The American College of Obstetricians and Gynecologists lists the vaccine as contraindicated in pregnancy and also recommends a 3-month interval before conception (ACOG 1993). In case of a significant exposure risk in a non-immune patient, a vaccination during the third trimester is suggested.

Mumps vaccine is also a live attenuated virus vaccine. Mumps occurring during pregnancy may result in an increased rate of first-trimester abortion. Although a fetal risk from the vaccine has not been confirmed, the vaccine should not be used during pregnancy because, in theory, fetal infection with the attenuated viruses might occur. Several publications dealt with the controversy over the alleged link between MMR vaccination in the child and autism, but this is now discredited in the eyes of most scientists.

> **Recommendation.** Both vaccines are contraindicated in pregnancy because, theoretically, fetal infection with the attenuated vaccines might occur. Because these vaccines are normally administered together with the rubella vaccine, its contraindications are similar. There is no indication for termination of pregnancy if vaccination has taken place in pregnancy. The manufacturer recommends avoiding pregnancy for 3 months following vaccination.

2.7.9   Meningococcal meningitis vaccine

The polyvalent meningococcal meningitis vaccine may be administered during pregnancy if the woman is entering an area where the disease is endemic. From the use of this vaccine, mostly in the third trimester of pregnancy, it is concluded that there are no indications for harm of the unborn (Letson 1998). Protecting antibodies have been found to cross the placenta. In breast milk and in the serum of the newborn, significantly higher IgA and IgG levels were found in 157 individuals vaccinated in the third trimester, in comparison with controls (Shahid 2002).

> **Recommendation.** Vaccination, if necessary, is not known to be associated with developmental disorders.

2.7.10   Pneumococcal vaccination

Pneumococcal vaccination during pregnancy was thought to be the way of preventing pneumococcal disease during the first month of life. From studies with 280 participants (Chaithongwongwatthana 2006), it was concluded that there was no adverse effect on pregnancy and on the health of the newborn. However, there was no evidence that pneumococcal vaccination during pregnancy reduced neonatal infection.

> **Recommendation.** There are no indications to vaccinate against neonatal pneumococcal infection during pregnancy. On the other hand, vaccination does not seem to be harmful for the fetus, and does not require any intervention.

2.7.11   Poliomyelitis vaccine

Oral polio vaccine (Sabin) contains attenuated live poliomyelitis viruses of all three poliovirus types. It is no longer recommended for routine vaccinations because in very rare cases it may cause poliomyelitis. The inactivated form of the vaccine (Salk), mostly in combinations with other vaccines (injection), is now preferred.

When there were outbreaks of poliovirus in Israel and Finland, mass oral polio vaccinations of the population, including pregnant women, were performed. Based on the observation of more than 15 000 pregnancies, there was no increased risk of spontaneous abortion and no increase in birth defects or prematurity (Harjulehto-Mervaala 1995, Ornoy 2006, 1993, 1990). The authors consider the oral poliovirus vaccine as safe for pregnant women; however, it should not be used in the last month of pregnancy, to avoid contamination of delivery rooms by the virus-shedding mother. Live attenuated poliovirus is no longer relevant as a result of practical extinction of the disease, at least in the developed world. Polio-like changes (damage to the anterior horn cells of the spinal cord) were noted in a fetus aborted at 21 weeks' gestation when the previously immune mother received oral polio vaccine at 18 weeks (Castleman 1964), but no similar effect has been published since.

> **Recommendation.** Immunization with inactivated polio vaccine can be performed when compellingly indicated. There is no reason to terminate a pregnancy when polio vaccination (with inactivated or attenuated virus vaccine) has been administered to a pregnant woman.

2.7.12   Rabies vaccine

The rabies vaccine contains attenuated live virus matter, which is produced nowadays from human cell cultures. This vaccine, which has been available since 1980, has, in contrast to earlier vaccines, virtually no side effects. Case reports on active and/or passive immunization during a pregnancy indicate an uncomplicated course of pregnancy (Chutivongse 1995, Chabala 1991, Fescharek 1989). A study was published regarding the safety and immunogenicity of purified vero cell rabies vaccine (PVRV) during pregnancy (Sudarshan 1999). Twenty-nine pregnant women exposed to rabies were vaccinated with PVRV, and none of the women experienced any adverse side effects to the vaccine. The intrauterine growth and development monitored by ultrasound examination was found to be normal, and the outcome of pregnancy was satisfactory. There were no congenital anomalies in any of the infants born, and they were healthy with normal growth and development during the 1-year follow-up period. The rabies-neutralizing antibody titers from day 14 to day 365 following vaccination in these women was adequate and well above the minimum protective level of 0.5 IU/ml serum. Protective levels of antibodies were also present in the serum of some of the babies tested, until 3 months of age. The mothers and infants followed for a 1-year period were doing well at the end of the study period.

> **Recommendation.** Since rabies is an illness with fatal consequences, a pregnant woman must always be simultaneously immunized (actively and passively) following a bite from an animal suspected to be rabid.

2.7.13   Rubella vaccine

Rubella immunization uses attenuated live virus vaccine. Antibody levels of 10–15 international units IgG/ml are considered protective. Naturally acquired rubella generally confers a lifelong and usually high degree of immunity against the disease for the majority of individuals. Rubella immunization is contraindicated shortly before and during pregnancy (Tookey 2001), despite the fact that in all surveillance studies to date (including more then 700 pregnancies) no child has been born with congenital rubella syndrome after vaccination of its seronegative mother during pregnancy (see, for example, Hamkar 2006, Enders 2005, Best 1991, Tookey 1991). A study led by the Motherisk Program of Toronto in Canada, quoted by Josefson (2001), compared the rates of fetal malformations in the infants of 94 women who mistakenly received rubella vaccinations while pregnant with 94 pregnant women who were not vaccinated during pregnancy. The rate of fetal anomalies was similar in both groups. In addition, no significant differences existed in miscarriage rates, birth weight or developmental milestones between the two groups. Hearing-test results were also equivalent across the groups. The only significant difference was the higher rate of abortions in the group who received vaccinations during pregnancy. In one case, a child was born with a congenital cataract discussed in association with maternal rubella vaccination (Fleet 1974). This case was not validated, and it is possible that the wild virus infected this mother just before she received the vaccination.

However, the rubella vaccine virus does cross the placenta and can infect the fetus (Hamkar 2006). In 2% of the cases studied there was a proof of rubella-specific IgM-antibodies in the newborn, and in 3–20% the vaccine virus could be isolated in abortion material (CDC 1989). In another publication, inadvertent immunization several weeks before and after conception of seronegative women with RA27/3 rubella virus live-attenuated vaccine was reported (Hofmann 2000). Whereas in five cases the vaccine virus was not transmitted vertically, in one case vaccination led to the development of persistent fetal infection with prolonged virus shedding for more than 8 months. Sequence analysis performed on isolates from amniotic fluid and from cord blood leukocytes, as well as from infantile urine, confirmed an infection by the vaccine strain. At birth, the newborn infant exhibited none of the symptoms compatible with the congenital rubella syndrome, and signs indicative for the development of late-onset disease were not apparent. This observation constitutes the first unequivocal documented case of rubella vaccine virus related to persistent fetal infection. In the US, the CDC changed the recommendation concerning the pregnancy interval after receiving rubella vaccination only, reducing it from 3 months to 1 month (CDC 2001).

Recommendation. The risk of congenital rubella syndrome from rubella vaccination is theoretical, and in any case is not comparable with the high risk of a rubella embryopathy when the wild virus has infected the mother. If a rubella vaccination has inadvertently been administered to a woman before or during pregnancy, there is no indication for termination of pregnancy or invasive diagnostic tests.

2.7.14   Tetanus and diphtheria vaccines

These vaccines are bacteriological vaccines that contain the relevant toxoids, and there are no indications of embryotoxic properties in these vaccines, which have been used for many decades – also in pregnant women. The suspicion of an increased risk of funnel thorax and clubfoot as a result of tetanus toxoid, suggested about 30 years ago and never confirmed, is of anecdotal character (Heinonen 1977). A large case-control pair analysis conducted in Hungary (Czeizel 1999) failed to detect any teratogenic effect of tetanus toxoid.

Recommendation. To protect against maternal illness and neonatal tetanus, sufficient immune protection should be guaranteed during the pregnancy. As a rule, basic immunization is given in childhood; afterwards, a booster immunization is recommended every 10 years. If the booster has been neglected, it can be made up in the second or third trimester. The mother may also be immunized in the first trimester if this is indicated.

2.7.15   Typhoid vaccine

There are two types of typhoid vaccine: the older, inactivated typhoid vaccine, administered parenterally, and the oral live typhoid vaccine with *Salmonella typhi* type 21a. The live vaccine does not protect against paratyphoid A and B, but has a lower rate of side effects than does the inactivated vaccine. When a typhoid infection occurs during pregnancy, the risk of miscarriage is increased as a result of typhoid septicemia. For this reason, neither of these vaccines is absolutely contraindicated during pregnancy, according to the Advisory Committee on Immunization Practices. No adverse reactions are known from the vaccine (Mazzone 1994).

> **Recommendation.** A preference for immunization with the oral typhoid vaccine has been expressed, because of its better efficacy and fewer adverse reactions, in particular fever.

2.7.16   Varicella vaccine

Varicella vaccine is a live attenuated viral vaccine that was licensed in 1995 in the US. Although indications of this vaccine in Europe are limited to children with deficient immunity of any cause, the problem of vaccination during pregnancy may arise in selected cases. A Pregnancy Registry for this vaccine was established in the US as a collaborative effort between the manufacturer (Merck Pregnancy Registry Program, 2000) and the Centers for Disease Control and Prevention because congenital varicella syndrome has occurred in newborns of women who experienced primary infection with natural chickenpox during the first half of their pregnancies (Ingardia 1999, Enders 1994). Congenital varicella syndrome is characterized by cutaneous scarring in a certain dermatome and/or hypoplasia of an extremity (Roberts 1990). Additional manifestations may include low birth weight, microcephaly, localized muscular atrophy, ocular anomalies, and neurological abnormalities.

The varicella vaccine registry obtained the outcomes of 362 prospectively registered pregnancies (Shields 2001). The rates of spontaneous abortions, late fetal deaths, and minor or major congenital anomalies were not increased. The reported defects showed no specific pattern. Timing of vaccine exposure and biologic plausibility do not support the assumption of a causal relationship between varicella vaccination and the congenital anomalies observed in the registry. Although the number of exposures is not sufficient to rule out a very low risk, data collected in the registry to date do not show congenital varicella syndrome in association with the vaccination.

> **Recommendation.** Varicella vaccination is not recommended during pregnancy, but inadvertent vaccination does not seem to be at high risk for the fetus and does not require any intervention.

2.7.17   Yellow fever vaccine

The yellow fever vaccine contains attenuated live viruses. Fifty-eight pregnancies followed by the European Network of Teratology Information Services (ENTIS) gave no substantial indication of embryo- or fetotoxic effect after first-trimester vaccination (Robert 1999). In a small number of women who received this vaccine during various stages of pregnancy there was no evidence of transplacental passage of the attenuated virus, although in most mothers who produced neutralizing antibodies these antibodies either crossed the placenta or were transferred to neonates through the colostrum. No adverse effects associated with prenatal exposure to this vaccine were observed at birth or during a 3- to 4-year follow-up period (Nasidi 1993). There is one report on congenital infection after first-trimester vaccination (Tsai 1993), but no other report has confirmed this potential risk. Finally, a small case-control study conducted in Brazil (Nishioka 1998) compared 39 women who attended a hospital after spontaneous abortion with 74 women attending the antenatal clinic of the same hospital. A non-significant risk for spontaneous abortion was found.

> **Recommendation.** Yellow fever vaccine should be avoided during pregnancy. However, since yellow fever can be life-threatening, a pregnant woman should be immunized – even in the first trimester – if a trip to a region where the disease is endemic cannot be postponed.

2.7.18   Immunoglobulins

Immunoglobulin solutions contain primarily immunoglobulin-G (IgG) antibodies, and are produced from pooled human plasma. The extent to which IgG antibodies pass through the placenta is dependent on the gestational age, the dosage, the length of treatment, and the kind of preparation given. However, Fab fragments do not pass (Miller et al. 2003). Immunoglobulins are used for different maternal or fetal indications – for example, in cases of antibody deficiency or infectious diseases (especially as a preventive measure), to improve the symptoms of some maternal autoimmune diseases, or to treat the symptoms of some fetal conditions (such as, for instance, heart block in the fetuses of mothers with lupus erythematosus).

Both immunoglobulins and hyperimmune sera against specific infections are not, as far as we know today, embryotoxic (review in Briggs 2005).

Non-specific risks via human blood products, such as the transfer of virus infections and anaphylaxis, cannot be ruled out completely, and can indirectly endanger the fetus.

A study of 93 children whose mothers had been given γ-globulin prophylaxis against hepatitis during pregnancy on known gestational dates showed significant dermatoglyphic changes on the fingertips of the children exposed prenatally (Ross 1996). This effect, which can hardly be considered to be a birth defect, only occurred when γ-globulin had been administered in the first 163 days of pregnancy. This anecdotal report does not modify the recommendation.

> **Recommendation.** Immunoglobulins – standard γ-globulin and hyperimmune sera – may be used in pregnancy for appropriate indications.

References

ACOG. Immunization during pregnancy. Technical Bulletin October 1991, No. 160. Intl J Gynecol Obstet 1993; 40: 69–79.

Anonymous. Sexually transmitted diseases treatment guidelines 2006. MMWR 2006 (55. www.fda.gov/bbs/topics/NEWS/2006/NEW01385.html).

Ayoola EA, Johnson AO. Hepatitis B in pregnancy: immunogenicity, safety and the transfer of antibodies to infants. Intl J Gynecol Obstet 1987; 25: 297–301.

Best JM. Rubella vaccines: past, present and future. Epidemiol Infect 1991; 107: 17–30.

Bigham M, Copes R. Thiomersal in vaccines: balancing the risk of adverse effects with the risk of vaccine-preventable disease. Drug Saf 2005; 28: 89–101.

Briggs GG, Freeman RK, Yaffe SJ. Drugs in Pregnancy and Lactation, 7th edn. Baltimore, MD: Lippicott, Williams & Wilkins, 2005.

Castleman B, McNeely BU. Case records of the Massachusetts General Hospital. Case 47–1964. Presentation of Case. N Engl J Med 1964; 271: 676–82.

CDC. Rubella vaccination in pregnancy. United States, 1971–1988. MMWR 1989; 38: 289–93.

CDC. Notice to readers: revised ACIP recommendations for avoiding pregnancy after receiving a rubella-containing vaccine. MMWR 2001; 50: 1117.

Chabala S, Williams M, Amenta R et al. Confirmed rabies exposure during pregnancy: treatment with human rabies immune globulin and human diploid cell vaccine. Am J Med 1991; 91: 423–41.

Chaithongwongwatthana S, Yamasmit W, Limpongsanurak S et al. Pneumococcal vaccination during pregnancy for preventing infant infections. Cochrane Database Syst Rev 2006; (1): CDC004903.

Chutivongse S, Wilde H, Benjavongkulchai M et al. Postexposure rabies vaccination during pregnancy: effect on 202 women and their infants. Clin Infect Dis 1995; 20: 818–20.

Czeizel AE, Rockenbauer M. Tetanus toxoid and congenital anomalies. Intl J Gynecol Obstet 1999; 64: 253–8.

Enders G, Miller E, Cradock-Watson J et al. Consequences of varicella zoster in pregnancy: prospective study of 1739 cases. Lancet 1994; 343: 1547–50.

Enders G. Accidental rubella vaccination at the time of conception and in early pregnancy [in German]. Bundesgesundheitsbl-Gesundheitsforsch-Gesundheitsschutz 2005; 48: 685–6.

Fescharek R, Quast U, Dechert G. Postexposure rabies vaccination during pregnancy: experience from post-marketing surveillance with 16 patients. Vaccine 1989; 7: 546–8.

Fleet WF Jr, Benz EW Jr, Karzon DT et al. Fetal consequences of maternal rubella immunization. J Am Med Assoc 1974; 227: 621–7.

Geelen SP. Adjustment of the hepatitis-B vaccination scheme for newborns born to hepatitis-B virus carriers as of 1 January 2006 [in Dutch]. Ned Tijdschr Geneeskd 2006; 150(8): 415–18.

Hamkar R, Jalilvand S, Abdolbaghi MH et al. Inadvertent rubella vaccination of pregnant women: evaluation of possible transplacental infection with rubella vaccine. Vaccine 2006; 24: 3558–63.

Harjulehto-Mervaala T, Hovi T, Aro T et al. Oral poliovirus vaccination and pregnancy complications. Acta Obstet Gynecol Scand 1995; 74: 262–5.

Hartret T, Neuzil K, Shintani A et al. Maternal morbidity and perinatal outcomes among pregnant women with repiratory hospitalizations during influenza season. Am J Obstet Gynecol 2003; 189: 1705–12.

Heinonen OP, Slone S, Shapiro S. Birth Defects and Drugs in Pregnancy. Littleton, MA: Publishing Sciences Group, 1977.

Hofmann J, Kortung M, Pustowoit B et al. Persistent fetal rubella vaccine virus infection following inadvertent vaccination during early pregnancy. J Med Virol 2000; 61: 155–8.

Ingardia CJ, Kelley L, Lerer T et al. Correlation of maternal and fetal hepatitis B antibody titers following maternal vaccination in pregnancy. Am J Perinatol 1999; 16(3): 129–32.

JCVI (Joint Committee on Vaccination and Immunity) UK 2006 (www.advisorybodies. doh.gov.uk/jcvi/mins-flu-090306.htm).

Josefson D. Rubella vaccine may be safe in early pregnancy. Br Med J 2001; 322: 695.

Lee C, Gong Y, Brok J et al. Effect of hepatitis B immunisation in newborn infants of mothers positive for hepatitis B surface antigen: systematic review and meta-analysis. Br Med J 2006; 332: 328–36.

Letson GW, Little JR, Ottman J. Meningococcal vaccine in pregnancy: an assessment of infant risk. Pediatr Infect Dis J 1998; 17: 261–3.

Levy M, Koren G. Hepatitis B vaccine in pregnancy: maternal and fetal safety. Am J Perinatol 1991; 8: 227–32.

Mazzone T, Celestini E, Fabi R et al. Oral typhoid vaccine and pregnancy. Reprod Toxicol 1994; 8: 278–9.

Miller RK, Mace K, Polliotti B, DeRita R, Hall W, Treacy G. Marginal transfer of ReoPro™ (Abciximab) compared with lmmunoglobulin G (F105), insulin and water in the perfused human placenta *in vitro*. Placenta 2003; 24: 727–38.

Munoz FM, Englund JA. Vaccines in pregnancy. Infect Dis Clin North Am 2001; 15: 253–71.

Munoz FM, Greisinger AJ, Wehmanen OA et al. Safety of influenza vaccination during pregnancy. Am J Obstet Gynecol 2005; 192: 1098–106.

Naleway AL, Smith WJ, Mullooly JP. Delivering influenza vaccine to pregnant women. Epidemiol Rev 2006; 28: 47–53.

Nasidi A, Monath TP, Vanderberg J et al. Yellow fever vaccination and pregnancy: a four-year prospective study. Trans R Soc Trop Med Hyg 1993; 87: 337–9.

2

Pregnancy

2.7 Vaccines and immunoglobulins

Nishioka SDA, Nunes-Araujo FRF, Pires WP et al. Yellow fever vaccination during pregnancy and spontaneous abortion: a case-control study. Trop Med Intl Health 1998; 3: 29–33.

Ornoy A, Arnon J, Feingold M et al. Spontaneous abortions following oral poliovirus vaccination in first trimester {Letter}. Lancet 1990; 31(335): 800.

Ornoy A, Ben Ishai P. Congenital anomalies after oral poliovirus vaccination during pregnancy {Letter}. Lancet 1993; 1(341): 1162.

Ornoy A, Tenenbaum A. Pregnancy outcome following infections by coxsackie, echo, measles, mumps, hepatitis, polio and encephalitis viruses. Reprod Toxicol 2006; 21: 446–57.

Reddy PA, Gupta I, Ganguly NK. Hepatitis-B vaccination in pregnancy: safety and immunogenic response in mothers and antibody transfer to neonates. Asia Oceania J Obstet Gynaecol 1994; 20: 361–5.

Robert E, Vial T, Schaefer C et al. Exposure to yellow fever vaccine in early pregnancy. Vaccine 1999; 17: 283–5.

Roberts RM. Fetal effects from varicella-zoster. In: ML Buyse (ed.), Birth Defects Encyclopedia. Cambridge, MA: Blackwell Scientific Publications, 1990, pp. 708–10.

Ross LJ. Dermatoglyphics in offspring of women given gamma globulin prophylaxis during pregnancy. Teratology 1996; 53: 285–9.

Shahid NS, Steinhoff MC, Roy E. Placental and breast transfer of antibodies after maternal immunization with polysaccharide meningococcal vaccine: a randomized, controlled evaluation. Vaccine 2002; 20: 2404–9.

Shields KE, Galil K, Seward J et al. Varicella vaccine exposure during pregnancy: data from the first 5 years of the pregnancy registry. Obstet Gynecol 2001; 98: 14–19.

Sudarshan MK, Madhusudana SN, Mahendra BJ. Post-exposure prophylaxis with purified vero cell rabies vaccine during pregnancy – safety and immunogenicity. J Commun Dis 1999; 31: 229–36.

Tanaka I, Shima M, Kubota Y et al. Vertical transmission of hepatitis A virus. Lancet 1995; 345: 397.

Tookey P, Jones G, Miller BH et al. Rubella vaccination in pregnancy. CDR (Lond Engl Rev) 1991; l: R86–88.

Tookey P. Pregnancy is contraindication for rubella vaccination still. Br Med J 2001; 322: 1489.

Tsai TF, Paul R, Lynberg MC et al. Congenital yellow fever virus infection after immunization in pregnancy. J Infect Dis 1993; 168: 1520–23.

Heart and circulatory system drugs and diuretics

2.8

Corinna Weber-Schöndorfer

There are enormous hemodynamic changes during pregnancy. By gestational week 5, the mother's blood volume has already risen; by the end of pregnancy, the increase is 50%. Vascular resistance and blood pressure drop, and the resting pulse rate rises 10–20 bpm, resulting in a 30–50 percent increase in cardiac output. During delivery, blood pressure rises and ejection volume further increases. Approximately 1–3 days after delivery, and sometimes as late as 1 week, the cardiac pre-pregnancy situation returns (Oakley 2003).

Heart disease is rare during pregnancy (<1 percent), but hypertonic and hypotonic regulatory disturbances are much more common and may require treatment.

2.8.1 Arterial hypertension and pregnancy

Different kinds of arterial hypertension should be distinguished from one another as follows (for pulmonary hypertension, see section 2.8.14):

- Chronic hypertension (with or without proteinuria) which was diagnosed before, during or after pregnancy
- Pre-eclampsia, eclampsia that is proteinuria (>300 mg/d), and newly diagnosed hypertension (edemas are no longer necessary symptoms)
- Pre-eclampsia in a pregnant woman with pre-existing chronic hypertension, which occurs in 20–25 percent of all pregnancies with chronic hypertension
- Pregnancy-induced hypertension (PIH) that occurs beyond 20 weeks without proteinuria and returns to normal 12 weeks after delivery; approximately half of these pregnant women develop pre-eclampsia.

Blood pressure of 140/90 mmHg is the threshold for hypertension in pregnancy. Treatment should only be initiated at levels higher than 160/110 mmHg, because below that there are no advantages in treatment for the outcome of mother and child. If a patient has no proteinuria, a blood pressure at threshold level, normal ECG and echocardiography, and no abnormalities at the examination, the outcome is usually favorable.

Complications of severe hypertension in pregnant women may include intracerebral bleeding, cardiac problems, and placental dysfunction. Placental detachment, prematurity, intrauterine growth restriction, and perinatal death are problems that may occur due to placental dysfunction. The risk for mother and child in any case of pre-eclampsia is high. It has been suggested that there is a deranged interaction between invasion of the trophoblast and decidua, followed by insufficient dilatation of the uterine spiral arteries, which leads to placental hypoperfusion. There is no other causal therapy in this case, except delivery. A conservative option for therapy is antihypertensive therapy at diastolic values beyond 110 mmHg, plus 100 mg per day acetylsalicylic acid, if there is to be strict control of this pregnancy. The HELLP syndrome (hemolysis, elevated liver enzymes, low platelet count) can be a life-threatening condition for mother and fetus.

A prospective study with almost 2000 pregnant women confirmed that the risk is strikingly higher in pre-eclampsia compared with other forms of hypertension (Ray 2001). A meta-analysis concerning anti-hypertensive drugs and the possible changes of fetal and neonatal heart rate stated that the data concerning nifedipine, hydalazine, labetalol, and methyldopa are insufficient for any conclusion to be drawn (Waterman 2004).

The drugs of choice for the treatment of hypertension in pregnancy are different from those used to treat non-pregnant patients, but despite many studies and experiences there are still no uniform recommendations for pregnant women. Controlled systematic large studies are rare. Drugs that have been on the market a long time tend to be used in preference to newer drugs because of lack of safety data for the fetus in the latter group.

In cases of chronic hypertension, the drug of first choice is methyldopa, followed by metoprolol, dihydralazine/hydralazine, and nifedipine.

If a pregnancy is complicated by any form of pre-eclampsia, dihydralazine, nifedipine and urapidil show good results. β-blockers are also acceptable, of which labetalol is the best proven one.

Hypertensive diseases in pregnancy require good control and diagnostic procedures in order to decide on the optimum therapy.

2.8.2   α-methyldopa

Pharmacology

Methyldopa is well-absorbed orally, and has a half-life of about 2 hours. The mechanism of action in the CNS is not known. It is activated by decarboxylation to α-methyl-noradrenaline, a false transmitter with a much weaker action than noradrenaline. Methyldopa is well suited for long-term use because it does not normally alter cardiac function. Cardiac minute output particularly, and blood flow to the kidney or uterus, is not changed, but peripheral total resistance is lowered. According to one study, α-methyldopa had no influence on the vascular resistance of the umbilical artery (Houlihan 2004). Günenç (2002) analyzed the effect of α-methyldopa in 24 pregnant women with pre-eclampsia using Doppler sonography: The vascular resistance in the uterine artery was reduced, but not in the umbilical artery or in the fetal middle cerebral artery.

Methyldopa is well-absorbed both by the intravenous (i.v.) and oral routes. The onset of action is delayed for 1–2 hours after i.v. administration and 4–6 hours after oral administration. It is effective for 6–12 hours. Methyldopa crosses the placenta, producing fetal serum concentrations similar to those in the mother (Jones 1978).

Toxicology

In a group of 242 children exposed in the first trimester, neither the frequency nor the type of birth defect was remarkable (Rosa, cited in Briggs 2005).

Concerns have been raised regarding the effect of methyldopa on brain development due to its effects on cerebral monoamine metabolism. Results of a 7.5-year follow-up study of children born to hypertensive women who had participated in a trial of methyldopa treatment during pregnancy produced inconclusive results (Ounsted 1980, Moar 1978, Redman 1976). The sons of mothers who had started treatment at 16–20 weeks' gestation were found to have smaller (about 1.3 cm) head circumferences than those born to untreated hypertensive mothers. This statistically significant difference was no longer seen at 6 and 12 months of age. There were no other differences, including in mean intelligence quotients, between the two groups at 4.5 and 7.5 years of age. A reduction in skull growth has not been confirmed by other workers, and no consistent adverse effect has been observed among children born to women treated with methyldopa late in pregnancy (Montan 1996, Pearson 1993, Fidler 1983). One recently published case report describes maternal hepatitis during pregnancy probably caused by methyldopa (Phadnis 2006). Another publication discusses the causal relationship between intrauterine long-term methyldopa exposure and neonatal suppurative parotitis (Todoroki 2006), which has been seen in adults previously.

Transient tremor, irritability, and mildly decreased systolic blood pressure (4–5 mmHg lower in the first 48 hours of life) have been reported in neonates whose mothers were treated with methyldopa either chronically or late in pregnancy (Sulyok 1991, Bodis 1982, Whitelaw 1981). No clinically significant long-term problems have been associated with these findings. In individual cases, hepatotoxic effects were observed following the use of methyldopa during pregnancy (Smith 1995).

> **Recommendation.** α-methyldopa is one of the preferred first-line drugs of choice for the treatment of hypertension in pregnancy.

2.8.3   β-adrenergic receptor blockers

Pharmacology

β-blockers (*acebutolol, alprenolol, atenolol, betaxolol, bisoprolol, celiprolol, carvedilol, esmolol, labetalol, metoprolol, nadolol, nebivolol, oxprenolol, pindolol, propranolol, sotalol,* and *timolol*) have a wide spectrum of activity, and are often used to treat hypertension. There are two types of β-receptors; β_1-receptors predominate in the heart, and β_2-receptors mediate relaxation (dilatation) of vascular and other smooth muscle (e.g. in the airways and blood vessels). Metoprolol is β_1-specific, whereas the classic β-blockers such as propranolol and oxprenolol have both β_1 and β_2 activity. Labetalol has both β- and α-receptor blocking activity, and has been successfully used in a number of pregnancies (Pickles 1992, Plouin 1990, 1987). All β-blockers cross the placenta.

Toxicology

To date, there is no clear evidence to indicate that β-blockers are teratogens (Magee 2000). There have been occasional reports of congenital anomalies following in utero exposure to β-blockers, but no causal relationship has been proven.

A report on 105 newborns exposed to atenolol in the first trimester described 12 infants with birth defects (Rosa, cited in Briggs 2005). However, there was no pattern of malformations, and the data have not been confirmed by other studies.

In the TIS in Berlin, we have analyzed more than 200 prospectively ascertained pregnancies which were exposed to metoprolol in the first trimester. Among 175 live births there were 7 with major malformations (4 percent): cleft palate ($n = 2$), atrial septal defect ($n = 2$), stenosis of pulmonary artery ($n = 1$), diaphragmatic hernia ($n = 1$), and polycystic kidney ($n = 1$).

Statistically significant growth restriction was described in a number of studies on atenolol (Tabacova 2003A, Easterling 1999A). Some of these investigations found a stronger effect of atenolol compared with acebutolol, pindolol, and labetalol. Growth restriction could not be confirmed when compared with a non-exposed control group (Lydakis 1999, Katz 1987), but there is a continuing debate whether other β-blockers might produce the same effects as atenolol (Magee 2003). It is difficult to determine whether atenolol itself or the underlying maternal disease has the potential to cause a reduction of placental perfusion. Intrauterine growth restriction may be attributed to reduced substrate availability due to the lowering of blood sugar as a result of β-receptor blockade. Postnatal growth in the first year of life and other developmental landmarks seem not to be adversely affected (Reynolds 1984).

Bayliss (2002) analyzed 491 pregnant hypertensive women, of whom 302 took at least one antihypertensive drug; the remaining 189 women, without medication, were the controls. Only those newborns who were exposed from conception or from the first trimester until birth ($n = 40$) had a significant lower birth weight.

Atenolol, only taken in the second trimester, did not produce such results. In any case, and independent of the mother's medication, pre-eclampsia led to growth restriction.

Some studies have compared i.v. labetalol for pre-eclampsia with nifedipine, and described a favorable outcome (Scardo 1999, Vermillion 1999). Meta-analysis revealed advantages of i.v. labetalol compared with dihydralazine or diazoxide in cases of severe late-onset hypertension in late pregnancy (Magee 2000).

There is insufficient experience of use in pregnancy of alprenolol, betaxolol, bopindolol, bupranolol, carazolol, carteolol, carvedilol, celiprolol, mepindolol, nadolol, nebivolol, penbutolol, talinolol, and tertatolol to determine their safety.

Although a significant teratogenic risk is not expected with β-blockers, there is a theoretical risk of neonatal β-receptor blockade – leading to neonatal bradycardia, hypotension, and hypoglycemia (Rubin 1983A, Dumez 1981). Respiratory distress and apnea have been reported following *in utero* exposure to propranolol until birth, but such adverse effects are rare (Turnstall 1969). There are conflicting opinions regarding the safety of stopping medication with β-blockers 24–48 hours before delivery. Neonatal symptoms of β-blockade are usually mild and improve within 48 hours of delivery with no long-term effects. Nevertheless, obstetricians, midwives, and pediatricians should be informed about maternal medication and made aware of the possibility of neonatal toxicity.

There is a theoretical risk of intensifying premature uterine contractions as a result of β-receptor blockers. However, no negative influence on inhibition of contractions was described as a result of giving β_1-receptor blockers during a tocolysis with β_2-sympathomimetics (Trolp 1980).

> **Recommendation.** β-receptor blockers such as labetalol, propranolol, and metoprolol, which have been in long-term use, are among the first-line drugs of choice for treating hypertension in pregnancy. Treatment with other β-blockers with less information on its safe use in pregnancy is not an indication for invasive diagnostic procedures or for termination of pregnancy. It is important to be aware of pharmacological effects such as decreased heart rate, hypoglycemia, and respiratory problems, particularly in premature neonates, when treatment with β-blockers continues until birth.

2.8.4   Hydralazine and dihydralazine

Pharmacology

Hydralazine and *dihydralazine* are structurally similar vasodilator drugs that have been used for the treatment of hypertension in pregnancy for over 40 years. Following oral administration, up to 80 percent absorption occurs, and approximately 66 percent of the drug is deactivated in the liver. The half-life is 2–8 hours. Hydralazine and dihydralazine cross the placenta well, and cord-blood drug concentrations may exceed those in the mother (Franke 1986). Although results from animal studies show an increase in uterine blood flow (Lipshitz 1987, Weiner 1986) after hydralazine administration, studies in hypertensive women indicate that changes in intervillous blood flow are, at best, variable or non-existent (Gudmundsson 1995, Grunewald 1993, Suionio 1986). In the past, hydralazine has been administered by intermittent intra-muscular injection or continuous intravenous infusion (Pritchard 1984, Sibai 1984, Garden 1982). Occasionally, continuous intra-venous infusion has resulted in a higher incidence of abnormal fetal heart rate tracings (Kirshon 1991, Spinnato 1986), which has led some clinicians to recommend that this route of administration be avoided (Kirshon 1991).

Toxicology

Parenteral hydralazine was the most widely used drug in the acute treatment of hypertensive emergencies during pregnancy in the past. A maternal symptom-complex including headache, flushing, palpitations, nausea, and vomiting may develop, mimicking imminent eclampsia. There is limited experience with prolonged use of hydralazine in pregnancy. Symptomatic neonatal thrombocytopenia, leukopenia, petechial bleeding, and hematomas have been reported after prenatal exposure (Widerlov 1980). Therefore, chronic use should be reserved for refractory patients.

There is little reported experience concerning first-trimester use of hydralazine in the human. The National Collaborative Perinatal Project identified eight infants exposed to hydralazine in the first trimester, none of whom had birth defects (Heinonen 1977). In another study of 40 pregnant women treated in the first trimester, there was only one infant with a birth defect (Rosa, cited in Briggs 2005). To date, there is no conclusive evidence of teratogenic effects in human pregnancy.

Most available information reports on the use of hydralazine in the third trimester to treat PIH. In some cases, liver toxicity was observed in pre-eclamptic patients (Hod 1986).

In patients with severe pre-eclampsia who are hypovolemic, the administration of hydralazine may induce a rapid fall of blood pressure and possibly worsen perinatal outcome if delivery occurs before 32 weeks' gestation. This is probably avoidable if the pre-existing hypovolemia is corrected prior to hydralazine administration (Derham 1990).

2

Pregnancy

2.8 Heart and circulatory system drugs and diuretics

Concerns have also been expressed that the administration of *dihydralazine* may decrease myocardial perfusion and increase the risk of maternal arrhythmias in eclampsia (Bhorat 1993). One case report described a temporal association between the maternal administration of hydralazine and fetal premature atrial contractions. The arrhythmia subsided spontaneously once hydralazine administration was discontinued (Lodeiro 1989).

There is also one case report of a woman treated with hydralazine for PIH in which the fetus died 36 hours after delivery from a pericardial effusion and cardiac tamponade (Yemini 1989). A postmortem examination suggested a lupus-like syndrome possibly due to maternal and fetal sensitivity to hydralazine.

Magee (2003) compared the maternal, fetal, and perinatal outcomes of pregnancies with severe hypertension, treated either by hydralazine or by other hypertensive drugs, mostly nifedipine or labetalol, in a meta-analysis. Therapy took place during the second and/or third trimesters. There are conflicting results, but it is clear that hydralazine is not the first-line drug of choice for severe hypertension in pregnancy.

Although there are numerous reports of successful intrapartum control of maternal blood pressure with hydralazine (Rosenfeld 1986, Spinnato 1986), there is a possibility that systemic vasodilatation may be accompanied by decreased placental perfusion resulting in fetal/neonatal bradycardia (Spinnato 1986). Theoretically, this complication is preventable by avoiding maternal hypotension.

> **Recommendation.** (Di)hydralazine may be used for the treatment of hypertension in pregnancy. In acute hypertensive crisis, it is used intravenously.

2.8.5   Nifedipine and other calcium antagonists

Pharmacology and toxicology

Nifedipine is a frequently prescribed calcium antagonist for the treatment of hypertension (Easterling 1999B, Levin 1994). A recent meta-analysis of trials involving 27 743 patients has shown that calcium antagonists are inferior to other types of antihypertensive drugs as first-line agents in reducing the major complications of hypertension, although they are equally effective in reducing blood pressure (Pahor 2000). Nifedipine and *verapamil* have been studied in the most detail. There is little experience with the use of *amlodipine,   diltiazem,   felodipine,   gallopamil,   isradipine, lercanidipine, nicardipine, nilvadipine, nimodipine, nisoldipine,* and *nitrendipine* in the first trimester of human pregnancies (Casele 1997).

Embryogenesis is a highly calcium-dependent process, and experimental findings indicate that early embryonic differentiation can be disturbed by this class of drugs. For example, digital defects (hypophalangism) have been observed in individual animal studies (Danielson 1989). In contrast to the results of animal experiments, there is no clear evidence that calcium antagonists cause a decrease in utero-placental perfusion in human pregnancy (Lindow 1988).

No treatment-related adverse effects on the infants of women treated with nifedipine in the second or third trimester of pregnancy have been reported in therapeutic trials and clinical series (Papatsonis 2001, Koks 1998, Brown 1997, Hill 1995, Kwawukume 1995, McCombs 1995, Ray 1995, Childress 1994, Levin 1994).

Nifedipine, like other calcium antagonists, is used as a tocolytic as well as in cases of coronary disease (Papatsonis 1997, Ray 1995, Childress 1994). Furthermore, nifedipine, often in combination with methyldopa, has been shown to be effective in the treatment of hypertension from different etiologies.

Although a distinctly higher rate of intrauterine growth restriction and cesarean births following nifedipine therapy has been described, no clear causal relationship has been established (Constantine 1987). It is difficult to distinguish the risk factors associated with either full-blown hypertension itself, or the potential adverse effects of the drug.

Combination therapy with magnesium can lead to a sharp drop in the mother's blood pressure with a disturbance of the utero-placental blood supply (Waismann 1988), which in individual cases may result in serious fetal hypoxia. There is also one case report of dramatic worsening of already impaired circulation with growth retardation in the fetus of a hypertensive woman who took 10 mg of nifedipine sublingually in the thirty-second week of pregnancy (Hata 1995).

Many studies have demonstrated the tocolytic effect of nifedipine. Prenatally exposed children who were followed to the ages of 5–12 months were reported to develop normally (Ray 1995). This was confirmed by another study that analyzed the long-term follow-up (until age of 9–12 years) of *in utero* nifedipine- or ritodrine-exposed children (Houtzager 2006). There is one case report of a myocardial infarction following the tocolytic use of nifedipine subsequent to the administration of ritodrine, but no clear causal relationship has been established (Oei 1999). Recently, the occurrence of acute pulmonary edema during *nicardipine* therapy for premature labor was reported in five complicated pregnancies: one triplet pregnancy associated with gestational diabetes, two twin pregnancies, one with insulin-dependent diabetes, and one with a history of mitral regurgitation. No fetal-related morbidity was seen (Vaast

2004). Pulmonary edema after tocolytic therapy has been reported so far only with the administration of β-adrenergic substances.

Apart from the treatment of maternal hypertension, verapamil has been used to treat fetal supraventricular tachycardia, but in some cases it has been associated with hyperprolactinemia and galactorrhea.

Overall, the range of well-documented reports involving calcium-antagonist treatment in the first trimester is limited in comparison to reports on its use later in pregnancy. No congenital anomalies were reported among about 25 infants whose mothers took vera-pamil during the first trimester of pregnancy in a study performed by a group of Teratogen Information Services (Magee 1996). In the Hungarian Case-Control Surveillance of Congenital Abnormalities, maternal verapamil use during pregnancy was no greater than expected among 20 830 children with various congenital anomalies (Czeizel 1997).

No adverse drug-related effects were observed among the infants of 137 hypertensive women treated with verapamil in late preg-nancy in two therapeutic trials (Marlettini 1990, Orlandi 1986). However, in one study a decrease in gestational age and average birth weight was reported in 296 infants whose mothers were treated with verapamil to inhibit premature labor (Czeizel 1998), but the premature labor itself may account for most of these findings.

There was no increased incidence of fetal/neonatal toxicity among 37 newborns exposed to nifedipine and 76 exposed to vera-pamil during the first trimester (Rosa, cited in Briggs 2005). In the same study, among 27 newborns whose mothers were treated with diltiazem, four (15 percent) had anomalies, two of which were car-diac anomalies. It is not clear whether this is a coincidental finding. Another two small prospective studies of calcium-channel blockers, mainly nifedipine and verapamil use in pregnancy, reported two birth defects of the extremities among some 100 infants (Sørensen 1998, Magee 1996). However, the authors did not exclude the pos-sibility that this could be due to the underlying maternal illness and other medication. The calcium-channel blockers taken by the affected mothers were diltiazem and nifedipine.

The largest controlled multicenter study to date with first-trimester exposure to calcium blockers analyzed 299 prospectively ascer-tained pregnancies and did not find an increased rate of all major malformations or of digital defects. Nifedipine ($n = 75$) and verapamil ($n = 61$) were taken most often, followed by diltiazem ($n = 39$) and amlodipin ($n = 38$). The premature birth rate was significantly higher in the exposed group. In some centers, a tendency to reduced birth weight was noted in newborns and prematures. This effect is probably due to placental perfusion problems caused by hyperten-sion, and not by the drugs themselves (Weber-Schöndorfer 2004).

There is a case report of a pregnant woman who was treated with verapamil for supra-ventricular tachycardia twice during the third trimester, and subsequently had an infant with severe congenital hypertrophic cardiomyopathy despite the fact that a fetal echocardiogram at 31 weeks' gestation was normal (Shen 1995). Although a causal relationship cannot be established on the basis of a single report, it is interesting that pregnant rats treated with twice the maximum human therapeutic dose of verapamil delivered offspring with myocardial hypertrophy (Pearce 1985) or other cardiovascular malformations, especially alterations of the aortic arch branching pattern (Scott 1997).

Recommendation. Nifedipine or verapamil, the best-studied calcium antagonists during pregnancy, are the preferred first-line drugs of choice in this group for the treatment of hypertension or cardiac arrhythmias in the second and third trimesters. In the first trimester, calcium antagonists are considered to be second-line therapy. If exposure with another calcium blocker has occurred during the first trimester, a detailed ultrasound diagnosis is advisable. Overall, exposure to a calcium antagonist during pregnancy is not an indication for either invasive diagnostic procedures or termination of pregnancy.

2.8.6   ACE inhibitors

Pharmacology and toxicology

Benazepril, captopril, cilazapril, enalapril, fosinopril, imidapril, lisinopril, moexipril, perindopril, quinapril, ramipril, spirapril, and *trandolapril* are angiotensin-converting enzyme inhibitors (ACE inhibitors) that inhibit the conversion of angiotensin I to angiotensin II. They are effective and generally well-tolerated, and in recent years there has been increasing use of these drugs. However, in general there is no clear advantage with respect to a lowering of mortality in comparison to the classic antihypertensives such as β-receptor blockers and thiazide diuretics.

There are conflicting results concerning teratogenicity. More than 600 evaluated pregnancies in case reports and case series indicate that exposure to ACE inhibitors in the first trimester do not appear to be associated with any increase in the incidence of malformations (Schaefer 2006, Burrows 1998, Gilstrap 1998, Barr 1997, de Moura 1995). Most of the data available refer to the use of captopril and enalapril.

Data from a prospective study indicate that there was no increase in any pattern of developmental anomalies in 86 newborns whose mothers had been treated with captopril in the first trimester. Similarly, in 4 of 40 children with a birth defect who had been exposed to enalapril, no specific pattern of malformations was observed (Rosa, cited by Briggs 2005). A recently published epidemiologic cohort study analyzed births and medical records and reported finding statistical indications of increased risk of cardiovascular and CNS malformations in infants whose mothers received a prescription for an ACE inhibitor during first trimester (209 mothers) (Cooper 2006). The cardiovascular defects consisted of 7 cases (atrial and/or septal defects and/or patent ductus arteriosus); the three cases classified as having CNS defects were spina bifida (1), microcephaly, undefined "eye anomaly" (1), and coloboma, which is not a true CNS defect. Adverse outcomes were found in a total of 18 infants. This study used prescription records as a surrogate for exposure, and did not exclude the possible confounding effects of diabetes mellitus. The results of this study provide a signal which has not been confirmed by other data. A large, prospective cohort study should be enrolled, to test especially whether there is an increased risk for heart or CNS malformations.

Lisinopril, a long-acting ACE inhibitor has been used to treat malignant hypertension in pregnancy (Tomlinson 2000). Tabacova (2003B) analyzed 110 pregnancies with abnormal outcome after exposure to enalapril, which have been reported to the FDA. Mainly when medication was taken beyond the first trimester, complications were noted as follows: oligohydramnios and resulting contractures, ossification defects, pulmonary hypoplasia, and renal insufficiency up to anuria.

The following reports of fetal and neonatal toxicity after exposure in the second half of pregnancy are typical: hypoxia, hypotension, renal tubular dysgenesis, oligohydramnios, and anuria requiring dialysis following the use of ACE inhibitors in late pregnancy (Murki 2005, Filler 2003, Gilstrap 1998, Lavoratti 1997). Hypoplasia of the skull bones (calvarial hypoplasia) has also been observed in six infants, which could be a consequence of limited perfusion and increased pressure on the skull caused by oligohydramnios (Barr 1994). If oligohydramnios is diagnosed in pregnancy while taking an ACE inhibitor, and medication is stopped, there is a chance that amniotic fluids will regenerate (Muller 2002).

The mechanism of toxicity is as follows. Fetal urine production and kidney function start at the end of the first trimester. Angiotensin-converting enzymes appear at about 26 weeks' gestation. ACE inhibitors reduce the tonus of kidney vessels, and as a consequence urine production is reduced, followed by an oligohydramnios, because beyond the sixteenth gestational week the fetal urine production is the main source for the amniotic fluid. Prasad (2003) describes a dysgenesia of renal tubules caused by hypoxia.

Similar developmental disturbances have also been observed in experimental animal studies with higher doses of ACE inhibitors.

Spontaneous abortions, intrauterine fetal deaths and premature births with hyaline membrane syndrome have also been reported following administration of ACE inhibitors, but it is not clear to what degree these adverse events can be attributed to the medication, or to the severe hypertension. This is also true in the case of persistent ductus arteriosus, which could theoretically be explained by drug-induced elevation of bradykinin.

No specific data were found on the use of benazepril, cilazapril, fosinopril, imidapril, perindopril, quinapril, ramipril, and trandolapril in pregnancy. Theoretically, these drugs have a similar potential for inducing adverse fetal and neonatal effects to other ACE inhibitors.

> **Recommendation.** ACE inhibitors are contraindicated throughout pregnancy, except in cases of severe illness that cannot be treated in any other way. Where clinically appropriate, medication should be changed to one of the antihypertensive drugs of choice. If exposure has occurred in the first trimester, a detailed ultrasound diagnosis is advisable. Whether fetal echocardiography should be recommended in any case of first-trimester exposure is a question of debate. Overall, exposure to an ACE inhibitor during pregnancy is not an indication for either invasive diagnostic procedures or termination of pregnancy. However, in cases involving long-term prenatal therapy in the second and/or third trimesters, the fetus should be monitored for the potential development of oligohydramnios, and fetal growth should be assessed with detailed ultrasound scans.

2.8.7   Angiotensin-II receptor antagonists

Pharmacology and toxicology

Candesartan, eprosartan, irbesartan, losartan, telmisartan, valsartan, olmesartan, and *tasosartan* competitively and selectively block the AT1 receptor, and therefore angiotensin II is inhibited.

The sartans are used as antihypertensives and in the case of cardiomyopathy. In the case of diabetes mellitus with renal complications, they decrease proteinuria and increase the glomerular filtration rate.

Only limited experience concerning first-trimester exposure exists: In the database of the Berlin TIS, we prospectively ascertained 65 pregnancies. Almost all of the 46 live births were healthy.

There were two heterogenous major malformations: one term growth-restricted newborn had a cleft palate, a persistant ductus arteriosus, a ventricular septal defect, and an aortic isthmus stenosis; another pregnancy was terminated because of exencephaly. A third pregnancy resulted in a stillbirth with no visible malformations (Schaefer 2003). Serreau (2005) reported on 10 cases with first-trimester exposure, three of which were exposed for a longer period:

- Four neonates were full terms and healthy.
- In a twin pregnancy, one twin died at 10 weeks' gestation, the other at 30 weeks'.
- Three pregnancies were terminated: the first an apparently healthy fetus in week 13, and the second in week 17 because of craniofacial dysmorphia, clinodactylia, and tubular dysplasia with microcysts. The third fetus was exposed until week 28, when a prenatal ultrasonography diagnosed oligohydramnios, macrocephaly, renal hyperechogenicity, and ventriculomegaly. The pregnancy was terminated 4 weeks later, and autopsy showed macrognathia, craniofacial dysmorphia, and cortical dysplasia with microcysts.
- In one pregnancy with losartan exposure until week 8, oligohydramnios and intrauterine growth restriction were diagnosed, but postnatal development was normal.
- A candesartan-exposed pregnancy until week 31 was complicated by oligohydramnios, hypocalvaria, and increased size of one kidney. A girl was born at 35 weeks' gestation with hypocalvaria and major renal tubular dysfunction. At four months, the child had a large fontanelle but normal growth and psychomotor development. Renal function was normal, although renal prognosis remains questionable.
- An oligohydramnios was diagnosed in a twin pregnancy (diamniotic, dichorionic) exposed to losartan until at least week 32. After spontaneous delivery in week 35 the infants presented severe hypotension and anuria, and died of respiratory failure shortly afterwards. Furthermore, growth retardation, hypoplastic skull bones, narrowed chest, and an enlarged colon was noted in one twin when an autopsy took place. The histological examination of the kidneys revealed severe lesions, including tubular dysgenesis associated with poorly developed vasa recta (Daika-Dahmane 2006).

The fetal complications, some of them are already described above, are strikingly similar to those previously seen in ACE inhibitors – namely, oligohydramnios, fetal renal failure, decreased calcification of the skull, lung hypoplasia, contractures of limbs, and stillbirths or dead as newborn. At least 19 case reports of these fetal effects have been published (Alwan 2005, Schaefer 2003, Briggs 2001,

Chung 2001, Martinovic 2001, Saji 2001). Exposure during the second and third trimesters produces the problem. There are two case reports, which indicate that after stopping medication the symptoms can be at least partially reversible (Bos-Thompson 2005, Berkane 2004).

> **Recommendation.** Angiotensin-II receptor antagonists are contraindicated throughout pregnancy, and are only acceptable when all other treatment regiments have been ineffective. If exposure has occurred in the first trimester, a detailed ultrasound diagnosis is advisable. Overall, exposure to an angiotensin-II receptor antagonist during pregnancy is not an indication for either invasive diagnostic procedures or termination of pregnancy. However, in cases involving long-term prenatal therapy in the second and/or third trimesters, the fetus should be monitored for the potential development of oligohydramnios, and fetal growth should be assessed with detailed ultrasound scans.

2.8.8   Clonidine

Pharmacology and toxicology

Clonidine is an antihypertensive that acts primarily as a central α-receptor antagonist. The drug is well-absorbed; the bioavailability is approximately 75 percent, and the half-life is 8.5 hours.

Clonidine does not appear to have teratogenic potential, based on the limited data available. No increase in the incidence of birth defects was reported in a group of 59 pregnant women treated in the first trimester (Rosa, cited in Briggs 2005). There are a few individual case reports of fetal and neonatal toxicity following clonidine exposure. Sudden fetal death has been observed (Heilmann 1970), and there is a report of one newborn infant with transient hypertension which was interpreted as a withdrawal symptom (Boutroy 1988). However, there are reports of over 200 pregnancies in which clonidine was well-tolerated and clinically effective (Horvarth 1985). In one study of children at 6 years of age, whose mothers had received clonidine monotherapy during pregnancy, hyperactive behavior and sleep disturbances were seen more often in the drug-exposed group than in the control group (Huisjes 1986). Although the results of this study are similar to those from experimental animal studies, they have not as yet been confirmed by other clinical studies.

> **Recommendation.** Clonidine should be considered as a second-line choice for the treatment of hypertension in pregnancy. Its use is not an indication for termination of the pregnancy or for invasive diagnostic procedures.

2.8 Heart and circulatory system drugs and diuretics

2.8.9   Diazoxide

Pharmacology and toxicology

Diazoxide is fully absorbed when given orally, and has a half-life of between 20 and 40 hours. It readily crosses the placenta, and fetal plasma concentrations are similar to those in the mother. After bolus injection, observable hypotensive states can be prevented with continual infusion, or repeated small doses (Duley 1995). Its use should be reserved for the treatment of hypertensive crises.

Diazoxide has a diabetogenic effect on the metabolism (Sweetman 2002). Case reports showed hyperglycemia not only in pregnant women, but also in their newborns (Milsap 1980, Neuman 1979). Therefore, the thiazide derivate, diazoxide, is also used as an oral antihypoglycemic.

Hyperuricemia, water retention, and inhibition of contractions have been observed in treated mothers. In newborns, alopecia, an increase in lanugo hair, and retarded bone development have been observed (Milner 1972).

> **Recommendation.** Diazoxide should only be used in exceptional circumstances to treat hypertensive crises in pregnant women. Great care should be exercised with bolus administration. Treatment with diazoxide is not an indication for invasive diagnostic procedures, or for termination of pregnancy.

2.8.10   Magnesium sulfate

Pharmacology and toxicology

Magnesium sulfate, although not actually an antihypertensive, has proven valuable in the treatment of pre-eclampsia. Magnesium sulfate is the drug of choice for treatment of seizures in eclampsia (Oettinger 1993). In a group of 31 fetuses where the mothers were administered the drug i.v. as an initial loading dose of 4–6 g, followed by an infusion of 2–3.5 g/h, magnesium sulfate was found not to be harmful (Gray 1994). A significantly lower risk of repeated convulsions in eclampsia was seen in a study of 1700 women given parenteral magnesium sulfate compared with those given phenytoin or diazepam (Duley 1995).

Magnesium sulfate also promotes improved uterine circulation and acts to inhibit contractions. In addition, cerebral paresis is reported to develop less often in extremely low birth weight newborns when magnesium is used prenatally to treat tocolysis or eclampsia (Nelson 1995).

In a comparative study of 400 pregnancies, neither magnesium sulfate nor phenytoin treatment for hypertension or prevention of eclampsia adversely affected the course of labor (Leveno 1998).

The effectiveness of parenteral magnesium in the treatment of premature labor has not yet been proven.

Magnesium, when used in higher doses, or when kidney function is limited, can cause marked muscle hypotonia in both mother and newborn. In extreme cases, especially when its effect is enhanced by a calcium antagonist such as nifedipine, a dangerous drop in maternal blood pressure can occur which may result in fetal hypoxia.

See also Chapter 2.14.

> **Recommendation.** Magnesium sulfate can be used for appropriate indications such as pre-eclampsia and eclampsia. It is the drug of choice for treatment of seizures in eclampsia.

2.8.11   Nitroprusside

Pharmacology and toxicology

Sodium nitroprusside is a fast-acting vasodilator that acts directly on arterial and venous smooth muscle. It crosses the placenta and reaches similar concentrations in the fetus to those in the mother. It is rapidly metabolized to potentially toxic substances such as cyanide and thiocyanate. However, the usual recommended therapeutic doses do not appear to cause excessive accumulation of cyanide in the fetal liver. Overall, there are insufficient data to determine whether or not sodium nitroprusside is fetotoxic or teratogenic in human pregnancy (Shoemaker 1984).

> **Recommendation.** Sodium nitroprusside is not recommended as a drug of choice in pregnancy. However, intravenous infusion can be effective in a hypertensive crisis. Inadvertent exposure, or use in specific clinical conditions, is no reason for additional diagnostic tests or for termination of pregnancy.

2.8.12   Reserpine

Pharmacology and toxicology

Reserpine, a sympatholytic that causes the depletion of catecholamines and serotonin in tissues throughout the body, is well-absorbed orally. In the past, reserpine was used frequently for long-term therapy in cases of hypertensive pregnancy complications (Towell 1966).

A number of case reports of fetal and neonatal toxicity have been reported following exposure in pregnancy, but no pattern of defects was observed and no causal relationship has been established. In contrast, there have been several reports of normal outcomes in pregnancies involving exposure to reserpine (Czeizel 1988, Heinonen 1977). Occasional breathing and sucking disturbances have been observed in newborns following exposure to reserpine in the third trimester of pregnancy.

Reserpine has been largely displaced by the newer classes of antihypertensives because of its numerous side effects, including postural hypotension, cardiac arrhythmias, gastric ulceration, and diarrhea. Depletion of brain amines and serotonin can also cause depression and behavioral changes, and chronic use may induce extrapyramidal effects.

> **Recommendation.** Reserpine is no longer considered to be a drug of choice for the majority of pregnant hypertensive women because of the numerous associated side effects and the possibility of alterations in fetal brain development; β-blockers such as metoprolol, α-methyldopa, (di)hydralazine, and nifidipine are less toxic to the mother and fetus and are the preferred drugs of choice. However, the inadvertent use of reserpine, or its use in specific clinical conditions, is no reason for termination of pregnancy or for additional diagnostic procedures in the absence of severe maternal toxicity.

2.8.13   Other antihypertensives

Pharmacology and toxicology

Prazosin, a peripheral α-receptor blocker with vasodilator properties, often used in combination with β-blockers, has been used successfully in individual cases of essential hypertension in late pregnancy without any apparent fetotoxic effects. No adverse effects attributable to prazosin were observed among 8 infants in one series, or 10 infants in another, whose mothers had been treated with this medication during the third trimester of pregnancy for hypertension (Bourget 1995, Rubin 1983B). Nevertheless, there are insufficient data on its potential reproductive toxicity to recommend its use during pregnancy under normal conditions. There is insufficient experience for use in pregnancy to assess the embryotoxic potential of other peripheral α-receptor blockers such as *bunazosin, doxazosin, indoramin, terazosin,* and *urapidil.*

However, i.v. urapidil has been recommended as an alternative to (di)hydralazine for the treatment of eclampsia by the International

Society for the Study of Hypertension in Pregnancy. Its advantage over dihydralazine appears to be that there is no increase in intra-cerebral pressure.

There is a lack of published data on the use of the centrally acting α-receptor blockers *moxonidine, guanfacine*, and *guanabenz* in human pregnancy. Therefore, no clear risk assessment can be made.

Minoxidil is a vasodilator that is used in cases of severe hypertension, usually in conjunction with a diuretic and a β-blocker. It can also be applied topically to promote hair growth in adults, and can cause fetal hypertrichosis (Kaler 1987). The excessive neonatal hair growth usually disappears gradually over the first 3 months of life. Individual case reports on newborns with different birth defects do not permit a differential assessment of teratogenic risk.

Similarly, there are insufficient data available on vasodilators such as *diisopropylamine* and *cicletanine*.

Phenoxybenzamine is an α-blocker which is used in the treatment of pheochromocytoma and of neurogenic disturbance of micturition. There are no publications on first-trimester exposure; in later pregnancy no fetal adverse effects have been described.

The serotonin antagonist *ketanserin* also acts as an antihypertensive drug. In the treatment of pre-eclampsia, no specific fetotoxic effects have been described so far.

Nesiritide is a new drug for heart failure, with no experience in pregnancy.

> **Recommendation.** Urapidil may be used in late pregnancy to treat pre-eclampsia, as a possible alternative to dihydralazine. Prazosin should only be discussed for second- or third-trimester use, if antihypertensive drugs of choice have failed. Phenoxybenzamine may be used in the treatment of pheochromocytoma. The other abovementioned antihypertensives are contraindicated in human pregnancy because of a lack of safety data. Better-studied drugs discussed in earlier sections are the drugs of choice. However, inadvertent use of this miscellaneous group of antihypertensive drugs, or their use in specific clinical conditions, is no reason for a termination of pregnancy or for invasive diagnostic procedures.

2.8.14   Pulmonary hypertension and its medication

Chronic pulmonary hypertensive diseases are characterized by permanently elevated pulmonary artery resistance (mean pulmonary arterial pressure above 25 mmHg at rest and above 30 mmHg during exercise). They have recently been reclassified at the World Health Organization Meetings, depending on the underlying disease and the location of the vascular lesion, into five different subgroups (subgroup 1: pulmonary artery hypertension).

The therapy consists of symptomatic measures like oxygen supply, diuretics (see sections 2.8.22–27), perhaps digitalis (see section 2.8.18), and specific steps. The target of therapy is the treatment of underlying disease, if possible, with the avoidance of local thrombosis by anticoagulation (for coumarins, see Chapter 2.7), treatment of vasoconstriction (for nifedipin/amlodipine/diltiazem see section 2.8.5), and the prevention of vascular remodeling. The physiological changes during pregnancy aggravate the disease, with the consequence of a high maternal mortality rate. Without specific treatment, this ranges between 30 and 50 percent. Therefore, such patients are counseled to avoid pregnancy or to interrupt pregnancy if it occurs. Nevertheless, there are women who decide to continue their pregnancy. Others discover pulmonary hypertensive disease for the first time during pregnancy. Pregnant patients with pulmonary hypertension should be managed in specialized centers. As well as late pregnancy, the period after delivery carries a high risk of maternal death (Weiss, 2000).

Pulmonary artery hypertension (PAH) (with the idiopathic, the familiar form, and others associated with, for example, autoimmune diseases as sclerodermia) is a rare, progressive condition.

In this section we introduce relatively new substances for the treatment of PAH; these have in common the fact that there is limited or no experience with treatment during pregnancy. Substances may be approved for different indications in different countries, and some are not licensed in all countries.

▶ Prostacyclin analog

Prostacyclin analogs currently used for the treatment of arterial pulmonary hypertension are *epoprostenol, treprostinil, beraprost*, and *iloprost*. They not only have vasodilatatory and antiplatelet properties, but also an anti-remodeling effect.

Epoprostenol is an instabile synthetic prostacyclin analog which has to be given continuously intravenously and has an extreme short half-life of 3 minutes. The disadvantages are severe adverse effects such as septic complications. Interruption of i.v. therapy can be life-threatening.

In experimental studies, there has been no evidence of teratogenicity. Placental transfer is unknown. Moodley (1992) described almost 50 cases of the use of epoprostenol during late pregnancy for the treatment of severe eclampsia. No specific fetal harm was reported; the reported complications were mainly due to prematurity or to severity of maternal disease. The use of epoprostenol for pulmonary hypertension in 10 pregnant women has been described (Avdalovic 2004, Bildirici 2004, Geohas 2003, Stewart 2001, Easterling 1999A), but only 3 of the women were exposed during the first trimester or for a longer period (Bendayan 2005, Badalian 2000). In one case report, epoprostenol was injected and/or inhaled. Overall there was a good success rate in treating pulmonary hypertension, and no hints of adverse fetal or embryonic effects. Although first-trimester experience is very limited, the maternal benefit in pulmonary hypertension outweighs any potential risk to the embryo/fetus.

Treprostinil has to be administered by continuous subcutaneous infusion. Local pain at the infusion site is a significant side effect in approximately 85 percent of subjects. There is no experience in human pregnancy.

Beraprost and *iloprost* are stable synthetic analogs of epoprostenol with similar activity. Beraprost can be given orally, but there are no data concerning use during pregnancy. Its elimination half-life is 35–40 minutes. Iloprost can be inhaled or administered intravenously. Its plasma half-life is 20–30 minutes. A publication describes its use in three pregnancies (Elliot 2005). The first woman started therapy at 8 weeks' gestation. In the beginning she inhaled iloprost, but as deterioration occurred, she was converted to iloprost i.v. She delivered a male premature infant without congenital anomalies at 26 weeks' gestation (650 g, Apgar scores of 8 at 1 min and 9 at 5 min). The second woman started iloprost treatment at 19 weeks' gestation and delivered a healthy male infant at 36 weeks. The third woman started nebulized iloprost at 17 weeks' gestation and delivered a healthy girl at 35 weeks' gestation.

Endothelin-receptor (ET) antagonists

Bosentan is highly (98 percent) bound to plasma albumin, and has an elimination half-life of about 5 hours. It is a neurohormone that binds specifically to endothelin receptors A and B, and acts as vasodilator.

It has been found to be teratogenic in rats at doses equal to or greater than twice the maximum recommended human dose, and showed carcinogenicity (product information, preclinical safety data). In the USA it is a restricted drug with substantial criteria for use, so that patients do not become pregnant: pregnancy must be excluded prior to therapy, reliable contraceptive methods are necessary, and monthly pregnancy tests are required. There is almost no experience concerning the use of bosentan during human pregnancy.

Inadvertent exposure to bosentan and sildenafil until gestational week 30, in a complicated pregnancy, has been reported. The growth-retarded female newborn had no malformations, initially developed normally, but then died of an RS virus infection when 6 months old (Molelekwa 2005). Elliot (2005) describes bosentan exposure in one case until at least 6 weeks of pregnancy; therapy was then changed immediately and the woman delivered a premature but healthy son.

Sitaxsentan and *ambrisentan*, as selective ET A blockers, are currently being investigated for efficacy in PAH.

▶ **Phosphodiesterase (PDE5) inhibitors**

Sildenafil is a selective phosphodiesterase type-5 inhibitor. Phosphodiesterase inhibition has been demonstrated to treat PAH by reducing cyclic guanosine monophosphate (cGMP) breakdown, making pulmonary vascular smooth muscle more sensitive to endogenous and administered nitric oxid, and thus has an acute pulmonary vasodilator effect. It was tested in an experimental study on human placentas where 27 normal placentas were compared with 12 from pregnancies with intrauterine growth retardation. The placental perfusion was only improved by sildenafil in those placentas from pregnancies with growth retardation (Wareing 2005). (Notice also the abovementioned case report regarding sildenafil and bosentan exposure.) Another publication reports on a 22-year-old nullipara who had an atrioventricular defect which was surgically closed because of Eisenmenger syndrome. Shortly afterwards she reported being 7 weeks' pregnant, and therapy with diltiazem and sildenafil was initiated. At 9 weeks' gestation, therapy with sildenafil was stopped because of the high cost. At 31 weeks' gestation, the patient deteriorated; sildenafil and *l-arginine* were initiated and diltiazem treatment was stopped. Finally, at 36 weeks' gestation, a male infant of 2290 g was delivered, having Apgar scores of 9 at 1 and 5 minutes (Lacassie 2004).

> **Recommendation.** Pulmonary hypertension is a life-threatening disease in pregnancy, and therefore interdisciplinary management in specialized centers is mandatory. The best medical regime for the mother's benefit should be chosen. Most experience in the specific treatment of chronic pulmonary hypertension during pregnancy exists with epoprostenol. Bosentan should be avoided in pregnancy, unless the severity of PAH overweighs the potential risk.

2.8.15   Hypotension and antihypotensives

Hypotension (low blood pressure) may occur in some healthy people with a normal heart and blood vessels. Symptoms usually occur only when the blood pressure is so low that blood flow to the brain is reduced, causing dizziness and fainting. The most common type of hypotension is postural hypotension, where symptoms occur after abruptly standing or sitting. Postural hypotension is sometimes an adverse effect of drug treatment (antidepressants), or may be due to illness (diabetes mellitus), or to nerve damage that disrupts the reflexes controlling blood pressure. In the majority of cases, treatment of hypotension depends on the underlying cause.

In the 1980s, particular attention was paid to the consequences of chronic hypotension in pregnancy. An increased rate of prematurity of up to 17 percent was attributed to untreated hypotension (Goeschen 1984), and treatment during pregnancy was advocated. *Dihydroergotamine* was considered to be more effective than the adrenergic substances, and use of this drug in hypotensive pregnant women has been reported in the German literature (Goeschen 1984). However, its use in pregnancy is controversial because of its potential oxytocic effects and adverse pregnancy outcomes associated with vascular injury (Raymond 1995).

2.8.16   Dihydroergotamine

Pharmacology and toxicology

Dihydroergotamine (DHE) is a semi-synthetic derivative of the ergot alkaloid ergotamine that is contraindicated in pregnancy. Hydrogenated DHE does not cross biomembranes easily, and is only absorbed to a limited extent after oral administration, with peak effectiveness reached within 2 hours. DHE is degraded by the liver, and the metabolites are excreted through the bile.

Embryotoxic effects and stimulation of uterine contractions are not likely to occur after oral therapeutic doses. However, the risk cannot be eliminated in the case of an overdose or after intravenous administration. There was a reduction in fetal weight among the offspring of pregnant guinea pigs treated chronically with dihydroergotamine in doses less than those used in humans. The clinical significance of this is unknown. An evaluation of data of the Swedish birth registry among 52 pregnant women who took dihydroergotamine in first trimester did not show major malformations (Källén 2001).

Premature labor has been reported after administration of DHE in late pregnancy (Lippert 1984). Therefore, most authorities consider DHE to be either contraindicated in pregnancy, or only to be used for specific indications in individual patients in whom other treatments have failed (see also Chapter 2.1).

2 Pregnancy

2.8 Heart and circulatory system drugs and diuretics

> **Recommendation.** Occasional oral use in low doses for migraine or vascular headaches seems not to have marked teratogenic effects, but idiosyncratic reactions may occur resulting in fetal damage. Dihydroergotamine may be used where severe hypotension has been resistant to other treatment regimens. It is contraindicated near term.

2.8.17   Adrenergic substances

Pharmacology and toxicology

The adrenergic substances *epinephrine* (*adrenaline*) and norepinephrine (*noradrenaline*) are vasoconstrictor drugs that may be used in acute hypotension. *Amezinium, etilefrine, gepefrin, midodrine, norfenefrine,* and *pholedrine* are also used as antihypotonics.

Vasoconstrictor sympathomimetics raise blood pressure transiently by acting at α-adrenergic receptors to constrict peripheral vessels. The danger of using vasoconstrictors is that they raise blood pressure at the expense of the perfusion of other vital organs, such as the kidney. In animal studies, adrenergic substances caused a reduction of uterine blood supply (Hohmann 1992).

Animals treated with high doses of amezinium by gavage during organogenesis showed no evidence of teratogenicity at the highest doses, despite the presence of severe maternal and fetal toxicity (Satoh 1988A, 1988B). Postnatal studies in rats revealed no adverse effects.

There are limited conflicting data concerning the frequency of congenital anomalies reported in the children of women treated with adrenaline during pregnancy (Czeizel 1998, Heinonen 1977). No reports were found of teratogenic effects within the therapeutic dose range in human pregnancy.

> **Recommendation.** When significant symptoms compel drug treatment of hypotension in pregnancy, adrenergic substances may be prescribed. Combination preparations should not be used because of the possibility of drug interaction.

2.8.18   Cardiac glycosides

Pharmacology and toxicology

Digoxin, a metabolic product of digitoxin, is the most widely used form of the digitalis cardiac glycosides. It is used in the treatment of atrial fibrillation and in some cases of heart failure.

Digitoxin is 90–100 percent absorbed in the gastrointestinal tract, and is excreted via the liver. It has a half-life of, on average, 7 days. Digoxin is widely distributed and extensively bound in varying degrees to tissues throughout the body, which results in an apparent high volume of distribution. It is excreted primarily through the kidneys, and has a half-life of about 40 hours.

Absorption from the gastrointestinal tract is about 80 percent for *methyldigoxin* and *acetyldigoxin*. Methyldigoxin is demethylated in the liver, whereas acetyldigoxin is deacetylated in the intestinal mucosa.

All digitalis glycosides cross the placenta, resulting in significant fetal levels (Gilstrap 1998). Cord levels are about 50–80 percent of maternal levels (Chan 1978). However, the myocardial sensitivity in the fetus appears to be less than it is in adults (Saarikoski 1978). There are, as yet, no known toxic effects on the fetus from digitalis glycosides. In some instances it has been used to treat fetal tachycardias (Hallak 1991, Rotmensch 1987).

> **Recommendation.** Digitalis glycosides can be used during pregnancy. There have been no reports linking digitalis glycosides with congenital malformations. They are indicated for some kinds of maternal and fetal tachycardia, and for some instances of chronic cardiac failure.

2.8.19   Antiarrhythmic therapy of the pregnant woman and of the fetus

The two different situations, therapy of the pregnant woman and of the fetus, should be distinguished. If the pregnant woman needs an antiarrhythmic therapy, a drug is recommended which passes via the placenta in low amounts. On the other hand, if the fetus is the patient, sufficient placental transfer is desirable in order to treat the fetus via the mother. Supraventricular extrasystoles and premature ventricular beats are not harmful, and neither the mother nor the fetus needs medical treatment.

Antiarrhythmic therapy of the pregnant woman

New onset of tachycardia in otherwise healthy women is seldom seen in pregnancy. If supraventricular tachycardia, atrial flutter, atrial fibrillation or ventricular tachycardia has led to an unstable hemodynamical situation, *electrocardioversion* is recommended as in ventricular flutter or fibrillation. This treatment does not affect the

2 Pregnancy

2.8 Heart and circulatory system drugs and diuretics

fetus, because the electrical threshold of fetal heart is high and the fetus is located outside of the stress field power flow. In the case of a stable hemodynamical situation, a drug-monitored cardioversion should be tried. Another indication for an antiarrhythmic therapy in pregnant women is to prevent a relapse. Bombelli (2003) reported on three cases of successful radiofrequency catheter ablation in drug-refractory maternal supraventricular tachycardia in late pregnancy. Nevertheless, the risk of X-ray exposure time should be taken into account. If treatment of bradycardia is necessary, a pregnant woman should also be fitted with a *pacemaker*.

▶ Antiarrhythmic therapy of the fetus

In a small percentage of all pregnancies (0.4–0.6 percent), fetal tachycardia, mainly supraventricular, can be found. Fetal tachycardia is defined as more than 180 beats per minute, and mostly occurs in late pregnancy. A majority of affected fetuses do not have a visible heart malformation. If symptoms are persistent, cardiac failure or cardiomyopathy with pleural or pericardial effusion and/or ascites can result and edema. Fetal hydrops is defined as fluid retention in two or more compartments, and can precede intrauterine death. The drug of first choice is digitalis, but in case of hydrops, fetal serum concentration of digitalis might not reach therapeutic levels. This could be the reason why, in cases of fetal hydrops caused by tachycardia, digitalis therapy is often not successful (Oudijk 2002). The drugs of second choice, in combination with or without digitalis, are sotalol and/or flecainide (Doherty 2003, Oudijk 2002). It takes at least 72 hours, sometimes up to 14 days, before flecainide can succeed in converting the rhythm to sinus rhythm (Krapp 2002). Athanssiadis (2004) advocates that verapamil is the drug of second choice, whereas others think that it is contraindicated (Oudijk 2002). Another possibility is to inject adenosine directly into the umbilical vein. If cardioversion has succeeded, hydrops fetalis can regress slowly (d'Souza 2002), which can take from 8 days (Porat 2003) to 4–6 weeks. There is a case report of a fetus treated via the mother with flecainide, where the fetal heart rate decreased without converting to sinus rhythm. Nevertheless, hydrops regressed (Krapp 2002). If there is no success prematurely, labor might be induced in order to try electrocardioversion of the newborn. In general, a healthy pregnant woman seldom suffers from adverse effects of the antiarrhythmic therapy of the fetus. Bradycardia as fetal side effect can occur, which is more likely after injection of adenosine into the umbilical vein than after other treatment. All antiarrhythmics can produce arrhythmias, at worst ventricular fibrillation of the fetus, which can lead to intrauterine death.

A fetal bradycardia can be at first compensated by an increase in cardiac output. However, a fetal heart rate below 55 bpm is insufficient, and heart failure with the consequence of fetal hydrops can result (Eronen 2001). The underlying fetal congenital atrioventricular block may have been caused by a congenital heart defect, or by placental passage of maternal autoantibodies (Maeno 2005). In the latter case, halogenated steroids can be tried unless heart block is not complete. Sometimes, sympathomimetics have been given. Induction of labor can be discussed to implant a pacemaker postnatally.

Pharmacology and toxicology

Antiarrhythmics are divided into different classes (IA, IB, IC, II, III and IV) which are used for the different forms of arrhythmias.

- Class IA – quinidine, ajmaline, detajmium, disopyramide, procainamide, and prajmalium
- Class IB – lidocaine (lignocaine), aprindine, mexiletine, phenytoin, and tocainide
- Class IC – flecainide, propafenone, encainide, and lorcainide
- Class II – includes β-receptor blockers
- Class III – amiodarone and the β-blocker sotalol; also bretylium, ibutilide, almokalant, and dofetilide
- Class IV – the calcium blockers verapamil, gallopamil, and diltiazem.

Adenosine does not belong to any of the classical categories.

Class IA

Quinidine is almost completely absorbed when given orally, and reaches its maximum serum concentration within 1–4 hours. About 20 percent is excreted by the kidneys and 80 percent via the liver. As a vagal antagonist, it can increase the heart rate slightly despite its depressive effect on the pacemaker cells. Quinidine is one of the oldest antiarrhythmics, and is apparently without any noteworthy teratogenic potential. It passes the placenta and reaches similar concentrations in the fetus as in the mother. Successful treatment of mother and of the fetus has been described.

Disopyramide is also thought to have a contraction-promoting effect (Tadmor 1990). There have been no published case reports of malformations after exposure to disopyramide or *procainamide*. Both cross the placenta. Procainamide has been used for cardioversion in cases of fetal supraventricular tachycardia. There is insufficient experience in pregnancy with prenatal tolerance for *ajmaline*, *detajmium*, and *prajmalium*.

Class IB

Lidocaine (*lignocaine*) has been used widely as an anesthetic drug during pregnancy (see Chapter 2.16). Since only about 30 percent is utilized after oral administration, due to metabolism in the liver, parenteral administration is necessary in cases of arrhythmia. There was one published case report describing successful therapy with lidocaine in a fetus with QT-prolongation in the ECG (Cuneo 2003), which suffered from ventricular tachycardia and incomplete atrioventricular heart block. There is no recognizable teratogenic effect in human pregnancies. Lidocaine crosses placenta in considerable amounts, and can lead to a depressed newborn if the serum concentration is high. A study from France reported about 50 pregnancies where lidocaine was injected into the umbilical vein in order to induce fetocide of malformed fetuses during gestational weeks 20–36. First sufentanil (5 μg) was injected, followed by 7–30 ml lidocaine (1%), which led to cardial asystolia (Senat 2003). *Phenytoin* is a teratogenic anticonvulsant drug (see Chapter 2.10). *Mexiletine* crosses the placenta. There have been a few case reports that have not revealed a teratogenic risk. There is insufficient experience regarding prenatal tolerance for aprindine and tocainide.

Class IC

Many case reports document the efficacy of *flecainide* in treating fetal arrhythmias (Krapp 2002). In particular with fetuses that already suffer from hydrops, flecainide is superior to digitalis. In order to minimize fetal adverse effects, close monitoring of the mother's serum concentration is recommended (Rasheed 2003). In one case report, hyperbilirubinemia of a newborn has been described as an adverse effect of flecainide therapy during pregnancy (Athanassiadis 2004). In contrast to animal data, there is, as yet, no recognizable teratogenic or fetotoxic effect in human pregnancy, but experience of first-trimester exposure is rare. With *propafenone*, there have not as yet been any indications of teratogenic potential from the 30 cases collected by the manufacturer.

Class II

For β-receptor blockers, see section 2.8.3.

Class III

Amiodarone has a long elimination half-life of 14–58 days. If fetal exposure is to be avoided, medication should have been stopped several months before conception. Amiodarone can cause fetal bradycardia and – because of its high iodine content (39 percent) – congenital hypothyroidism (Lomenick 2004, Grosso 1998). In order to treat fetal hypothyreoidism, injection of thyroxine into the amniotic fluid might be an option, as described in some case reports. Among 27 children who were treated by amiodarone *in utero* (Pradhan 2006), 5 had hypothyroidism after delivery. A sixth baby with ongoing therapy developed hypothyroidism postnatally at the age of 3 months (Strasburger 2004). Bartelena (2001) analyzed 64 cases that had already been published; there was a maternal indication for antiarrhythmic therapy in 56 cases. A dozen children were diagnosed having transient hypothyroidism; two of them also had congenital goiter. Some of the hypothyroid and even some of the euthyroid children showed discrete neuropsychological anomalies. Therefore, a direct neurotoxic effect of amiodarone is suggested. Occasionally a QT-prolongation in the ECG of newborns was noted. Other children had intrauterine growth restriction, although several causes could account for this: exposure to amiodarone or to the co-medication, mostly β-receptor blockers, or the underlying disease of the mother. To date, most of the exposed children have been healthy – even those who initially suffered from hypothyroidism developed normally (Magee 1999). Experience of first-trimester exposure is limited to approximately 20 pregnancies (Magee 1995), of which 2 resulted in children with congenital anomalies (Ovadia 1994); this might be coincidental.

Sotalol crosses the placenta in considerable amounts; therefore, this is a potent drug for treating fetal arrhythmias. In a case series of 18 fetuses with tachycardia, an accumulation of the drug was found in the amniotic fluid but not in the fetuses themselves. Conversion to sinus rhythm succeeded in 13 of 14 cases with monotherapy, but two fetuses had a relapse. One intrauterine death occurred. Treatment in two of four fetuses that also received digitalis was successful (Oudijk 2003). There is no recognizable teratogenic or fetal effect in human pregnancies to date. A risk of neonatal β-receptor blockade, e.g. neonatal bradycardia, hypotension, and hypoglycemia, should be taken into account (see Chapter 2.8.3).

Bretylium and *ibutilide* have to be injected intravenously – bretylium in case of ventricular fibrillation or ventricular tachycardia, ibutilide in case of atrial fibrillation. There is one published case report describing the use of bretylium throughout a whole pregnancy, resulting in an uneventful outcome (Gutgesell 1990). In animal studies, ibutilide, *almokalant*, and *dofetilide* demonstrated a cluster of malformations similar to phenytoin (Danielsson 2001). Experience during human pregnancies does not exist.

Class IV

For risk analysis with longer-term use of calcium antagonists such as *verapamil* and *diltiazem*, see section 2.8.5. Although animal data indicate teratogenic developmental disturbances of distal phalanges, similar effects have not been observed in human pregnancies.

Adenosine has a very short half-life of less than 2 seconds. It has to be injected intravenously. No specific fetal adverse effects have been described so far, whether the pregnant woman or the fetus is the patient (Hubinot 1998).

The same applies for electrocardioversion, including implanted defibrillators (Joglar 1999) (see above).

Recommendation. Antiarrhythmics themselves can cause arrhythmia, and therefore, provoke a life-threatening situation. For this reason, it is important critically to evaluate the indication, especially during pregnancy. Drugs of choice for the treatment of pregnant women:

- Class IA – quinidine
- Class IB – lidocaine
- Class IC – propafenone and/or, in the second or third trimester, flecainide
- Class IIB – β-blockers for long-term use.

If Class III antiarrhythmics are absolutely necessary, sotalol should be chosen. In Class IV, verapamil and diltiazem are acceptable. Because of its proven teratogenicity, phenytoin is contraindicated at least in the first trimester. However, if a pregnant woman has been treated with a drug that is not recommended above, or if such a drug is absolutely necessary for the mother (or fetus), this does not necessitate termination of pregnancy. In cases of first-trimester exposure, especially with phenytoin, a detailed ultrasound diagnosis should be offered; however, this is not necessary if a longer-term use β-blocker or calcium-blocker was given. If treatment with amiodarone was administered beyond the twelfth week (when the fetal thyroid begins to function), adverse effects on the fetal thyroid development should be ruled out with an ultrasound scan, and the thyroid status in the newborn monitored.

The drug of first choice for treatment of fetal supraventricular tachycardia is digitalis; the second choice is sotalol or flecainide. Because of its possible adverse effects on the thyroid, amiodarone should be considered as reserve drug.

2.8.20 Nitrates and other so-called vasodilators

Pharmacology and toxicology

Organic nitrates are available in many forms, but all relax vascular smooth muscle by releasing nitric oxide (also known as endothelium-derived relaxing factor) which acts via cyclic GMP.

Glyceryl trinitrate (GTN), *isosorbide mononitrate*, and *isosorbide dinitrate* are used as coronary dilators, therapeutically after a heart attack and to prevent cardiac spasms in pregnancy. In addition, they have been used successfully for gall bladder colic, and attempts have been made to use them to lower blood pressure in pre-eclampsia. They have also been used for inhibiting contractions (Lees 1994).

Toxic effects on the fetus have not been reported. The two principal side effects of nitrates are hypotension (with dizziness and fainting) and a throbbing headache.

The use of other so-called vasodilators, such as *amrinon, dipyridamole*, and *molsidomin*, are controversial with respect to their effectiveness. There is insufficient experience with their use in pregnancy for them to be recommended. Dipyridamole is said to intensify myocardial schemia. Molsidomin is carcinogenic in animal studies, and the formation of methemoglobin was observed following the use of high doses.

> **Recommendation.** Nitrates may be used in pregnancy for appropriate indications. Dipyridamole, molsidomine, and other so-called vasodilators are contraindicated. However, inadvertent exposure is no reason for termination of pregnancy, or for additional diagnostic procedures.

2.8.21 Cardiovascular drugs

Pharmacology and toxicology

Pentoxifylline/oxpentifylline, naftidrofuryl, and *inositol nicotinate* have been prescribed for peripheral vascular disorders such as intermittent claudication due to occlusion of vessels, either by spasm or sclerotic plaque, although their effectiveness has not been clearly demonstrated.

Pentoxifylline belongs to the methylxanthines, from which caffeine and theophylline are also derived. There are no large epidemiological studies on the use in pregnancy of either naftidrofuryl or pentoxifylline. However, up until now experience in clinical practice and the pharmacology of these substances argue against any noteworthy teratogenic potential.

Inositol nicotinate is a derivative of nicotinic acid; no reports of its use in human pregnancy were found.

Gingko biloba is being prescribed more frequently in some countries. From the limited data available, there is no clear evidence of specific teratogenic effects in human pregnancy. However, as there have been no systematic studies, a differential risk assessment is not possible (see Chapter 2.19).

Hydroxy ethyl starch is a plasma expander which is occasionally infused as a means of enhancing circulation and for hemodilution.

2 Pregnancy

2.8 Heart and circulatory system drugs and diuretics

Apart from anaphylactic reactions, there is no apparent risk for the embryo. This is also true for the other common means for volume substitution.

There is no experience available for the other so-called cardio-vascular drugs.

> **Recommendation.** If treatment with cardiovascular drugs is unavoidable, pentoxifylline, naftidrofuryl or hydroxy ethyl starch can be used. The use of other substances is not an indication for termination of pregnancy. In cases of doubt, a detailed ultrasound diagnosis can be performed to confirm normal morphological development.

2.8.22   Diuretics

Diuretics are only rarely indicated during pregnancy, in cases such as, for instance, heart failure or lung edema. Accepted indications have changed in comparison to earlier years, and are different from those for non-pregnant patients. Since the causes of pre-eclampsia have been better understood (see section 2.8.1), hypertension, ede-mas, and, in particular, pre-eclampsia are no longer treated with these drugs. Diuretics can reduce the plasma volume and lead to a reduced perfusion of the placenta (Sibai 1984, Lammintausta 1978).

2.8.23   Thiazide diuretics

Pharmacology and toxicology

Hydrochlorothiazide, chlorthalidone, mefruside, bemetizide, ben-droflumethiazide, butizide, chlorazanil, clopamide, indapamide, metolazone, polythiazide, quinethazone, trichlormethiazide, and *xipamide* are benzthiazide derivatives whose action depends on the inhibition of absorption of sodium and chloride in the distal tubule area. These drugs cause a potassium loss and lead to a reduction in the plasma volume. In addition, they inhibit the excretion of uric acid. Benzthiazides are well-absorbed in the intestinal tract and are excreted unchanged in the urine. They cross the placenta and, when they are given sub partu, can lead to electrolyte changes (hyponatremia, hypokalemia), to thrombopenia, and to reactive hypoglycemia in the newborn as a result of their diabetogenic effect on the mother. In addition, prolonged labor has been described as a result of the inhibitory action on the smooth muscles.

In patients with severe pre-eclampsia, the intravasal volume is reduced in most cases. Benzthiazide derivatives would lower it even further (Sibai 1984). In addition, a reduction in placental perfusion has been observed, which leads to intrauterine growth restriction because of its effect on fetal blood supply. Published experience on over 5000 treated pregnant women has given no indication, to date, of teratogenicity (embryo/fetotoxicity) from this group of saluretics.

The best-studied among these is *hydrochlorothiazide*. In a group of 567 pregnant women treated in the first trimester, neither an increase in particular anomalies nor an overall increase in birth defects was found (Rosa, cited in Briggs 2005). Moreover, neither the frequency nor the kind of anomalies among 46 newborns exposed to *indapamide* during the first trimester was remarkable (Rosa, cited in Briggs 2005).

Olesen (2001) analyzed the birth registries of Denmark and Scotland and found 232 and 31 cases, respectively, where a thiazide diuretic drug was prescribed at least once during pregnancy. Among 35 first-trimester exposed fetuses, there were three with malformations. The birth weight was significantly lower, and premature deliveries occurred more often. There were methodical deficiencies.

> **Recommendation.** See section 2.8.27.

2.8.24   Furosemide and other high-ceiling diuretics

Pharmacology and toxicology

Azosemide, bumetanide, ethacrynic acid, etozolin, piretanide, and *torasemide*, like *furosemide*, are high-ceiling diuretics and forced-action natriuretics.

The action of *furosemide* as the prototype of high-ceiling diuretics wears off in about 2–4 hours. It can lead to a reduction in the intravasal volume in the mother, and to a decline in the utero-placental circulation, which can affect the fetus (Sibai 1984). It can also cause potassium loss. Taken orally, furosemide is well-absorbed and is excreted almost unchanged in both the urine and feces. It reaches the fetus and can stimulate its urine production for a short time. Mediated by prostaglandin E2, an inhibitory action on the physiological closure of the ductus arteriosus in the premature baby, with resultant respiratory distress syndrome, has been discussed in one study (Green 1983). An ototoxic action has been described, particularly in combination with aminoglycosides (Brown 1991, Salamy 1989). The frequency of birth defects was not elevated among 350 newborns exposed during the first trimester (Rosa, cited in Briggs 2005).

In one case report, inner ear damage after treatment with ethacrynic acid and kanamycin, which is also ototoxic, in the third trimester was reported (Jones 1973). As yet, there have not been any other substantial indications of embryo- or fetotoxic damage in human beings. The number of documented experiences is insufficient for a differentiated risk assessment.

Following treatment with *bumetanide* in the first trimester, two children with heart defects were born to mothers in a group of 44 (Rosa, cited in Briggs 2005).

There is insufficient documented experience with the other high-ceiling diuretics.

However, there has been no indication of specific teratogenic action identified with any of the medications mentioned.

Olesen (2001) analyzed the birth registries of Denmark and Scotland and found 315 and 73 cases, respectively, where a diuretic drug was prescribed at least once during pregnancy. High-ceiling diuretics were found in 83 and 31 cases, respectively. Among 43 first-trimester exposed fetuses, there were five with malformations. Premature deliveries occurred more often. It should be noted that there were methodical deficiencies.

> **Recommendation.** See section 2.8.27.

2.8.25 Aldosterone antagonists

Pharmacology and toxicology

Spironolactone is the most important representative of the aldosterone antagonists, in which the diuretic action depends on the inhibition of receptors for aldosterone and other mineral corticoids in the tubule cells. An antiandrogen action is also recognized, which can be used in women who suffer from hirsutism and in boys who have pubertas praecox. For men, treatment with spironolactone can cause gynecomastia.

In contrast to the saluretics discussed above, spironolactone leads to potassium retention. For this reason, a typical side effect for spironolactone is hyperkalemia. In animal experiments, carcinogenic properties have been observed. There are, as yet, no indications of any clinical relevance of this finding for human beings. Among 31 newborns exposed in the first trimester, there were no signs of any specific birth defects (Rosa, cited in Briggs 2005). A case report describes a woman who took spironolactone during a triplet pregnancy and delivered three healthy children (one boy and two girls). They were also unremarkable with respect to any anti-androgen effects. The oldest child was followed to the age of 13 years (Groves 1995).

Eplerenon is a new aldosterone antagonist which is used as co-drug for patients, after myocardial infarction, who suffer from heart failure. It diminishes the risk of cardiovascular morbidity and mortality. There is no experience with use in human pregnancies.

> **Recommendation.** See section 2.8.27.

2.8.26   Amiloride and triamterene

Pharmacology and toxicology

Amiloride and the folic acid antagonist *triamterene* are among the potassium-saving diuretics in which the action depends on directly influencing the tubular transport. In contrast to spironolactone, they are not aldosterone antagonists. In one report, 318 newborns exposed to triamterene in the first trimester and 28 exposed to amiloride were described. No increase in birth defects was observed (Rosa, cited in Briggs 2005). Additional case reports on amiloride, mainly on the use in Bartter syndrome, have described healthy newborns (Deruelle 2004, Almeida 1989). No specific teratogenic action of either amiloride or triamterene has been recognized to date.

> **Recommendation.** See section 2.8.27.

2.8.27   Mannitol

Pharmacology and toxicology

Mannitol is the most frequently used osmotic diuretic. It is administered intravenously, excreted unchanged by the kidneys, and leads to a rapid reduction of interstitial fluid volume while at the same time increasing the intravasal fluid, thus resulting in hemodilution.

In the past there were reports about the positive action of mannitol used during pregnancy. Today it no longer plays a decisive role in pre-eclampsia therapy.

2 Pregnancy

2.8 Heart and circulatory system drugs and diuretics

> **Recommendation.** Diuretics are no longer part of the standard therapy for hypertension and edema during pregnancy; they should only be used for particular indications. In such cases, hydrochlorothiazide is the diuretic of choice. Furosemide can also be given when treatment of heart or renal failure requires a diuretic. When therapy is long term, the mother's electrolytes and hematocrit should be monitored and the development of oligohydramnios ruled out. If treatment is continued throughout the pregnancy, hypoglycemia in the newborn should be determined. Mannitol may be used during pregnancy when an osmotic diuretic is necessary. Other benzthiazide derivatives, ethacrynic acid, amiloride, triamterene, and aldosterone antagonists should be avoided during pregnancy. If therapy with aldosterone antagonists is absolutely necessary, spironolactone should be chosen. None of the diuretics is an indication for interrupting the pregnancy.

References

Almeida OD Jr, Spinnato JA. Maternal Bartter's syndrome and pregnancy. Am J Obstet Gynecol 1989; 160: 1225–6.

Alwan S (A), Polifka JE, Friedman JM. Angiotensin II receptor antagonist treatment during pregnancy. Birth Def Res A 2005; 73: 123–30.

Athanassiadis AP, Dadamogias C, Netskos D et al. Fetal tachycardia: is digitalis still the first-line therapy? Clin Exp Obstet Gynecol 2004; 31: 293–5.

Avdalovic M, Sandrock C, Hoso A et al. Epoprostenol in pregnant patients with secondary pulmonary hypertension. Treat Respir Med 2004; 3: 29–34.

Badalian SS, Silverman RK, Aubry RH et al. Twin pregnancy in a woman on long-term epoprostenol therapy for primary pulmonary hypertension. J Reprod Med 2000; 45: 149–52.

Bar J, Hod M, Merlob P. Angiotensin converting enzyme inhibitors use in the first trimester of pregnancy. Int J Risk Safety Med 1997; 10: 23–6.

Barr M Jr. Teratogen update: angiotensin-converting enzyme inhibitors. Teratology 1994; 50: 399–409.

Bartalena L, Bogazzi F, Braverman E et al. Effects of amiodarone administration during pregnancy on neonatal thyroid function and subsequent neurodevelopment. J Endocrinol Invest 2001; 24: 116–30.

Bayliss H, Churchill D, Beevers M et al. Anti-hypertensive drugs in pregnancy and fetal growth: evidence for "pharmacological programming" in the first trimester? Hypertens Pregnancy 2002; 21: 161–74.

Bendayan D, Hod M, Oron G et al. Pregnancy outcome in patients with pulmonary arterial hypertension receiving prostacylin therapy. Obstet Gynecol 2005; 106: 1206–10.

Berkane N, Carlier P, Verstraete L et al. Fetal toxicity of valsartan and possible reversible adverse side effects. Birth Def Res A 2004; 70: 547–9.

Bhorat IE, Naidoo DP, Rout CC et al. Malignant ventricular arrhythmias in eclampsia: a comparison of labetalol with dihydralazine. Am J Obstet Gynecol 1993; 168: 1292–6.

Bildirici I, Shumway JB. Intravenous and inhaled epoprostenol for primary pulmonary hypertension during pregnancy and delivery. Obstet Gynecol 2004; 103: 1102–5.

Bodis J, Sulyok E, Ertl T et al. Methyldopa in pregnancy hypertension and the newborn. Lancet 1982; 2: 498–9.

Bombelli F, Lagona F, Salvati A et al. Radiofrequency catheter ablation in drug refractory maternal supraventricular tachycardias in advanced pregnancy. Obstet Gynecol 2003; 102: 1171–3.

Bos-Thompson MA, Hillaire-Buys D, Muller F et al. Fetal toxic effects of angiotensin II receptor antagonists: case report and follow-up after birth. Ann Pharmacother 2005; 39: 157–61.

Bourget P, Fernandez H, Edouard D et al. Disposition of a new rate-controlled formulation of prazosin in the treatment of hypertension during pregnancy: transplacental passage of prazosin. Eur J Drug Metab Pharmacokinet 1995; 20(3): 233–41.

Boutroy MJ, Gisonna CR, Legagneur M et al. Placental transfer and neonatal adaption. Early Hum Dev 1988; 17: 275–86.

Briggs GG, Nageotte MP. Fatal fetal outcome with the combined use of valsartan and atenolol. Ann. Pharmacother 2001; 35: 859–61.

Briggs GG, Freeman RK, Yaffe SJ. Drugs in Pregnancy and Lactation, 7th edn. Baltimore, MD: Williams & Wilkins, 2005.

Brown DR, Watchko JF, Sabo D. Neonatal sensorineural hearing loss associated with furosemide: a case-control study. Dev Med Child Neurol 1991; 33: 816–23.

Brown MA, McCowan LME, North RA et al. Withdrawal of nifedipine capsules: jeopardising the treatment of acute severe hypertension in pregnancy? Med J Aust 1997; 166: 640–43.

Burrows RF, Burrows EA. Assessing the teratogenic potential of angiotensin-converting enzyme inhibitors in pregnancy. Aust NZ J Obstet Gynaecol 1998; 38: 306–11.

Casele HL, Windley KC, Prieto IA et al. Felodipine use in pregnancy. Report of three cases. J Reprod Med 1997; 42: 378–81.

Chan V, Tse TF, Wong V. Transfer of digoxin across the placenta and into breast milk. Br J Obstet Gynaecol 1978; 85: 605–9.

Childress CH, Katz VL. Nifedipine and its indications in obstetrics and gynecology. Obstet Gynecol 1994, 83: 616–24.

Chung NA, Lip GY, Beevers M et al. Angiotensin-II-receptor inhibitors in pregnancy. Lancet 2001; 357: 1620–21.

Constantine G, Beevers DG, Reynolds AL et al. Nifedipine as a second line antihypertensive drug in pregnancy. Br J Obstet Gynaecol 1987; 94: 1136–42.

Cooper WO, Hernandez-Diaz S, Arbogast PG et al. Major congenital malformations after first-trimester exposure to ACE inhibitors. N Engl J Med 2006; 354: 2443–51.

Cuneo BF, Ovadia M, Strasburger JF et al. Prenatal diagnosis and in utero treatment of torsades de pointes associated with congenital long QT syndrome. Am J Cardiol 2003; 91: 1395–8.

Czeizel AE. Reserpine is not a human teratogen. J Med Genet 1988; 25: 787.

Czeizel AE, Rockenbauer M. Population-based case-control study of teratogenic potential of corticosteroids. Teratology 1997; 56: 335–40.

Czeizel AE, Toth M. Birth weight, gestational age and medications during pregnancy. Int J Gynaecol Obstet 1998; 60: 245–9.

Daika-Dahmane F, Levy-Beff E, Jugie M et al. Foetal kidney maldevelopment in maternal use angiotensin II type I receptor antagonists. Pediatr Nephrol 2006; 21: 729–32.

Danielsson BR, Reicand S, Rundquist E et al. Digital defects induced by vasodilating agents: Relationship to reduction in uteroplacental blood flow. Teratology 1989; 40: 351–8.

2 Pregnancy

2.8 Heart and circulatory system drugs and diuretics

Danielsson BR, Skold AC, Azarbayjani F. Class III antiarrhythmics and phenytoin: teratogenicity due to embryonic cardiac dysrhythmia and reoxygenation damage. Curr Pharm Des 2001; 7: 787–802.

de Moura R, Lopes MA. Effects of captopril on the human foetal placental circulation: an interaction with bradykinin and angiotensin I. Br J Clin Pharmacol 1995; 39: 497–501.

Derham RJ, Robinson J. Severe pre-eclampsia: is vasodilation therapy with hydralazine dangerous for the preterm fetus? Am J Perinatal 1990; 7(3): 239–14.

Deruelle P, Dufour P, Magnenant E et al. Maternal Bartter's syndrome in pregnancy treated by amiloride. Eur J Obstet Gynecol Reprod Biol 2004; 115:106–7.

Doherty G, Bali S, Casey F. Fetal hydrops due to supraventricular tachycardia – successful outcome in a difficult case. Ir Med J. 2003; 96: 52–3.

d'Souza D, MacKenzie WE, Martin WL. Transplacental flecainide therapy in the treatment of fetal supraventricular tachycardia. J Obstet Gynaecol. 2002; 22: 320–2.

Duley L. Which anticonvulsant for women with eclampsia? Evidence from the collaborative eclampsia trial. Lancet 1995; 345: 1455.

Dumez Y, Tchobroutsky C, Hornych H et al. Neonatal effects of maternal administration of acebutolol. Br Med J Clin Res 1981; 283: 1077–9.

Easterling TR (A), Brateng D, Schmucker B et al. Prevention of pre-eclampsia: a randomized trial of atenolol in hyperdynamic patients before onset of hypertension. Obstet Gynecol 1999; 93: 725–33.

Easterling TR (B), Ralph DD, Schmucker BC. Pulmonary hypertension in pregnancy: treatment with pulmonary vasodilators. Obstet Gynecol 1999; 93: 494–8.

Elliot CA, Stewart P, Webster VJ et al. The use of iloprost in early pregnancy in patients with pulmonary arterial hypertension. Eur Respir J 2005; 26: 168–73.

Eronen M, Heikkila P, Teramo K. Congenital complete heart block in the fetus: hemodynamic features, antenatal treatment, and outcome in six cases. Pediatr Cardiol 2001; 22: 385–92.

Fidler J, Smith V, Fayers P et al. Randomized controlled comparative study of methyldopa and oxprenolol in treatment of hypertension in pregnancy. Br Med J Clin Res 1983; 18: 1927–30.

Filler G, Wong H, Condello A et al. Early dialysis in a neonate with intrauterine lisinopril exposure. Arch Dis Child Fetal Neonatal Ed 2003; 88: F154–6.

Franke G, Pietsch P, Schneider T et al. Studies on the kinetics of and distribution of dihydralazine in pregnancy. Biol Res Pregnancy Perinatal 1986; 7: 300–33.

Garden A, Davey DA, Dommisse I. Intravenous labetabol and intravenous dihydralazine in severe hypertension of pregnancy. Clin Exp Hypertens 1982; 1: 371–83.

Geohas C, McLaughlin VV. Successful management of pregnancy in a patient with Eisenmenger syndrome with epoprostenol. Chest 2003; 124: 1170–73.

Gilstrap LC, Little BB. Drugs & Pregnancy, 2 ed. New York: Chapman & Hall, 1998.

Goeschen K, Jäger A, Saling E. Value of treatment with dihydroergotamine for hypotension in pregnancy [in German]. Geburtsh Frauenheilk 1984; 44: 351–5.

Gray SE, Rodis J, Lettieri L et al. Effect of intravenous magnesium sulfate on the biophysical profile of the healthy preterm fetus. Am J Obstet Gynecol 1994; 170: 1131–5.

Green TP, Thompson TR, Johnson DE et al. Furosemide promotes patent ductus arteriosus in premature infants with the respiratory-distress syndrome. N Engl J Med 1983; 308: 743–8.

Grosso S, Berardi R, Cioni M et al. Transient neonatal hypothyroidism after gestational exposure to amiodarone: a follow-up of two cases. J Endocrinol Invest 1998; 21: 699–702.

Groves TD, Corenblum B. Spironolactone therapy during human pregnancy. Am J Obstet Gynecol 1995; 172: 1655–6.

Grunewald C, Carlstrom K, Lunell N et al. Dihydralazine in pre-eclampsia: acute effects on atrial natriuretic peptide concentration and feto-maternal hemodynamics. J Maternal-Fetal Investig 1993; 3: 21–4.

Gudmundsson S, Gennser G, Marsal K. Effects of hydralazine on placental and renal circulation in preeclampsia. Acta Obstet Gynecol Scand 1995; 74: 415–18.

Günenç O, Çiçek N, Gorkemli H et al. The effect of methyldopa treatment on uterine, umblical and fetal middlecerebral artery blood flows in pre-eclamptic patients. Arch Gynecol Obstet 2002; 266: 141–4.

Gutgesell M, Overholt E, Boyle R. Oral bretylium tosylate use during pregnancy and subsequent breastfeeding: a case report. Am J Perinatol 1990; 7: 144–5.

Hallak M, Neerhof MG, Perry R et al. Fetal supraventricular tachycardia and hydrops fetalis: combined intensive, direct, and transplacental therapy. Obstet Gynecol 1991; 78: 523–5.

Hata T, Manabe A, Hata K et al. Changes in blood velocities of fetal circulation in association with fetal heart rate abnormalities: effect of sub-lingual administration of nifedipine. Am J Perinatol 1995; 12: 80–1.

Heilmann L, Kurz E. The therapy of the hypertensive form of late gestosis {in German; author's transl}. Geburtsh Frauenheilk 1970; 38: 1348.

Heinonen OP, Slone D, Shapiro S (eds). Birth Defects and Drugs in Pregnancy. Littleton, MA: Publishing Sciences Group, 1977.

Hill WC. Risks and complications of tocolysis. Clin Obstet Gynecol 1995; 38(4): 725–45.

Hod M, Friedman S, Schoenfeld A et al. Hydralazine-induced hepatitis in pregnancy. Int J Fertil 1986; 31: 352–5.

Hohmann M, Kunzel W. Dihydroergotamine causes fetal growth retardation in guinea pigs. Arch Gynecol Obstet 1992; 251: 187–92.

Horvath JS, Phippard A, Korda A et al. Clonidine hydrochloride, a safe and effective antihypertensive agent in pregnancy. Obstet Gynecol 1985; 66: 634–8.

Houlihan DD, Dennedy MC, Ravikumar N et al. Anti-hypertensive therapy and the feto-placental circulation: effects on umbilical artery resistance. J Perinatal Med 2004; 32: 315–19.

Houtzager BA, Hogendoorn SM, Papatsonis DNM et al. Long-term follow-up of children exposed in utero to nifedipine or ritodrine for the management of preterm labour. Br J Obstet Gynaecol 2006; 113: 324.

Hubinont C, Debauche C, Bernard P et al. Resolution of fetal tachycardia and hydrops by a single adenosine administration. Obstet Gynecol 1998; 92: 718.

Huisjes HJ, Hadders-Algra M, Touwen BCL. Is clonidine a behavioural teratogen in the human? Early Hum Dev 1986; 41: 431–88.

Joglar JA, Page RL. Treatment of cardiac arrhythmias during pregnancy. Drug Saf 1999; 20: 85–94.

Jones HC. Intrauterine ototoxicity. A case report and review of the literature. J Natl Med Assoc 1973; 65: 201–3.

Jones MRH, Cummings AJ. A study of the transfer of α-methyldopa to the human foetus and newborn infant. Br J Clin Pharmacol 1978; 6: 432–4.

Kaler SG, Patrinos ME, Lambert GH et al. Hypertrichosis and congenital anomalies associated with maternal use of minoxidil. Pediatrics 1987; 79(3): 434–6.

Källén B, Lygner PE. Delivery outcome in women who used drugs for migraine during pregnancy with special reference to sumatriptan. Headache 2001; 41: 351–6.

Katz V, Blanchard G, Dingman C et al. Atenolol and short umbilical cords. Am J Obstet Gynecol 1987; 63: 1271–2.

Kirshon B, Wasserstrum N, Cotton DB. Should continuous hydralazine infusions be utilized in severe pregnancy-induced hypertension? Am J Perinatol 1991; 8: 206–8.

Koks CAM, Brolmann HAM, de Kleine MJK et al. A randomized comparison of nifedipine and ritodrine for suppression of preterm labor. Eur J Obstet Gynecol Reprod Biol 1998; 77: 171–6.

Krapp M, Baschat AA, Gembruch U et al. Flecainide in the intrauterine treatment of fetal supraventricular tachycardia. Ultrasound Obstet Gynecol 2002; 19: 158–64.

Kwawukume EY, Ghosh TS. Oral nifedipine therapy in the management of severe pre-eclampsia. Int J Gynecol Obstet 1995; 49: 265–9.

Lacassie HJ, Germain AM, Valdés G et al. Management of Eisenmenger syndrome in pregnancy with sildenafil and l-arginine. Obstet Gynecol 2004; 103: 1118–20.

Lammintausta R, Erkkola R, Eronen M. Effect of chlorothiazide treatment of renin-aldosterone system during pregnancy. Acta Obstet Gynecol Scand 1978; 57: 389–92.

Lavoratti G, Seracini D, Fiorini P et al. Neonatal anuria by ACE inhibitors during pregnancy. Nephron 1997; 76: 235–6.

Lees C, Campbell S, Jaunlaux E et al. Arrest of preterm labour and prolongation of gestation with glyceryl trinitrate, a nitric oxide donor. Lancet 1994; 343: 1325–6.

Leveno KJ, Alexander JM, McIntire DD et al. Does magnesium sulfate given for prevention of eclampsia affect outcome of labor? Am J Obstet Gynecol 1998; 178: 707–12.

Levin AC, Doering PL, Hatton RC. Use of nifedipine in the hypertensive diseases of pregnancy. Ann Pharmacother 1994; 28: 1371–8.

Lindow SW, Davies N, Davey DA et al. The effect of sublingual nifedipine on utero-placental blood flow in hypertensive pregnancy. Br J Obstet Gynaecol 1988; 95: 1276–81.

Lippert TH, Bohm HR. Risk of treatment with dihydroergotamine in pregnancy (in German). Geburtshilfe Frauenheilkd 1984; 44: 403–5.

Lipshitz J, Ahokas RA, Reynolds SL. The effect of hydralazine on placental perfusion in the spontaneously hypertensive rat. Am J Obstet Gynecol 1987; 156: 356–9.

Lodeiro JG , Feinstein SJ, Lodeiro SB. Fetal premature atrial contractions associated with hydralazine. Am J Obstet Gynecol 1989; 160: 105–7.

Lomenick JP, Jackson WA, Backeljauw PF. Amiodarone-induced neonatal hypothyroidism: a unique form of transient early-onset hypothyroidism. J Perinatol 2004; 24: 397–9.

Lydakis C, Lip GY, Beevers M et al. Atenolol and fetal growth in pregnancies complicated by hypertension. Am J Hypertens 1999; 12: 541–7.

Maeno Y, Himeno W, Saito A et al. Clinical course of fetal congenital atrioventricular block in the Japanese population: a multicentre experience. Heart 2005; 91: 1075–9.

Magee LA, Downar E, Sermer M et al. Pregnancy outcome after gestational exposure to amiodarone in Canada. Am J Obstet Gynecol 1995; 172: 1307–11.

Magee LA, Schick B, Sage SR et al. The safety of calcium channel blockers in human pregnancy: a prospective, multicenter cohort study. Am J Obstet Gynecol 1996; 174: 823–8.

Magee LA, Nulman I, Rovet JF et al. Neurodevelopment after in utero amiodarone exposure. Neurotoxicol Teratol 1999; 21: 261–5.

Magee LA, Elran E, Bull SB et al. Risks and benefits of beta-receptor blockers for pregnancy hypertension: overview of the randomized trials. Eur J Obstet Gynecol Reprod Biol 2000; 88: 15–26.

Magee LA, Cham C, Waterman EJ et al. Hydralazine for treatment of severe hypertension in pregnancy: meta-analysis. Br Med J 2003; 25(327): 955–60.

Marlettini MG, Crippa S, Morselli-Labate AM et al. Randomized comparison of calcium antagonists and beta-blockers in the treatment of pregnancy-induced hypertension. Curr Ther Res 1990; 48(4): 684–92.

Martinovic J, Benachi A, Laurent N et al. Fetal toxic effects and angiotensin-II-receptor antagonist. Lancet 2001; 358: 241–2.

McCombs M. Update on tocolytic therapy. Ann Pharmacother 1995; 29: 515–22.

Milner RDG, Chouksey SK. Effects of fetal exposure to diazoxide in man. Arch Dis Child 1972; 47: 537–43.

Milsap RL, Auld PA. Neonatal hyperglycemia following maternal diazoxide administration. J Am Med Assoc 1980; 243: 144–5.

Moar VA, Jefferies MA, Mutch LM et al .Neonatal head circumference and the treatment of maternal hypertension. Br J Obstet Gynaecol 1978; 85: 933–7.

Molelekwa V, Akhter P, McKenna P et al. Eisenmenger's syndrome in a 27 week pregnancy – management with bosentan and sildenafil. Ir Med J 2005; 98: 87–8.

Montan S, Anandakumar C, Arulkumaran S et al. Randomised controlled trial of methyldopa and isradipine in preeclampsia – effects on uteroplacental and fetal hemodynamics. J Perinatal Med 1996; 24: 177–84.

Moodley J, Gouws E. A comparative study of the use of epoprostenol and dihydralazine in severe hypertension in pregnancy. Br J Obstet 1992; 99: 727–30.

Muller PR, James A. Pregnancy with prolonged fetal exposure to an angiotensin-converting enzyme inhibitor. J Perinatol 2002; 22: 582–4.

Murki S, Kumar P, Dutta S et al. Fatal neonatal renal failure due to maternal enalapril ingestion. J Matern Fetal Neonatal Med 2005; 17: 235–7.

Nelson KB, Grether JK. Can magnesium sulfate reduce the risk of cerebral palsy in very low birth-weight infants? Pediatrics 1995; 95: 263–9.

Neumann J, Weiss B, Rabello Y et al. Diazoxide for the acute control of severe hypertension complicating pregnancy : a pilot study. Obstet Gynecol 1979; 53: 50–55.

Oakley C, Child A, Jung B et al. Expert consensus document on management of cardiovascular diseases during pregnancy. Eur Heart J 2003; 24: 761–81.

Oei SG, Oei SK, Brolmann HAM. Myocardial infarction during nifedipine therapy for preterm labor. N Engl J Med 1999; 340: 154.

Oettinger M, Perlitz Y. Asymptomatic paroxysmal atrial fibrillation during intravenous magnesium sulfate treatment in pre-eclampsia. Gynecol Obstet Invest 1993; 36: 244–6.

Olesen C, de Vries CS, Thrane N et al. Effect of diuretics on fetal growth: a drug effect or confounding by indication? Pooled Danish and Scottish cohort data. Br J Clin Pharmacol 2001; 51: 153–7.

Orlandi C, Marlettini MG, Cassani A et al. Treatment of hypertension during pregnancy with the calcium antagonist verapamil. Curr Ther Res 1986; 39(6): 884–93.

Oudijk MA, Ruskamp JM, Ambachtsheer BE et al. Drug treatment of fetal tachycardias. Pediatr Drugs 2002; 4: 49–63.

Oudijk MA, Ruskamp JM, Ververs FF et al. Treatment of fetal tachycardia with sotalol: transplacental pharmacokinetics and pharmacodynamics. J Am Coll Cardiol 2003; 42: 765–70.

Ounsted MK, Moar VA, Good FJ et al. Hypertension during pregnancy with and without specific treatment; the development of the children at the age of four years. Br J Obstet Gynaecol 1980; 87: 19–24.

2

Pregnancy

2.8 Heart and circulatory system drugs and diuretics

Ovadia M, Brito M, Hoger GL et al. Human experience with amiodarone in the embryonic period. Am J Cardiol 1994; 73: 316–17.

Pahor M, Psaty B, Alderman MH et al. Health outcomes associated with calcium antagonists compared with other first-line antihypertensive therapies: a meta-analysis of randomised controlled trials. Lancet 2000; 356(9246): 1949–54.

Papatsonis DN, Van Geijn HP, Ader HJ et al. Nifedipine and ritodrine in the management of preterm labor: a randomized multicenter trial. Obstet Gynecol 1997; 90: 230–34.

Papatsonis DN, Lok CA, Bos JM et al. Calcium channel blockers in the management of preterms labor and hypertension in pregnancy. Eur J Obstet Gynecol Reprod Biol 2001; 97: 122–40.

Pearce PC, Hawkey C, Symons C et al. Role of calcium in the induction of cardiac hypertrophy and myofibrillar disarray. Experimental studies of a possible cause of hypertrophic cardiomyopathy. Br Heart J 1985; 54: 420–27.

Pearson G, Bradley S. Pharmacologic management of hypertension in pregnancy. OCP 1993; 20(2): 38–44.

Phadnis SV, Sangay MR, Sanusi FA. Alpha-methyldopa-induced acute hepatitis in pregnancy. R Aust NZ Coll Obstet Gynaecol 2006; 46: 254–60.

Pickles CJ, Pipkin FB, Symonds EM. A randomized placebo controlled trial of labetalol in the treatment of mild to moderate pregnancy induced hypertension. Br J Obstet Gynaecol 1992; 99: 964–8.

Plouin PF, Breart G, Maillard F et al. Maternal effects and perinatal safety of labetalol in the treatment of hypertension in pregnancy. Comparison with methyldopa in a randomized cooperative trial. Arch Mal Coeur 1987; 80: 952–5.

Plouin PF, Breart G, Llado J et al. A randomized comparison of early with conservative use of antihypertensive drugs in the management of pregnancy-induced hypertension. Br J Obstet Gynaecol 1990; 97: 134–11.

Porat S, Anteby EY, Hamani Y et al. Fetal supraventricular tachycardia diagnosed and treated at 13 weeks of gestation: a case report. Ultrasound Obstet Gynecol 2003; 21: 302–5.

Pradhan M, Manisha, Singh R et al. Amiodarone in treatment of fetal supraventricular tachycardia. Fetal Diagn Ther 2006; 21: 72–6.

Prasad N, Gulati S, Jain M et al. An unusual case of neonatal anuria. Indian Pediatr 2003; 40: 258–60.

Pritchard JA, Cunningham FG, Pritchard SA. The Parkland Memorial Hospital protocol for treatment of eclampsia: evaluation of 245 cases. Am J Obstet Gynecol 1984; 148: 951–63.

Rasheed A, Simpson J, Rosenthal E. Neonatal ECG changes caused by supratherapeutic flecainide following treatment for fetal supraventricular tachycardia. Heart 2003; 89: 70.

Ray D, Dyson D. Calcium channel blockers. Clin Obstet Gynecol 1995; 38(4): 713–21.

Ray JG, Vermeulen MJ, Burrows EA et al. Use of antihypertensive medications in pregnancy and the risk of adverse perinatal outcomes: McMaster Outcome Study of Hypertension In Pregnancy 2 (MOSHIP 2). BMC Pregnancy Childbirth 2001; 1: 6.

Raymond GV. Teratogen update: ergot and ergotamine. Teratology 1995; 51: 344–7.

Redman CWG, Beilin LJ, Bonnar J et al. Fetal outcome in trial of antihypertensive treatment in pregnancy. Lancet 1976; 2: 753–6.

Reynolds B, Butters L, Evans J et al. First year of life after the use of atenolol in pregnancy associated hypertension. Arch Dis Child 1984; 59: 1061–3.

Rosenfeld J, Bott-Kanner G, Boner G et al. Treatment of hypertension during pregnancy with hydralazine monotherapy or with combined therapy with hydralazine and pindolol. Eur J Obstet Gynecol Reprod Biol 1986; 22: 197–204.

Rotmensch HH, Rotmensch S, Elkayam U. Management of cardiac arrhythmias during pregnancy. Current Concepts Drug 1987; 33: 363.

Rubin PC (A), Butters L, Kelman AW et al. Labetalol disposition and concentration – effect relationships during pregnancy. Br J Clin Pharmacol 1983; 15: 465–70.

Rubin PC (B), Butters L, Low RA et al. Clinical pharmacological studies with prazosin during pregnancy complicated by hypertension. Br J Clin Pharmacol 1983; 16: 543–7.

Saarikoski S. Placental transfer and fetal uptake of 3H-digoxin in humans. Br J Obstet Gynaecol 1978; 85: 605–9.

Saji H, Yamanaka M, Hagiwara A et al. Losartan and fetal toxic effects. Lancet 2001; 357: 363.

Salamy A, Eldredge L, Tooley WH. Neonatal status and hearing loss in high-risk infants. J Pediatr 1989; 114: 847–52.

Satoh T (A), Narama I. Reproduction studies of amezinium emtilsulfate(3) – teratogenicity study in rats. Yakuri to Chiryo 1988; 16: 1557–72.

Satoh T (B), Narama I. Reproduction studies of Amezinium metisulfate(4) – teratogenicity study in rabbits. Yakuri to Chiryo 1988; 16: 1573–83.

Scardo JA, Vermillion ST, Newman RB et al. A randomized, double-blind, hemodynamic evaluation of nifedipine and labetalol in preeclamptic hypertensive emergencies. Am J Obstet Gynecol 1999; 181: 862–6.

Schaefer C. Angiotensin II-receptor-antagonists: further evidence of fetotoxicity but not teratogenicity. Birth Def Res A 2003; 67: 591–4.

Schaefer C, Weber-Schöndorfer C. ACE-inhibitors during early pregnancy. Presentation at the 16th Annual ENTIS Conference, 2006, Abano, Italy.

Scott WJ Jr, Resnick E, Hummler H et al. Cardiovascular alterations in rat fetuses exposed to calcium channel blockers. Reprod Toxicol 1997; 11(2/3): 207–14.

Senat MV, Fischer C, Bernard JP et al. The use of lidocaine for fetocide in late termination of pregnancy. Br J Obstet Gynecol 2003; 110: 296–300.

Serreau R, Luton D, Macher M-A et al. Developmental toxicity of the angiotensin II type 1 receptor antagonists during human pregnancy: a report of 10 cases. Br J Obstet Gynaecol 2005; 112: 710–12.

Shen O, Entebi E, Yagel S. Congenital hypertrophic cardiomyopathy associated with in utero verapamil exposure. Prenat Diagn 1995; 15(11): 1088–9.

Shoemaker CT, Meyers M. Sodium nitroprusside for control of severe hypertensive disease of pregnancy: a case report and discussion of potential toxicity. Am J Obstet Gynecol 1984; 149: 171–3.

Sibai BM, Spinnato JA, Watson DL et al. Pregnancy outcome in 303 cases with severe pre-eclampsia. Obstet Gynecol 1984; 64: 319–25.

Sibai BM, Grossman RA, Grossman HG. Effects of diuretics on plasma volume in pregnancies with long-term hypertension. Am J Obstet Gynecol 1985; 150: 831–5.

Smith GN, Piercy WN. Methyldopa hepatotoxicity in pregnancy: a case report. Am J Obstet Gynecol 1995; 172: 222–4.

Sørensen HT, Steffensen FH, Olesen C et al. Pregnancy outcome in women exposed to calcium channel blockers. Reprod Toxicol 1998; 12: 383–4.

Spinnato JA, Sibai BM, Anderson GD. Fetal distress after hydralazine therapy for severe pregnancy-induced hypertension. South Med J 1986; 79: 559–62.

Stewart R, Tuazon D, Olsen G et al. Pregnancy and primary pulmonary hypertension. Chest 2001; 119: 973–5.

Strasburger JF, Cuneo BF, Michon MM et al. Amiodarone therapy for drug-refractory fetal tachycardia. Circulation 2004; 109: 375–9.

Suionio S, Saarikoski S, Tahvanainen K et al. Acute effects of dihydralazine mesylate, furosemide, and metoprolol on maternal hemodynamics in pregnancy-induced hypertension. Am J Obstet Gynecol 1986; 155: 122–5.

2

Pregnancy

2.8 Heart and circulatory system drugs and diuretics

Sulyok E, Bodis J, Hartman G et al. Neonatal effects of methyldopa therapy in pregnancy hypertension. Acta Paediatr Hung 1991; 31(1): 53–63.

Sweetman, S. (ed.) Martindale: The Complete Drug Reference, 33rd edn. London: Pharmaceutical Press, 2002.

Tabacova S (A), Kimmel CA, Wall K et al. Atenolol developmental toxicity: animal-to-human comparisons. Birth Def Res A 2003; 67: 181–92.

Tabacova S (B), Little R, Tsong Y et al. Adverse pregnancy outcomes associated with maternal enalapril antihypertensive treatment. Pharmacoepidemiol Drug Saf 2003; 12: 633–46.

Tadmor OP, Keren A, Rosenak D et al. The effect of disopyramide on uterine contractions during pregnancy. Am J Obstet Gynecol 1990; 162: 482–6.

Todoroki Y, Tsukahara H, Kawatani M et al. Neonatal suppurative parotitis possibly associated with congenital cytomegalovirus infection and maternal methyldopa administration. Pediatr Int 2006; 48: 185–6.

Tomlinson AJ, Campbell J, Walker JJ et al. Malignant primary hypertension in pregnancy treated with lisinopril. Ann Pharmacother 2000; 34: 180–82.

Towell ME, Hyman Al. Catecholamine depletion in pregnancy. J Obstet Gynaecol Br Commonw 1966; 73: 431–8.

Trolp R, Inner M, Bernius U. Efficency of tocoylsis by fenoterol and fenoterol in combination with a beta-1-blocking compound {in German; author's translation}. Geburtsh Frauenheilk 1980; 40: 602–9.

Turnstall ME. The effect of propranolol on the onset of breathing at birth. Br J Anaesth 1969; 41: 792.

Vaast P, Dubreucq-Fossaert S, Hofflin-Debarge V et al. Acute pulmonary oedema during nicardipine therapy for premature labour report of five cases. Eur J Obstet Gynecol 2004; 113: 98–9.

Vermillion ST, Scardo JA, Newman RB et al. A randomized, double-blind trial of oral nifedipine and intravenous labetalol in hypertensive emergencies of pregnancy. Am J Obstet Gynecol 1999; 181: 858–61.

Waisman GD, Mayorga LM, Camera MJ et al. Magnesium plus nifedipine: potentiation of hypotensive effect in preeclampsia? Am J Obstet Gynecol 1988; 159: 308–9.

Wareing M, Myers JE, O'Hara M et al. Sildenafil citrate (Viagra) enhances vasodilation in fetal growth restiction. J Clin Endocrinol Metab 2005; 90: 2550–55.

Waterman EJ, Magee LA, Lim KI et al. Do commonly used oral antihypertensives alter fetal or neonatal heart rate characteristics? A systematic review. Hypertens Pregnancy 2004; 23: 155–69.

Weber-Schöndorfer C. Pregnancy outcome after exposure to calcium-channel blockers during first trimester. Presentation at the 14th Annual ENTIS Conference, 2004, Prague.

Weiner CP, Herring J, Wang J et al. Chronic measurement, using a Doppler probe, of uterine artery flow in the gravid guinea-pig. J Reprod Fertil 1986; 77: 247–56.

Weiss BM, Hess OM. Pulmonary vascular disease and pregnancy: currrent controversies, management strategies, and perspectives. Eur Heart J 2000; 21: 104–115.

Whitelaw A. Maternal methyldopa treatment and neonatal blood pressure. Br Med J 1981; 283: 471.

Widerlov E , Karlmann I, Storsater J. Hydralazine-induced neonatal thrombocytopenia. N Engl J Med 1980; 303: 1235–8.

Yemini M, Shoham (Schwartz) Z, Dgani R et al. Lupus-like syndrome in a mother and newborn following administration of hydralazine: a case report. Eur J Obstet Gynaecol Reprod Biol 1989; 30: 193–7.

Anticoagulant and fibrinolytic drugs

2.9

Minke Reuvers

2.9.1   Pregnancy and coagulation

During pregnancy and the immediate puerperium, the risk for
venous thromboembolism (VTE) is substantially increased. As
described historically by Virchow, there are, in his opinion, three
factors that predispose an individual to the development of venous
thrombosis: hypercoagulability, vascular damage, and stasis. As

higher estrogen levels stimulate hepatic protein synthesis, plasma levels increase for most of the procoagulant proteins, including fibrinogen, Factor VIII, and vitamin K-dependent factors. Fibrinolytic activity decreases due to the increased levels of plasminogen activator inhibitors produced by the placenta. These changes represent the physiological preparation for the hemostatic challenge of delivery (Greer 1999, Dizon-Townson 1998). In addition, venous flow decreases from the lower extremities (stasis), and delivery and placental separation create vascular damage (Dizon-Townson 1998). The true incidence of VTE associated with pregnancy is not exactly known, but deep vein thrombosis (DVT) and pulmonary embolism (PE) remain the leading causes of maternal morbidity and mortality in developed countries (Bates 2004, McColl 2004, Dizon-Townson 1998). Women with previous VTE might have an increased risk, but the true risk is unknown, and the estimates range from 0% to 13% (Bates 2004).

Growing evidence suggests that thrombophilia is also associated with an increased risk of VTE and adverse pregnancy outcomes (early and late pregnancy loss, pre-eclampsia, placental abruption, and intrauterine growth restriction (IUGR)) (Dudding 2004). Thrombophilia is either an inherited or an acquired thrombotic tendency. The most common inherited thrombophilias are the factor V Leiden mutation, the prothrombin gene mutation, methylenetetrahydrofolate reductase (MTHFR) polymorphism, and deficiencies of antithrombin, protein C or protein S. Antiphospholipid syndrome belongs to the acquired thrombophilias (Adelberg 2002). However, the absolute risk of VTE and serious adverse outcomes remains low. Management of pregnant women with thrombophilias is still subject to debate in the recent literature (see section 2.9.2). Universal agreement regarding thromboprophylaxis during pregnancy has not been established to date, because of the lack of reliable data on the specific risks and the efficacy of thromboprophylaxis. A prior thrombotic event or thrombophilia is not currently viewed by all clinicians as an indication for thromboprophylaxis during pregnancy (see section 2.9.2).

Most recommendations include the following indications:

- thromboprophylaxis in patients with an established increased risk, including patients with malignancies, postoperative patients, long-term immobilization
- prevention and treatment of VTE
- prevention and treatment of systemic embolism in patients with valvular heart disease and/or mechanical heart valves
- prevention of pregnancy loss in women with antiphospholipid antibodies and previous pregnancy losses.

2.9.2   Heparins

Pharmacology

Heparins are sulfated, long-chain acidic mucopolysaccharides, and their molecular weight ranges from 4000 to 30 000 daltons, with a mean of about 15 000 daltons. Heparins prevent thrombus formation and limit thrombus extension. They act as an antithrombin III cofactor, thereby increasing its ability to neutralize the hemostatic enzymes, most importantly factor Xa and thrombin (factor IIa). When administered in prophylactic, low dosages (subcutaneous), it is mainly factor Xa that is neutralized; in higher therapeutic dosages, thrombin will also be neutralized. Heparins can initiate plasminogen activator release by endothelial cells, and this accounts for their fibrinolytic activity. Heparins are broken down in the gut, and require a parenteral route of administration (intravenous or subcutaneous). They have a poor bioavailabilty (10%), are metabolized in the liver, and have a half-life of about 4–6 hours. Heparin does not cross the placental barrier due to its high molecular weight and its negative charge.

Low molecular-weight heparins (LMWHs) are increasingly preferred to unfractioned heparin (UH) for thromboprophylaxis, as well as for the treatment of VTE, and in the pregnant patient. They are heparin fragments produced by chemical or enzymatic depolymerization, and their molecular weight ranges from 4000–6000 daltons. They specifically inhibit factor Xa. Their advantage lies in a longer half-life (injecting once a day), their better bioavailability (85%), and their association with a lower incidence of osteoporosis, allergy, and heparin-induced thrombocytopenia (HIT), which may cause thrombotic events. There is evidence that LMWH, just like UH, do not cross the placenta.

Toxicology

Based upon safety data, UH was previously considered to be the anticoagulant drug of choice during pregnancy for most indications. Maternal disadvantages include the risk of HIT, allergy, and osteoporosis. Long-term heparin therapy (>1 month) may be associated with increased bone loss, particularly during pregnancy, which is probably a cause of reversible bone demineralization in itself. UH can cause maternal bleeding; the same probably also applies to LMWH (Lindqvist 2000).

Low molecular-weight heparins have now largely replaced unfractioned heparin, because of their improved safety profile. The risks of HIT, allergy, and osteoporosis appear lower. Skin reactions have been reported; switching to another LMWH can be helpful. Like UH, LMWHs do not cross the human placenta, so there is no risk of teratogenesis or fetal hemorrhage. This was confirmed in several publications, which included the use of *enoxaparin, dalteparin, nadroparin, tinzaparin*, and *certoparin*. LMWHs are used for prophylaxis as well as for treatment (adjusted dose) of VTEs in pregnancy (Greer 2005, Bates 2004, McColl 2004, Sørensen 2000, Sanson 1999). In high-risk pregnant women with inherited thrombophilias, preliminary non-randomized studies suggest a benefit for prophylaxis with heparin (UH or LMWH) with or without low-dose aspirin, but controlled studies, assessing the specific risks and the benefits from possible interventions, are not sufficient to provide for definitive conclusions (Robertson 2005, Brenner 2005, Huxtable 2005, Vossen 2004, Kujovich 2004). At present, thromboprophylaxis during pregnancy is still controversial (Cetin 2005, Bates 2004, Greer 2003, Brenner 2003, Gebhardt 2003). However, consensus has been reached on thromboprophylaxis for recurrent pregnancy loss in patients with antiphospholipid syndrome. Although reports of LMWH use in pregnant women with prosthetic heart valves are starting to appear, data are not sufficient to make definitive recommendations. There is still concern regarding the efficacy of UH and LMWH in preventing thromboembolic complications. If used, aggressive adjusted dosing is recommended (Bates 2004).

Recommendation. Low molecular-weight heparins (LMWH) may be regarded as the anticoagulant drugs of choice for thromboprophylaxis and for the treatment of VTE during pregnancy. The combination of LMWH and low-dose aspirin is recommended for the prevention of pregnancy loss in women with phospholipid antibodies and previous pregnancy loss. No definitive recommendations can be given for the treatment of pregnant women with inherited thrombophilias or with mechanical heart valves.

2.9.3   Protamines

Pharmacology and toxicology

Protamines are simple (alkaline) proteins found in the sperm of several species. Protamin-HCl and protamine sulfate are anticoagulants used as an antidote for heparin, with which (heparins being strongly acid) they form an inactive complex, neutralizing the anticoagulant activities of both drugs. The protamine–heparin complex is eliminated by the kidneys. In cases of LMWH overdose, its efficacy as an antidote seems to be less.

> **Recommendation.** Protamines can be used during pregnancy in cases of heparin (or LMWH) overdose.

2.9.4   Low-dose aspirin (LDA)

Pharmacology and toxicology

Low-dosage treatment with 75–300 mg *acetylsalicylic acid* daily is prescribed for thrombosis prophylaxis and for the prevention of pre-eclampsia.

This therapy (preferably in combination with low molecular-weight heparins) is found to be effective in preventing recurrent pregnancy loss and other pregnancy complications in women with antiphospholipid syndrome, as in systemic lupus erythematosus (see also Chapter 2.9.2). Many studies indicate a benefit of low-dose aspirin, in combination with LMWHs or alone, in the treatment of high-risk thrombophilic pregnant women; other studies do not confirm these findings. In one meta-analysis, aspirin treatment seemed to have, for women with moderate and high risk, a small but significant effect on reducing the rate of preterm birth, but it did not reduce the rate of perinatal death (Kozer 2003). The use of low-dose aspirin for preventing recurrent pregnancy loss and other serious obstetrical complications in women with thrombophilia remains a subject for debate (Robertson 2005, Bates 2004, Gris 2004, Brenner 2003).

Many studies have looked at the use of 'low-dosage' treatment to prevent high blood pressure in pregnancy, and its consequences – such as, for instance, intrauterine growth delays (see Chapter 2.1.2 for further details). No adverse effects in the mother, fetus or newborn in association with the use of low-dose aspirin were observed.

> **Recommendation.** 'Low-dose' treatment with acetylsalicylic acid can be used for appropriate indications.

2.9.5   Other non-coumarin antithrombotic drugs

Pharmacology and toxicology

Hirudin-like compounds are *lepirudine* and *desirudin. Danaparoid* is a heparinoid with a molecular weight of about 6500 daltons, and, based upon molecular weight and similar compounds, it is likely that it will not cross the placenta. These compounds are used in cases of heparin intolerability, such as heparin-induced thrombocytopenia (HIT). In a recent review, use in pregnancy was evaluated; no indications of increased risk of adverse fetal outcome were observed (Lindhoff-Last 2005).

Dipyridamol, primarily indicated as a coronary vasodilator (see Chapter 2.8), is also used as a synergistic antithrombotic agent when administered with aspirin, or heparin, in patients with prosthetic heart valves. It has, combined with other anticoagulants, also been investigated in women with essential thrombocythemia, in attempts to reduce the incidence of recurrent abortions and fetal growth retardation. Unfortunately, data are insufficient for an opinion about its safety (Eliyahu 1997).

Abciximab, clopidogrel, eptibatide, ticlopidine, and *tirofiban* antagonize platelet aggregation. No data are available about their use during pregnancy. However, it was demonstrated that abciximab did not cross the *in vitro* perfused human placental lobule because it was degraded by the placenta since it is a chimearic Fab fragment (Miller 2003).

Recommendation.   In cases of heparin-induced thrombocytopenia (HIT), danaparoid may be prescribed. When one of the other abovementioned antithrombotics has been used during the first trimester, the termination of pregnancy or invasive diagnostics are not required.

2.9.6   Vitamin K antagonists

Pharmacology

Coumarin derivatives (4-hydroxycoumarin compounds) are oral anticoagulants (OA) that prevent vitamin K from acting as a cofactor in the hepatic synthesis of the vitamin K-dependent coagulation factors II, VII, IX, and X (as well as the anticoagulants, proteins C and S). They are also called vitamin K antagonists (VKA). Available coumarin derivatives are *acenocoumarol, phenprocoumon,* and *warfarin*. Apart from coumarins, the *indanediones, fluindione* and *phenidione*, are used as a VKA for the same purpose.

Coumarin derivatives are nearly totally resorbed in the gut and are bound to albumin by more than 95%. Because the action of the drug is based on inhibition of the synthesis of the coagulation factors, it takes 1–3 days before blood concentrations are effectively lowered and the drug becomes effective. Coumarins are oxidized in the liver and excreted by the kidneys. The elimination half-time is

24 hours for acenocoumarol, 36 hours for warfarin, and 150 hours for phenprocoumon. Interaction with other drugs can occur through competition, oxidating enzymes in the liver as well as binding to plasma proteins.

2

Toxicology

Pregnancy

The embryotoxic properties of coumarins have been established in humans. Coumarins readily cross the placenta and will reach the fetus. Coumarin therapy during pregnancy is implicated in two major adverse effects. Coumarins can produce a characteristic pattern of malformations, coumarin or warfarin embryopathy, central nerve system (CNS) abnormalities, and fetal bleeding. The rate of spontaneous abortion is also increased (Schaefer 2006, Blickstein 2002, Bates 1997, Pauli 1993, Hall 1980).

To estimate the prevalence of congenital anomalies associated with coumarin exposure during pregnancy, van Driel (2002A) reviewed 17 studies describing a total of 979 pregnancies, of which 449 involved acenocoumarol, 327 warfarin, and 203 an unspecified coumarin). From the 979 pregnancies, 689 children were born alive. Twenty-three children had skeletal anomalies, interpreted as indicative for coumarin embryopathy, of 394 children born alive to mothers using coumarins throughout pregnancy (6%).

Warfarin is by far the most discussed vitamin K antagonist (VKA) in scientific literature with respect to teratogenicity. Considering the pathogenetic mechanisms discussed in the context of warfarin, it can be assumed that all coumarins and indanediones have a similar teratogenic and fetotoxic potential. Van Driel et al. (2002A) summarized 57 reports published since 1955, describing 63 cases of congenital anomalies after exposure to VKAs. Of the 63 cases, 51 (81%) had skeletal anomalies. The most consistent clinical feature was mid-face hypoplasia ($n = 47$), including a depressed nasal bridge, underdevelopment or absence of the nasal septum, a small, upturned nose with grooves between the tip of the nose and the alae nasi, micrognathia, a prominent forehead, and a flat appearance of the face. Stippling in the epiphyseal regions (chondrodysplasia punctata) was described in 32 of the 63 cases, mostly along the axial skeleton, at the proximal femora and in the calcanei (Hall 1980). The possible mechanisms for this effect are thought to be the inhibition of the enzyme arylsulfatase and inhibition of the synthesis of vitamin K-dependent (non-coagulant) proteins, thus interfering with normal bone and cartilage development. This radiological finding apparently resolves as the epiphyses calcify. Limb hypoplasia, primarily involving the distal digits, may be seen in up to one-third of children with warfarin embryopathy (Pauli 1993). Other abnormalities that have been associated with the coumarin embryopathy are

2.9 Anticoagulant and fibrinolytic drugs

summarized by van Driel (2002A). Abnormalities described include abnormalities of the central nervous system, e.g. agenesis of the corpus callosum, schizencephaly, meningocele, Dandy-Walker malformation, and optic atrophy, as well as microcephaly, cerebral atrophy, hydrocephaly or ventriculomegaly, hearing loss, retardation, or slow development. Furthermore, there were a few cases reporting dysgenesis of the eye, cardiac defects (tetralogy of Fallot, persistent truncus arteriosus, and atrial septal defects), asplenia syndrome, absence of a kidney, cleft lip and palate, hypoplasia of the lungs with absence of the right diaphragm, and situs inversus. In addition, 13 cases of minor physical anomalies were reported, including low-set or poorly developed ears, a high-arched palate, hypertelorism, antimongoloid palpebral fissures, and widely spaced nipples.

Most publications state that the sensitive time for causing teratogenic effects (coumarin embryopathy) is in weeks 6–9, without clearly defining whether this is counted from conception or LMP, or evaluate those case reports exclusively exposed before week 9. A critical review of all published reports, however, does not provide evidence for a highly sensitive period until week 8 after LMP (week 6 postconception). Those five case reports cited in the literature as indicative for an embryopathy risk associated with exposure exclusively at ≤ week 8 were either calculated in weeks after conception (Hall 1989, Balde 1988), or causality was doubtful (Ruthnum 1987, Cox 1977) and/or additional contributing factors were reported (Lapiedra 1986).

CNS abnormalities are thought to result from intracerebral hemorrhages and subsequent scarring, and are associated with exposure at any time during pregnancy – mostly the second trimester. The sequelae of intracerebral bleeding appear to be more debilitating than those of the coumarin embryopathy; intracranial bleeding during delivery is especially to be feared.

To study long-term effects, van Driel (2003B, 2001) and Wesseling and co-workers (2001, 2000) compared a coumarin exposed cohort of about 300 children aged from 7.6 to 15.1 years with a control group consisting of some 260 non-exposed children, with respect to their neurological, behavioral, and cognitive development. There were only two children in the exposed cohort with signs of coumarin embryopathy. They were normally developed at 9.2 and 13.1 years, respectively (van Driel 2002B). The mean height and overall growth of exposed children did not differ from those of the unexposed children. None of the children was found to be neurologically abnormal. However, there was a slightly increased risk for minor neurological dysfunction after exposure during the second or third trimester (Wesseling 2001). There were no differences in mean IQ, but 11 of the exposed children versus 3 unexposed children measured an IQ of < 80. These 11 children were only exposed during the second and third trimesters. There were no differences in clinically relevant problem behavior. However, less favorable task-oriented and social–emotional behavior was observed among the exposed cohort (van Driel 2001). Three other follow-up studies with a total of 72 children could not find significant differences in physical or mental development (Olthof 1994, Wong 1993, Chong 1984). These data suggest that the risk of a healthy newborn developing late onset teratogenic effects of first-trimester VKA exposure is remote.

The largest controlled, prospective study until now includes 666 pregnancies with 670 exposures to different vitamin K antagonists. In this multicenter study, pregnancies were compared, with respect to their outcome, with 1049 controls. In most cases, treatment occurred from the beginning. This study confirmed the teratogenicity of coumarins, and revealed a three-fold miscarriage rate after first-trimester treatment. The rate of elective terminations was also higher. Live births occurred in only 53%. Prematurity was more frequent. The rate of major birth defects was significantly increased (OR 3.86; 95% CI 1.86–8.00). There were only two coumarin embryopathies observed among 356 live births (0.6%), and exposure to a vitamin K antagonist in these cases was later than 6 weeks postconception. The risk for coumarin embryopathy seems to be small, however, and the outcomes of this study confirmed that when exposure was limited to the first 6 (postconceptional) weeks, the risk of major malformations did not appear to be substantially increased (Peters 2006, Schaefer 2006).

Adverse outcome was suggested to be dose-dependent (more than 5 mg/day) in a small study of 52 patients with mechanical heart valves who had been exposed to warfarin during 71 pregnancies (Cotrufo 2002).

Several studies indicate that the choice of anticoagulant regimens for mechanical heart valve thromboprophylaxis during pregnancy should be made by balancing two risks: maternal morbidity and mortality from thromboembolic complications on the one hand, and fetal loss and embryopathy on the other – which means choosing between coumarin therapy throughout pregnancy, or substitution with adjusted-dose heparin between weeks 6 and 12. The dosage necessary to keep satisfactory levels of anticoagulation and thrombotic risks associated with specific valves are parameters to be reckoned with (Bates 2004, Cotrufo 2002, Chan 2000, Vitale 2000): maternal risk should be weighed against a possible fetal risk.

Recommendation. In view of possible fetal embryopathy and other adverse effects, coumarin derivatives are not recommended in the first trimester or at the end of pregnancy, and generally are not recommended

2

Pregnancy

2.9 Anticoagulant and fibrinolytic drugs

for use during pregnancy. Patients on coumarin derivatives who are planning a pregnancy should preferably be put on heparin (UH or LMWH) prior to pregnancy or, at the latest, prior to the sixth week after conception, which warrants adequate pregnancy testing. In high-risk patients with mechanical heart valves, an exception may be necessary because of maternal health requirements; here, oral anticoagulants throughout pregnancy until near term may need to be considered. The risk for coumarin embryopathy is small, in particular when therapy during the first trimester did not take place later than week 8 after the first day of last menstruation; therefore, elective termination of a wanted pregnancy is not recommended if (inadvertent) exposure took place in early pregnancy. Close follow-up by the obstetrician, including level II ultrasound, should be recommended in any case of vitamin K antagonist exposure during pregnancy.

2.9.7   Vitamin K

Pharmacology and toxicology

Vitamin K refers to a group of fatty substances important in the synthesis of coagulation factors. Vitamin K_1 (*phytomenadione, phytonadione, phylloquinone*) is found in plants; vitamin K_2 is synthesized from vitamin K_1 by various bacteria in adult intestines; vitamin K_3 (*menadione*) is a synthetic analog of vitamin K_1; and vitamin K_4 is the water-soluble form of menadione. Vitamin K is used as an antidote in treatment with coumarins. Under normal conditions, there is no need for the administration of vitamin K in pregnant women because gastrointestinal bacteria supply adequate amounts. Women who are taking certain drugs or antibiotics (such as anticonvulsants, rifampin, isoniazid) may be vitamin K-deficient due to the enhanced degradation or alterations in bowel flora. In such women, supplementation with vitamin K has been recommended.

Vitamin K is also used in neonates to treat the increased physiological bleeding risk. This phenomenon is caused by the relative deficiency of vitamin K, due on the one hand to the absence of intestinal bacteria to form sufficient amounts of vitamin K, and on the other hand for the deficient capability of the neonatal liver to synthesize those (vitamin K-dependent) proteins that are important for the coagulation process.

Published human experience with the use of vitamin K during pregnancy is limited to the third trimester.

Vitamin K_1 does not seem to cross the placenta readily (Shearer 1982). The transfer of vitamin K to the fetus or the amelioration of neonatal hemostasis has not been reported convincingly to date (Anai 1993). Prenatal menadione exposure has been associated with neonatal hyperbilirubinemia. Former concerns that parenteral vitamin K application in neonates may increase the risk of childhood cancer have not been confirmed in the literature, and are generally refuted (Roman 2002).

For prophylaxis with vitamin K, oral administration of 1–2 mg directly after birth is recommended. Parenteral administration is advised in neonates at high risk.

> **Recommendation.** Newborns should routinely receive 1–2 mg of vitamin K directly after birth. In those cases where the mother was treated with vitamin K-antagonizing drugs (such as the antiepileptics carbamazepine, phenobarbital, phenytoin or primidone, or with rifampicin or coumarin derivatives), parenteral administration directly after birth is advised, and the neonate should be given 1–2 mg vitamin K orally two to three times a week during the first 2 weeks after birth.

2.9.8   Fibrinolysis

Fibrinolytic drugs are used to dissolve thrombotic blocking. Fibrin, an end product of coagulation, is a polymer that is broken up into water-soluble parts by plasmin, a peptidase. These fibrin parts then dissolve along with the thrombus. Plasmin is formed from plasminogen, an endogenous glycoprotein, under the influence of endogenous activators like *urokinase* and *tissue-plasminogen activator*. Apart from these, exogenous substances such as *streptokinase* can enhance the forming of plasminogen. In the case of a hemorrhage as a result of fibrinolytic therapy, synthetic inhibitors like *tranexamic acid* and *para-aminomethyl-benzoic acid* (*PAMBA*) will have rapid hemostatic action.

2.9.9   Streptokinase

Pharmacology and toxicology

Streptokinase is a plasminogen activator isolated from hemolytic streptococci. Through the forming of plasmin, it will have fibrinolytic effects on recently formed (not older than a few hours) thrombi. Probably no more than trace amounts of streptokinase will cross the placenta; maternal treatment has not caused fibrinolytic effects in exposed fetuses (Turrentine 1995). The half-life of streptokinase is only 20 minutes. Data on the use of streptokinase during pregnancy are limited. In several articles (Usta 2004, Nassar 2003, Turrentine 1995, Ludwig 1973), some 170 women were reported to have been treated with streptokinase during pregnancy; there were no fetal complications, and a direct or indirect risk to the fetus was not established. There have been rare reports of retroplacental hematoma and placental abruption. Being an antigen, streptokinase is capable of evoking the formation of maternal antibodies, which cross the placenta and can cause a passing sensitization of the fetus.

> **Recommendation.** Streptokinase can be used during pregnancy in life-threatening circumstances. Care is needed when using streptokinase during the intrapartum period, because of an increased risk of maternal hemorrhage.

2.9.10   Other fibrinolytics

Pharmacology and toxicology

Urokinase is a plasminogen activator that is normally found in mammalian blood and urine. It plays an important role in the solution of physiologic clotting – for instance, in menstrual bleeding. It also is thought to play a role in preventing microthrombi in the placental circulation. There are insufficient data on the use of urokinase during pregnancy. In a few cases, the therapeutic use of urokinase during pregnancy was followed by the delivery of a healthy infant (la Valleur 1996, Turrentine 1995).

Alteplase (tissue-plasminogen activator) is an endogenous factor from endothelial cells that exerts its activity mainly in contact with the fibrin from thrombi. It is questionable whether this new fibrinolytic agent from gentechnology will surpass the older ones. There are no data on its use during pregnancy.

Regarding *antistreptase*, *reteplase*, and *acetylized-plasminogen-streptokinase-activator-complex* (APSAC), there is no information about their use during pregnancy.

> **Recommendation.** Urokinase, alteplase, antistreptase, and APSAC should only be used during pregnancy in life-threatening circumstances. Special precaution is needed when using them during the intrapartum period, because of the risk of increased maternal bleeding. Inadvertent use during the first trimester does not require the termination of pregnancy, or invasive diagnostic procedures.

2.9.11   Inhibitors of fibrinolysis

Pharmacology and toxicology

Aprotinin is a polypeptid that inhibits many proteinases – among others, plasmin and plasminogen activators – which explains its antifibrinolytic properties. As a foreign protein, it can induce sensitization. There is no information on its use during pregnancy.

Epsilon-aminocaproic acid is an inhibitor of fibrinolysis. The use of this agent is associated with an increased risk of thrombosis and embolism, with possible renal failure from thrombosis in glomerular capillary arteries. It was reported not to be teratogenic in rabbits. No information is available regarding its use during pregnancy.

Para-aminomethyl-benzoic acid and *tranexamic acid* are synthetically derived antifibrinolytic agents. They act like epsilon-aminocaproic acid, and are used for the treatment of coagulopathies with increased fibrinolytic activity.

> **Recommendation.** There are no specific indications for the use of aprotinin, epsilon-aminocaproic acid, para-aminomethyl-benzoic acid or tranexamic acid during pregnancy. Inadvertent use during the first trimester does not require the termination of pregnancy or invasive diagnostic procedures.

2.9.12   Volume expanders

Volume expanders are dextrans, gelatin derivatives, hydroxy ethyl starch, and human albumin solutions. They may be used during pregnancy only for appropriate indications, such as circulatory shock; they are not indicated for the purpose of hemodilution, which can be achieved with electrolyte solutions.

Because of the risks of viral contamination (HIV, hepatitis B and C, cytomegaly), blood transfusions should only be administered during pregnancy when there is a vital indication.

▶ Dextrans

Dextrans are glucopolysaccharides used as volume expanders. They are available with a mean molecular weight of 60 000/70 000 (dextran 60/dextran 70) and with a mean molecular weight of 40 000 (dextran 40). Dextran 60 (70) has a half-life of 24 hours and dextran 40 has a half-life of 6 hours. They have thrombocyte aggregation-inhibiting properties. Dextrans may cause serious anaphylactoid reactions that can be prevented by injecting 20 ml of the low molecular-weight (1000) hapten dextran (dextran 1) before a dextran infusion. Specific embryo- or fetotoxic effects have not been observed to date. An anaphylactic reaction may be of concern, though, because it endangers the fetus.

> **Recommendation.** Dextrans can be used as volume expanders in pregnancy in cases of emergency.

► **Gelatins**

Gelatin derivatives, such as *polygeline* and *modified gelatin,* are polypeptides used as plasma substitutes in the form of polymers with a mean molecular weight of about 35 000 in a 4% solution. Specific embryo- or fetotoxic effects have not been observed to date.

> **Recommendation.** Gelatin derivatives can be used as volume expanders in cases of emergency.

► **Hydroxy ethyl starch**

Hydroxy ethyl starch (HES) is, just like dextran, a network of polysaccharides. The mean molecular weight lies between 70 000 and 200 000, depending on the compound. Low molecular-weight hydroxy ethyl starch may enhance the liquid properties of blood. Anaphylactic reactions may occur. Apart from possible precipitation in the placenta, no embryo- or fetotoxic effects have been observed.

> **Recommendation.** Hydroxy ethyl starch can be used as a volume expander in pregnancy in cases of emergency or to improve microcirculation.

► **Albumin**

Albumin (human) is formed from the blood of healthy donors, and should be free from HIV and hepatitis virus. Human albumin is administered in cases of albumin deficiency, to raise the osmotic pressure in cases of edema and intravascular hypovolemia. Human albumin cannot cross the placenta. There are no known embryo- or fetotoxic effects. In cases of significant proteinuria, as an indication of renal disturbances, none of the mentioned substances is certain to maintain or act upon osmotic pressure.

> **Recommendation.** Human albumin can be used during pregnancy as a volume expander, and in cases of albumin deficiency.

References

Adelberg AM, Kuller JA. Thrombophilias and recurrent miscarriage. Obstet Gynecol Surv 2002; 57: 703–9.

Anai T, Hirota Y, Yoshimatsu J et al. Can prenatal vitamin K1 (phylloquinone) supplementation replace prophylaxis at birth? Obstet Gynecol 1993; 81: 251–4.

Balde MD, Breitbach GP, Wettstein A et al. Tetralogy of Fallot following coumarin administration in early pregnancy – an embryopathy? {in German}. Geburtshilfe Frauenheilkd 1988; 48: 182–3.

Bates SM, Ginsberg JS. Anticoagulants in pregnancy: fetal effects. Baillieres Clin Obstet Gynaecol 1997; 11: 479–88.

Bates SM, Greer IA, Hirsh J et al. Use of Antithrombotic Agents during Pregnancy: The Seventh ACCP Conference on Antithrombotic and Thrombolytic Therapy. Chest 2004; 126(Suppl 3): S627–44.

Blickstein D, Blickstein I. The risk of fetal loss associated with Warfarin anticoagulation. Intl J Gynaecol Obstet 2002; 78: 221–5.

Brenner B, Kupferminc MJ. Inherited thrombophilia and poor pregnancy outcome. Best Pract Res Clin Obstet Gynecol 2003; 17: 427–39.

Brenner B, Hoffman R, Carp H et al. Efficacy and safety of two doses of enoxaparin in women with thrombophilia and recurrent pregnancy loss: the LIVE-ENOX study. J Thromb Haemost 2005; 3: 227–9.

Cetin I. Is it time for clinical use of LMWH in women with adverse pregnancy outcome or do we need large-scale prospective studies? J Thromb Haemost 2005; 3: 791–2.

Chan WS, Anand S, Ginsberg JS. Anticoagulation of pregnant women with mechanical heart valves – a systematic review of the literature. Arch Intern Med 2000; 160: 191–6.

Chong MK, Harvey D, de Swiet M. Follow-up study of children whose mothers were treated with warfarin during pregnancy. Br J Obstet Gynaecol 1984; 91: 1070–73.

Cotrufo M, De Feo M, De Santo L et al. Risk of warfarin during pregnancy with mechanical valve prostheses. Obstet Gynecol 2002; 99: 35–40.

Cox DR, Martin L, Hall BD. Asplenia syndrome after fetal exposure to warfarin. Lancet 1977; 26: 1134.

Dizon-Townson D, Branch DW. Anticoagulant treatment during pregnancy: an update. Semin Thromb Hemost 1998; 24(Suppl 1): 55–62.

Dudding TE, Attia J. The association between adverse pregnancy outcomes and maternal factor V Leiden genotype: a meta-analysis. Thromb Haemost 2004; 91: 700–11.

Eliyahu S, Shalev E. Essential thrombocythemia during pregnancy. Obstet Gynecol Surv 1997; 52: 243–7.

Gebhardt GS, Hall DR. Inherited and acquired thrombophilias and poor pregnancy outcome: should we be treating with heparin? Curr Opin Obstet Gynecol 2003; 15: 501–6.

Greer IA. Thrombophilia: implications for pregnancy outcome. Thromb Res 2003; 109: 73–81.

Greer IA, Nelson PC. Low-molecular-weight heparins for thromboprophylaxis and treatment of venous thromboembolism in pregnancy: a systematic review of safety and efficacy. Blood 2005; 106: 401–7.

Gris JC, Mercier E, Quere I et al. Low-molecular-weight heparin versus low-dose aspirin in women with one fetal loss and a constitutional thrombophilic disorder. Blood 2004; 103: 3695–9.

Hall BD. Warfarin embryopathy and urinary tract anomalies: possible new association {Letter}. Am J Med Genet 1989; 34: 292–3.

Hall JG, Pauli RM, Wilson KM. Maternal and fetal sequelae of anticoagulation during pregnancy. Am J Med 1980; 68: 122–40.

Huxtable LM, Tafreshi MJ, Ondreyco SM. A protocol for the use of enoxaparin during pregnancy: results from 85 pregnancies including 13 multiple gestation pregnancies. Clin Appl Thromb Hemostasis 2005; 11: 171–81.

Kozer E, Costei AM, Boskovic R et al. Effects of aspirin consumption during pregnancy on pregnancy outcomes: meta-analysis. Birth Def Res B 2003; 68: 70–84.

Kujovich JL. Thrombophilia and pregnancy complications. Am J Obstet Gynecol 2004; 191: 412–24.

Lapiedra OJ, Bernal JM, Ninot S et al. Open heart surgery for thrombosis of a prosthetic mitral valve during pregnancy. Fetal hydrocephalus. J Cardiovasc Surg (Torino) 1986; 27: 217–20.

la Valleur J, Molina E, Williams PP et al. Use of urokinase in pregnancy. Two success stories. Postgrad Med 1996; 99: 269–70, 272–3.

Lindhoff-Last E, Kreutzenbeck HJ, Magnani HN. Treatment of 51 pregnancies with danaparoid because of heparin intolerance. Thromb Haemost 2005; 93: 63–9.

Lindqvist PG, Dahlback B. Bleeding complications associated with low molecular weight heparin prophylaxis during pregnancy. Thromb Haemost 2000; 84: 140–41.

Ludwig H. Results of streptokinase therapy in deep venous thrombosis during pregnancy. Postgrad Med J 1973; 49(Suppl): 65–7.

McColl MD, Greer IA. Low-molecular-weight heparin for the prevention and treatment of venous thromboembolism in pregnancy. Curr Opin Pulmon Med 2004; 10: 371–5.

Miller RK, Mace K, Polliotti B et al. Marginal transfer of ReoPro™ (abciximab) compared with immunoglobulin G (F105), inulin and water in the perfused human placenta. In vitro. Placenta; 24: 727–38.

Nassar AH, Abdallah ME, Moukarbel GV et al. Sequential use of thrombolytic agents for thrombosed mitral valve prosthesis during pregnancy. J Perinatal Med 2003; 31: 257–60.

Olthof E, De Vries TW, Touwen BC et al. Late neurological, cognitive and behavioural sequelae of prenatal exposure to coumarins: a pilot study. Early Hum Dev 1994; 38: 97–109.

Pauli RM, Haun JM. Intrauterine effects of coumarin derivatives. Dev Brain Dysfunct 1993; 6: 229–47.

Peters PWJ. Vitamin K antagonists in pregnancy – an overestimated risk? Thromb Haemost 2006; 95: 922–3.

Robertson L, Wu O, Langhorne P et al. Thrombophilia in pregnancy: a systematic review. Br J Haematol 2006; 132: 171–96.

Roman E, Fear NT, Ansell P et al. Vitamin K and childhood cancer: analysis of individual patient data from six case-control studies. Br J Cancer 2002; 86: 63–9.

Ruthnum P, Tolmie JL. Atypical malformations in an infant exposed to warfarin during the first trimester of pregnancy. Teratology 1987; 36: 299–301.

Sanson BJ, Lensing AWA, Prins MH et al. Safety of low-molecular-weight heparin in pregnancy: a systematic review. Thromb Haemost 1999; 81: 668–72.

Schaefer C, Hannemann D, Meister R et al. Vitamin K antagonists and pregnancy outcome – a multi-centre prospective study. Thromb Haemost 2006; 95: 949–57.

Shearer MJ, Rahim S, Barkhan et al. Plasma vitamin K1 in mothers and their newborn babies. Lancet 1982; 2: 460–63.

Sørensen HT, Johnsen SP, Larsen H et al. Birth outcomes in pregnant women treated with low-molecular-weight heparin. Acta Obstet Gynecol Scand 2000; 79: 655–9.

Turrentine MA, Braems G, Ramirex MM. Use of thrombolytics for the treatment of thromboembolic disease during pregnancy. Obstet Gynecol Surv 1995; 50: 534–41.

Usta IM, Abdallah M, El Hajj M et al. Massive subchorionic hematomas following thrombolytic therapy in pregnancy. Obstet Gynecol 2004; 103(5 Pt 2): 1079–82.

Van Driel D, Wesseling J, Sauer JJ et al. In utero exposure to coumarins and cognition at 8 to 14 years old. Pediatrics 2001; 107: 123–9.

Van Driel D (A), Wesseling J, Sauer PJJ et al. Teratogen update: fetal effects after in utero exposure to coumarins overview of cases, follow-up findings, and pathogenesis. Teratology 2002; 66(3): 127–40.

Van Driel D (B), Wesseling J, de Vries TW et al. Coumarin embryopathy: long-term follow-up of two cases. Eur J Pediatr 2002; 161: 231–2.

Vitale N, de Freo M, de Santo LS et al. Dose-dependent fetal complications of warfarin in pregnant women with mechanical heart valves. J Am Coll Cardiol 1999; 33: 1637–41.

Vossen CY, Preston FE, Conard J et al. Hereditary thrombophilia and fetal loss: a prospective follow-up study. J Thromb Haemost 2004; 2: 592–6.

Wesseling J, van Driel D, Heymans HS et al. Behavioural outcome of school-age children after prenatal exposure to coumarins. Early Hum Dev 2000: 58: 213–24.

Wesseling J, van Driel D, van der Veer E et al. Neurological outcome in school-age children after prenatal exposure to coumarins. Early Hum Dev 2001: 63: 83–95.

Wong V, Cheng CH, Chan KC. Fetal and neonatal outcome of exposure to anticoagulants during pregnancy. Am J Med Genet 1993; 45: 17–21.

Antiepileptics

2.10

Elisabeth Robert-Gnansia and
Christof Schaefer

2.10.1 Epilepsy and antiepileptic drugs in pregnancy

It has been known for several decades that infants of epileptic mothers are at an increased risk of major and minor malformations. This is mainly attributable to the teratogenicity of antiepileptic drugs (AED), the disease in itself increasing the risk mildly, if at all (Morrow 2006, Artama 2005, Fried 2004, Holmes 2001). No epidemiological technique, though, is ideal to separate the effects of the disease from those of the drugs on the fetus. Few epileptic patients can live without treatment, and it might be questioned whether those who can are indeed actually epileptic. Lindhout and Omtzigt (1992) described a marked increase in malformations amongst infants exposed to first-trimester seizures. However, most investigators have found that maternal seizures during pregnancy had no impact on the frequency of malformations (Canger 1999, Kaneko 1999, Dansky 1991), or on the development of infant epilepsy or febrile convulsions (Dansky 1991). There have been reports of maternal seizures during pregnancy being associated with an increased risk of miscarriage, preterm labor, intracranial hemorrhage, and fetal hypoxia with bradycardia. Adab (2004) showed that five or more tonic–clonic seizures in pregnancy were predictive of a lower IQ, after adjustment for confounding factors. There is no compelling epidemiological evidence that positively correlates the duration of antiepileptic drug therapy prior to conception with an increased risk for an adverse pregnancy outcome (Dansky 1991). In a study by Holmes (2000), 57 children whose mothers had a history of epilepsy, but did not have any antiepileptic medication or seizures during their pregnancies, were evaluated. When compared with a matched control group, there was no difference between the two groups of children in either IQ scores or physical features (facial dysmorphia or digit hypoplasia).

Several dysmorphic syndromes have been described related to classical antiepileptic drugs (AEDs), i.e. *phenytoin, valproic acid, trimethadione, carbamazepine, phenobarbital*, and *primidone*. The developmental anomalies resemble each other, and may be referred to as an anticonvulsant or epilepsy syndrome, instead of a phenytoin, barbiturate, carbamazepine or valproic acid (VPA) syndrome. Reactive epoxide metabolites of the anticonvulsants are regarded as a cause of the embryotoxic effects (Raymond 1995, Omtzigt 1993, Buehler 1990).

> ### AEDs and folic acid

Among others, folic acid deficiency has been discussed as a possible teratogenic pathway for anticonvulsants (Lindhout 1992, Seip 1976). Blake (1978) showed in rats that folic acid treatment during pregnancy prevented the decrease in phenytoin hydroxylase-specific activity, and thus may prevent the embryotoxic effects. El Mazar (1992) made a study in mice, supporting the view that VPA-induced teratogenesis may be mediated via an interaction with folate metabolism. Although folinic acid and vitamin B_6 + vitamin B_{12} could effectively reduce valproate-induced malformations, the protection was not complete, which may suggest the involvement of other factors. A study on folic acid antagonists (including anticonvulsants) and the risk of birth defects (Hernandez-Diaz 2000) did not demonstrate a protective effect of periconceptional folic acid supplementation, and another had the same conclusions (Craig 1999). Nevertheless, as a minimum of 0.4 mg folic acid per day is now recommended for any woman, epileptic patients should be given daily supplementations according to national recommendations – at least until the eighth week of pregnancy. A higher dosage of 4–5 mg is recommended by most authors.

Recommendations for anticonvulsant therapy. Because treatment with antiepileptics increases the risk of fetal anomalies, the following recommendations for anticonvulsant therapy are made:

- The importance of planned pregnancies with effective birth control should be emphasized, with consideration of the effects of the enzyme-inducing AEDs lowering the efficacy of hormonal contraceptive medications (Zupanc 2006): carbamazepine, felbamate (a mild inducer), oxcarbazepine (a mild inducer), phenobarbital, phenytoin, primidone, and topiramate (a mild inducer). Careful patient management, including the use of an intrauterine device (IUD) or hormonal contraceptives with an increased anti-ovulatory dosage in patients receiving enzyme-inducing AEDs, may further minimize the risk of unintended pregnancies.
- Antiepileptics are not to be used for other indications than epilepsy – e.g. bipolar disorder – when a pregnancy is planned.
- Before pregnancy occurs, the patient's diagnosis and treatment regimen should be reassessed. It is important to verify whether the individual patient continues to require medications, and whether she is taking the most appropriate AED to balance control of her seizures with teratogenic risks. For most women who have epilepsy, withdrawal of all AEDs before pregnancy is not a realistic option.
- A decision to undergo a trial while not taking AEDs before a planned pregnancy should be based on the same principles used for AED withdrawal in any person who has epilepsy. The trial should be completed at least 6 months before planned conception to provide some reassurance that seizures are not going to recur.
- A woman with epilepsy must be informed that the risk of a congenital malformation for her child is increased two- to three-fold. On the other

hand, she has a better than 90% chance of bringing a child without major birth defects into the world.

- Differential risks among AEDs should be considered. Changing the treatment of a woman with well-controlled epilepsy in cases of medication with a potential teratogenic risk may be a risk for inducing seizures. In the absence of alternative medication, phenytoin and carbamazepine may be continued when pregnancy is planned. When a woman is treated with valproic acid, efforts should be made to change her medication for another anticonvulsant.
- If a woman who has epilepsy definitely requires AEDs for seizure control, then monotherapy should be used, if possible (Kaneko 1999, Samrén 1999, Bertollini 1987, Källén 1986). If large daily doses are needed, then frequent smaller doses (three or four doses a day) or extended-release formulations may be helpful to avoid high blood peak levels. Dosages should be kept as low as can be justified therapeutically. To achieve this, regular monitoring of maternal serum levels should be considered.
- A treatment including a combination of anticonvulsants (polytherapy) is not an indication for the termination of pregnancy. In this case, the therapy should be reviewed critically, and the dosage cautiously reduced to as low as is therapeutically justified.
- Pregnant epileptic women treated with AEDs should be offered prenatal diagnosis. In spite of studies which did not discover an increased risk of malformations in children of untreated women with epilepsy (such as Holmes 2001), such women should also be offered prenatal diagnosis as a precaution. This should include a detailed anatomical fetal ultrasound with an experienced clinician during the second trimester, to rule out major disturbances of structural development.

In this chapter, sections 2.10.2–9 discuss the classical antiepileptic drugs, while sections 2.10.10–19 concentrate on the newer antiepileptics.

2.10.2   Benzodiazepines

Pharmacology

Benzodiazepines are used as AEDs, tranquilizers, and hypnotics. In the following pages, only those representatives of this group which are currently used for antiepileptic therapy will be discussed (for details on benzodiazepines, see also Chapter 2.11). *Diazepam* and *clonazepam* have proven themselves as AEDs. They inhibit the spread of pathological excitation, but not focal activities. Following oral administration, diazepam is quickly absorbed and is primarily bound to plasma proteins. It is hydroxylated in the liver and metabolized to the still active desmethyldiazepam, which is excreted through the kidneys after glucuronidation. The half-life is between 1 and 2 days; in newborns it is considerably longer because of the diminished clearance. Diazepam crosses the placenta easily. During birth, the concentration in the cord blood is up to three times the level in the maternal blood (Bakke 1982).

Clonazepam and *clobazam* are similar to diazepam, chemically and structurally.

Toxicology

Earlier publications have described an increased risk of cleft lip and cleft palate with *diazepam* treatment (Saxen 1975). This could not be substantiated in a later trial (Rosenberg 1983). In view of one case report describing an oblique facial cleft in a newborn of a mother who attempted suicide in early pregnancy with 50 tablets of diazepam (Rivas 1984), and given the rarity of this malformation, an increased risk with extremely high dosages can be suspected. Other birth defects, i.e. inguinal hernia, were described but could not be confirmed. The question was reviewed in a meta-analysis (Dolovitch 1998): pooled data from cohort studies demonstrated no association between fetal exposure to benzodiazepines and the risk of major malformations or oral cleft. Case-control studies, however, indicated increased rates of major birth defects, in particular isolated oral clefts.

Laegreid (1989) reported on eight children whose mothers had abused prescription drugs during their pregnancies, taking at least 30 mg of diazepam and 75 mg of oxazepam per day. All the children had facial anomalies; in addition, some of them were microcephalic, had toxic symptoms (apnea), and showed signs of withdrawal postpartum. Later, mental retardation, attention deficits, and hyperkinetic disorders were observed to varying degrees. However, these case descriptions have been criticized on the grounds that the kind of exposure and its scope are not adequately documented and, in one case, that Zellweger syndrome was not ruled out. In follow-up studies on the children at about 18 months, an improvement in the symptoms was established (Laegreid 1992).

In a number of animal studies (Kellogg 1985, Simmons 1984), it is has been demonstrated that diazepam at low dosages can modify selected behaviors based upon permanent modification of the downstream responses to the benzodiazepine receptors. The results of these studies support the hypothesis that *in utero* exposure to drugs targeted for action on the central nervous system, including diazepam, can induce long-lasting alterations to the neural substrates of behavior of the offspring, with resulting functional consequences.

Benzodiazepine therapy does not seem, according to the current state of knowledge, to have as high a teratogenic risk as the other anticonvulsants. However, the risk of functional disturbances in newborns is to be considered when benzodiazepines are used in high doses during the birth process, or when 15–20 mg is taken regularly over a prolonged period, including during the last trimester. On the one hand, respiratory depression must be expected after high doses pre-partum – for example, for treatment of seizures during eclampsia. On the other hand, after continuous exposure, withdrawal symptoms like restlessness, tremors, muscular hypertonia, vomiting, diarrhea, and convulsions can occur in the neonatal period. A "floppy infant syndrome", with muscle flacidity, lethargy, disturbances of temperature regulation, and weak sucking, lasting from a week to many months, has been described. A dose–response relationship is likely, because the frequency of newborn complications rises when doses exceed 30–40 mg or when diazepam is taken for extended periods, allowing accumulation to occur (Gillberg 1977, Haram 1977, Scanlon 1975). However, because it accumulates in the fetus, daily doses of even 6 mg of diazepam may lead to symptoms in neonates.

In the newborn, diazepam can dislodge bilirubin from its binding with albumin and – at least theoretically – at high dosages can intensify the neonatal icterus.

There are about 175 documented pregnancies with exposure to *clonazepam* in pregnancy (Lin 2004, Vajda 2003, Weinstock 2001, Ornoy 1998). Although tetralogy of Fallot, microcephaly, and dysmorphic features were observed, no particular pattern of anomalies can be defined, and data do not show a significant increase in major birth defects.

There is insufficient information on *clobazam* in pregnancy with respect to fetal outcome. Structural teratogenic effects are just as unlikely as they are with other benzodiazepines. In the neonatal period, the same complications as with diazepam would seem to be possible.

> **Recommendation.** Should there be an indication for low doses of diazepam or clonazepam, treatment is permitted even during the first trimester. After long-term treatment, especially during the third trimester, withdrawal effects in the newborn must be expected, and the child should be observed closely during the first days of life. This applies also to those cases where high dosages were used shortly before or during delivery, when neonatal respiratory depression is possible.
>
> Exposure to benzodiazepines is not an indication for a termination of the pregnancy. In cases of abuse or long-term treatment with high dosages during organogenesis, a detailed fetal anatomical ultrasound examination should be offered. If such exposure has occurred during later pregnancy, observations of fetal motor patterns can be performed by ultrasound.

2.10 Antiepileptics

2.10.3   Carbamazepine

Pharmacology

Carbamazepine has structural similarities to tricyclic antidepressants, and is used for grand-mal epilepsy, focal and psychomotor seizures, and trigeminal neuralgia. The anticonvulsive action of carbamazepine, similar to that of other AEDs, can be explained as a membrane-stabilizing action. Carbamazepine is well-absorbed when given orally, binds strongly to proteins, and has a plasma half-life of 1–2 days. In the fetus, carbamazepine reaches 50–80% of the maternal concentration.

Toxicology

Carbamazepine is teratogenic in human beings. Monotherapy was found to increase the malformation rate about a two-fold by several authors (Matalon 2002, Ornoy 2000, Canger 1999, Kaneko 1999, Samrén 1999, 1997), while others do not find increased rates of birth defects (Morrow 2006, Artama 2005, Kaaja 2003). A single group of investigators described a fetal carbamazepine syndrome, with dysmorphic features – e.g. upslanting palpebral fissures, epicanthal folds, short nose, long philtrum, distal digit hypoplasia, and microcephaly (Jones 1989). Carbamazepine increases the risk of spina bifida, microcephaly, and hypospadias. The risk of spina bifida is increased about ten-fold – i.e. it occurs in about 1% of exposed newborns. Apart from spina bifida, there have been additional reports of hypospadias, microcephaly, some facial dysmorphic features, and the absence of hypoplastic distal phalanges (Källén 1994, Robert 1994, Little 1993, Rosa 1991, Jones 1989). Dean (2002) observed cases of facial dysmorphology and developmental delay.

After an association between carbamazepine and congenital eye malformations (i.e. anophthalmia, microphthalmia, and coloboma) in children was proposed by Sutcliffe (1998), who reported four cases, a Dutch group from EUROCAT (Kroes 2002) checked all of their cases with eye malformations for carbamazepine use by the mother, and also reviewed 13 studies in the literature. The analysis did not support Sutcliffe's hypothesis.

Kaaja (2003) prospectively followed up 970 pregnancies in women with epilepsy at a single maternity clinic. The occurrence of major malformations was associated with various anticonvulsants, but not with carbamazepine monotherapy.

The teratogenic effect of carbamazepine seems to be associated with noticeably reduced activity of the enzyme, epoxide hydrolase. This enzyme defect – apparently attributable to a genetic predisposition – may be measured in the fetal amniocytes, but a test for routine clinical use is as yet not available.

Postnatal development

The risk of cognitive disturbances with carbamazepine monotherapy was reported in subsequent studies (Ornoy 1996), and observed especially in children who also have facial dysmorphia. On the contrary, in a study by Gaily (2004), the intelligence of 182 children of mothers with epilepsy (study group) and 141 control children was tested in a blinded setting at preschool or school age. Data on maternal antiepileptic treatment and seizures during pregnancy were gathered prospectively. Of these children, 107 were exposed to antiepileptic monotherapy, among them 86 to carbamazepine. Thirty children were exposed to polytherapy; 23 cases included carbamazepine. The median maternal doses and blood levels of carbamazepine during the second half of pregnancy were 600 mg and 26 μmol/l. The mean verbal and non-verbal IQ scores in the children exposed *in utero* to carbamazepine monotherapy did not differ from those in the control subjects. The authors concluded that carbamazepine monotherapy with maternal serum levels within the reference range does not impair intelligence in prenatally exposed offspring. Exposures to polytherapy and to another drug (valproate) during pregnancy were associated with significantly reduced verbal intelligence.

Carbamazepine can induce vitamin K deficiency, resulting in coagulation disturbances in the neonate (Howe 1999), like all enzyme-inducing AEDs (see also section 2.10.6).

Recommendation. Carbamazepine may be used in pregnancy to treat epilepsy, keeping in mind the risks mentioned. Monotherapy is desirable. The drug concentration should be monitored regularly, and the daily dose kept as low as can be justified therapeutically. Liver and kidney function, as well as hematological parameters, should be checked regularly.

Exposure to carbamazepine does not require termination of pregnancy. However, as an additional preventive measure, a detailed ultrasound diagnosis should be conducted in the second trimester as well as an α-fetoprotein determination in the maternal serum around week 16, especially to detect neural tube defects.

To decrease the risk of coagulation disturbances in the fetus and newborn, the newborn should receive 1 mg of vitamin K (preferably intramuscularly) at birth and 1 mg orally every 3 days in the first 2 weeks of life (see also section 2.10.6).

2.10.4   Ethosuximide and other succimides

Pharmacology

Ethosuximide is only effective with petit-mal seizures. It seems to facilitate the transfer of glucose in the brain and, under experimental conditions, it raises the seizure threshold.

Ethosuximide is well-absorbed when taken orally, and reaches a maximum concentration in the blood after 3–4 hours. It binds to protein plasma only to a limited extent. Plasma concentrations of 40–100 μg/ml are required to prevent petit-mal seizures.

Toxicology

There are only a few reports of ethosuximide therapy during pregnancy. No typical pattern of birth defects has been observed in the infants of 57 treated women (Lindhout 1992). In a series of 18 fetuses exposed during the first trimester, there were no birth defects (Rosa 1993, cited in Briggs 2005). No adverse effect was detected either among 13 exposures (Samrén 1997). Although the available reports are in no way sufficient for a differentiated risk assessment, there does not seem to be a teratogenic risk comparable to the other anticonvulsants. There is a report of neonatal hemorrhage following *in utero* exposure to ethosuximide, indicating a vitamin K antagonistic potential (Speidel 1974).

There is insufficient experience with the other succinimides, *mesuximide* and *phensuccimide*, to assess their risks in pregnancy.

> **Recommendation.** Ethosuximide belongs to the drug of choice for petit-mal seizures in pregnancy. Mesuximide and phensuccimide are less well-studied, and are therefore not recommended.
>
> Exposure to succimide derivatives does not require a termination of pregnancy. However, detailed ultrasound diagnosis around week 20 should confirm normal development of the fetus.
>
> To decrease the risk of coagulation disturbances in the fetus and newborn, the newborn should receive 1 mg of vitamin K (preferably intramuscularly) at birth and 1 mg orally every 3 days in the first 2 weeks of life (see also section 2.10.6).

2.10.5   Oxazolidine anticonvulsants

Pharmacology and toxicology

Trimethadione used to be the best known of the oxazolidine derivatives. Currently, this drug is no longer used because of its numerous side effects and because of the availability of better medications.

Oxazolidine was used to treat petit-mal seizures. Experience is limited, depending primarily on 36 documented pregnancies in 9 families, and suggesting a comparatively high teratogenic risk. Among the signs of "trimethadione syndrome", similar to those connected to other anticonvulsants, are pre- and postnatal growth retardation, mental developmental delays, speech defects, craniofacial signs such as deformed, low-set ears, palate deformities including clefts, microcephaly, epicanthus and dental anomalies, broad nasal bridge, V-shaped eyebrows, and developmental disturbances of the heart, the extremities, and the urogenital tract (reviewed by Briggs 2005).

2

Pregnancy

> **Recommendation.** Oxazolidine anticonvulsants are contraindicated in pregnancy because better-tolerated anticonvulsants are available. Nevertheless, when there has been exposure, termination of pregnancy is not indicated. However, an expanded prenatal diagnosis with a detailed fetal ultrasound during the second trimester should be conducted to identify any major disturbances of structural development.

2.10.6   Phenobarbital and primidone

Pharmacology

Among barbiturates, *phenobarbital* and *primidone* have proven themselves as AEDs. These probably achieve their anticonvulsant effect by stabilizing the neuron membranes.

Primidone is converted to the metabolites phenobarbital and phenylethylmalonamide, which have an anticonvulsant action. Because the indications, effectiveness, half-lives, and undesirable side effects of primidone and phenobarbital in pregnancy are similar, only phenobarbital will be described extensively. Barbiturates used as hypnotics during pregnancy are also described in Chapter 2.11.

Barbexaclone is phenobarbital combined with *levopropylhexedrine*, a psychostimulant that can counteract sedation.

Phenobarbital and primidone are very effective in focal epilepsy and grand-mal seizures. Phenobarbital has been used as a sedative and anticonvulsant since the beginning of the twentieth century (Hauptmann 1912). Phenobarbital is well-absorbed when given orally. Up to 50% is protein-bound. About 25% is excreted unchanged via the kidney, and the remainder is excreted after oxidative metabolism. It has a long half-life of 2–6 days. As a result of its induction of drug-metabolizing enzymes in the liver, phenobarbital influences the metabolization of other selected drugs – and thus the effectiveness of other medications given at the same time can be altered. Phenobarbital reaches the fetus quickly, and results in an increase in fetal liver enzyme activity, especially in the perinatal period. Such applies to the glucuronidating enzymes that are responsible for the excretion of bilirubin (Tavoloni 1983).

2.10 Antiepileptics

Toxicology

Among 1415 pregnant women treated with phenobarbital during the first trimester, there was neither an increased rate of birth defects nor a specific pattern of anomalies (Heinonen 1977). According to studies from the same authors, cardiovascular birth defects occurred somewhat more frequently than expected when the less common barbiturates were used. In another case series of 334 newborns exposed during the first trimester, the birth defect rate was 6% – i.e. higher than the spontaneous rate of 2–3%. A possible association with cardiovascular defects was discussed, but a distinctive pattern was not found (Rosa 1993, cited in Briggs 2005). Similarly, data from the North American Registry of Pregnancies Exposed to AED demonstrated that, among 77 infants of mothers prospectively enrolled prior to the first prenatal echography, and treated with phenobarbital as monotherapy, the incidence of congenital anomalies was 6.5% – i.e. four times that in a similar analogous population-based cohort of suitable women (Holmes 2004).

In two studies, malformation rates of about 5% were observed for phenobarbital monotherapy (Canger 1999, Kaneko 1999). A syndrome of facial dysmorphia, characteristic also for other anticonvulsants, was described in 15% of 46 children exposed to phenobarbital: epicanthal folds, hypertelorism, broad, flat nasal bridge, upturned nasal tip, and wide prominent lips. Distal digital hypoplasia was observed in 24% of the children, and developmental delay in 3 of the 16 children that were examined in later life (Jones 1992).

In the 1970s, these features, including intrauterine and postnatal growth retardation, were described by some authors in pregnant patients treated with phenobarbital during pregnancy. The clinical features were similar to those seen with *in utero* exposure to both phenytoin and alcohol. The authors felt that it should not be classified as a separate syndrome (Seip 1976). There have been reports that a combination of phenobarbital and caffeine may increase the malformation rate: Samrén (1999) reported five infants with major malformations exposed to this combination, but did not draw any conclusion on the role of caffeine.

Phenobarbital therapy can affect the metabolism of steroids, vitamin D, and vitamin K, and, at least theoretically, can cause hypocalcemia and coagulation disturbances in the newborn (Kaaja 2002, Friis 1977). To decrease the risk of coagulation disturbances in the fetus and the newborn, daily administration of vitamin K (10–20 mg orally) in the last 4 weeks of pregnancy has been recommended, according to several guidelines (Choulika 2004). However, the efficacy of this procedure is debatable. Probably, it is more efficient to administer vitamin K to the neonate (Hey 1999, Howe 1999, Eller 1997, Malone 1997).

There is much less documented experience with *primidone* during pregnancy. However, similar effects to those of phenobarbital can be anticipated (Rating 1982, Myhree 1981). A primidone embryopathy has been suggested with hirsute foreheads, thick nasal roots, anteverted nostrils, a long philtrum, straight thin upper lip, distal digital hypoplasia, intrauterine growth restriction, and an increased risk for psychomotor retardation and heart defects (Gustavson 1985, Rudd 1979).

In contrast to long-term anticonvulsant use, single doses of barbiturates (such as in painkillers or as part of narcosis) have never been associated with being teratogenic.

Postnatal development

Withdrawal symptoms were observed in newborns whose mothers had taken 60–300 mg of phenobarbital daily in the last months of pregnancy. Hyperirritability and tremors may, in such cases, appear later in neonatal life – i.e. 3–14 days postpartum. High doses, administered shortly before delivery, can result in neonatal respiratory depression.

From a developmental point of view, the results are rather contradictory. In the study by Adams (2004), children *in utero* exposed to phenobarbital monotherapy had scores on the general, verbal, and non-verbal indices of neurodevelopment 10 to 14 points lower than controls. On the contrary, Dean (2002) found that infants exposed *in utero* to phenobarbital monotherapy had not more often developmental delay than controls.

Van der Pol (1991) reported that the cognitive development of children who had been exposed *in utero* to phenobarbital alone, or in combination with carbamazepine, was significantly impaired in comparison with children of non-epileptic mothers.

Recommendation. Phenobarbital and primidone may be used therapeutically in pregnancy for focal epilepsy, grand-mal seizures, and less severe forms of pre-eclampsia. The teratogenic risk of anticonvulsive medication should be emphasized. Phenobarbital treatment during the first trimester may increase the malformation rate to up to twice the background rate. Treatment with barbiturates is not an indication for terminating a pregnancy. However, an anatomical ultrasound should be considered to rule out major disturbances of structural development.

When treatment continues until delivery, the newborn should be observed for clinical signs of drug withdrawal. To decrease the risk of coagulation disturbances in the fetus and newborn, the newborn should receive 1 mg of vitamin K (preferably intramuscularly) at birth and 1 mg orally every 3 days in the first 2 weeks of life. A preventive effect of phenobarbital on brain bleeding and kernicterus in the newborn has not been established (Shankaran 2002).

Pregnancy

2.10 Antiepileptics

2.10.7 Phenytoin

Pharmacology

Phenytoin is the most widely used hydantoin derivative with an antiepileptic effect. It has been used therapeutically since 1938. Phenytoin has a marked seizure-inhibiting effect, and is effective with grand-mal seizures, focal epilepsy, sensory and psychomotor seizures, and in status epilepticus, without demonstrating any sedative or hypnotic properties. It has been used for the treatment of eclampsia (Friedman 1993).

Phenytoin inhibits the spread of spinal cord reflexes and has a stabilizing influence on peripheral nerves and heart muscle cells. For this reason, it is also used as an antiarrhythmic.

Phenytoin is rapidly absorbed in the small intestine. Inactivation occurs via hydroxylation in the liver. The main metabolite is excreted through the kidneys. The half-life of phenytoin varies considerably, from 20 to 50 hours.

Phenytoin accumulates in fat tissues. Plasma concentrations are lower in pregnant than in non-pregnant women. In the last trimester of pregnancy, this is partially compensated by the fact that the phenytoin which is not bound to the plasma proteins increases. Also, the lowered plasma concentrations are seen as the cause for the higher seizure tendency during pregnancy. Co-medication – especially with other AEDs – may further reduce the efficacy of phenytoin. Phenytoin may reduce the efficacy of hormonal contraceptives.

Toxicology

The teratogenic potential of phenytoin has been known since 1964 (Janz 1964). Originally, the anomalies observed were called "fetal hydantoin syndrome" (Hanson 1975, Loughnan 1973). Among these developmental disturbances are craniofacial dysmorphia, anomalies of the distal phalanges, pre- and postnatal growth retardation, and cardiac defects. Limitations in cognitive development have frequently been observed (Scolnik 1994, Vanoverloop 1992). The most prominent developmental anomalies of the skull, face, and extremities are broad nasal bridge, wide fontanels, low-set hair, hypertelorism, low-set ears, epicanthus, ptosis, iris coloboma, cleft lip and palate, microcephaly, short neck, hypoplasia of nails and distal phalanges in the fingers and toes, finger-like thumbs, and hip dysplasia. Digital effects are often subtle and easily overlooked by inexperienced examiners or only visible after radiologic examination (Lu 2000). However, in most cases of affected children, only a few of these mentioned anomalies (also reported after exposure to other AEDs) are observed.

With phenytoin monotherapy, the risk of a birth defect is thought to be two to three times the basic risk in untreated, non-epileptic pregnant women. Additional studies do not all confirm the increased risk of malformations after phenytoin monotherapy (Canger 1999, Samrén 1999). A disproportional increase in the embryotoxic risk (up to more than 50%) was observed after combination therapy with two additional anticonvulsants (Lindhout 1984). What must be considered in these cases, however, is that the mothers had a particularly severe form of epilepsy. Other authors also observed increased malformation rates after combination therapies with phenytoin (Kaneko 1999, Samrén 1999). Holmes (2001) found that the frequency of at least one of the following features was increased in the 87 infants exposed to phenytoin alone, compared to unexposed control infants: major malformations, microcephaly, growth retardation, hypoplasia of the mid-face and fingers.

Newborns exposed to phenytoin, similarly to those exposed to barbiturates, may have coagulation disturbances due to vitamin K deficiency (see also section 2.10.6).

Genetic susceptibility

Bustamante and Stumpff (1978) described trizygotic triplets who were affected to varying degrees with growth retardation, and mid-facial, nail, and digital phalangeal hypoplasia. While all three triplets were affected after exposure *in utero* to both phenytoin and phenobarbital, only one had a cleft lip and palate (triplet C). Only triplet B had craniosynostosis, indicating the differences in susceptibility to specific malformations expressed by genetically diverse siblings who shared approximately comparable uterine environments. The case history of a heteropaternal (two fathers) dizygotic twin pregnancy with one healthy and one 'phenytoin' baby also supports the thesis that the genetically determined activity of epoxide hydrolase in the embryo is decisive over an accumulation of teratogenically effective epoxides (Raymond 1995, Phelan 1982). Buehler (1990) demonstrated that infants with low detoxification capacities that were exposed to phenytoin *in utero* were at increased risk for the "fetal hydantoin syndrome", compared with similarly exposed individuals with normal epoxide hydrolase activity. Lyon (2003) suggested after a case report that the malformations observed may sometimes be the result of vascular disruption after episodes of bradyarrhythmia in the fetus.

Postnatal development

Dean (2002) found that the frequency of developmental delay in children exposed *in utero* to phenytoin was significantly higher than in controls (p = 0.005). However, Adab and colleagues, who

2

Pregnancy

2.10 Antiepileptics

had a small number (21) of women with phenytoin included in their study, found no major risk of cognitive impairment and a relatively low risk for major malformations (Adab 2004).

Briggs (2005) reviewed the possible risk of transplacental carcinogenesis of phenytoin exposure, and described 12 children, exposed prenatally, who developed neuroectodermal tumors, including six neuroblastomas. Satgé (1998) also carried out a systematic review of child tumors described in association with exposure to drugs during pregnancy, although they concluded that the number of cases still is too small to establish a causal relationship between phenytoin and neuroblastoma.

> **Recommendation.** When epilepsy is well-controlled with phenytoin, therapy should be continued. Monotherapy should definitely be the goal. The selection of the daily dose, supported by regular determinations of plasma concentrations, should be as low as possible. While planning a pregnancy, the question should, above all, be discussed whether, after years of freedom from seizures, anticonvulsant medication is still necessary.
>
> Treatment with phenytoin is not an indication for terminating a pregnancy. However, as a precaution an expanded prenatal diagnosis should be considered, including anatomical ultrasound diagnosis to rule out major disturbances of structural development. To decrease the risk of coagulation disturbances in the newborn, the child should receive 1 mg of vitamin K (preferably intramuscular) at birth and 1 mg orally every 3 days during the first 2 weeks of life (see also section 2.10.6).

2.10.8   Sultiam

Pharmacology and toxicology

A case series from more than 30 years ago described 11 pregnancies, 3 of which were spontaneously aborted. Birth defects were not reported.

> **Recommendation.** A risk assessment is not possible due to a lack of experience. There is no reason today to terminate a pregnancy which has occurred during treatment. As is the case with other anticonvulsants, especially with combination therapies, an increased rate of birth defects is to be expected. An expanded prenatal diagnosis with a detailed fetal ultrasound during the second trimester should be performed to rule out major disturbances of structural development.

2.10.9   Valproic acid

Pharmacology

Valproic acid (valproate, VPA) is effective for different forms of epilepsy, and apparently leads to an increase in the concentration of the inhibiting transmitter substance, γ-amino butyric acid (GABA), in the brain.

Valproic acid is well-absorbed after oral intake, and up to 95% is found in the plasma bound to the proteins. The lipophilia explains valproic acid's ability to cross the blood–brain barrier and the placenta. Towards the end of pregnancy, valproic acid is metabolized rapidly via the liver. At the same time, the unbound portion in the plasma increases. The processes balance each other, and thus the available active substance remains about the same (Nau 1981).

The concentration in the cord blood at birth is higher than in the mother's plasma. Because their liver enzymes are not yet mature, newborns have delayed excretion of valproic acid. The half-life can be extended from 8–15 hours to 15–60 hours.

Toxicology

With valproic acid monotherapy, the overall risk of birth defects is two to three times higher than the basic risk of untreated, non-epileptic pregnant women, and also higher than with other antiepileptic drugs in monotherapy (e.g. Meador 2006). Di Liberti (1984) defined dysmorphic features in children exposed to valproic acid *in utero* as a syndrome. These children have inferior epicanthal folds, a flat nasal bridge, an upturned nasal tip, a thin vermilion border, a shallow philtrum, and a downturned mouth. Long, thin, overlapping fingers and toes, and hyper-convex nails have also been described. Several cases of radial ray anomalies have been reported after fetal valproate exposure (Rodriguez-Pinilla 2000, Sharony 1993, Robert 1992, Jäger-Roman 1986).

A comprehensive review of the literature from 1978 to 2000 was carried out by Kozma (2001), who identified 69 cases that were solely exposed to valproic acid with adequate phenotypic description. The clinical manifestations of the fetal valproate syndrome encompass a wide spectrum of abnormalities, including consistent facial phenotype, multiple systemic and orthopedic involvement, central nervous system dysfunction, and altered physical growth. The facial appearance is described, as in di Liberti's paper, as a small, broad nose, small ears, flat philtrum, a long upper lip with shallow philtrum, and micro/retrognathia. In this review, 62% of the patients had musculoskeletal abnormalities, 30% had minor skin defects, 26% had cardiovascular abnormalities, 22% had genital abnormalities, and 16%

had pulmonary abnormalities. Less frequently encountered abnormalities included brain, eye, kidney, and hearing defects. Of the affected children, 12% died in infancy, and 29% of those that survived had developmental deficits/mental retardation. Although 15% of patients had growth retardation, an overgrowth pattern was seen in 9%. Neural tube defects were seen in 3% of the sample, which is typical for valproic acid, with an at least 20-fold increased risk of spina bifida or other neural tube defects (Dansky 1991, Bjerkedal 1982, Robert 1982). These anomalies are constituted between the seventeenth and twenty-eighth days after conception.

Other major malformations significantly associated with valproic acid are trigonocephaly (Källén 2005, Malm 2002, Lajeunie 2001, Ardinger 1988) and hypospadias (Källén 2004). In a study using a surveillance system (MADRE) of infants with malformations and maternal first-trimester drug exposure (Arpino 2000), classical malformations associated with valproic acid were found (spina bifida, cardiac malformations, hypospadias, limb-reduction defects), but also less classical ones – porencephaly and other specified anomalies of the brain, anomalies of the face, coarctation of aorta.

The UK Epilepsy and Pregnancy Registry (Morrow 2006) reported a higher malformation rate with valproate, at 5.9% (95% CI 4.3–8.2), than with carbamazepine, at 2.3% (1.4–3.7), and lamotrigine, at 2.1% (1.0–4.0). Most of the more recent cohort studies, reviewed by Tomson (2004), have also identified a non-significant trend toward a higher teratogenicity with valproate.

Other more recent papers have confirmed the increased risk for major malformations, and valproic acid seems to be the most teratogenic antiepileptic drug (Artama 2005, Wide 2004).

Duncan (2001) reported two women taking moderate doses of VPA who repeatedly bore children with neural tube defects, despite folate supplementation. This suggests a pharmacogenetic susceptibility to the teratogenic effects of VPA.

A dose–response relationship was found in some recent studies. Women receiving daily doses of 1000 mg VPA or more, or having plasma levels exceeding 70 µg/ml, were at a significantly increased risk for having a child with a major malformation (Vajda 2005, Kaneko 1999, Samrén 1999).

Glover (2002) also found an increased risk of visual defects: in a retrospective study conducted in England on 46 children exposed to AED *in utero*, of which 37 were exposed to VPA (29 in monotherapy); myopia was noticed in 50% of the cases exposed to VPA in monotherapy. Eye defects occurred in the entire group exposed to AED: strabism, 20%; astigmatism, 24%; and anisometropia (difference of the power of refraction of the two eyes), 11%.

Children exposed to valproate *in utero* also appear to be at greater risk for perinatal distress (43%) and low Apgar scores (28%), postnatal growth deficiency, and microcephaly (Ardinger 1988, Jäger-Roman 1986). In rare cases, neonatal liver cell necroses have been described (Legius 1987), sometimes resulting in neonatal death.

Postnatal development

Whereas most studies in the 1990s concentrated on the increased risk of major congenital malformations from prenatal valproic acid exposure, the effects on cognitive and behavioral development are increasingly being explored. A clinical study was reported, describing 57 children with anticonvulsant syndrome, 46 of which had been exposed to valproic acid *in utero*. Of these children 80% had behavioral problems, including attention deficit and hyperactivity disorder, autistic features, or Asperger's syndrome (Moore 2000); this was confirmed in five additional patients (Williams 2001). Examining neonatal behavior and later neurologic functions in a study of 40 children exposed *in utero* to a single AED, those exposed to valproic acid were the most compromised. Valproic acid serum concentrations at birth correlated with the degree of neonatal hyperexcitability and neurologic dysfunction at the age of 6 years (Koch 1996). In another study (Rasalam 2005) aimed at evaluating the clinical features and frequency of autistic disorder or Asperger's syndrome in children exposed to anticonvulsant medication *in utero*, it was concluded that sodium valproate was the drug most commonly associated with this kind of disorder: 5 of 56 (8.9%). In this study, fetal anticonvulsant syndrome associated with autistic disorder was characterized by an even sex ratio, the absence of regression or skill loss, and language delay in the absence of global delay.

In the study by Gaily (2004), the intelligence of 182 children of mothers with epilepsy (study group) and 141 control children was tested in a blinded setting at preschool or school age. Data on maternal antiepileptic treatment and seizures during pregnancy were gathered prospectively. Of the children, 107 were exposed to antiepileptic monotherapy, among them 13 to valproate; 30 children were exposed to polytherapy, among them 17 included valproate. The median maternal doses and blood levels of valproate in monotherapy during the second half of pregnancy were 1200 mg and 370 μmol/l. Compared with the other study group children and control subjects, exposures to polytherapy and to valproate during pregnancy were associated with significantly reduced verbal IQ scores: in children exposed to valproate, mean 82; 95% CI 78–87, in those exposed to polytherapy, mean 85; 95% CI 80–90.

Similar results were obtained in a retrospective study of children born to mothers with epilepsy, and performed in epilepsy clinics in

Liverpool and Manchester, UK (Adab 2004). A total of 249 children aged 6 and over were studied: 41 were exposed to sodium valproate. Mean verbal IQ was significantly lower in the valproate group compared to unexposed and other monotherapy groups. Multiple regression analysis showed that both valproate exposure and frequent (>5) tonic–clonic seizures in pregnancy were significantly associated with a lower verbal IQ, despite adjusting for other confounding factors. There was a significant negative correlation between dysmorphic features and verbal IQ in children exposed to valproate. The same group confirmed a significant correlation between the verbal intelligence quotient and dysmorphic facial features in the valproate-exposed children (Kini 2006).

Another study (Eriksson 2005) included 39 children aged 6.6–13.4 years, identified through a population-based pregnancy registry. Mothers with carbamazepine monotherapy and mothers with epilepsy but without antiepileptic treatment during pregnancy, and their age and gender-matched children, served as controls. Hospital records were reviewed and neuropsychological assessment of children was performed evaluator-blinded. The prevalence of low IQ (<80) was 19% (4 of 21), and of very low IQ (<70) was 10% (2 of 21) in valproate monotherapy exposed children. The mothers using valproate scored significantly lower in intelligence tests, and also had a significantly lower educational level. Altogether, 21% (8 of 39) of the children had minor neurological dysfunctions.

In summary, inheritance and cumulative environmental factors may partly explain the increased prevalence of neurocognitive symptoms in children exposed to valproate *in utero*, although concern about the possible long-term effects of intrauterine valproate exposure does exist.

Recommendation. There should be caution in prescribing valproate to women considering becoming pregnant if suitable treatment alternatives (see below), and with less teratogenic potential, are available. Any attempt to change treatment should be accomplished prior to conception. The importance of maintained seizure control must also be kept in mind, and the woman who needs valproate to control her seizures should not be discouraged from pregnancy, provided that current informed counseling is given. When epilepsy is well-controlled with valproic acid, if no possibility exists to replace it by one of the novel anticonvulsants, and if the woman wants to become pregnant, therapy may be continued during pregnancy. Monotherapy is preferred, as for any anticonvulsant. VPA should be given in three to four doses per day, and kept as low as possible while not exceeding 1000 mg daily. Plasma levels should be controlled regularly and not exceed 70 μg/ml.

Treatment with valproic acid is not an indication for termination of pregnancy. However, an expanded prenatal diagnosis with an α-fetoprotein determination in maternal blood around the sixteenth week of pregnancy and detailed fetal ultrasound in the second trimester should be conducted to rule out major disturbances of structural development, especially neural tube defects. The woman should be informed of the risks for both structural and behavioural anomalies.

Sections 2.10.10–19 discuss the newer antiepileptic drugs.

2.10.10   Felbamate

Pharmacology and toxicology

There were seven pregnancies exposed to felbamate reported to the drug company. The outcome was uneventful in four cases, two pregnancies were terminated, and one was spontaneously aborted.

Recommendation. A risk assessment for felbamate is not possible due to a lack of experience. There is no reason to terminate a pregnancy which has occurred during treatment. As is the case with other anticonvulsants, especially with combination therapies, an increased rate of birth defects is to be expected. An expanded prenatal diagnosis with a detailed fetal ultrasound during the second trimester should be performed to rule out major disturbances of structural development.

2.10.11   Gabapentin

Pharmacology and toxicology

Gabapentin is 1-(aminomethyl)cyclohexaneacetic acid; it inhibits dopamine release in parts of the central nervous system.

Morrow (2006) reported 31 informative pregnancy outcomes with exposure to gabapentin monotherapy, and observed 1 congenital malformation (ventriculoseptal defect). Moreover, 51 pregnancies were reported to the company (Montouris 2003), and a similar number of cases was gathered in a prescription study (Wilton 2002) performed within the Australian Epilepsy Register. Four different birth defects were observed among these prospective and retrospective data, all with polytherapy including gabapentin. Chambers (2005) reported one newborn with facial dysmorphy after monotherapy.

Recommendation. Available human and experimental data do not indicate a substantial teratogenic risk of gabapentin monotherapy. However, definite risk assessment is not possible due to a lack of experience. There is no reason to terminate a pregnancy which has occurred during treatment. As is the case with other anticonvulsants, especially with combination therapies, an increased rate of birth defects is to be expected. An expanded prenatal diagnosis with a detailed fetal ultrasound during the second trimester should be performed to rule out major disturbances of structural development. Gabapentin should not be used for treatment of non-epileptic diseases (neuropathic pain, psychiatric diseases) when pregnancy cannot be ruled out.

2.10.12   Lamotrigine

Pharmacology and toxicology

Lamotrigine, another "add-on" supplementary anticonvulsive, is used for adults with partial and secondary generalized tonic–clonic seizures.

Lamotrigine seems to increase the probability of getting pregnant compared to valproate: in a study by Isojärvi (1998), lamotrigine was substituted for valproate because of frequent occurrence of polycystic ovaries and hyperandrogenism associated with weight gain and hyperinsulinemia in women taking valproate. Twelve such patients were observed for 12 months, and the total number of polycystic ovaries in these women decreased from 20 during valproate medication to 11, 1 year after replacing valproate with lamotrigine. Lamotrigine also seems to interact with hormonal contraception: Sabers (2001) reported seven cases in which the plasma levels of lamotrigine were significantly decreased by oral contraceptives (mean 49%, range 41–64%). The interaction was of clinical relevance in most of the patients, who either experienced increased seizure frequency/recurrence of seizures after oral contraceptives had been added, or adverse effects following withdrawal of oral contraceptives. Because the drug has a specific kinetic during pregnancy, i.e. an up to 300% increase of clearance, there is a risk of seizures due to decreased rates of the lamotrigine blood level in pregnant patients (Petrenaite 2005, Pennell 2004). Such a seizure increase was described in nine pregnancies on lamotrigine monotherapy by de Haan (2004); this was probably related to a gradual decline of the drug level-to-dose ratio to 40% of baseline.

Case reports are available on a small number of successful pregnancies with exposure to lamotrigine in monotherapy (Cissoko 2002, Jovic 1999). In a review by Battino (2002), 10 newborns with congenital anomalies were observed out of 135 exposed to lamotrigine. The available (but still unpublished) prospective case observations of the manufacturer on 989 pregnancies with exposure to lamotrigine in monotherapy during the first trimester do not indicate a teratogenic risk in human beings: 26 major malformations were observed among 908 eligible outcomes (2.9%). No specific malformation was associated with the drug, but an increased rate of major birth defects was seen in cases of combination with valproic acid (15 of 133 = 11.3%; GlaxoSmithKline 2007).

The UK Epilepsy and Pregnancy Registry Belfast (Morrow 2006) reported 647 informative pregnancy outcomes with exposure to lamotrigine monotherapy, and observed 21 major congenital malformations (3.2%, 95% CI 2.1–4.9), which does not significantly differ from the background population rate. A positive dose-response was observed nevertheless, with a rate of 5.4% (95% CI 3.5–7.3) for total daily doses of more than 200 mg; the types of malformations were not dissimilar from those with other anticonvulsants, although hypospadias and gastrointestinal atresias seem to be overrepresented. However, no dose-effect at least at daily doses up to 400 mg was found in the registry of the manufacturer (GlaxoSmithKline 2007). Sabers (2004) reported 1 major birth defect among 51 pregnancies documented in a Danish registry.

Of 791 pregnant women enroled by the North American AED registry and exposed to lamotrigine as monotherapy and who gave birth between January 1997 and June 2006, 684 could be evaluated (Holmes 2006). Eighteen children had major malformations (2.8%). All the mothers had taken folic acid periconceptionally. Among the major malformations were 5 oral clefts: 2 cleft lip and palate (doses: 400 mg and 125 mg), and 3 cleft palate (doses: 300, 500, 100 mg). The data suggest a risk of cleft of 1 in 137 – i.e. 7.3 per 1000 – vs 0.6 per 1000 in the comparison group. Data from other registries (GlaxoSmithKline, Swedish and Australian registries) show that 4 newborns had clefts among 1623 exposed – i.e. 2.5 per 1000 (Holmes 2006, personal communication).

This constitutes a signal for a potential risk of cleft in case of *in utero* exposure to lamotrigine, but no clear conclusion can be drawn because the rate in the unexposed group was particularly low, because the cleft rate is highly variable among populations, and because of the risk due to maternal epilepsy itself. It should be mentioned that, in contrast with classical antiepileptic drugs, no dysmorphic features have been reported to date.

Recommendation. With respect to newer antiepileptics in pregnancy, most documented experience exists for lamotrigine. If comparable therapeutic efficacy can be assumed, lamotrigine may be used instead of a classic

Pregnancy

2.10 Antiepileptics

antiepileptic drug. If possible, the daily dosage should not exceed 200 mg. After treatment in the first trimester, termination of pregnancy is not indicated. As is the case with other anticonvulsants, especially with combination therapies, an expanded prenatal diagnosis with a detailed ultrasound testing during the second trimester should be performed to rule out major disturbances of structural development. Because the pharmacokinetic changes display marked inter-patient variation, frequent lamotrigine-level monitoring and appropriate dose adjustments are advised in the period before and during pregnancy and after delivery.

2.10.13   Levetiracetam

Pharmacology and toxicology

Levetiracetam is the S-isomer of etiracetam. Of 21 women who became pregnant on levetiracetam during clinical trials, 2 had babies with abnormalities, but both women were exposed to other anticonvulsants as well. Case reports are available for three pregnancies with exposure to levetiracetam in monotherapy with no adverse outcomes (Long 2003). A report on 11 pregnancies exposed to levetiracetam (Ten Berg 2005) reported no congenital malformations, but 3 of 9 babies had low birth weight (1 pregnancy miscarried and 1 was terminated). The largest case series published so far (Morrow 2006) reported 22 pregnancy outcomes with exposure to levetiracetam monotherapy, and observed no case of congenital malformation. The case series by Ten Berg (EURAP Netherlands) was enlarged in 2006, and now contains 39 exposed pregnancies that resulted in 28 liveborn babies (Ten Berg 2006). One had an inguinal hernia. Nine of the mothers had monotherapy, and none of their infants had malformations. Six (21%) of the newborns were small for date; all of them were exposed to polytherapy. An interaction between levetiracetam and other anticonvulsants was proposed as a mechanism for growth retardation.

Recommendation. A risk assessment for this drug is not possible due to a lack of experience. There is no reason today to terminate a pregnancy which has occurred during treatment. As is the case with other anticonvulsants, especially with combination therapies, an increased rate of birth defects is to be expected. An expanded prenatal diagnosis with a detailed fetal

2

Pregnancy

ultrasound during the second trimester should be performed to rule out major disturbances of structural development.

2.10.14   Oxcarbazepine

Pharmacology

Oxcarbazepine is similar to carbamazepine in chemical structure, but it is not metabolized through the arene oxide metabolite pathway to epoxides. Oxcarbazepine and its active metabolite 10-hydroxy-10,11-dihydrocarbamazepine (10-OH-CBZ) cross the human placenta to the fetus, and can be found in cord blood at delivery (Pienimaki 1997).

Toxicology

Oxcarbazepine is teratogenic in rats but not in rabbits. Among 37 documented pregnancies (Andermann 1994, Friis 1993, Bulau 1988), the following outcomes were observed: 3 spontaneous abortions, 2 infants with mild dysmorphic features that disappeared later in life, 1 infant with spina bifida (mother also received valproate), 1 newborn with "amniotic bands", and 31 normal infants, including a pair of twins. An extensive literature review (Montouris 2005) identified a total of 248 pregnancies involving maternal exposure to oxcarbazepine monotherapy and 61 involving adjunctive therapy. There were six malformations among the monotherapy group – i.e. a malformation rate of 2.4%, no different from the malformation rate reported in the general population (2–4%). There were four malformations associated with oxcarbazepine adjunctive therapy – i.e. a malformation rate of 6.6%. With additional cases documented by Artama (2005), Meischenguiser (2004), Sabers (2004), and Kaaja (2003), more than 300 pregnancies were documented; two-thirds of them were exposed to monotherapy.

Recommendation. Available human data do not indicate a substantial teratogenic risk of oxcarbazepine monotherapy. However, data are insufficient to rule out such a risk. Oxcarbazepine may be continued during pregnancy if effective in controlling seizures. Exposure to oxcarbazepine does not require termination of pregnancy. However, as an additional preventive measure, a detailed ultrasound diagnosis should be conducted in the second trimester as well as an α-fetoprotein determination in the maternal serum

2.10 Antiepileptics

around the sixteenth week. To decrease the risk of coagulation disturbances in the fetus and newborn, the newborn should receive 1 mg of vitamin K (preferably intramuscularly) at birth and 1 mg orally every 3 days in the first 2 weeks of life (see also section 2.10.6).

2.10.15   Pregabalin

There is insufficient experience for a risk assessment of *pregabalin* in pregnancy. Clinical trials covering a few women with first-trimester exposure have not as yet indicated substantial terato-genicity. There were indications for skeletal abnormalities and neural tube defects in some animal experiments.

Recommendation. Exposure to pregabalin does not require termination of pregnancy. However, as an additional preventive measure, a detailed ultrasound diagnosis should be conducted in the second trimester.

2.10.16   Tiagabine

Pharmacology and toxicology

Tiagabine is a GABA-uptake inhibitor. Of 22 exposed pregnancies reported by Leppik (1999), 9 were carried to term. The only mentioned anomaly was a hip dislocation in a breech birth. Additional case reports did not observe birth defects (for example, Vajda 2003).

Recommendation. A risk assessment is not possible due to a lack of experience. There is no reason to terminate a pregnancy which has occurred during treatment. As is the case with other anticonvulsants, especially with combination therapies, an increased rate of birth defects is to be expected. An expanded prenatal diagnosis with a detailed fetal ultrasound during the second trimester should be performed to rule out major disturbances of structural development.

2.10.17 Topiramate

Pharmacology and toxicology

Hoyme (1998) reported on a growth-retarded girl with hirsutism and dysmorphic features of the nose and distal phalanges, whose mother took 700 mg *topiramate* twice daily throughout the whole pregnancy. In the post-marketing surveillance system of the company, 38 exposed pregnancies (17 of them monotherapy) were registered; 3 of the polytherapy-exposed infants had congenital anomalies. Yerby (2003) mentioned 5 cases of hypospadias among 110 pregnancies reported to the drug company without details. Additional case reports with normal outcomes were reported by Öhman (2002), and Vajda (2003). The UK registry data (Morrow 2006) include 28 pregnancy outcomes with exposure to topiramate monotherapy, and 2 major congenital malformations (cleft lip and palate, hypospadias) were observed.

In summary, about 150 exposed pregnancies so far have a documented outcome, but this experience is insufficient to rule out a moderate risk, given the fact that topiramate is teratogenic in animal experiments, sometimes with an equivalence of only 20% of the human dosage (per surface area).

> **Recommendation.** A risk assessment is not possible due to a lack of experience. There is no reason today to terminate a pregnancy which has occurred during treatment. As is the case with other anticonvulsants, especially with combination therapies, an increased rate of birth defects is to be expected. An expanded prenatal diagnosis with a detailed fetal ultrasound during the second trimester should be performed to rule out major disturbances of structural development.

2.10.18 Vigabatrin

Pharmacology and toxicology

Vigabatrin, a so-called "add-on" or supplementary antiepileptic, irreversibly inhibits the GABA-aminotransferase and thereby increases the concentration of the inhibiting neurotransmitter, GABA, in the central nervous system. As a result, abnormal discharges, which cause seizure activity, are suppressed.

Neuropathological effects have been reported in the developing rat brain (Qiao 2000). Transplacental passage of vigabatrin has been demonstrated in animal experiments (Aboulrazzaq 2001). In the few reported instances of human fetal exposure to vigabatrin monotherapy, no congenital malformations have resulted. Cases of diaphragmatic hernia (Kramer 1992) and hypospadias (Lindhout 1994) were reported in children also exposed to carbamazepine. Two cases of hypocalcemia were also mentioned. Vajda (2003) found no teratogenic effects among 8 pregnancies reported to the Australian Epilepsy Register. Congenital anomalies have been reported in 14.5% (of these, two-thirds were major malformations) of 196 pregnancies exposed to vigabatrin (Committee for Proprietary Medicinal Products 1999), but most cases were polytherapies. Vigabatrin is under discussion because it has been found to cause concentric visual-field defects in 30–40% of the users (Spencer 2003, Kälviäinen 1999), but there is insufficient information available on visual-field defects in children who have been exposed prenatally (Sorri 2005).

> **Recommendation.** There is, to date, insufficient experience with humans to rule out a teratogenic effect of vigabatrin. When vigabatrin treatment occurs in the first trimester, termination of pregnancy is not indicated. As with other anticonvulsants, especially with combination therapy, an increased risk of birth defects must be anticipated. An expanded prenatal diagnosis with a detailed fetal ultrasound during the second trimester should be performed to rule out major disturbances of structural development. To decrease the risk of coagulation disturbances in the fetus and newborn, the newborn should receive 1 mg of vitamin K (preferably intramuscularly) at birth and 1 mg orally every 3 days in the first 2 weeks of life (see also section 1.10.6).

2.10.19 Zonisamid

A case series describes 26 pregnancies exposed to *zonisamid*, 4 with monotherapy. There were no birth defects after monotherapy; however, 2 infants among those who had been exposed to combination therapy (valproate and/or phenytoin) had birth defects (1 atrioseptal defect and 1 anencephaly) (Kondo 1996). Two additional cases under anticonvulsant combination therapy were reported, both healthy newborns (Kawada 2002).

> **Recommendation.** A risk assessment is not possible due to a lack of experience. There is no reason today to terminate a pregnancy which has occurred during treatment. As is the case with other anticonvulsants, especially with combination therapies, an increased rate of birth defects is to be

expected. An expanded prenatal diagnosis with a detailed fetal ultrasound during the second trimester should be performed to rule out major disturbances of structural development.

References

Aboulrazzaq YM, Padmanabhan B, Bastari SMA et al. Placental transfer of vigabatrin and its effect on concentration of amino acids in the embryo of TO mice. Teratology 2001; 63: 127–33.

Adab N, Kini U, Vinten J et al. The longer-term outcome of children born to mothers with epilepsy. J Neurol Neurosurg Psychiatry 2004; 75: 1575–83.

Adams J, Holmes LB, Janulewicz P. The adverse effect profile of neurobehavioral teratogens: phenobarbital. Birth Defects Res A 2004; 70: 280.

Andermann E. Oxcarbazepine: experience and future role. Epilepsia 1994; 35(Suppl 3): S26.

Ardinger HH, Atkin JF, Blackston RD et al. Verification of the fetal valproate syndrome phenotype. Am J Med Genet 1988; 29: 171–85.

Arpino C, Brescianini S, Robert E et al. Teratogenic effects of antiepileptic drugs: use of an international database on malformations and drug exposure (MADRE). Epilepsia 2000; 41: 1436–43.

Artama M, Auvinen A, Raudaskoski T et al. Antiepileptic drug use of women with epilepsy and congenital malformations in offspring. Neurology 2005; 64: 1874–8.

Bakke OM, Haram K. Time-course of transplacental passage of diazepam: influence of injection-delivery interval on neonatal drug concentrations. Clin Pharmacokinet 1982; 7: 353–62.

Battino D, Mamoli D, Messina S et al. Malformations in the offspring of pregnant women with epilepsy. Presentation of an International Registry of Antiepileptic Drugs and Pregnancy (EURAP). Rev Neurol 2002; 34: 476–80.

Bertollini R, Källén B, Mastroiacovo P et al. Anticonvulsant drugs in monotherapy. Effect on the fetus. Eur J Epidemiol 1987; 3: 164–71.

Bjerkedal T, Czeizel A, Goujard J et al. Valproic acid and spina bifida {letter}. Lancet 1982; 2: 1096.

Blake DA, Collins JM, Miyasaki BC et al. Influence of pregnancy and folic acid on phenytoin metabolism by rat liver microsomes. Drug Metab Dispos 1978; 6: 246–50.

Briggs GG, Freeman RK, Yaffe SJ. Drugs in Pregnancy and Lactation, 7th edn. Baltimore, MD: Williams & Wilkins, 2005.

Buehler BA, Delimont D, Van Waes M et al. Prenatal prediction of risk of the fetal hydantoin syndrome. N Engl J Med 1990; 322: 1567–72.

Bulau P, Paar WD, von Unruh GE. Pharmacokinetics of oxcarbazepine and 10-hydroxy-carbazepine in the newborn child of an oxcarbazepine-treated mother. Eur J Clin Pharmacol 1988; 34: 311–13.

Bustamante SA, Stumpff LC. Fetal hydantoin syndrome in triplets. A unique experiment of nature. Am J Dis Child 1978; 132: 978–9.

Canger R, Battino D, Canevini MP et al. Malformations in offspring of women with epilepsy: a prospective study. Epilepsia 1999; 40: 1231–6.

2

Pregnancy

2.10 Antiepileptics

Chambers CD, Kao KK, Felix RJ et al. Pregnancy outcome in infants prenatally exposed to newer anticonvulsants {Abstract}. Birth Defects Res A 2005; 73: 316.

Choulika S, Grabowski E, Holmes LB. Is antenatal vitamin K prophylaxis needed for pregnant women taking anticonvulsants? Am J Obstet Gynecol 2004; 190: 882–3.

Cissoko H, Jonville-Bera AP, Autret-Leca E. New antiepileptic drugs in pregnancy: outcome of 12 exposed pregnancies {in French}. Thérapie 2002; 57: 397–401.

Committee for Proprietary Medicinal Products. Opinion following an article 12 referral. Vigabatrin. (CPMP-report/1357/99). The European Agency for the Evaluation of Medicinal Products, 1999.

Craig J, Morrison P, Morrow J et al. Failure of periconceptional folic acid to prevent a neural tube defect in the offspring of a mother taking sodium valproate. Seizure 1999; 8: 253–4.

Dansky LV, Finnell RH. Parental epilepsy, anticonvulsant drugs, and reproductive outcome: epidemiologic and experimental findings spanning three decades; 2: Human studies. Reprod Toxicol 1991; 5: 301–35.

Dean JCS, Hailey H, Moore SJ et al. Long-term health and neurodevelopment in children exposed to antiepileptic drugs before birth. J Med Genet 2002; 39: 251–9.

de Haan GJ, Edelbroek P, Segers J et al. Gestation-induced changes in lamotrigine pharmacokinetics: a monotherapy study. Neurology 2004; 63: 571–3.

di Liberti JH, Farndon PA, Dennis NR et al. The fetal valproate syndrome. Am J Med Genet 1984; 19: 473–81.

Dolovitch LR, Addis A, Régis Vaillancourt JM et al. Benzodiazepine use in pregnancy and major malformation or oral cleft: meta analysis of cohort and case-control studies. BMJ 1998; 317: 838–43.

Duncan S, Mercho S, Lopes-Cendes I et al. Repeated neural tube defects and valproate monotherapy suggest a pharmacogenetic abnormality. Epilepsia 2001; 42: 750–53.

Eller DP, Patterson CA, Webb GW. Maternal and fetal implications of anticonvulsive therapy during pregnancy. Obstet Gynecol Clin North Am 1997; 24: 523–34.

Eriksson K, Viinikainen K, Mönkkönen A et al. Children exposed to valproate in utero – population based evaluation of risks and confounding factors for long-term neurocognitive development. Epilepsy Res 2005; 65: 189–200.

Fried S, Kozer E, Nulman I et al. Malformation rates in children of women with untreated epilepsy. A meta-analysis. Drug Saf 2004; 27: 197–202.

Friedman SA, Lim KH, Baker CA et al. Phenytoin versus magnesium sulfate in pre-eclampsia: a pilot study. Am J Perinatol 1993; 10: 233–8.

Friis B, Sardemann H. Neonatal hypocalcaemia after intrauterine exposure to anticonvulsant drugs. Arch Dis Child 1977, 52: 239–41.

Friis ML, Kristensen O, Boas J et al. Therapeutic experiences with 947 epileptic outpatients in oxcarbazepine treatment. Acta Neurol Scand 1993; 87: 224–7.

Gaily E, Kantola-Sorsa E, Hiilesmaa V et al. Normal intelligence in children with prenatal exposure to carbamazepine. Neurology 2004; 13(62): 28–32.

Gillberg C. "Floppy infant syndrome" and maternal diazepam. Lancet 1977; 2: 244.

GlaxoSmithKline. Lamotrigine Pregnancy Registry. Interim Report, 1 September 1992 through 30 September 2006, issued January 2007.

Glover SJ, Quinn AG, Barter P et al. Ophthalmic findings in fetal anticonvulsant syndrome(s). Ophthalmology 2002; 109: 942–7.

Gustavson EE, Chen H. Goldenhar syndrome, anterior encephalocele and aqueductal stenosis following fetal primidone exposure. Teratology 1985; 32: 13–18.

Hanson JW, Smith DW. The fetal hydantoin syndrome. J Pediatr 1975; 87: 285–90.

Haram K. "Floppy infant syndrome" and maternal diazepam. Lancet 1977; 2: 612–13.

Hauptmann A. Luminal bei epilepsie. München Med Wochenschr 1912; 59: 1907–8.

Heinonen OP, Slone D, Shapiro S. Birth Defects and Drugs in Pregnancy. Littleton, MA: Publishing Sciences Group, 1977.

Hernandez-Diaz S, Werler MM, Walker AM et al. Folic acid antagonists and the risk of birth defects. N Engl J Med 2000; 343: 1608–14.

Hey E. Effect of maternal anticonvulsant treatment on neonatal blood coagulation. Arch Dis Child Fetal Neonatal Ed 1999; 81: F208–10.

Holmes LB, Rosenberger PB, Harvey EA et al. Intelligence and physical features of children of women with epilepsy. Teratology 2000; 61: 196–202.

Holmes LB, Harvey EA, Coull BA et al. The teratogenicity of anticonvulsant drugs. N Engl J Med 2001; 344: 1132–8.

Holmes LB, Wyszynski DF, Lieberman E. The AED (antiepileptic drug) pregnancy registry: a 6-year experience. Arch Neurol 2004; 61: 673–8.

Holmes LB, Wyszynski DF, Baldwin EJ et al. Increased risk for non-syndromic cleft palate among infants exposed to lamotrigine during pregnancy {Abstract}. Birth Defects Res A 2006; 76: 318.

Howe AM, Oakes DJ, Woodman PDC et al. Prothrombin and PIVKA-II levels in cord blood from newborns exposed to anticonvulsants during pregnancy. Epilepsia 1999; 40: 980–84.

Hoyme HE, Hauck L, Quinn D. Minor anomalies accompanying prenatal exposure to topiramate. J Invest Med 1998; 46: 119A.

Isojärvi JIT, Rättya J, Myllylä VV. Valproate, lamotrigine, and insulin-mediated risks in women with epilepsy. Ann Neurol 1998; 43: 446–51.

Jäger-Roman E, Deichl A, Jakob S et al. Fetal growth, major malformations, and minor anomalies in infants born to women receiving valproic acid. J Pediatr 1986; 108: 997–1004.

Janz D, Fuchs U. Are antiepileptic drugs harmful when given during pregnancy? German Med Monthly 1964; 9: 20–22.

Jones KL, Lacro RV, Johnson KA et al. Pattern of malformations in the children of women treated with carbamazepine during pregnancy. N Engl J Med 1989; 320: 1661–6.

Jones KL, Johnson KA, Chambers CC. Pregnancy outcome in women treated with phenobarbital monotherapy. Teratology 1992; 45: 452.

Jovic NJ. Lamotrigine in the treatment of pregnancy patients with Juvenile Myoclonic Epilepsy. Epilepsia 1999; 40 (Suppl 2): 283.

Kaaja E, Kaaja R, Matila R et al. Enzyme-inducing antiepileptic drugs in pregnancy and the risk of bleeding in the neonate. Neurology 2002; 58: 549–53.

Kaaja E, Kaaja R, Hiilesmaa V. Major malformations in offspring of women with epilepsy. Neurology 2003; 60: 575–9.

Källén B. A register study of maternal epilepsy and delivery outcome with special reference to drug use. Acta Neurol Scand 1986; 73: 253–7.

Källén B. Maternal carbamazepine and infant spina bifida. Reprod Toxicol 1994; 8: 203–5.

Källén B. Valproic acid is known to cause hypospadias in man but does not reduce anogenital distance or causes hypospadias in rats. Basic Clin Pharmacol Toxicol 2004; 94: 51–4.

Källén B, Robert-Gnansia E. Maternal drug use, fertility problems, and infant craniostenosis. Cleft Palate Craniofac J 2005; 42: 589–93.

Kälviäinen R, Nousiainen I, Mäntyjärvi M et al. Vigabatrin a gabaergic antiepileptic drug causes concentric visual field defects. Neurology 1999; 53: 922–6.

Kaneko S, Battino D, Andermann E et al. Congenital malformations due to antiepileptic drugs. Epilep Res 1999; 33: 145–58.

Kawada K, Itoh S, Kusaka T et al. Pharmacokinetics of zonisamide in perinatal period. Brain Dev 2002; 24: 95–7.

Kellogg CK, Simmons RD, Miller RK et al. Prenatal diazepam exposure in rats: long-lasting functional changes in the offspring. Neurobehav Toxicol Teratol 1985; 7: 483–8.

Kini U, Adab N, Vinten J et al. Dysmorphic features: an important clue to the diagnosis and severity of fetal anticonvulsant syndromes. Arch Dis Child Fetal Neonatal Ed 2006; 91: 90–95.

Koch S, Jäger-Roman E, Losche G et al. Antiepileptic drug treatment in pregnancy: drug side effects in the neonate and neurological outcome. Acta Paediatr 1996; 85: 739–46.

Kondo T, Kaneko S, Amano Y et al. Preliminary report on teratogenic effects of zonisamide in the offspring of treated women with epilepsy. Epilepsia 1996; 37: 1242–4.

Kozma C. Valproic acid embryopathy: report of two siblings with further expansion of the phenotypic abnormalities and a review of the literature. Am J Med Genet 2001; 98: 168–75.

Kramer G. Vigabatrin: Wirksamkeit und Verträglichkeit bei Epilepsie im Erwachsenenalter. Akt Neurol 1992; 19: S28–40.

Kroes HY, Reefhuis J, Cornel MC. Is there an association between maternal carbamazepine use during pregnancy and eye malformations in the child? Epilepsia 2002; 43: 929–31.

Laegreid L, Olegard R, Walstrom J et al. Teratogenic effects of benzodiazepine use during pregnancy. J Pediatr 1989; 114: 126–31.

Laegreid L, Hagberg G, Lundberg A. Neurodevelopment in late infancy after prenatal exposure to benzodiazepines – a prospective study. Neuropediatrics 1992; 23: 60–67.

Lajeunie E, Barcik U, Thorne J et al. Craniosynostosis and fetal exposure to sodium valproate. J Neurosurg 2001, 95: 778–82.

Legius E, Jaeken J, Eggermont E. Sodium valproate, pregnancy, and infantile fatal liver failure. Lancet 1987; 2: 1518–19.

Leppik IE, Gram L, Deaton R et al. Safety of tiagabine: summary of 53 trials. Epilepsy Res 1999; 33: 235–46.

Lin AE, Peller AJ, Westgate MN et al. Clonazepam use in pregnancy and the risk of malformations. Birth Def Res A 2004; 70: 534–6.

Lindhout D, Hoeppener RJEA, Meinardi H. Teratogenicity of antiepileptic drug combinations with special emphasis on epoxidation (of carbamazepine). Epilepsia 1984; 25: 77–83.

Lindhout D, Omtzigt JG. Pregnancy and the risk of teratogenicity. Epilepsia 1992; 33(Suppl 4): S41–8.

Little BB, Santos-Ramos R, Newell JF et al. Megadose carbamazepine during the period of neural tube closure. Obstet Gynecol 1993; 82(4 Pt 2 Suppl): 705–8.

Long L. Levetiracetam monotherapy during pregnancy: a case series. Epilepsy Behav 2003; 4: 447–8.

Loughnan PM, Gold H, Vance JC. Phenytoin teratogenicity in man. Lancet 1973; 1: 70–72.

Lu MCK, Sammel MD, Cleveland RH et al. Digit effects produced by prenatal exposure to antiepileptic drugs. Teratology 2000; 61: 277–83.

Lyon HM, Holmes LB, Huang T. Multiple congenital anomalies associated with in utero exposure of phenytoin: possible hypoxic ischemic mechanism? Birth Defects Res A 2003; 67: 993–6.

Malm H, Kajantie E, Kivirikko S et al. Valproate embryopathy in three sets of siblings: further proof of hereditary susceptibility. Neurology 2002; 59: 630–33.

Malone FD, d'Alton ME. Drugs in pregnancy: anticonvulsants. Seminars Perinatal 1997; 21: 114–23.

Matalon S, Schechtman S, Goldzweig G et al. The teratogenic effect of carbamazepine: a meta-analysis of 1255 exposures. Reprod Toxicol 2002; 16: 9–17.

Meador KJ, Baker GA, Finnell RH et al. In utero antiepileptic drug exposure: fetal death and malformations. Neurology 2006; 67: E6–7.

Meischenguiser R, d'Giano CH, Ferraro SM. Oxcarbazepine in pregnancy: clinical experience in Argentina. Epilepsy Behav 2004; 5: 163–7.

Montouris G. Gabapentin exposure in human pregnancy: results from the Gabapentin Pregnancy Registry. Epilepsy Behav 2003; 4: 310–17.

Montouris G. Safety of the newer antiepileptic drug oxcarbazepine during pregnancy. Curr Med Res Opin 2005; 21: 693–701.

Moore SJ, Turnpenny P, Quinn A et al. A clinical study of 57 children with fetal anticonvulsant syndrome. J Med Genet 2000; 37: 489–97.

Morrow J, Russell A, Guthrie E et al. Malformation risks of antiepileptic drugs in pregnancy: a prospective study from the UK Epilepsy and Pregnancy Register. J Neurol Neurosurg Psychiatry 2006; 77: 193–8.

Myhree SA, Williams R. Teratogenic effects associated with maternal primidone therapy. J Pediatr 1981; 99: 160–62.

Nau H, Rating D, Koch S et al. Valproic acid and its metabolites: placental transfer, neonatal pharmacokinetics, transfer via mother's milk and clinical status in neonates of epileptic mothers. J Pharmacol Exp Ther 1981; 219: 768–77.

Öhman I, Vitols S, Luef G et al. Topiramate kinetics during delivery, lactation, and in the neonate: preliminary observations. Epilepsia 2002; 43: 1157–60.

Omtzigt JG, Los FJ, Meijer JW et al. The 10,ll-epoxide-10,ll-diol pathway of carbamazepine in early pregnancy in maternal serum, urine, and amniotic fluid: effect of dose, comedication, and relation to outcome of pregnancy. Ther Drug Monit 1993; 15: 1–10.

Ornoy A, Cohen E. Outcome of children born to epileptic mothers treated with carbamazepine during pregnancy. Arch Dis Child 1996; 75: 517–20.

Ornoy A, Arnon J, Shechtman S et al. Is benzodiazepine use during pregnancy really teratogenic? Reprod Toxicol 1998; 12: 511–15.

Ornoy A, Shechtman S, Arnon J et al. Is carbamazepine administration during pregnancy teratogenic? A prospective controlled study on pregnancy outcome in 229 exposed women {Abstract}. Teratology 2000; 61: 440.

Pennell PB, Newport DJ, Stowe ZN et al. The impact of pregnancy and childbirth on the metabolism of lamotrigine. Neurology 2004; 62: 292–5.

Petrenaite V, Sabers A, Hansen-Schwartz J. Individual changes in lamotrigine plasma concentrations during pregnancy. Epilepsy Res 2005; 65: 185–8.

Phelan MC, Pellock JM, Nance WE. Discordant expression of fetal hydantoin syndrome in heteropaternal dizygotic twins. N Engl J Med 1982; 307: 99–101.

Pienimaki P, Lampela E, Hakkola J et al. Pharmacokinetics of oxcarbazepine and carbamazepine in human placenta. Epilepsia 1997; 38: 309–16.

Qiao M, Malisza KL, Del Bigio MR et al. Effect of long-term vigabatrin administration on the immature rat brain. Epilepsia 2000; 41: 655–65.

Rasalam AD, Hailey H, Williams JH et al. Characteristics of fetal anticonvulsant syndrome associated autistic disorder. Dev Med Child Neurol 2005; 47: 551–5.

2

Pregnancy

2.10 Antiepileptics

Rating D, Nau H, Jäger-Roman E et al. Teratogenic and pharmacokinetic studies of primidone during pregnancy and in the offspring of epileptic women. Acta Paediatr Scand 1982; 71: 301–11.

Raymond GV, Buehler BA, Finnell RH et al. Anticonvulsant teratogenesis: 3. Possible metabolic basis {Letter}. Teratology 1995; 51: 55–6.

Rivas F, Hernandez A, Cantu JM. Acentric craniofacial cleft in a newborn female prenatally exposed to a high dose of diazepam. Teratology 1984; 30: 179–80.

Robert E, Guibaud P. Maternal valproic acid and congenital neural tube defects. Lancet 1982; 2: 937.

Robert E, Jouk PS. Preaxial limb defects after valproic acid exposure during pregnancy. In: P. Mastroiacovo, B. Källén, E. Castilla (eds), Proceedings of the First International Meeting of the Genetic and Reproductive Epidemiology Research Society (GRERS). Rome: Ghedini Editore, 1992, pp. 101–5.

Robert E, Källén B. In utero exposure to carbamazepine. Effects on the fetus. Issues Rev Teratol 1994; 7: 37–55.

Rodriguez-Pinilla E, Arroyo I, Fondevilla J et al. Prenatal exposure to valproic acid during pregnancy and limb deficiencies: a case-control study. Am J Med Genet 2000; 90: 376–81.

Rosa FW. Spina bifida in infants of women treated with carbamazepine during pregnancy. N Engl J Med 1991; 324: 674–7.

Rosenberg L, Mitchell AA, Parsells JL et al. Lack of relation of oral clefts to diazepam use during pregnancy. N Engl J Med 1983; 309: 1282–5.

Rudd NL, Freedom RM. A possible primidone embryopathy. J Pediatr 1979; 94: 835–7.

Sabers A, Buchholt JM, Uldall P et al. Lamotrigine plasma levels reduced by oral contraceptives. Epilepsy Res 2001; 47: 151–4.

Sabers A, Dam M, a-Rogvi-Hansen B et al. Epilepsy and pregnancy: lamotrigine as main drug used. Acta Neurol Scand 2004; 109: 9–13.

Samrén EB, van Duijn CM, Koch S et al. Maternal use of antiepileptic drugs and the risk of major congenital malformations: a joint European prospective study of human teratogenesis associated with maternal epilepsy. Epilepsia 1997; 38: 981–90.

Samrén EB, van Duijn CM, Christiaens GCM et al. Antiepileptic drug regimens and major congenital abnormalities in the offspring. Ann Neurol 1999; 46: 739–46.

Satgé D, Sasco AJ, Little J. Antenatal therapeutic drug exposure and fetal/neonatal tumours: review of 89 cases. Paediatr Perinat Epidemiol 1998; 12: 84–117.

Saxen I, Saxen L. Association between maternal intake of diazepam and oral clefts {Letter}. Lancet 1975; 13: 498.

Scanlon JW. Effect of benzodiazepines in neonates. N Engl J Med 1975; 292: 649.

Scolnik D, Nulman I, Rovet J et al. Neurodevelopment of children exposed in utero to phenytoin and carbamazepine monotherapy program. J Am Med Assoc 1994; 271: 767–70.

Seip M. Growth retardation, dysmorphic facies and minor malformations following massive exposure to phenobarbital in utero. Acta Paediatr Scand 1976; 65: 617–21.

Shankaran S, Paille L, Wright L et al. Neurodevelopmental outcome of premature infants after antenatal phenobarbital exposure. Am J Obstet Gynecol 2002; 187: 171–7.

Sharony R, Garber A, Viskochil D et al. Preaxial ray reduction defects as part of valproic acid embryofetopathy. Prenat Diagn 1993; 13: 909–18.

Simmons RD, Miller RK, Kellogg CK. Prenatal exposure to diazepam alters central and peripheral responses to stress in adult rat offspring. Brain Res 1984, 307: 39–46.

Sorri I, Herrgard E, Viinikainen K et al. Ophthalmologic and neurologic findings in two children exposed to vigabatrin in utero. Epilepsy Res 2005; 65: 117–20.

Speidel BD, Meadow SR. Epilepsy, anticonvulsants and congenital malformations. Drugs 1974; 8: 354–65.

Spencer EL, Harding GFA. Examining visual field defects in the pediatric population exposed to vigabatrin. Doc Ophthalmol 2003; 107: 281–7.

Sutcliffe AG, Jones RB, Woodruff G. Eye malformations associated with treatment with carbamazepine during pregnancy. Ophthalmic Genet 1998; 19: 59–62.

Tavoloni N, Wittman R, Jones MJ et al. Effect of low-dose phenobarbital on hepatic microsomal UDP-glucuronyl transferase activity. Biochem Pharmacol 1983; 32: 2143–7.

Ten Berg K, Samren EB, van Oppen AC et al. Levetiracetam use and pregnancy outcome. Reprod Toxicol 2005; 20: 175–8.

Ten Berg K, van Oppen AC, van Donselaar CA et al. Outcome of human pregnancy with levetiracetam exposure {Abstract}. Birth Def Res A 2006; 76: 318.

Tomson T, Perucca E, Battino D. Navigating toward fetal and maternal health: the challenge of treating epilepsy in pregnancy. Epilepsia 2004; 45: 1171–5.

Vajda FJ, O'Brien TJ, Hitchcock A et al. The Australian registry of anti-epileptic drugs in pregnancy: experience after 30 months. J Clin Neurosci 2003; 10: 543–9.

Vajda FJ, Eadie MJ. Maternal valproate dosage and foetal malformations. Acta Neurol Scand 2005; 112: 137–42.

van der Pol MC, Hadders-Algra M, Huisjes HJ et al. Antiepileptic medication in pregnancy: late effects on the children's central nervous system development. Am J Obstet Gynecol 1991; 164: 121–8.

Vanoverloop D, Schnell RR, Harvey EA et al. The effects of prenatal exposure to phenytoin and other anticonvulsants on intellectual function at 4 to 8 years of age. Neurotoxicol Teratol 1992; 14: 329–35.

Weinstock L, Cohen LS, Bailey JW et al. Obstetrical and neonatal outcome following clonazepam use during pregnancy: a case series. Psychother Psychosom 2001; 70: 158–62.

Wide K, Windbladh B, Källén B. Major malformations in infants exposed to antiepileptic drugs in utero with emphasis on carbamazepine and valproic acid: a nation-wide population-based register study. Acta Paediatr 2004; 93: 174–6.

Williams G, King J, Cunningham M et al. Fetal valproate syndrome and autism: additional evidence of an association. Dev Med Child Neurol 2001; 43: 202–6.

Wilton LV, Shakir S. A postmarketing surveillance study of gabapentin as add-on therapy for 3100 patients in England. Epilepsia 2002; 43: 983–92.

Yerby MS. Clinical care of pregnant women with epilepsy: neural tube defects and folic acid supplementation. Epilepsia 2003; 44(Suppl 3): 33–40.

Zupanc ML. Antiepileptic drugs and hormonal contraceptives in adolescent women with epilepsy. Neurology 2006; 66: S37–45.

Pregnancy

2.10 Antiepileptics

Psychotropic drugs

2.11

Hanneke Garbis and Patricia R. McElhatton

There is accumulating evidence that psychiatric illness can adversely affect pregnancy outcome and child development. The available data have been summarized by Levey (2004), Bonari (2004), and Cott (2003). Untreated psychiatric disorders during pregnancy may cause spontaneous abortions, pre-eclampsia, placental abnormalities, decreased fetal growth, preterm labor, preterm delivery, low birth weight, small for gestational age babies, and perinatal and birth complications. In addition, a study by Hansen (2000) suggests that excessive emotional stress during organogenesis can cause congenital malformations, particularly those of the cranial neural crest. Jablensky (2005) reports a higher incidence of any birth defects, especially defects of the cardiovascular system, in pregnant women with schizophrenia.

Psychiatric illness should always be treated with psychotherapy or appropriate medication if needed. Abrupt discontinuation of psychotropic drugs can lead to serious adverse effects, such as discontinuation symptoms and recurrence of the primary psychiatric disorder (Einarson 2001A). Cohen (2006) reports a high rate of depression relapse among pregnant women who discontinued their medication before becoming pregnant, compared to women who maintained their medication. On the other hand, many women of reproductive age and even pregnant women are prescribed long-term antidepressant therapy for minor mood disorders that could be treated with non-medical therapies.

2.11.1   Tricyclic and tetracyclic antidepressants

Pharmacology and toxicology

Tricyclic antidepressants (TCAs) inhibit the reuptake of the neurotransmitters, noradrenaline and serotonin, in the adrenergic neurones, which results in increased concentrations of those neurotransmitters at the receptor.

Imipramine, a tertiary amine, is the prototype of a TCA. Other members of this group are *amitriptyline, clomipramine, dibenzepin, dosulepine, dothiepin, doxepin, imipramine, lofepramine, protriptyline*, and *trimipramine. Desipramine* and *nortriptyline* are secondary amines, which have less parasympatholytic properties.

Monitoring of maternal serum levels is recommended due to altered pharmacokinetics during pregnancy, especially in the second and third trimesters. TCA subtherapeutic levels have been associated with depressive relapse. Thus, the usual therapeutic dose may not be sufficient to keep the mother stable, and it may need to be readjusted (Gold 1999, Wisner 1993).

TCAs are highly lipid-soluble, and therefore can easily cross the placenta. Fetal exposure can be considerable, as has been demonstrated for nortriptyline and clomipramine (Loughhead 2006).

Congenital malformations (limb and heart malformations, polydactyly, and hypospadias) were occasionally reported during the 1970s and 1980s, but so far no causal relationship has been established between *in utero* exposure to TCAs and congenital malformations (Simon 2002, Ericson 1999, McElhatton 1996, Brunel 1994, Patuszak 1993). An increased risk for cardiovascular defects after maternal use of clomipramine has recently been reported by Källén (2006). The odds ratio was 1.87 (95% CI; 1.16–2.99). Further studies are needed to confirm this.

Maternal exposure to antidepressants may be associated with a risk for spontaneous abortions. However, the underlying depression could also be a contributing factor (Hemels 2005). Källén (2004) reports an increased risk for preterm birth and low birth weight.

Short-term withdrawal symptoms such as jitteriness, irritability, myoclonus, and convulsions have been reported in the neonate after chronic maternal use, especially near term (Källén 2004, Bloem 1999, Bromiker 1994, Schimmell 1991). Sanz (2005) found an association between maternal use of TCAs and neonatal withdrawal syndrome and convulsions only for clomipramine, and not for the other TCAs. In the study of Källén (2004), 90% of the women had used clomipramine and 10% had used amitriptyline.

Nulman (2002, 1997) found that *in utero* exposure to TCAs did not affect the neurodevelopment (cognitive, language, and behavioral development) in preschool children.

There are no or limited data for *dosulepine, doxepin, lofepramine*, and *trimipramine*.

Desipramine and *nortriptyline* are preferred by some investigators, since they are less anticholinergic and the least likely to exacerbate the orthostatic hypotension which occurs during pregnancy (Nonacs 2002).

Maprotiline is a tetracyclic antidepressant and a derivative of imipramine. It inhibits the reuptake of noradrenaline in the synapses, and has mood-enhancing properties. No adverse effects were reported following the use of maprotiline during pregnancy in a small number of women (McElhatton 1996).

Recommendation. The older TCAs, such as amitriptyline, clomipramine, desipramine, imipramine, and nortriptyline, belong to the group of drugs of choice in the treatment of depression during pregnancy. Monitoring of maternal serum levels is recommended, and if necessary the daily dose should be adjusted. The use of other drugs from this group for which fewer data are available is not an indication for termination of pregnancy or specific prenatal diagnostics. Furthermore, a pregnant patient who is stable with a second-choice antidepressant should not be changed to another drug, because this may worsen her health. However, a detailed fetal ultrasonography may be offered. Regular psychiatric and obstetric care is recommended to diagnose in time a relapse or pregnancy complications (intrauterine growth retardation, premature contractions). Observation of the neonate for withdrawal symptoms or adaptation problems for at least 2 days is recommended when TCAs have been used up to delivery. To prevent neonatal adaptation disorders, dose reduction or even treatment interruption in the days immediately preceding delivery can be discussed with the patient if the clinical course allows. However, to prevent a relapse at this vulnerable stage, pre-pregnancy dosage should be started immediately after delivery.

2.11.2   Selective serotonin reuptake inhibitors (SSRIs)

Pharmacology and toxicology

SSRIs such as *citalopram, escitalopram, fluoxetine, fluvoxamine, paroxetine*, and *sertraline* selectively inhibit the presynaptic reuptake of serotonin. They have only negligible effects on noradrenaline and dopamine uptake.

SSRIs are equally effective but are better tolerated by some patients than TCAs. The SSRIs are also safer than other antidepressants for the mother and fetus in women with suicidal ideation. Fluoxetine is a long-acting SSRI. The half-lives of fluoxetine and the metabolite norfluoxetine are several days and 14 days, respectively. The half-life of citalopram is 36 hours; fluvoxamine, paroxetine, and sertraline have half-lives of less than 24 hours.

Heikkinen (2003, 2002) report that during pregnancy maternal drug concentrations of citalopram and fluoxetine may be lower than in non-pregnant women, and could lead to therapeutic failure. In a study with small numbers, Hostetter (2000) found that more than half of the pregnant women using fluoxetine, paroxetine or sertraline required an increase in their daily dose.

Hendrick (2003A) studied the placental passage of SSRIs and their metabolites. Umbilical cord concentrations were lower than maternal concentrations. The mean ratios of umbilical cord to maternal serum concentrations ranged from 0.29 to 0.89, and were lowest for paroxetine and sertraline and highest for citalopram and fluoxetine. The fetus appears to be able to metabolize and eliminate the drugs to some extent. Maternal use of those drugs does not lead to accumulation in the fetus. Infant fluoxetine and norfluoxetine concentrations are high at delivery and during the early postnatal period, and are only slowly eliminated by the infant. Norfluoxetine concentrations were still detectable at the age of 2 months in most of the infants (Heikkinen 2003). Only fluoxetine and norfluoxetine, and not paroxetine, sertraline or O-desmethylsertraline, could be detected in infant serum by Rampono (2004).

Many investigators, using different methods and study designs, have studied the pregnancy outcome after maternal use of SSRIs. Some studies involve SSRIs as a group; other studies involve a single SSRI, mostly fluoxetine. The outcome of several thousands of pregnancies is known for citalopram, fluoxetine, paroxetine, and sertraline; of several hundreds for fluvoxamine. There are insufficient data for escitalopram.

Congenital malformations

The majority of the studies did not find an increased incidence of major congenital malformations after first-trimester exposure to SSRIs as a group (Hallberg 2005, Malm 2005, Hendrick 2003B, Simon 2002, Ericsson 1999, Kulin 1998, McElhatton 1996, Brunel 1994), and to the single SSRIs fluoxetine (Cohen 2000, Goldstein 1997, Chambers 1996, Patuszak 1993), citalopram (Sivojelezova 2005), and sertraline (Chambers 1999). Rates of congenital malformations were within the normal range in all studies. Only Chambers (1996) reported an increased incidence of three or more minor malformations, but further details are not given, which makes the clinical significance of the data difficult to assess.

Most of those studies were performed with relatively small numbers of pregnancies; four studies report on larger numbers. Hallberg (2005) summarized the data available from the Swedish Medical Birth Registry, which gives information on 4291 children born to mothers exposed to SSRIs (citalopram $n = 1696$, fluoxetine $n = 574$, paroxetine $n = 708$, sertraline $n = 1067$) in early pregnancy. The reported incidence of congenital malformations was 2.9%, which does not differ from the expected rate among unexposed infants. Malm (2005) performed a population-based study of 1782 women exposed to SSRIs during pregnancy, 1398 of them in the first trimester (citalopram $n = 554$, fluoxetine $n = 525$, fluvoxamine $n = 65$, paroxetine $n = 152$, sertraline $n = 118$). Congenital malformations were not more common in the SSRI group when compared with the control group. Major malformations were more common in women exposed to fluoxetine in the first trimester, but after adjusting for confounders the association did not reach statistical significance. Among them were 12 cases of isolated cardiovascular anomalies, of which 8 were ventricular septal defects. This is nearly three-fold more than the prevalence of cardiovascular malformations generally in Finland. Goldstein (1997) has summarized the outcomes of 796 fluoxetine-exposed pregnancies during the first trimester from the Pregnancy Registry of Eli Lilly. In a prospective controlled study of the European Network of Teratology Information Services (ENTIS), the pregnancy outcome of 1987 SSRI-exposed women was investigated (citalopram $n = 244$, fluoxetine $n = 460$, fluvoxamine $n = 214$, paroxetine $n = 871$, sertraline $n = 198$). No increased incidence of major congenital malformations was found (McElhatton, personal communication).

In a population-based cohort study from Denmark on women who filled prescriptions for SSRIs from 30 days before conception to the end of the first trimester, an increased risk of congenital malformations (RR of 1.84; CI 1.25–2.71) was found among women with prescriptions during the second or third month of pregnancy. There was no evidence that the association was specific to particular malformations (Wogelius 2006).

In 2005, concerns were raised after the publication of some studies suggesting an association between first-trimester exposure to paroxetine and cardiovascular anomalies – in particular, ventricular and atrial septum defects (Källén 2006, Diav-Citrin 2005A). However, the individual risk is small, and further studies are needed to verify this association. Cardiac septal defects are recorded as major malformations, but they often spontaneously close. The chance of detecting such a small defect by echocardiography is small.

In a preliminary study, Alwan (2005), using the Birth Defects Surveillance Systems in the USA, found that women using SSRIs in the first trimester were more likely to have an infant with omphalocele than those who did not use SSRIs at this time. The effect was strongest with paroxetine. They also suggest an association between exposure to any SSRI and having an infant with craniosynostosis. The results have to be confirmed in other datasets.

Over 20% of all cases of congenital malformations in infants of mothers using citalopram during pregnancy reported to the FDA were represented by eye abnormalities (optical nerve and retinal defects). Signals of eye malformations have also been reported in other countries (Tabacova 2004).

Adverse obstetric outcome

Maternal exposure to antidepressants may be associated with a risk for spontaneous abortion. However, the underlying depression could also be a contributing factor (Hemels 2005).

Several investigators have found an increased incidence of preterm birth when SSRIs have been used throughout pregnancy or in the last half of pregnancy (Källén 2004, Costei 2002, Simon 2002, Ericsson 1999, Chambers 1996, Goldstein 1995). Here, too, the underlying depression could be a contributing factor. In most studies, there was no control for the impact of maternal depression. The data from Simon (2002), however, suggest that maternal use of SSRIs rather than maternal depression has a specific effect on lower gestational age, with a consequent effect on birthweight, as tricyclic antidepressants had no such effect.

A decrease in birth weight has also been reported by other authors. Simon (2002) found that by 6 months of age, the infant weight was normal again.

Neonatal adaptation disorders

There is increasing evidence that exposure to SSRIs late in pregnancy is associated with neonatal withdrawal symptoms. Moses-Kolko and colleagues have reviewed most of the data about potential adverse events in neonates exposed *in utero* to SSRIs (Moses-Kolko 2005). Data concern case reports, case series, and cohort studies published in literature. Reported symptoms are jitteriness, shivering, tremors, increased muscle tone, feeding and sleep disturbances, irritability, agitation, respiratory distress, and excessive crying. Symptoms are usually mild and transient, but may need treatment in special neonatal care units. Levinson-Costiel (2006) found neonatal withdrawal symptoms in 30% of 60 neonates after long-term *in utero* exposure to SSRIs; symptoms were severe in 8 cases. The onset of symptoms is 12 hours to 5 days after birth, but they may also occur immediately at birth, suggesting acute neonatal toxicity (Nordeng 2005, Isbister 2001). Other authors have reported additional cases or case series of neonatal withdrawal symptoms for citalopram (Tabacova 2005), fluoxetine (Rampono 2004), paroxetine (Haddad 2005, Rampono 2004, Jaiswal 2003), and sertraline (Santos 2004).

Neonatal withdrawal symptoms are most commonly reported for paroxetine. There are case reports of neonatal convulsions after late *in utero* exposure to paroxetine (Sanz 2005).

Oberlander (2004) reports significantly elevated paroxetine levels in infants showing withdrawal symptoms whose mothers had used both paroxetine and clonazepam, compared with paroxetine only. Clonazepam appeared to have altered paroxetine metabolism, leading to increased drug levels and risk for transient neonatal symptoms. Laine (2004) suggests that the poor metabolizer genotype of CYP2D6 may be a risk factor for perinatal complications in infants exposed to SSRIs late in pregnancy.

In a small cohort study, Chambers (1996) found that 2 of 73 infants exposed to fluoxetine in late pregnancy had persistent pulmonary hypertension (normal incidence is 1–2 per 1000). Data from a case-control study of Chambers (2006) support an association between the maternal use of SSRIs in late pregnancy and persistent pulmonary hypertension in the offspring, the absolute risk probably being relatively low (6–12 per 1000). Further studies are needed to confirm these findings.

Two infants, one with prolonged Q-interval and one with cardiac arrhythmia after *in utero* exposure to fluoxetine, have been reported (Dubnov 2005, Abebe-Campino 2002).

Bleeding disorders and hematomas have been associated with the use of SSRIs in adults. Gestational exposure to SSRIs appears to reduce substantially platelet serotonin uptake in the fetus. Such exposure may have physiologic effects (Anderson 2004). Four case reports of intraventricular hemorrhage in the newborn after exposure to paroxetine ($n = 3$) and fluoxetine ($n = 1$) late in pregnancy have been summarized by Nordeng (2005). Pediatricians should be aware of an increased hemorrhagic tendency in infants exposed to SSRIs.

Neurodevelopment

Neurodevelopment of infants who have been exposed to SSRIs during pregnancy has not been extensively studied. Several studies with small numbers have been published. Neurobehavioral, cognitive, and language development in infants and children born to mothers who took fluoxetine or other SSRIs during pregnancy was similar to that of non-exposed children (Mattson 2004, 1999, Casper 2003, Nulman 2002, 1997). Mattson (2004) and Casper (2003) found a slight delay in motor development and motor control.

Recommendation. SSRIs have not been associated with an increased risk of major congenital malformations in most studies. Further studies are needed to verify the association between first-trimester maternal exposure to paroxetine and infant cardiac defects, as suggested in some recent studies. The average safety profile seems to be better for sertraline and citalopram than for fluoxetine and paroxetine. Fluvoxamine is probably safe, but data on pregnancy outcome are fewer. Appropriate treatment of the depression must always be a primary consideration when evaluating the risks and benefits to the mother and the infant. Inadvertent use of any SSRI does not require termination of pregnancy. Furthermore, a pregnant patient who is stable with a second-choice antidepressant should not be changed to another drug, because this may worsen her health. However, a detailed fetal ultrasonography may be offered. Regular psychiatric and obstetric care is recommended to diagnose in time a relapse or pregnancy complications (intrauterine growth retardaton, premature contractions). Observation of the neonate for withdrawal symptoms or adaptation problems for at least 2 days is recommended when SSRIs have been used up to delivery. To prevent neonatal adaptation disorders, dose reduction or even treatment interruption in the days immediately preceding delivery can be discussed with the patient if the clinical course allows. However, to prevent a relapse at this vulnerable stage, pre-pregnancy dosage should be started immediately after delivery. After SSRI treatment near term, it is important to be aware of an increased hemorrhagic tendency in the newborn.

2.11.3   Monoaminoxidase inhibitors (MAOIs)

Pharmacology and toxicology

MAOIs inhibit the enzyme, monoaminoxidase, which is responsible for the metabolism of neurotransmitters. The inhibition is either reversible, as with the newer MAOIs (e.g. *moclobemide*), or irreversible, as with the older MAOIs (e.g. *isocarboxazid, phenelzine,* and *tranylcypromine*).

MAOIs have been associated with a high incidence of toxicity in man. There is a possible interaction between tyramine (which is present in high-protein food and drinks) and MAOIs, which may manifest itself as an acute hypertensive crisis.

An increased risk of congenital malformations was reported in a small group of 21 women with first-trimester exposure to MAOIs, mainly *phenelzine* and *tranylcypromine* (Heinonen 1977). A recent case report again discussed the association between hypertelorism, cardiac and other defects with *tranylcypromine* exposure (Kennedy 2000). However, as the number of cases is so small, no clear causal relationship could be established.

No data were found on the use of moclobemide in pregnancy, and only very limited data on *isocarboxazid.*

Hypertension is a common complication of pregnancy, and is often insidious in onset. MAOIs can exacerbate this condition and may lead to alterations in placental blood flow, particularly placental hypoperfusion, which may have serious consequences for fetal growth and development (Mortola 1989).

In situations where premature labor occurs, tocolysis with a betamimetic may be indicated, but is not possible because of the potential interaction with MAOIs. Anesthetic management in labor may also be complicated because of potential interactions with narcotic analgesics in these patients.

> **Recommendation.** The limited data available on the safety of MAOI use in pregnancy and the potential for interacting with other medication and certain food substances mean that MAOIs are not recommended for use during pregnancy. They can exacerbate hypertension, and may interfere with drugs used at delivery. They should be avoided unless all other treatments have failed. Nevertheless, exposure to MAOIs in the first 3 months of pregnancy is not an indication for termination of a pregnancy. Detailed fetal ultrasonography may be offered in such cases to control normal development. Furthermore, a pregnant patient who is stable with these drugs should not be changed to another drug, because this may worsen her health. Regular psychiatric and obstetric care is recommended to diagnose in time a relapse or pregnancy complications (intrauterine growth retardaton, premature contractions). Observation of the neonate for withdrawal symptoms or adaptation problems for at least 2 days is recommended when MAOIs have been used up to delivery. To prevent neonatal adaptation disorders, dose reduction or even treatment interruption in the days immediately preceding delivery can be discussed with the patient if the clinical course allows. However, to prevent a relapse at this vulnerable stage, pre-pregnancy dosage should be started immediately after delivery.

2.11.4   Other antidepressants

Pharmacology and toxicology

The antidepressants *amineptine, amoxapine, atomoxetine, bupropion, duloxetine, iprindole, medifoxamine, mianserin, mirtazapine, nefazodone, oxitriptan, reboxetine, tianeptine, trazodone, venlafaxine,* and *viloxazine* are not structurally related to TCAs, SSRIs or MAOIs.

Atomoxetine selectively inhibits noradrenaline, and was recently introduced to the market to treat attention deficit and hyperactivity syndrome. There is no experience in pregnancy to date.

Bupropion is an aminoketone antidepressant which acts on noradrenergic and dopaminergic systems. The drug was developed as an antidepressant, but was found to support weaning from cigarette smoking as well. In the Bupropion Pregnancy Registry of GlaxoSmithKline (2006), 783 prospective cases with bupropion exposure during pregnancy are registered, 621 with exposure during the first trimester. The preliminary results have not confirmed an increased incidence of congenital malformations or a consistent pattern of defects, although a higher than expected rate of cardiac anomalies had been discussed. Chun-Fai-Chan and colleagues also did not find an increased incidence of congenital malformations or other adverse pregnancy outcomes after intrauterine first-trimester exposure among 136 pregnancies (Chun-Fai-Chan 2005). They found higher rates of spontaneous abortions, but these were similar to those in other studies examining the safety of antidepressants during pregnancy.

There is insufficient experience with the noradrenaline and the serotonin reuptake inhibitor *duloxetine*. In animal studies, cardio-vascular and skeletal defects were induced in dosages below the upper therapeutic level in human.

Mirtazapine inhibits the reuptake of seotonin and noradrenaline. No teratogenic effects were reported following its use during pregnancy in about 200 pregnancies, mainly exposed during the first trimester (e.g. Djulus 2006, Yaris 2004A, Biswas 2003, Kesim 2002, Saks 2001). Mirtazapin was also used to treat hyperemesis gravdarum (Guclu 2005, Rohde 2003, Dorn 2002, Saks 2001).

Nefazodone and *trazodone* are related phenylpiperazine antidepressants which inhibit the reuptake of noradrenaline and serotonin and block the serotonin receptors in the synapses. There was no indication for teratogenicity in about 100 published pregnancies, most of them exposed to nefazodone during the first trimester (Yaris 2004A, Einarson 2003).

Trazodone has sedative properties and is also used as a hypnotic. Approximately 70 pregnancies, mainly exposed during the first trimester, were evaluated. No indication of teratogenicity was observed (Einarson 2003, McElhatton 1996).

In a multicenter prospective controlled study by Einarson and colleagues, about 150 pregnancies were covered with exposure to *venlafaxine*, a so-called bicyclic antidepressant that is unrelated to other antidepressants and inhibits the reuptake of serotonin and noradrenaline (Einarson 2001B). Yaris (2004A) reports the outcome of a small case series of prospectively followed pregnancies in which venlafaxine, nefazodone, and mirtazapine had been used by the mother. All in all, there have been almost 300 exposed pregnancies evaluated in published studies and case reports, and as yet there is no indication of a substantial teratogenic risk (see also di Gianantonio 2006, Okotore 1999, Ellingrod 1994). A case of neonatal withdrawal symptoms following late use in pregnancy of venlafaxine has been reported by de Moor (2003). In a recent study, 32 children prenatally exposed to venlafaxine were compared to control groups with exposure to other antidepressants, unexposed siblings, and healthy mothers. Healthy controls scored significantly higher than the venlafaxine group and the other control groups in full-scale IQ, performance IQ, and verbal IQ, indicating that other factors than the antidepressant drug, such as maternal disease or the social environment, may be associated with the child's cognitive abilities (Nulman 2006).

Fewer or no data are available for *amineptine, amoxapine, medifoxamine, mianserin, oxitriptan*, and *viloxazine* (McElhatton 1996, Brunel 1994).

Hypericin (hypericum; St. John's Wort, SJW) is a herbal medicine which is used as an antidepressant. SJW may interact with a number of drugs, including antidepressants (see Chapter 2.19).

> **Recommendation.** As there is insufficient experience with the use of most of these drugs during pregnancy, they are drugs of second choice (in the cases of mirtazapine, venlafaxine) or should be avoided if possible. The use in the first 3 months of pregnancy is not an indication for termination of pregnancy. Furthermore, a pregnant patient who is stable with these drugs should not be changed to another drug because this may worsen her health. However, a detailed fetal ultrasonography may be offered after their use in the first trimester. Regular psychiatric and obstetric care is recommended to diagnose in time a relapse or pregnancy complications (intrauterine growth retardation, premature contractions). Observation of the neonate for withdrawal symptoms or adaptation problems for at least 2 days is recommended when these antidepressants have been used up to delivery. To prevent neonatal adaptation disorders, dose reduction or even treatment interruption in the days immediately preceding delivery can be discussed with the patient if the clinical course allows. However, to prevent a relapse at this vulnerable stage, pre-pregnancy dosage should be started immediately after delivery.

2.11.5 Antipsychotic drugs and pregnancy – "classical" or atypical antipsychotics?

Neuroleptic agents probably act by blocking cerebral dopamine receptors. They have mood-changing properties, and do not affect intellectual ability. The group of neuroleptic drugs includes phenothiazines (low and high potency), thioxanthenes, butyrophenones, and atypical antipsychotics. Pregnancy outcome is known to be poorer in psychotic women, especially if inadequately treated. Most data on their use during pregnancy are available for phenothiazines and haloperidol. These drugs have been on the market for decades. These are indications that atypical antipsychotics have less extrapyramidal side effects, including tardive dyskinesia, compared to haloperidol or other classical antipsychotics. However, there is still a controversial debate about the superiority of atypicals with respect to a patient's tolerability in comparison to haloperidol (at least when used in dosages <10 mg/d; Henke 2005, Davis 2004, Rosenheck 2003) or to phenothiazines like perphenazin (Lieberman 2005). The choice of antipsychotic drugs should be made individually, considering the broad experience with phenothazines during pregnancy and the potentially lower risk for neurological side effects of atypical antipsychotics when a woman of reproductive age needs therapy. Due to the lower prolactin increase of most atypical antipsychotics, a change from phenothiazines to atypical neuroleptics may consequently result in an unwanted pregnancy. A pregnant patient who is stable with an antipsychotic with insufficient experience in pregnancy should not be changed to another drug, because this may worsen her health.

2.11.6   Phenothiazines and thioxanthenes

Pharmacology and toxicology

Phenothiazines are effective in the treatment of psychosis and of hyperemesis, as they also block histamine receptors. They readily cross the placenta; elimination is much slower by the fetus and the neonate than by adults. *Chlorpromazine* is the prototype of phenothiazines, and is structurally related to *promethazine*, which is used as an antihistaminic. Phenothiazines block the dopamine receptors in the basal ganglia, the hypothalamus, and the limbic system. Due to their effect on dopamine metabolism, they may cause extrapyramidal effects. Phenothiazines also have antiemetic and antiallergic properties (see Chapters 2.2 and 2.4).

Data on use during pregnancy are available for *alimemazine, chlorpromazine, dixyrazine, fluphenazine, levomepromazine, pericyazine, perphenazine, prochlorperazine, promazine, thioridazine, trifluoperazine*, and *triflupromazine*. The data on pregnancy outcome are conflicting. Case reports of malformations have been reported (e.g. microcephaly, syndactyly, cardiac malformations), but most larger studies have failed to demonstrate a significant risk for congenital malformations (Altshuler 1996, McElhatton 1992). Most information is available from studies in which pregnant women had been treated for hyperemesis gravidarum. For this indication, smaller doses are used than those needed to treat psychosis.

Phenothiazines may cause dose-dependent withdrawal symptoms or transient extrapyramidal symptoms in the neonate which may last for several weeks (McElhatton 1992).

Few or no data are available for the thioxanthenes *chlorprothixene, clopenthixol, flupenthixol, metofenazate, perazine, prothipendyl, zotepine*, and *zuclopenthixol*.

2

Pregnancy

Recommendation. Phenothiazines may be used during pregnancy when treatment of acute psychosis or chronic psychotic illness is necessary. Most experience is available with alimemazine, chlorpromazine, fluphenazine, levomepromazine, promazine, and thioridazine. If needed to treat extrapyramidal side effects, biperiden can be added to the medication. Treatment with other phenothiazines is not an indication for termination of pregnancy. Regular psychiatric and obstetric care is recommended to diagnose in time a relapse or pregnancy complications (intrauterine growth retardaton, premature contractions). Observation of the neonate for adaptation problems, extrapyramidal, and withdrawal symptoms, for at least 2 days, is recommended when neuroleptics have been used up to delivery. To prevent neonatal adaptation disorders, dose reduction or even treatment interruption in the days immediately preceding delivery can be discussed with the patient if the clinical course allows. However, to prevent a relapse at this vulnerable stage, pre-pregnancy dosage should be started immediately after delivery.

2.11.7   Butyrophenones

Pharmacology and toxicology

Haloperidol is the oldest and most important drug in this group. There are two old case reports of limb-reduction defects after first-trimester exposure to haloperidol. In total, there are more than 400 prospectively ascertained pregnancies exposed to haloperidol, mainly during the first trimester and in retrospective case-control studies (e.g. Diav-Citrin 2005B). These data do not confirm an increased rate of congenital malformations after first-trimester exposure. The largest study (Diav-Citrin 2005B) evaluated 188 pregnancies with haloperidol treatment and 27 with *penfluridol*. Among the reported malformations, this study found two cases of limb defects, one after haloperidol and one after penfluridol exposure. Fewer data are available on other butyrophenones, such as *benperidol, bromperidol, droperidol, melperone, pipamperone*, and *trifluperidol*, or the structurally related drugs, *fluspirilen* and *pimozide*. Teratogenic effects have not been seen, but data are insufficient to exclude an increased risk of malformations.

2.11 Psychotropic drugs

Extrapyramidal symptoms and withdrawal symptoms such as sedation, feeding problems, and restlessness have been reported in the neonate after chronic maternal use of high doses near term. There are isolated cases of neonatal dyskinesia and severe hyperthermia after maternal treatment with haloperidol (Collins 2003, Mohan 2000).

> **Recommendation.** Haloperidol may be used during pregnancy when treatment of acute psychosis or chronic psychotic illness is necessary. If needed to treat extrapyramidal side effects, biperiden can be added to the medication. Treatment with other butyrophenones is not an indication for termination of pregnancy. Detailed fetal ultrasonography may be offered, with special emphasis on the limbs, after maternal use of a butyrophenone in the first trimester. Regular psychiatric and obstetric care is recommended to diagnose in time a relapse or pregnancy complications (intrauterine growth retardaton, premature contractions). Observation of the neonate for adaptation problems for at least 2 days is recommended when butyrophenones have been used up to delivery. To prevent neonatal adaptation disorders dose reduction or even treatment interruption in the days immediately preceding delivery can be discussed with the patient if the clinical course allows. However, to prevent a relapse at this vulnerable stage, pre-pregnancy dosage should be started immediately after delivery.

2.11.8   Atypical antipsychotic drugs

Pharmacology and toxicology

Amisulprid, aripiprazole, clozapine, olanzapine, quetiapine, risperidon, and *ziprasidone* are called atypical or second-generation antipsychotics. Compared with "classical" antipsychotics (butyrophenones, phenothiazines), they have fewer neurological side effects (extrapyramidal or dyskinetic symptoms) and most of them have a relatively higher affinity for serotonin receptors than for dopamine receptors, resulting (apart from amisulprid and, as a transient effect, in risperidon) in a lower or insignificant prolactin increase. Therefore, a change from phenothiazines to atypical neuroleptics may result in an unwanted pregnancy. An increased risk of hyperglycemia or glucose intolerance in pregnant women who are using clozapine or olanzapine has been observed. Weight increase may result with these drugs, and with quetiapine and risperidone (Gentile 2004). Glucose intolerance and excessive weight increase are risk factors for the outcome of pregnancy. On the other hand, a lower birth weight was reported in association with atypical antipsychotics (McKenna 2005). As with other psychotropic drugs, atypical antipsychotics may cause withdrawal symptoms or adaptation disorders in the newborn; seizures have also been reported in a few cases.

Mendhekar and colleagues report normal pregnancy outcome after use of *aripiprazole* in two women (Mendhekar 2006A, 2006B). One was exposed during the first 8 weeks and in the second half of pregnancy; the other one from week 29 until 6 days prior to delivery in week 37.

Clozapine (*Clozaril*) was the first atypical antipsychotic drug, and consists of an aromatic tricyclic dibenzodiazepine and a moiety similar to phenothiazines. Clozapine can induce immunoallergic agranulocytosis and myocarditis as well as seizures, and is therefore only used in patients refractory to other antipsychotics. Leukocyte and differential blood counts should be normal before starting treatment, and monitored for the first 18 weeks of therapy, then at least fortnightly for up to 1 year for patients on long-term therapy. Patients with stable blood counts who continue to take clozapine for more than 1 year should have blood counts monitored every 4 weeks, and for 4 weeks after discontinuation of treatment.

Barnas (1994) found that clozapine accumulates in fetal serum. Negative effects on neonatal white blood cell levels have not been reported so far. There are reports of pregnancies in which exposure to clozapine has occurred (McKenna 2005, Gupta 2004, Stoner 1997, Lieberman 1992). All of these pregnancies resulted in the birth of normal, healthy infants. The outcome of another 176 pregnancies has been reviewed by Gentile (2004). These data, as well as about 500 exposed pregnancies registered by the producer, do not suggest an association between prenatal clozapine exposure and congenital anomalies. There have been reports of decreased fetal heart-rate modulation (Yogev 2002), sedation, jitteriness or other withdrawal symptoms in the newborn (Gentile 2004).

There are reports on more than 200 pregnancies exposed to *olanzapine* (McKenna 2005, Levinson 2003, Ernst 2002, Mendhekar 2002, Biswas 2001, Malek-Ahmadi 2001, Nagy 2001, Neumann 2001, Goldstein 2000, Kirchheiner 2000, registry data of the producer), none of which indicate teratogenicity. There were three retrospective reports with neonatal seizures after exposure until the end of pregnancy (Goldstein 2000, observations of the authors). Glucose intolerance and onset of gestational diabetes have also been reported after the use of olanzapine in pregnancy (Gentile 2004). Olanzapine has also been associated with pre-eclampsia (Yonkers 2004, Kirchheiner 2000).

Based on about 40 published case observations and 150 pregnancies registered by the producer, there is no indication to date for

2

Pregnancy

2.11 Psychotropic drugs

teratogenic effects of *quetiapine* (McKenna 2005, Pace, cited in Gentile 2004, Yaris 2004B, Taylor 2003, Tényi 2002).

There are about 60 pregnancies exposed to *risperidone* in the published literature (McKenna 2005, Yaris 2004B, Ratnayake 2002, MacKay 1998), and approximately 200 pregnancies collected by the producer, none of which indicate teratogenic effects.

With respect to *amisulpride* and *ziprasidone*, there is insufficient experience with their use in pregnancy. However, up to now there are no reports indicating a specific teratogenic potential in humans.

> **Recommendation.** Atypical antipsychotics may be used during pregnancy when treatment of acute psychosis or chronic psychotic illness is necessary. If possible, olanzapine or quetiapine are preferred because these have the most documented experience in pregnancy. Treatment with other atypicals is not an indication for termination of pregnancy. Furthermore, a pregnant patient who is stable with one of the less well-known antipsychotics should not be changed to another drug, because this may worsen her health. However, a detailed fetal ultrasonography may be offered after their use in the first trimester. Regular psychiatric and obstetric care is recommended to diagnose in time a relapse or pregnancy complications (intrauterine growth retardation, premature contractions). Observation of the neonate for withdrawal symptoms or adaptation problems for at least 2 days is recommended when atypical antipsychotics have been used up to delivery. To prevent neonatal adaptation disorders, dose reduction or even treatment interruption in the days immediately preceding delivery can be discussed with the patient if the clinical course allows. However, to prevent a relapse at this vulnerable stage, pre-pregnancy dosage should be started immediately after delivery.

2.11.9   Other neuroleptic drugs

Pharmacology and toxicology

There are insufficient data on pregnancy use of *clothiapin, loxapine, remoxipride, sertindole, sulpiride*, and *tiapride*. Most of them are benzamide derivatives and selective dopamine antagonists. *Tiapride* has only weak neuroleptic properties, and is used for the treatment of tardive dyskinesia caused by neuroleptic drugs (see section 2.11.18).

Recommendation. These neuroleptics should not be used, due to lack of experience in pregnancy. However, their use is not an indication for termination of pregnancy. Furthermore, a pregnant patient who is stable with these drugs should not be changed to another drug because this may worsen her health. However, a detailed fetal ultrasonography may be offered after their use in the first trimester. Regular psychiatric and obstetric care is recommended to diagnose in time a relapse or pregnancy complications (intrauterine growth retardation, premature contractions). Observation of the neonate for withdrawal symptoms or adaptation problems for at least 2 days is recommended when neuroleptics have been used up to delivery. To prevent neonatal adaptation disorders, dose reduction or even treatment interruption in the days immediately preceding delivery can be discussed with the patient if the clinical course allows. However, to prevent a relapse at this vulnerable stage, pre-pregnancy dosage should be started immediately after delivery.

2.11.10 Lithium and other mood-stabilizers/ antimanic agents

Pharmacology and toxicology

Lithium salts are the first-choice agents in the treatment of bipolar disorders. They are well-absorbed from the gastrointestinal tract, and are excreted by the kidneys. The half-life is 24 hours. Lithium crosses the placenta, and fetal plasma concentrations are similar to or higher than maternal plasma concentrations. In pregnant women, renal excretion of lithium is increased by 50–100%.

Based on their findings, Viguera and colleagues suggest that clinicians managing women with bipolar disorders who are planning to conceive should consider the high risk of relapse associated with lithium discontinuation in the overall risk/benefit assessment (Viguera 2000).

In the 1970s, lithium treatment during pregnancy was strongly associated with congenital heart malformations, especially Ebstein's anomaly, in the child. Ebstein's anomaly is a defect of the tricuspid valve, and can be detected with fetal echocardiography. Other defects ascribed to lithium were anomalies of the external ear, CNS, ureter, and the endocrine system (survey in Kozma 2005). The teratogenic risk of first-trimester lithium use now appears to be lower than previously suggested (Yonkers 2004, Viguera 2002, Cohen 1994, Jacobson 1992, Zalzstein 1990). If an association does exist, it is a weak one – i.e. only 1 in 1000 fetuses exposed during the first trimester is affected (Shepard 2002).

Other adverse effects which have been reported occasionally are polyhydramnios after fetal polyuria, stillbirth, fetal and neonatal

2

Pregnancy

2.11 Psychotropic drugs

arrhythmia, neonatal jaundice, and maternal and neonatal goiter (Pinelli 2002).

During delivery, the renal clearance of lithium decreases considerably, possibly resulting in toxicity for both the mother and the neonate. A "floppy infant syndrome" was described in this context, characterized by lethargy, poor sucking, tachypnea, tachycardia, respiratory stress syndrome, cyanosis, and hypotonia (Kozma 2005). Therefore, lithium should be discontinued prior to delivery (or the dose should be decreased by 30–50%). Immediately after delivery the pre-pregnancy dose should be reinstituted in order to prevent relapse.

Some authors recommend controlling thyroid function in both the pregnant woman and the neonate (Frassetto 2002, Llewellyn 1998).

The pharmacological treatment of bipolar disorders also includes the known teratogens *valproic acid* and *carbamazepine*, and some of the newer anticonvulsants, such as *gabapentin* and *lamotrigine*. First-trimester use of carbamazepine and of valproate is associated with an increased risk of spina bifida of 0.5–1% and 1–2% respectively (see Chapter 2.10 for more detailed information on anticonvulsants).

> **Recommendation.** Exposure to lithium is not an indication for termination of pregnancy. Women who need lithium therapy may continue the drug during pregnancy, but they should be closely monitored. Lithium should be given in small, divided doses (i.e. slow-release preparations). Monthly monitoring of maternal serum levels of lithium is recommended, weekly during the last month of pregnancy, and every 2 days perinatally. If necessary, the dose should be adjusted. Salt-restricted diets and diuretics should be avoided. A detailed fetal echocardiography should be offered. Ultrasound monitoring may control for polyhydramnios. Lithium should be decreased or discontinued when delivery is expected, and reinstituted immediately after delivery. The thyroid function in both the pregnant woman and the neonate should be controlled, as well as toxic symptoms in the neonate. Valproic acid and carbamazepine should only be used for bipolar disorders during pregnancy if lithium, other psychopharmaceuticals, and newer antiepileptics have failed.

2.11.11   Barbiturates as sedative-hypnotic agents

Pharmacology and toxicology

Several groups of drugs are available for the treatment of sleeping disorders. These drugs have sedative or hypnotic properties, depending on the dose used. Long-term use of these drugs is not recommended. Barbiturates were the most important hypnotics on the market, prior to the introduction of the benzodiazepines. Today, only *phenobarbitone* (*phenobarbital*) is still in regular use.

Most experience with the use of barbiturates during pregnancy comes from women with epilepsy (see Chapter 2.10). Short-term use of barbiturates for sleeping disorders or for anesthesia is probably safe. When phenobarbitone is given near delivery, respiratory depression can occur in the neonate (Desmond 1972).

> **Recommendation.** Phenobarbitone is not recommended as a hypnotic during pregnancy. Sedating antihistamines such as diphenhydramine (see Chapters 2.2 and 2.4) or benzodiazepines are preferred for the treatment of sleeping disorders. Short-term use of phenobarbitone is not an indication for a termination of pregnancy, and does not require specific prenatal diagnostic procedures. Observation of the neonate for withdrawal symptoms or adaptation problems for at least 2 days is recommended when barbiturates have been used up to delivery.

2.11.12   Benzodiazepines

Pharmacology and toxicology

Benzodiazepines are among the most commonly used anxiolytic drugs by women of reproductive age and pregnant women. They have anxiolytic, anticonvulsant, hypnotic-sedating, and muscle-relaxing properties. They are structurally related, and act on specific benzodiazepine receptors. The half-life may vary considerably, and depends mainly on the biologic activity of the metabolites, which are formed in the liver via oxidation.

Benzodiazepines cross the placenta. The rate of metabolism in the neonate is very low, and accumulation may occur.

Benzodiazepines with a very short half-life (<6 hours), such as *brotizolam*, *midazolam*, and *triazolam*, are used in anesthesia and in the treatment of insomnia.

Benzodiazepines with a short half-life (6–24 hours), such as *alprazolam*, *bromazepam*, *clotiazepam*, *lorazepam*, *loprazolam*, *lormetazepam*, *metaclazepam*, *oxazepam*, and *temazepam*, are used as sedatives and hypnotics.

Benzodiazepines with a longer half-life (up to several days), such as *chlordiazepoxide*, *clobazam*, *clorazepate*, *diazepam*, *flunitrazepam*, *flurazepam*, *ketazolam*, *medazepam*, *nitrazepam*, *nordazepam*, and *prazepam*, are used mainly as sedatives and anxiolytics.

There is controversy about the risk of malformations after exposure to benzodiazepines in the first trimester. Reviews of prenatal exposure to benzodiazepines indicate that some studies showed an association with cardiac malformations, facial clefts, and multiple malformations (Iqbal 2002, McElhatton 1994). Also, a recent case-control study found weak but statistical significant associations with oral clefts, intestinal atresia, and microcephaly after first-trimester exposure (Rodriguez-Pinilla 1999). However, other studies do not confirm this association (Erös 2002, Dolovich 1998, Ornoy 1998, Patuszak 1996).

In a population-based case-control study, Czeizel (2003) did not find a detectable teratogenic risk to the fetus after maternal short-term use (during approximately 3 weeks) of *diazepam* in the first trimester. For *chlordiazepoxide*, a somewhat higher risk of congenital cardiovascular malformations after intrauterine exposure in the second and third months cannot be excluded, according to Czeizel (2004). In a French registry of congenital malformations, 262 malformed infants with intrauterine exposure to benzodiazepines were found. Among them were six cases of anal atresia, five of which had been exposed to *lorazepam*. The authors state that this finding should be regarded as preliminary until it is confirmed in other data sets (Bonnot 2001).

Limited data on *alprazolam* do not suggest a significant association with fetal malformations (Schick-Boschetto 1992, St Clair 1992). About 100 pregnancies exposed to *clonazepam*, 18 to *medazepam*, 18 to *nitrazepam*, and 13 to *tofisopam* were evaluated, but did not indicate teratogenicity (Lin 2004, Erös 2002).

The regular use of benzodiazepines in the third trimester up to delivery may cause the "floppy infant syndrome" (sedation, muscular hypotonia, sucking problems, apnea, cyanosis, and hypothermia) and neonatal withdrawal symptoms (e.g. hypertonia, hyperreflexia, restlessness, sleeping disorders, and tremors), especially if larger doses are used to control severe pre-eclampsia/eclampsia. However, because of accumulation in the fetus, even low doses (e.g. <10 mg diazepam) may cause neonatal symptoms (Peinemann 2001). Data on the long-term effects are scarce.

Recommendation. When strictly indicated, benzodiazepines are among the drugs of first choice for the treatment of anxiety and sleeping disorders during pregnancy. They should be given at the lowest possible dose for the minimum amount of time. For long-term treatment, antidepressants are preferred. Long-acting benzodiazepines should be avoided. Observation of the neonate for respiratory depression, withdrawal symptoms or adaptation problems is recommended when benzodiazepines have been used up to delivery.

2.11.13   Zaleplon, zolpidem, and zopiclone

Pharmacology and toxicology

Zaleplon, zolpidem, zopiclone, and *eszopiclone* are newer drugs with sedative-hypnotic properties, which have an agonistic effect on central benzodiazepine receptors. Chemically, they are not related to benzodiazepines. They usually have a short half-life. A prospective controlled study on 40 first-trimester *zopiclone*-exposed women found no increased rate of major malformations (Diav-Citrin 1999). There was a normal outcome among 18 *zolpidem*-exposed pregnancies (e.g. Wilton 1998). Data for *zaleplon* and *eszopiclone* are insufficient to assess the safety in pregnancy.

> **Recommendation.** These drugs should not be prescribed for pregnant women. Their inadvertent use is not grounds for termination of pregnancy. Detailed fetal ultrasonography may be considered after first-trimester exposure. The drugs of first choice for sleeping disorders are sedating antihistamines and benzodiazepines.

2.11.14   Other anxiolytic drugs

Pharmacology and toxicology

Buspirone binds to serotonin and dopamine receptors, *opipramol* is a dibenzazepine derivative, and *kavain* is a cavalactone that is present in the roots of *Piper methysticum* (Cava-Cava). In the USA, cava was also used in "health foods"; in some countries it was removed from the market because of hepatotoxicity. No data are available for the use of any of these drugs during pregnancy (see also Chapter 2.19).

Hydroxyzine is an antihistamine with sedative and anxiolytic properties. Several studies covering about 240 pregnancies have been published (e.g. Diav-Citrin 2003, Einarson 1997, Schatz 1997). No increased incidence of malformations has been found, but more data are needed to exclude a possible teratogenic risk.

Meprobamate is one of the oldest tranquilinizers on the market. Since the introduction of benzodiazepines, there are very few indications for its use in pregnant women. In the 1970s, the use of meprobamate in the first trimester was associated with a possible increase in cardiac defects and polydactyly, observed, for example,

Pregnancy

2.11 Psychotropic drugs

in a study of Milkovich (1974) covering 400 pregnancies. However, no causal relationship could be established.

> **Recommendation.** If anxiolytic therapy is required, benzodiazepines are the drugs of choice. Buspirone, kavain, hydroxyzine, meprobamate, and opipramol should be avoided during pregnancy. Inadvertent use is not an indication for a termination of pregnancy or invasive diagnostic procedures. A detailed fetal ultrasonography should be offered.

2.11.15   Chloral hydrate

Pharmacology and toxicology

Chloral hydrate is one of the oldest hypnotic drugs on the market. Chloral hydrate is quickly metabolized to trichloroethanol and trichloroacetic acid. There are few data on its use in pregnancy, but to date no increased incidence of congenital malformations has been reported (Heinonen 1977).

> **Recommendation.** Chloral hydrate should not be prescribed to pregnant women. Its inadvertent use is not grounds for termination of pregnancy or for additional diagnostic procedures. The drugs of first choice for sleeping disorders are sedating antihistamines and benzodiazepines.

2.11.16   Other sedative-hypnotic drugs

Some H1-antihistamines, such as *diphenhydramine* and *doxylamine*, have sedative properties (see Chapters 2.2 and 2.4).

Valerian is an herbal medicine. Data on its use during pregnancy are not available, but there is no indication of prenatal toxicity in humans with this broadly used substance. However, there is substantial controversy concerning its use during pregnancy (see also Chapter 2.19).

Clomethiazole, melperone, promethazine (see also section 2.11.6), and *scopolamine* are not recommended as hypnotics. *Clomethiazole* is used to treat withdrawal symptoms after chronic abuse of alcohol. There are insufficient data on the use of these drugs in human pregnancy.

Tryptophane is an amino acid, and is given as a sleep aid. Chronic use of tryptophane during pregnancy has been associated with increased fetal breathing movements.

> **Recommendation.** Clomethiazol, melperone, promethazine, scopolamine, and tryptophane should not be prescribed to pregnant women with sleeping disorders. Inadvertent use of these drugs during pregnancy is not grounds for termination of pregnancy, or for invasive diagnostic procedures. The drugs of first choice for sleeping disorders are sedating antihistamines such as diphenhydramine, valerian, or benzodiazepines.

2.11.17   Psychoanaleptic drugs

Pharmacology and toxicology

The most commonly used analeptics, e.g. *amphetamines*, *amphetaminil*, *fenetylline*, and *methylphenidate*, are derivatives of phenylethylamine. The prototype is the centrally acting drug, amphetamine, which can lead to addiction.

In about 50 pregnancies where *methylphenidate* had been used, no substantial indication for teratogenicity was found (e.g. Golub 2005, DeBooy 1993). However, only some of them were exposed during the first trimester. An increased incidence of prematurity and growth retardation as well as neonatal withdrawal symptoms have been reported in infants of mothers abusing methylphenidate together with other substances (DeBooy 1993). It is important to be aware that this drug is increasingly prescribed not only during childhood but also to women of reproductive age for attention deficit and hyperactivity syndrome.

Modafinil, with a different mode of action from amphetamines, is used for narcolepsy. *Pemolin* is an oxazolidine that has been used for attention deficit disorder.

Data are insufficient for risk evaluation of these drugs during pregnancy.

> **Recommendation.** Psychoanaleptic drugs are contraindicated during pregnancy. Inadvertent use of these drugs during pregnancy is not grounds for termination of pregnancy, or for invasive diagnostic procedures. Detailed fetal ultrasonography may be performed after recurrent or high-dose exposure in the first trimester. If drug treatment for narcolepsy is required, methylphenidate is recommended.

2.11.18 Parkinson drugs

Pharmacology and toxicology

Parkinsonism is mainly seen in older patients, and is not normally a disease in pregnant women. Parkinson drugs which are given also for juvenile parkinsonism and restless leg syndrome are *l-dopa/benserazide*. Some 15 exposed pregnancies have been reported, with uneventful delivery of normal children (e.g. Arai 1997, Nomoto 1997, von Graeventiz 1996).

Parkinson drugs such as the dopamine agonists *bromocriptine, cabergoline,* α-*dihydroergocryptine, lisuride,* and *pergolide,* are used in women of reproductive age to inhibit prolactin secretion. For information on these drugs, see Chapter 2.15.

Additional Parkinson drugs, some of them used for extrapyramidal symptoms caused by "classical" neuroleptic drugs, are the virustatic *amantadine, biperiden, benzatropin, bornaprin, budipin, carbidopa, dexetimid, entacapon, metixen, pergolide, pramipexol, pridinol, procyclidine, ropinirol, tiapride,* and *trihexyphenidyl,* as well as the monoaminooxydase-B- (MAO-B-) inhibitors *selegilin* and *rasigilin.* With the exception of the broadly used ergotamine derivatives, data are insufficient for risk assessment in pregnancy. There is a case report of a woman treated with high doses of *pramipexol* during pregnancy (Mucchiut 2004).

> **Recommendation.** Combined treatment of a neuroleptic drug with biperiden is acceptable in pregnancy when indicated. For restless leg syndrome, better-evaluated drug groups should be used. Inadvertent use of a Parkinson drug not belonging to the broadly used ergotamine derivatives is not grounds for termination of pregnancy, or for invasive diagnostic procedures. Detailed fetal ultrasonography may be considered where first-trimester exposure to less-used drugs has occurred.

References

Abebe-Campino G, Offer D, Stahl B et al. Cardiac arrhythmia in a newborn infant associated with fluoxetine use during pregnancy. Ann Pharmacother 2002; 36: 533–4.

Altshuler LL, Cohen L, Szuba MP et al. Pharmacologic management of psychiatric illness during pregnancy: dilemmas and guidelines. Am J Psychiatry 1996; 153: 592–606.

Alwan S, Reefhuis J, Rasmussen S et al. Maternal use of selective serotonin re-uptake inhibitors and risk for birth defects. Birth Defects Res A 2005; 73: 291.

Anderson GM, Czarkowski K, Ravski N. Platelet serotonin in newborns and infants: ontogeny, heritability and effect on in utero exposure to selective serotonin reuptake inhibitors. Pediatr Res 2004; 56: 418–22.

Arai H, Shinotoh H, Hattori T. L-dopa/benserazide during pregnancy in a patient with juvenile parkinsonism. Clin Neurol 1997; 37: 264–5.

Barnas C, Bergant A, Hummer M et al. Clozapine concentrations in maternal and fetal plasma, amniotic fluid and breast milk. Am J Psychiatry 1994; 151: 945.

Biswas PN, Wilton LV, Pearce GL et al. The pharmacovigilance of olanzapine: results of a post-marketing surveillance study on 8858 patients in England. J Psychopharmacol 2001; 15: 265–71.

Biswas PN, Wilton LV, Shakir SAW. The pharmacovigilance of mirtazapine: results of a prescription event monitoring study on 13 554 patients in England. J Psychopharmacol 2003; 17: 121–6.

Bloem BR, Lammers GJ, Roofthooft DW et al. Clomipramine withdrawal in newborns. Arch Dis Child Fetal Neonatal Ed 1999; 81: F77.

Bonari L, Pinto N, Ahn E et al. Perinatal risks of untreated depression during pregnancy. Can J Psychiatry 2004; 49: 726–34.

Bonnot O, Vollset SE, Godet PF et al. Maternal exposure to lorazepam and anal atresia in newborns: results from a hypothesis-generating study of benzodiazepines and malformations. J Psychopharmacol 2001; 21: 456–8.

Briggs GG, Freeman RK, Yaffe SJ. Drugs in Pregnancy and Lactation, 7th edn. Baltimore, MD: Williams & Wilkins, 2005.

Bromiker R, Kaplan M. Apparent intrauterine fetal withdrawal from clomipramine hydrochloride. J Am Med Assoc 1994; 272: 1722–3.

Brunel P, Vial T, Roche I et al. Suivi de 151 grossesses exposées á un traitement antidepresseur (IMAO exclus) au cours de l'organogenése. Thérapie 1994; 49: 117–22.

Casper RC, Fleischer BE, Lee-Ancajas JC et al. Follow-up of children of depressed mothers exposed or not exposed to antidepressant drugs during pregnancy. J Pediatrics 2003; 142: 402–8.

Chambers CD, Johnson KA, Dick LM et al. Birth outcomes in pregnant women taking fluoxetine. N Engl J Med 1996; 335: 1010–15.

Chambers CD, Dick LM, Felix RJ et al. Pregnancy outcome in women who use sertraline. Teratology 1999; 59: 6.

Chambers CD, Hernandez-Diaz S, van Marter LJ et al. Selective serotonin-reuptake inhibitors and risk of persistent pulmonary hypertension of the newborn. N Engl J Med 2006; 354: 579–87.

Chun-Fai-Chan B, Koren G, Fayez I et al. Pregnancy outcome of women exposed to bupropion during pregnancy: a prospective comparative study. Am J Obstet Gynecol 2005; 192: 932–6.

Cohen LS, Friedman JM, Jefferson JW et al. A re-evaluation of risk of in utero exposure to lithium. J Am Med Assoc 1994; 271: 146–50.

Cohen LS, Heller VL, Bailey JW et al. Birth outcomes following prenatal exposure to fluoxetine. Biol Psychiatry 2000; 48: 996–1000.

Cohen LS, Altshuler LL, Harlow BL et al. Relapse of major depression during pregnancy in women who maintain or discontinue antidepressant treatment. J Am Med Assoc 2006; 295: 499–507.

Collins KO, Comer JB. Maternal haloperidol therapy associated with dyskinesia in a newborn. Am J Health-Syst Pharm 2003; 60: 2253–5.

Costei AM, Kozer E, Ho T et al. Perinatal outcome following third-trimester exposure to paroxetine. Arch Pediatr Adolesc Med 2002; 156: 1129–32.

Cott AD, Wisner KL. Psychiatric disorders during pregnancy. Intl Rev Psychiatry 2003; 15: 217–30.

Czeizel AE, Erös E, Rockenbauer M et al. Short-term oral diazepam treatment during pregnancy. A population-based teratological case-control study. Clin Drug Invest 2003; 23: 451–62.

Czeizel AE, Rockenbauer M, Sørensen HT et al. A population-based case-control study of oral chlordiazepoxide use during pregnancy and risk of congenital abnormalities. Neurotoxicol Teratol 2004; 26: 593–8.

Davis JM, Chen N. Dose response and dose equivalence of antipsychotics. J Clin Psychopharmacol 2004; 24: 192–208.

DeBooy VD, Seshia MM, Tenenbein M et al. Intravenous pentazocine and methylphenidate abuse during pregnancy. Maternal lifestyle and infant outcome. Am J Dis Child 1993; 147: 1062–5.

Desmond MM, Schwanecke RP, Wilson GS et al. Maternal barbiturate utilization and neonatal withdrawal symptomatology. J Pediatr 1972; 80: 190–97.

Diav-Citrin O, Okotore B, Lucarelli K et al. Pregnancy outcome following first-trimester exposure to zopiclone: a prospective controlled cohort study. Am J Perinatal 1999; 16: 157–60.

Diav-Citrin O, Shechtman S, Aharonovich A et al. Pregnancy outcome after gestational exposure to loratadine or other antihistamines: a prospective controlled cohort study. J Allergy Clin Immunol 2003; 111: 1239–43.

Diav-Citrin O (A), Shechtman S, Weinbaum D et al. Paroxetine and fluoxetine in pregnancy: a multicenter, prospective, controlled study. Reprod Toxicol 2005; 20: 459.

Diav-Citrin O (B), Shechtman S, Ornoy S et al. Safety of haloperidol and penfluridol in pregnancy: a multicenter, prospective, controlled study. J Clin Psychiatry 2005; 66: 317–22.

di Gianantonio E, Petrella M, Andrisani A et al. Venlafaxine in pregnancy: a prospective controlled study {Abstract}. Reprod Toxicol 2006; 22: 269.

Djulus J, Koren G, Einarson TR et al. Exposure to mirtazapine during pregnancy: a prospective, comparative study of birth outcomes. J Clin Psychiatry 2006; 67: 1280–84.

Dolovich LR, Addis A, Regis Vaillancourt et al. Benzodiazepine use in pregnancy and major malformations or oral cleft: meta-analysis of cohort and case-control studies. Br Med J 1998; 317: 839–43.

Dorn C, Pantlen A, Rohde A. Mirtazapin (Remergil®): Behandlungsoption bei therapieresistenter Hyperemesis gravidarum? – ein Fallbericht. Geburtsh Frauenheilk 2002; 62: 1–4.

Dubnov G, Fogelman R, Merlob P. Prolonged Q interval in an infant of a fluoxetine treated mother. Arch Dis Child 2005; 90: 972–3.

Einarson A, Bailey B, Jung G et al. Prospective controlled study of hydroxyzine and cetirizine in pregnancy. Ann Allergy Asthma Immunol 1997; 78: 183–6.

Einarson A (A), Selby P, Koren G. Abrupt discontinuation of psychotropic drugs during pregnancy: fear of teratogenic risk and impact of counseling. J Psychiatry Neurosci 2001; 26: 44–8.

Einarson A (B), Fatoye B, Sarkar M et al. Pregnancy outcome following gestational exposure to venlafaxine: a multicenter prospective controlled study. Am J Psychiatry 2001; 158: 1728–30.

Einarson A, Bonari L, Voyer-Lavigne S et al. A multicentre prospective controlled study to determine the safety of trazodone and nefazodone use during pregnancy. Can J Psychiatry 2003; 48: 106–10.

Ellingrod VL, Perry PJ. Venflaxine: a hetercyclic antidepressant. Am J Hosp Pharm 1994; 51: 3033–46.

Ericsson A, Källén B, Wiholm BE. Delivery outcome after the use of antidepressants in early pregnancy. Eur J Clin Pharmacol 1999; 55: 503–8.

Ernst LC, Goldberg JF. The reproductive safety profile of mood stabilizers, atypical antipsychotics, and broad-spectrum psychotropics. J Clin Psychiatry 2002; 63: 42–55.

Erös E, Czeizel AE, Rockenbauer M et al. A population-based case-control study of nitrazepam, medazepam, tofisopam, alprazolam and clonazepam treatment during pregnancy. Eur J Obstet Gynecol Reprod Biol 2002; 101: 147–54.

Frassetto F, Tourneur-Martel F, Barjhoux C-L. Goiter in a newborn exposed to lithium in utero. Ann Pharmacother 2002; 36: 1745–8.

Gentile S. Clinical utilization of atypical antipsychotics in pregnancy and lactation. Ann Pharmacother 2004; 38: 1265–71.

GlaxoSmithKline. Bupropion Pregnancy Registry – Interim Report, 1 September 1997 through 28 February 2006. Issued: June 2006.

Gold LH. Treatment of depression during pregnancy. J Women's Health Gender-Based Med 1999; 8: 601–7.

Goldstein DJ. Effects of third trimester fluoxetine exposure on the newborn. J Clin Psychopharmacol 1995; 15: 417–20.

Goldstein DJ, Corbin LA, Sundell KL. Effects of first-trimester fluoxetine exposure on the newborn. Obstet Gynecol 1997; 89: 713–18.

Goldstein DJ, Corbin LA, Fung MC. Olanzapine-exposed pregnancies and lactation: early experience. J Clin Psychopharmacol 2000; 20: 399–403.

Golub M, Costa L, Crofton K et al. NTP-CERHR Expert Panel Report on the reproductive and developmental toxicity of methylphenidate. Birth Defects Res B 2005; 74: 300–81.

Guclu S, Gol M, Dogan E, Saygili U. Mirtazapine use in resistant hyperemesis gravidarum: report of three cases and review of the literature. Arch Gynecol Obstet 2005; 272: 298–300.

Gupta N, Grover S. Safety of clozapine in 2 successive pregnancies. Can J Psychiatry 2004; 49: 865.

Haddad PM, Pal BR, Clarke P et al. Neonatal symptoms following maternal paroxetine treatment: serotonin toxicity or paroxetine discontinuation syndrome? J Psychopharmacol 2005; 19: 554–7.

Hallberg P, Sjöblom V. The use of selective serotonin reuptake inhibitors during pregnancy and breast-feeding: a review and clinical aspects. J Clin Psychopharmacol 2005; 25: 59–73.

Hansen D, Lou HC, Olsen J. Serious life events and congenital malformations: a national study with complete follow-up. Lancet 2000; 356: 875–80.

Heikkinen T, Ekblad U, Kero P et al. Citalopram in pregnancy and lactation. Clin Pharmacol Ther 2002; 72: 184–91.

Heikkinen T, Ekblad U, Palo P et al. Pharmacokinetics of fluoxetine and norfluoxetine in pregnancy and lactation. Clin Pharmacol Ther 2003; 73: 330–37.

Heinonen OP, Slone D, Shapiro S. Birth Defects and Drugs in Pregnancy. Littleton, MA: Publishing Science Group, 1977.

Hemels MEH, Einarson A, Koren G et al. Antidepressant use during pregnancy and the rates of spontaneous abortions: a meta-analysis. Ann Pharmacother 2005; 39: 803–9.

Hendrick V (A), Stowe ZN, Altshuler LL et al. Placental passage of antidepressant medications. Am J Psychiatry 2003; 160: 993–6.

2

Pregnancy

2.11 Psychotropic drugs

Hendrick V (B), Smith LM, Suri R et al. Birth outcomes after prenatal exposure to antidepressant medication. Am J Obstet Gynecol 2003; 188: 812–15.

Henke M, Schmidt KG. Aktuelle Arzneitherapie der Schizophrenie: Empfehlungen für den Allgemeinarzt. Arzneiverordnung in der Praxis 2005; 32: 20–22.

Hostetter A, Stowe ZN, Strader JR et al. Dose of selective serotonin reuptake inhibitors across pregnancy: clinical implications. Depress Anxiety 2000; 11: 51–7.

Iqbal MM, Sobhan T, Ryals T. Effects of commonly used benzodiazepines on the fetus, the neonate, and the nursing infant. Psychiatric Services 2002; 53: 39–49.

Isbister GK, Dawson A, Whyte I et al. Neonatal paroxetine withdrawal syndrome or actually serotonin syndrome? Arch Dis Child Fetal Neonatal Ed 2001; 85: F147–8.

Jablensky AV, Morgan V, Zubrick et al. Pregnancy, delivery and neonatal complications in a population cohort of women with schizophrenia and major affective disorders. Am J Psychiatry 2005; 162: 79–91.

Jacobson SJ, Jones K, Johnson K et al. Prospective multicentre study of pregnancy outcome after lithium exposure during first trimester. Lancet 1992; 339: 530–33.

Jaiswal S, Coombs RC, Isbister GK. Paroxetine withdrawal in a neonate with historical and laboratory confirmation. Eur J Pediatr 2003; 162: 723–4.

Källén B. Neonate characteristics after maternal use of antidepressants in late pregnancy. Arch Pediatr Adolesc 2004; 158: 312–16.

Källén B, Otterblad Olausson P. Antidepressant drugs during pregnancy and infant congenital heart defect. Reprod Toxicol 2006; 21: 221–2.

Kennedy DS, Evans N, Wang I et al. Fetal abnormalities associated with high-dose tranylcypromine in two consecutive pregnancies {Abstract}. Teratology 2000; 61: 441.

Kesim M, Yaris F, Kadioglu M et al. Mirtazapine use in two pregnant women. Is it safe? Teratology 2002; 66: 204.

Kirchheiner J, Berghofer A, Bolk-Weischedel D. Healthy outcome under olanzapine treatment in a pregnant woman. Pharmacopsychiatry 2000; 33: 78–80.

Kozma C. Neonatal toxicity and transient neurodevelopment deficits following prenatal exposure to lithium: another clinical report and a review of the literature. Am J Med Genet 2005; 132A: 441–4.

Kulin NA, Patuszak A, Sage SR et al. Pregnancy outcome following maternal use of the new selective serotonin reuptake inhibitors. J Am Med Assoc 1998; 279: 609–10.

Laine K, Kytölä J, Bertilsson L. Severe adverse effect in a newborn with two defective CYP2D6 alleles after exposure to paroxetine during late pregnancy. Ther Drug Monit 2004; 26: 685–7.

Levey L, Ragan K, Hower-Hartley A et al. Psychiatric disorders in pregnancy. Neurol Clin 2004; 22: 863–93.

Levinson AJ, Zipursky RB. Antipsychotics and the treatment of women with psychosis. In: M Steiner, G Koren (eds), Handbook of Female Psychopharmacology. London: Martin Dunitz, 2003, p. 63.

Levinson-Costiel R, Merlob P, Linder N et al. Neonatal abstinence syncrome after in utero exposure to selective serotonin reuptake inhibitors in term infants. Arch Pediatr Adolesc Med 2006; 160: 173–6.

Lieberman J, Safferman AZ. Clinical profile of clozapine: adverse reactions and agranulocytosis. In: Y Lapierre, B Jones (eds), Clozapine in Treatment Resistant Schizophrenia: A Scientific Update. London: Royal Society of Medicine, 1992.

2

Pregnancy

Lieberman J, Stroup S, McEvoy J et al. Clinical antipsychiotic trials of intervention effectiveness (CATIE) investigators. Effectiveness of antipsychotic drugs in patients with chronic schizophrenia. N Engl J Med 2005; 353: 1209–23.

Lin AE, Peller AJ, Westgate M-N et al. Clonazepam use in pregnancy and the risk of malformations. Birth Defects Res A 2004; 70: 534–6.

Llewellyn A, Stowe ZN, Strader JR. The use of lithium and management of women with bipolar disorder during pregnancy and lactation. J Clin Psychiatry 1998; 59(Suppl 2): 57–64.

Loughhead AM, Stowe ZN, Newport et al. Placental passage of tricyclic antidepressants. Biol Psychiatry 2006; 59: 287–90.

MacKay FJ, WIlton LV, Pearce GL et al. The safety of risperidone: a post-marketing study on 7684 patients. Hum Psychopharmacol Clin Exp 1998; 12: 413–18.

Malek-Ahmadi P. Olanzapine in pregnancy. Ann Pharmacother 2001; 35: 1294–5.

Malm H, Klaukka T, Neuvonen P. Risks associated with selective serotonin reuptake inhibitors in pregnancy. Obstet Gynecol 2005; 106: 1289–96.

Mattson SN, Eastvold KL, Jones JA et al. Neurobehavioral follow-up of children prenatally exposed to fluoxetine. Teratology 1999; 59: 376.

Mattson SN, Calarco KE, Kao KK et al. Neurodevelopmental outcome of infants and toddlers exposed prenatally to selective serotonin reuptake inhibitors. Birth Defects Res A 2004; 70: 261.

McElhatton PR. The use of phenothiazines during pregnancy and lactation. Reprod Toxicol 1992; 6: 475–90.

McElhatton PR. The effects of benzodiazepine use during pregnancy and lactation. Reprod Toxicol 1994; 8: 461–75.

McElhatton PR, Garbis HM, Eléfant E. et al. The outcome of pregnancy in 689 women exposed to therapeutic doses of antidepressants. A Collaborative Study of the European Network of Teratology Information Services (ENTIS). Reprod Toxicol 1996; 10: 285–94.

McKenna K, Koren G, Tetelbaum M et al. Pregnancy outcome of women using atypical antipsychotic drugs: a prospective comparative study. J Clin Psychiatry 2005; 66: 444–9.

Mendhekar DN, War L, Sharma JB et al. Olanzapine and Pregnancy. Pharmacopsychiatry 2002; 35: 122–3.

Mendhekar DN (A), Sharma JB, Srilakshmi P. Use of aripiprazole during late pregnancy in a woman with psychotic illness. Ann Pharmacother 2006; 40: 575.

Mendhekar DN (B), Sunder KR, Andrade C. Aripiprazole use in a pregnant schizoaffective woman. Bipolar Disord 2006; 8: 299–300.

Milkovich L, van den Berg BJ. Effects of prenatal meprobamate and chlordiazepoxide hydrochloride on human embryonic and fetal development. N Engl J Med 1974; 291: 1268–71.

Mohan MS, Patole SK, Whitehall JS. Severe hypothermia in a neonate following antenatal exposure to haloperidol. J Paediatr Child Health 2000; 36: 412.

Moor RA, Mourad L, Haar J et al. Withdrawal symptoms in a neonatal infant following exposure to venlafaxine during pregnancy. Ned Tijdschr Geneesk 2003; 147: 1370–72.

Mortola JF. The use of psychotropic agents in pregnancy and lactation. Psychiatric Clin North Am 1989; 12: 69–87.

Moses-Kolko EL, Bogen D, Perel J et al. Neonatal signs after late in utero exposure to serotonin reuptake inhibitors. Literature review and implications for clinical applications. J Am Med Assoc 2005; 293: 2372–83.

Mucchiut M, Belgrado E, Cutuli D et al. Pramipexole-treated Parkinson's disease during pregnancy. Mov Disord 2004; 19: 1114–15.

2.11 Psychotropic drugs

Nagy A, Tényi T, Lenard K et al. Olanzapine and pregnancy {in Hungarian}. Orv Hetil 2001; 142: 137–8.

Neumann NU, Frasch K. Olanzapine and pregnancy. 2 case reports {in German}. Nervenarzt 2001; 72: 876–8.

Nomoto M, Kaseda S, Iwata S et al. Levodopa in pregnancy {Letter}. Mov Disord 1997; 12: 261.

Nonacs R, Cohen LS. Depression during pregnancy: diagnosis and treatment options. J Clin Psychiatry 2002; 63(Suppl 7): 24–30.

Nordeng H, Spigset O. Treatment with selective serotonin reuptake inhibitors in the third trimester of pregnancy. Drug Saf 2005; 28: 565–81.

Nulman I, Rovet J, Stewart DE et al. Neurodevelopment of children exposed in utero to antidepressant drugs. N Engl J Med 1997; 336: 258–62.

Nulman I, Rovet J, Stewart DE et al. Child development following exposure to tricyclic antidepressants or fluoxetine throughout fetal life: a prospective controlled study. Am J Psychiatry 2002; 159: 1889–95.

Nulman I, Knittel-Keren D, Valo S et al. Child neurodevelopment following exposure to venlafaxine in utero, unexposed siblings as comparison group: preliminary results {Abstract}. Reprod Toxicol 2006; 22: 280.

Oberlander TF, Misri S, Fitzgerald CE et al. Pharmacologic factors associated with transient neonatal symptoms following prenatal psychotropic medication exposure. J Clin Psychiatry 2004; 65: 230–37.

Okotore B, Einarson A, Chambers CD et al. Pregnancy outcome following gestational exposure to venlafaxine: a multicenter prospective controlled study. Teratology 1999; 59: 439.

Ornoy A, Arnon J, Shechtman S et al. Is benzodiazepine use during pregnancy really teratogenic? Reprod Toxicol 1998; 12: 511–15.

Patuszak A, Schick-Boschetto B, Zuber C et al. Pregnancy outcome following first-trimester exposure to fluoxetine (Prozac). J Am Med Assoc 1993; 269: 2246–8.

Patuszak A, Milich V, Chan S et al. Prospective assessment of pregnancy outcome following first trimester exposure to benzodiazepines. Can J Clin Pharmacol 1996; 3: 167–71.

Peinemann F, Daldrup T. Severe and prolonged sedation in five neonates due to persistence of active diazepam metabolites. Eur J Pediatr 2001; 160: 378–81.

Pinelli JM, Symington AF, Cunningham KA et al. Case report and review of the perinatal implications of maternal lithium use. Am J Obstet Gynecol 2002; 187: 245–9.

Rampono J, Proud S, Hackett P et al. A pilot study of newer antidepressant concentrations in cord and maternal serum and possible effects in the neonate. Intl J Neuropsychopharmacol 2004; 7: 329–34.

Ratnayake T, Libretto SE. No complications with risperidone treatment before and throughout pregnancy and during the nursing period. J Clin Psychiatry 2002; 63: 76–7.

Rodriguez-Pinilla E. Prenatal exposure to benzodiazepines: a case-control study. Presentation at the 10th Annual Conference of the European Network of Teratology Information Services, 1999.

Rohde A, Dembinski J, Dorn C. Mirtazapine (Remergil®) for treatment resistant hyperemesis gravidarum: rescue of a twin pregnancy. Arch Gynecol Obstet 2003; 268: 219–21.

Rosenheck R, Perlick D, Bingham S et al. Effectiveness and cost of olanzapine and haloperidol treatment of schizophrenia. J Am Med Assoc 2003; 290: 2693–702.

Saks BR. Mirtazapine: treatment of depression, anxiety, and hyperemesis gravidarum in the pregnant patient. A report of 7 cases. Arch Womens Ment Health 2001; 3: 165–70.

Santos RP, Pergolizzi JJ. Transient neonatal jitteriness due to maternal use of sertraline. J Perinatol 2004; 24: 392–4.

Sanz EJ, de las Cuevas C, Kiuru A et al. Selective serotonin reuptake inhibitors in pregnant women and neonatal withdrawal syndrome: a database analysis. Lancet 2005; 365: 482–7.

Schatz M, Petitti D. Antihistamines and pregnancy. Ann Allergy Asthma Immunol 1997; 78: 157–9.

Schick-Boschetto B, Zuber C. Alprazolam exposure during early human pregnancy. Teratology 1992; 45: 460.

Schimmell MS, Katz EZ, Shaag Y et al. Toxic neonatal effects following clomipramine therapy. J Toxicol Clin Toxicol 1991; 29: 479–84.

Shepard TH, Brent RL, Friedman JM et al. Update on new developments in the study of human teratogens. Teratology 2002; 65: 153–61.

Simon GE, Cunningham ML, Davis RL. Outcomes of prenatal antidepressant exposure. Am J Psychiatry 2002; 159: 2055–61.

Sivojelezova A, Shushaiber S, Sarkissian L et al. Citalopram use in pregnancy: prospective comparative evaluation of pregnancy and fetal outcome. Am J Obstet Gynecol 2005; 193: 2004–9.

St Clair SM, Schirmer RG. First-trimester exposure to alprazolam. Obstet Gynecol 1992; 80: 843–6.

Stoner SC, Sommi RW, Marken PA et al. Clozapine use in two full-term pregnancies. J. Clin Psychiatry 1997; 58: 364.

Tabacova SA, McCloskey CA, Fisher JR. Adverse developmental events reported to FDA in association with maternal citalopram treatment in pregnancy. Birth Defects Res A 2004; 70: 361.

Tabacova SA, McCloskey CA, Fisher JR. Withdrawal-type adverse events reported to FDA in association with maternal citalopram treatment in pregnancy. Birth Defects Res A 2005; 73: 299.

Taylor TM, O'Toole MS, Ohlsen RI et al. Safety of quetiapine during pregnancy. Am J Psychiatry 2003; 160: 588–9.

Tényi T, Trixler M, Keresztes Z. Quetiapine and pregnancy. Am J Psychiatry 2002; 159: 674.

Viguera AC, Nonacs R, Cohen LS et al. Risk of recurrence of bipolar disorder in pregnant and nonpregnant women after discontinuing lithium maintenance. Am J Psychiatry 2000; 157: 179–84.

Viguera AC, Cohen LS, Baldessarini RJ et al. Managing bipolar disorder during pregnancy: weighing the risks and the benefits. Can J Psychiatry 2002; 47: 426–36.

von Graeventiz KS, Shulman LM, Revell SP. Levodopa in pregnancy. Mov Disord 1996; 11: 115–16.

Wilton LV, Pearce GL, Martin RM et al. The outcomes of pregnancy women exposed to newly marketed drugs in general practice in England. Br J Obstet Gynaecol 1998; 105: 882–9.

Wisner KL, Perel JM, Wheeler SB. Tricyclic dose requirements across pregnancy. Am J Psychiatry 1993; 150: 1541–2.

Wogelius P, Norgaard M, Gislum M et al. Maternal use of selective serotonin reuptake inhibitors and risk of congenital malformations. Epidemiology 2006; 17: 701–4.

Yaris F (A), Kadioglu M, Kesim M et al. Newer antidepressants in pregnancy: prospective outcome of a case series. Reprod Toxicol 2004; 19: 235–8.

Yaris F (B), Yaris E, Kadioglu M et al. Use of polypharmacotherapy in pregnancy: a prospective outcome in a case. Progress Neuropharmacol Biol Psychiatry 2004; 28: 603–5.

Yogev Y, Ben-Haroush A, Kaplan B. Maternal clozapine treatment and decreased fetal heart rate variability. Intl J Gynecol Obstet 2002; 79: 259–60.

Yonkers KA, Wisner KL, Stowe et al. Management of bipolar disorder during pregnancy and the postpartum period. Am J Psychiatry 2004; 161: 608–20.

Zalzstein I, Koren G, Einarson T et al. A case-control study on the association between first trimester exposure to lithium and Ebstein's anomaly. Amer J Cardiol 1990; 65: 817–18.

Immunomodulators

2.12

Corinna Weber-Schöndorfer

2.12.1 Immunomodulators in general

Immunomodulators include immunosuppressive and immunostimulatory agents. Chemically defined immunosuppressants, such as *azathioprine, cyclosporine A, mycophenolate mofetil,* and *tacrolimus, sirolimus,* and *everolimus* should be distinguished from monoclonal antibodies. This group includes *basiliximab, bevacizumab, daclizumab, muromonab-CD3, natalizumab, ranibizumab,* and *palivizumab. Adalimumab, etanercept, bevacizumab,* and *infliximab* are monoclonal antibodies against human tumor necrosis factor (TNF) α. Corticosteroids also belong to the immunosuppressant drugs (see Chapter 2.15). The group of immunostimulatory agents includes the *interferons,* colony-stimulating factors, and Copolymer 1 (i.e. *glatiramer acetate*).

Most clinical experience involves pregnancies after kidney and liver transplantation. Long-term therapies include azathioprine, cyclosporine, and tacrolimus in combination with glucocorticoids (usually prednisolone). If no rejection has occurred and if the transplantation has been performed more than 2 years before conception, the outcome of the pregnancy is likely to be good. Women with immunosuppressant therapy are more frequently delivered by cesarean section. More premature births, more children with intrauterine growth retardation and transient neonatal renal function disorders have been reported. However, there is no substantial indication for an elevated risk for congenital malformations or persistent functional deficits in prenatally-exposed infants.

A study compared pregnancy outcome several years before and after transplantation. It was striking that some complications occurred in both groups with similar percentages – i.e. pre-eclampsia (22%), premature births (46%), lower birth weights (31%), small for gestational age (16%), and infant mortality rate (5%). Only the abortion rate was higher prior to transplantation than afterwards, but the adjusted odd ratios did not differ significantly. In neither of the two groups was there an increased rate of congenital malformations (Källén 2005). Therefore, it is conclusive that the complications are mainly due to the severity of maternal disease. The transplantation or the immunosuppressive therapy plays a minor part.

2.12.2   Azathioprine

Azathioprine (AZA) is an immunosuppressant extensively metabolized to the purine analog 6-mercaptopurine (6 MP) (see Chapter 2.13). Azathioprine is well-absorbed from the gastrointestinal tract when given by mouth (47%), whereas 6-mercaptopurine is less well-absorbed (only 16%). Both agents are bound to plasma proteins (30%). The risk evaluation for the two agents is comparable for the immunosuppressive dose. AZA can pass through the human placenta. De Boer (2006) describes three patients with Crohn's disease where the thiopurine metabolites were measured in the red blood cells (RBC) of mother and infant directly after delivery. The metabolite 6-methylmercaptopurine (responsible for hepatotoxicity) could not be detected in the RBC in any of the three infants. The metabolite 6-thioguaninenucleotides (responsible for myelotoxicity) was found in the infants, but in lower concentrations than in their mothers.

AZA is mutagenic in bacteria tests and teratogenic in animal experiments (Polifka 2002). However, approximately 40 studies and case series which total more than 1000 pregnancies and case reports involving 120 pregnancies have not demonstrated an increased malformation rate (Berkovitch 2005, Moskovitz 2004,

Armenti 2003, Francella 2003, Polifka 2002). Only Nørgård (2003) concluded from 10 exposed pregnancies in the Danish Medical Birth Registry that there was an increased risk for major malformations, for perinatal mortality, and for prematurity.

A risk of low birth weight and prematurity after *in utero* exposure to AZA has been reported (e.g. Berkovitch 2005), but this could be a consequence of the disease itself or of the associated therapy using glucocorticoids. Additionally, occasional leukopenia or pancytopenia has been reported. It was suggested that inhibition of neonatal hematopoiesis is predicted by whether or not maternal leukopenia is observed during the third trimester (Davison 1985).

Nulman (2004) evaluated the prenatal effects of a combination of cyclosporine and AZA on children's neurodevelopment, and compared it with unexposed children. The 20 exposed children (aged 3–13 years) were not significantly different from the unexposed regarding global, verbal, and performance IQ scores, compared with the control children. The exposed children appear to have language scores in the upper range of normal.

If the father took AZA or 6-MP at conception, no substantial risk for intrauterine development has been reported (see Chapter 1).

> **Recommendation.** Immunosuppression with azathioprine has not been associated with an increased risk of teratogenesis in approximately 1000 cases. Its use does not require termination of pregnancy. A detailed fetal ultrasound examination should be offered to confirm normal morphologic development in cases of first-trimester exposure. If the pregnant woman suffers from leukopenia in the third trimester, dose reduction must be considered to prevent leukopenia in the newborn.

2.12.3   Cyclosporine A

Cyclosporine A (CsA) originates from fungal cultures, and is used after organ transplantation or for treating immunological diseases. It is fetotoxic in animals at high doses, but no major teratogenic effect has been demonstrated experimentally (Brown 1985, Mason 1985).

There are more than 1000 case reports on renal and other transplant patients receiving cyclosporine who became pregnant and delivered a normal child (Ghanem 2005, Armenti 2003, Bar-Oz 2001, Rayes 1998, Wu 1998, Lamarque 1997).

Growth restriction has been observed in human pregnancies involving cyclosporine; however, several of these cases also included gestational exposure to corticosteroids, which may have contributed to stunting fetal growth. In a meta-analysis, the rate of low birth weight in cyclosporine-exposed pregnancies was increased compared with the rate in pregnancies in transplanted women who were not on cyclosporine (49% versus 38%), but no increased risk of malformations or prematurity was associated with the use of CsA during pregnancy in the population studied (Bar-Oz 1999).

After the first year, six infants had functional impairment of their B- and T-lymphocytes as well as natural killer cells; however, these deficits were not clinically apparent (di Paola 2000). In an earlier study by Baarsma (1993), prenatal cyclosporine was not associated with effects on the immune responses of infants up to 2 years. A cohort of 14 children exposed prenatally to cyclosporine and prednisone were followed to a mean age of 54 ± 32 months and evaluated to determine whether there were any detectable long-term immunologic and neurodevelopmental effects associated with these exposures. Test scores for this group did not differ significantly from those of a non-exposed control group (Rieder 1997). Nulman (2004) found similar results in 20 prenatally-exposed children.

In one case report (Roll 1997), a hepatoblastoma was reported in a 2-year-old who was exposed to cyclosporine (and prednisolone) throughout gestation. Although this association may be coinciden-tal, there is concern that chronic immunosuppressive therapy may increase the risk of tumor development in transplant patients. This case may indicate such a risk for fetuses exposed *in utero*.

CsA has a well-known nephrotoxic side effect, not only in trans-planted kidneys but also in normal kidneys. In 26 intrauterine exposed children, there was no evidence of nephrotoxicity when they were followed to an average age of 39 months after their birth (Shaheen 1993). Similarly, no impairment of renal function at 1 to 7 years of age was found among 12 children born to women who had been treated with cyclosporine during pregnancy (Cochat 2004).

> **Recommendation.** In more than 1000 pregnancies no substantial terato-genic effect was recognizable in human fetuses exposed to cyclosporine *in utero*. Its use does not require termination of pregnancy. A detailed fetal ultrasound examination should be offered to confirm normal morphologic development in case of first-trimester exposure.

2.12.4 Selective immunosuppressants

Tacrolimus is a macrolide obtained from Streptomyces, and is widely used as an immunosuppressant in transplant medicine. Skin diseases such as neurodermatitis are another indication; this will be discussed elsewhere (see Chapter 2.17). Certain advantages and disadvantages of tacrolimus in pregnancy are discussed compared to cyclosporine: rejection and hypertension are less common with tacrolimus, and the necessary dosage of prednisolone is lower. On the other hand, gestational diabetes occurs more often, as does transient hyperkalemia and transient reduction of kidney function in the newborn. Jain (1997) even reported on a newborn with anuria which lasted 36 hours. As with other immunosuppressant drugs, pre-eclampsia, prematurity, low birth weight, and cesarian births were seen at greater incidence.

More than 200 exposed pregnancies are documented, where tacrolimus was given together with prednisolone or other immunosuppressants. This is based on retrospectively ascertained case reports or case series (Jabiry-Zieniewicz 2006, Garcia-Donaire 2005, Jain 2004, Rayes 1998), on a small prospective study (Jain 2003), and on the National Transplantation Registry (Armenti 2003), which was started by the pharmaceutical industry in 1991.

In the prospective study, the outcome of 49 children of 37 liver-transplanted mothers was analyzed (Jain 2003). Two premature babies and one child with multiple anomalies died; one newborn had a unilateral cystic kidney without urine production. In a retrospective analysis of 100 pregnancies with 68 live-born children, there were four with different malformations (Kainz 2000). Retrospective cases report premature twins of 32 weeks' gestation. Both suffered from cardiomyopathy, of which one of them died (Vyas 1999). Among nine tacrolimus-exposed pregnancies, there were two with a small ventricular septal defect (Nagy 2003). An otherwise healthy premature baby who was exposed *in utero* to tacrolimus and mycophenolate mofetil demonstrated hypoplastic fingernails and short fifth fingers on both hands (Pergola 2001). There are rare case reports on the use of tacrolimus during pregnancy for other indications, such as refractory inflammatory bowel disease (Baumgart 2005).

No substantial teratogenic risk can be concluded from this data. Note that the above-mentioned adverse effects have been reported by almost all authors.

For tacrolimus as an ointment, see Chapter 2.17.

The macrolide *sirolimus* inhibits the proliferation of T-cells. Information on its use in human pregnancy is limited to a few case reports (Guardia 2006, Armenti 2003). *Everolimus* has not been evaluated for its use during pregnancy. *Pimecrolimus* is only available for dermatic use (see Chapter 2.17).

Mycophenolate mofetil (MMF) increases birth defects in experimental animal studies. In the National Transplantation Registry (Armenti 2003), no teratogenic effects have been reported in approximately 20 pregnancies. On the other hand, there is one case report of multiple congenital anomalies in a fetus which was exposed to MMF, tacrolimus, and prednisone (le Ray 2004); another child of a liver transplanted mother was born with atresia of the esophagus, and malformations of the heart and iris (Källén 2005). The premature baby with hypoplastic fingernails and short fifth fingers (Pergola 2001) is already mentioned above.

> **Recommendation.** The occurrence of gestational diabetes should be considered with tacrolimus therapy. In cases involving long-term prenatal therapy in the second and/or third trimesters, the newborn should be monitored for transient renal insufficiency and hyperkalemia. This applies to tacrolimus, everolimus, and sirolimus. There are insufficient data concerning the safety of first-trimester use of sirolimus, everolimus, and mycophenolate mofetil. From the 200 pregnancies exposed to tacrolimus no substantial teratogenic risk can be concluded. However, the use of these drugs does not require termination of pregnancy. A detailed fetal ultrasound examination should be offered to confirm normal morphologic development in cases of first-trimester exposure. Whether the immunosuppressant therapy of a transplanted woman who is stable on her medication should be changed is a question of risk–benefit assessment, because there is little experience in human pregnancies.

2.12.5   Monoclonal antibodies as part of an immunomodulatory therapy

Infliximab is a monoclonal antibody against human tumor necrosis factor (TNF) α. It is mainly used for the treatment of Crohn's disease, but is also prescribed for rheumatoid arthritis. The product is a chimeric antibody with a human constant region and a mouse variable region, produced by recombinant DNA technology in cultured cells. The Food and Drug Administration (FDA) reported a three-fold higher incidence of lymphoma after therapy with infliximab. An analysis of more than 60 mostly retrospective ascertained pregnancies with infliximab use in Crohn's disease did not reveal a teratogenic risk (Kimme 2006, Mahadevan 2005, Katz 2004). Unfortunately, no controlled studies have been reported.

Etanercept is a fusion protein consisting of a portion of the human tumor necrosis factor (TNF) receptor and a portion of human immunoglobin 1. Clinicians have collected reports on more than 20 pregnancies with exposure to etanercept – mostly only in the first trimester – and normal pregnancy outcomes (Kimme 2006, Chakravarty 2003, Wallace 2003, Sills 2001). VATER association in a child exposed throughout gestation to etanercept *in utero* may be coincidental, but has to be discussed in the future (Carter 2006).

Adalimumab is a recombinant human immunoglobin G_1 monoclonal antibody targeting TNF that is approved for rheumatoid arthritis as well as psoriatic arthritis. There are four reported cases with adalimumab treatment throughout pregnancy and healthy children (Kimme 2006, Mishkin 2006, Vesga 2005).

There are almost no data concerning the following monoclonal antibodies and their use in human pregnancies: *basiliximab, daclizumab, efalizumab, muromonab-CD3,* and *palivizumab.* The same applies for bevacizumab and ranibizumab, which are antibodies against the vascular endothelial growth factor and used for the treatment of macula degeneration.

Natalizumab is a humanized antibody against α_4-β_1-integrin, which hinders the infiltration of lymphocytes into the CNS. Because of the occurrence of progressive multifocal leukencephalopathy in two patients with multiple sclerosis and in one with Crohn's disease, the FDA withdrew it from the market. In March 2006, it was again approved for multiple sclerosis by the FDA. There are no published data on natalizumab during pregnancy.

> **Recommendation.** Monoclonal antibodies are contraindicated in pregnancy. Inadvertent use does not justify termination of pregnancy or invasive diagnostic procedures. A detailed fetal ultrasound examination should be offered to confirm normal morphologic development in cases of first-trimester exposure.

2.12.6   Interferons

Interferons are naturally occurring protein-like macromolecules with antiviral activity, which are used to stimulate the defense reactions of the organism.

Interferons include at least four classes of antigenically and physicochemically distinct proteins: *interferons α, -β, -γ* (gamma), and -τ (tau). They are present in embryonal, fetal, and adult tissues (Martinez-Maza 1984). Genetic engineering techniques have made specific interferons available in quantities sufficient to investigate their use as therapeutic agents. Both interferon-α and interferon-γ play a role in ovarian function (Grasso 1992). Because of these new observations, the interferons have been characterized as reproductive hormones. It is not clear whether or not interferons have a role in cell proliferation and differentiation, as well as other aspects of reproduction, such as the maternal recognition of pregnancy (Bazer 1997, Roberts 1996).

Interferon-α, including *interferon-α_{2a}, interferon-α_{2b}, interferon alpha-n3* and *interferon-alfacon-1*, seem to be important in maintaining human pregnancy (Chard 1991). Interferon-α is used as a therapeutic for chronic active hepatitis B and C, as well as for chronic granulocytic leukemia, hairy cell leukemia, other malignancies, and essential thrombocythemia. *Pegylated interferon-α_{2a}* and *pegylated interferon-α_{2b}* are modified forms of interferon in which polyethylene glycol is covalently bound to the compound to slow its inactivation and excretion, and are indicated for chronic hepatitis B and C (for ribavirine, see Chapter 2.6).

Interferon-α is not transferred across the placenta in significant amounts (Pons 1995). Several case reports have described successful pregnancies in women who received interferon-α during the first trimester, or throughout gestation (Regierer 2006, al Kindi 2005, Mesquita 2005, Al Bahar 2004, Mubarak 2002). A pregnant 15-year-old who suffered from thrombocythemia took interferon-α_{2a} throughout her pregnancy. Her female premature child was growth-retarded and showed signs of a neonatal lupus-like syndrome, like her mother, but was otherwise healthy (Fritz 2005).

Interferon-β is marketed for severe viral diseases; *interferon-β_{1a}* and *interferon-β_{1b}* are used for multiple sclerosis. So far, no specific risk has been proven. There is a small prospective study (Boskovic 2005) with 23 pregnancies complicated mostly by multiple sclerosis and interferon-β exposure. It was concluded that β-interferon therapy in the first trimester appears to be associated with an increased risk for fetal loss and low birth weight, but the small number of cases restricts this statement. Another study with interferon-β_{1a} therapy in 40 exposed pregnancies and 22 live births reported 1 newborn with hydrocephalus among otherwise healthy babies (Sandberg-Wollheim 2005). In the database of the Berlin TIS, we can overview 53 prospective ascertained interferon-β exposed pregnancies to date. They resulted in 8 ETOPs, 6 spontaneous abortions, and 39 live births; of these, one newborn had severe hip dysplasia and one had a minor malformation (an accessory ear tag).

Interferon-γ_{1b} is marketed for the prevention of serious infections with septic granulomatosis.

Administration of interferons has been associated with pyrexia, leukopenia, hypotension, fatigue, and anorexia (Mannering 1986, Vilcek 1984). It is possible that one of these adverse effects (in particular pyrexia) or the underlying disease itself might be associated with adverse reproductive effects. In summary, available information is

Recommendation. Interferon therapy during pregnancy is acceptable if no other similarly effective and better-proven drugs are available. Its inadvertent use does not justify termination of pregnancy or invasive diagnostic procedures. A detailed fetal ultrasound examination should be offered to confirm normal morphologic development in cases of first-trimester exposure.

insufficient for a detailed risk evaluation, but a significant teratogenic risk seems unlikely.

2.12.7   Thalidomide

Thalidomide became approved for use in the USA in 1998 for acute treatment of erythema nodosum leprosum, a cutaneous manifestation of leprosy.

Thalidomide was the first drug that was clearly shown to be a human teratogen, in the early 1960s, and probably has caused more known severe malformations in humans than any other drug. In view of the growing interest in treatment of several different diseases with thalidomide (Calabrese 2000), there is grave concern regarding its risk of teratogenicity. Comprehensive regulatory programs, such as STEPS (a program developed by the manufacturer, http://www.thalomid. com), have been instigated to minimize that risk. Thalidomide is contraindicated in women who do not meet the specific requirements of the STEPS (System for Thalidomide Education and Prescribing Safety) program (Teratology Society 2000) – the requirements being that women of childbearing age must use two reliable methods of contraception for 1 month before starting therapy, and for 1 month after stopping therapy. The STEPS program was developed by the manufacturer to limit the prescribing and use of thalidomide to tightly controlled situations, and to prevent inadvertent exposure of pregnant women. There are serious concerns that it will be increasingly prescribed for other inflammatory or immunologic diseases, such as ulcerating HIV-associated skin diseases, Behcet's disease, graft-versus-host reaction, etc. (Teratology Society 2000).

A study published in 1988 reviewed the history of thalidomide embryopathy, and gathered 4336 cases (constituting a minimal estimate) that had been identified throughout the world (Lenz 1988). In a 1996 report, 34 children with thalidomide embryopathy who were born in Latin America after 1965 were identified by the Latin American Collaborative Study of Congenital Malformations (ECLAMC) in endemic areas for leprosy (Castilla 1996). The real number is presumably much higher. Recently, information was obtained from the Teratology Information Center in Porto Allegre (Schüler, personal communication 2006) that women in early pregnancy occasionally take thalidomide, prescribed for another family member for leprosy, for minor complaints, not knowing the risk of the drug. In particular, those who are illiterate are not reached by programs such as STEPS.

Thalidomide causes different types of musculoskeletal defects, including the well-known phocomelia. Anomalies of the thumb (especially triphalangism) have been frequently reported. In addition, central nervous system anomalies (mainly cranial nerve palsy or crocodile tears), impairment of major organ systems (ocular, respiratory, gastrointestinal, cardiovascular, and genitourinary), and anomalies of neurological development (epilepsy, autism, learning disorders) were reported (Strömland 2000, Miller 1999). The risk of malformations after exposure during the sensitive period of organogenesis has been estimated to be between 20% and 50%.

The teratogenic mechanism of thalidomide is still a topic of debate. Thirty hypotheses were evaluated (Stephens 2000); 14 were rejected, and 16 were grouped into six categories, not mutually exclusive: DNA synthesis or transcription, synthesis and/or function of growth factors, integrins, angiogenesis, chondrogenesis, or cell death/injury.

The offspring of "thalidomide patients" have been examined, too. A hypothesis postulated that these would also have a higher risk for congenital anomalies, because thalidomide additionally was thought to have a mutagenic effect. Strömland (2000), as well as others, disproved this hypothesis. Apparently, there was a coincidence of a genetic anomaly, which looked very much like thalidomide embryopathy, with the fact of being offspring of a thalidomide-harmed mother.

Regarding thalidomide intake of the father and risk evaluation, see Chapter 1.

> **Recommendation.** Thalidomide is absolutely contraindicated in pregnancy, because it is the most powerful known human teratogen.

2.12.8   Other immunomodulators

Copolymer 1 (*glatiramer acetate*) is a mixture of synthetic polypeptides composed of four amino acids. It has been approved for use in the treatment of multiple sclerosis. The manufacturer reports that experimental reproduction studies did not uncover signs of adverse effects on fetal development (Johnson 1995). A poster presenting data of clinical trials and post-marketing surveillance from the manufacturer showed six healthy full-term infants and one with congenital anomaly during clinical trials. During post-marketing surveillance, 6 of 161 live-born had anomalies ("failure to thrive", finger abnormalities, cardiomyopathy, urethrostenosis, adrenal cyst, and anencephaly) (Coyle 2003). Among more than 30 live-borns there was one infant with clubfeet (unpublished experience of the European Network of Teratology Information Services, ENTIS).

There is insufficient experience of safety of use in pregnancy for the granulocyte colony-stimulating factors (G-CSF) such as *lenograstim, molgramostim, nartograstim,* and *pegfilgastrim*. Granulocyte colony-stimulating factor is normally present during pregnancy, and therefore a teratogenic risk seems to be unlikely.

There are more than 70 reports of the use of the recombinant G-CSF *filgastrim*, a glykoprotein cytokine, during pregnancy (Sangalli 2001); only a few first-trimester exposures were noted. Most children were healthy. Filgastrim crosses the placenta in amounts sufficient to produce a biological effect, and is therefore also indicated for prophylaxis of neonatal infections of premature babies (Calhoun 1996).

No data concerning *inosine pranobex* and pregnancy are available. *Levamisole* is used as an immunomodulator in combination with fluorouracil in the management of colorectal cancer, and as a veterinary anthelmintic. It is similar to metronidazole. Kazy (2004) reported on 11 pregnant women, 4 of which were first-trimester exposures, who had taken levamisole. Their offspring were healthy for as long as they were followed.

> **Recommendation.** The experiences in pregnancy with the substances mentioned above are limited. An inadvertent use in the first trimester does not justify termination of pregnancy, or invasive diagnostic procedures. A detailed fetal ultrasound examination should be offered to confirm normal morphologic development in cases of first-trimester exposure.

References

Al Bahar S, Pandita R, Nath SV. Pregnancy in chronic myeloid leukemia patients treated with alpha interferon. Int J Gynaecol Obstet 2004; 85: 281–2.

Al Kindi S, Dennison D, Pathare A. Imatinib in pregnancy. Eur J Haematol 2005; 74: 535–7.

Armenti VT, Radomski JS, Moritz MJ et al. Report from the national transplantation pregnancy registry (NTPR): outcomes of pregnancy after transplantation. Clin Transpl 2003; 131–41.

Baarsma R, Kamps WA. Immunological responses in an infant after cyclosporine A exposure during pregnancy. Eur J Pediatr 1993; 152: 476–7.

Bar-Oz B, Ma J, Tsao S et al. The effects of ciclosporine therapy on pregnancy outcome in organ transplanted women: a meta-analytical review. Teratology 1999; 59: 440.

Bar-Oz B, Ma J, Hackman R et al. Pregnancy outcome after cyclosporine therapy during pregnancy: a meta-analysis. Transplant 2001; 71: 1051–5.

Baumgart DC, Sturm A, Wiedemann B et al. Uneventful pregnancy and neonatal outcome with tacrolimus in refractory ulcerative colitis. Gut 2005; 54: 1822–3.

Bazer FW, Spencer TE, Ott TL. Interferon tau: a novel pregnancy recognition signal. Am J Reprod Immunol 1997; 37: 412–20.

Berkovitch M, Goldstein LH, Dolinsky G et al. Pregnancy outcome of women exposed to azathioprine during pregnancy: a prospective multicenter study {Abstract}. Reprod Toxicol 2005; 20: 454.

Boskovic R, Wide R, Wolpin J et al. The reproductive effects of beta interferon therapy in pregnancy. Neurology 2005; 65: 807–11.

Brown PAJ, Gray ES, Whiting PH et al. Effects of cyclosporine A on fetal development in the rat. Biol Neonate 1985; 48: 172–80.

Calabrese L, Fleischer AB. Thalidomide: current and potential clinical applications. Am J Med 2000; 108: 487–95.

Calhoun DA, Rosa C, Christensen RD. Transplacental passage of recombinant human granulocyte colony-stimulating factor in women with an imminent preterm delivery. Am J Obstet Gynecol 1996; 174: 1306–11.

Carter JD, Valeriano J, Vasey FB. Tumor necrosis factor-α inhibition and VATER association: a causal relationship? J Rheumatol 2006; 33: 1014–17.

Castilla E E, Ashton-Prolla P, Barreda-Mejia E et al. Thalidomide, a current teratogen in South America. Teratology 1996; 54: 273–7.

Chakravarty EF, Sanchez-Yamamoto D, Bush TM. The use of disease modifying antirheumatic drugs in women with rheumatoid arthritis of childbearing age: a survey of practice patterns and pregnancy outcomes. J Rheumatol 2003; 30: 241–6.

Chard T. Interferon-alpha is a reproductive hormone. J Endocrinol 1991; 131: 337–8.

Cochat P, Decramer S, Robert-Gnasia E et al. Renal outcome of children exposed to cyclosporine in utero. Transplant Proc 2004; 36: 208–10.

Coyle PK, Johnson K, Pardo L et al. Pregnancy outcome in patients with multiple sclerosis treated with glatiramer acetate {Poster}. J Neurol Neurosurg Psychiatry 2003; 74: 443.

Davison JM, Dellagrammatikas H, Parkin JM. Maternal azathioprine therapy and depressed haematopoiesis in the babies of renal allograft patients. Br J Obstet Gynaecol 1985; 92: 233–9.

De Boer NK, Jarbandhan SV, de Graaf P et al. Azathioprine use during pregnancy. Am J Gastroenterol 2006; 101: 1390.

Di Paola S, Schena A, Morrone LF et al. Immunologic evaluation during the first year of life of infants born to ciclosporine-treated female kidney transplant recipients: analysis of lymphocyte subpopulations and immunoglobulin serum levels. Transplantation 2000; 69: 2049–54.

Francella A, Dyan A, Bodian C et al. The safety of 6-mercatopurine for childbearing patients with inflammatory bowel disease: a retrospective cohort study. Gastroenterology 2003; 124: 9–17.

Fritz M, Vats K, Goyal RK. Neonatal lupus and IUGR following alpha-interferon therapy during pregnancy. J Perinatol 2005; 25: 442–4.

Garcia-Donaire JA, Acevedo M, Gutiérrez MJ et al. Tacrolimus as basic immunosuppression in pregnancy after renal transplantation. A single-center experience. Transplant Proc 2005; 37: 3754–5.

Ghanem ME, El-Baghdadi LA, Badawy AM et al. Pregnancy outcome after renal allograft transplantation. Eur J Obstet Gynecol Reprod Biol 2005; 121: 178–81.

Grasso G, Muscettola M. Possible role of interferon-gamma in ovarian function. Ann NY Acad Sci 1992; 650: 191–6.

Guardia O, Rial M del C, Casadei D. Pregnancy under sirolimus-based immunosuppression. Transplantation 2006; 81: 636.

Jabiry-Zieniewicz Z, Kaminski P, Pietrzak B et al. Outcome of four high-risk pregnancies in female liver transplant recipients on tacrolismus immunosuppression. Transplant Proc 2006; 38: 255–7.

Jain A, Venkataramanan R, Fung JJ et al. Pregnancy after liver transplantation under tacrolimus. Transplantation 1997; 64: 559–65.

Jain A, Reyes J, Marcos A et al. Pregnancy after liver transplantation with tacrolimus immunosuppression: a single center's experience: update at 13 years. Transplantation 2003; 76: 827–32.

Jain A, Shapiro R, Scantlebury VP et al. Pregnancy after kidney and kidney-pancreas transplantation under tacrolimus: a single center's experience. Transplantation 2004; 77: 897–902.

Johnson KP, Brooks BR, Cohen JA. Copolymer 1 reduces relapse rate and improves disability in relapsing-remitting multiple sclerosis: results of a phase III multicenter, double-blind, placebo-controlled trial. Neurology 1995; 45: 1268–76.

Kainz A, Harabacz I, Cowlrick IS et al. Review of the course and outcome of 100 pregnancies in 84 women treated with tacrolimus. Transplantation 2000; 70: 1718–21.

Källén B, Westgren M, Åberg A et al. Pregnancy outcome after maternal organ transplantation in Sweden. Br J Obstet Gynaecol 2005; 112: 904–9.

Katz JA, Antoni C, Keenan GF et al. Outcome of pregnancy in women receiving infliximab for the treatment of Crohn's disease and rheumatoid arthritis. Am J Gastroenterol 2004; 99: 2385–92.

Kazy Z, Puhó E, Czeisel AE. Levamisole (Decartis®) treatment during pregnancy. Reprod Toxicol 2004; 19: 3.

Kimme L, Hyrich, Deborah PM et al. Pregnancy outcome in women who were exposed to anti-tumor necrosis factor agents. Arthritis Rheum 2006; 54: 2701–2.

Lamarque V, Leleu MF, Monka C et al. Analysis of 629 pregnancy outcomes in transplant recipients treated with Sandimmun. Transplant Proc 1997; 29: 2480.

Lenz W. A short history of thalidomide embryopathy. Teratology 1988; 38: 341–51.

le Ray, C, Coulomb A, Eléfant E et al. Mycophenolate mofetil in pregnancy after renal transplantation: a case of major fetal malformations. Obstet Gynecol 2004; 103: 1091–4.

Mahadevan U, Kane S, Sandborn WJ et al. Intentional infliximab use during pregnancy for induction of maintenance of remission in Crohn's disease. Aliment Pharmacol Ther 2005; 21: 733–8.

Mannering GJ, Deloria LB. The pharmacology and toxicology of the interferons: an overview. Ann Rev Pharmacol Toxicol 1986; 26: 455–515.

Martinez-Maza O, Andersson U, Andersson J et al. Spontaneous production of interferon-gamma in adult and newborn humans. J Immunol 1984; 132: 251–5.

Mason RJ, Thomson AW, Whiting PH et al. Cyclosporine-induced fetotoxicity in the rat. Transplantation 1985; 39: 162–8.

Mesquita MM, Pestana A, Mota A. Successful pregnancy occurring with interferon-alpha therapy in chronic myeloid leukemia. Acta Obstet Gynecol Scand 2005; 84: 300–301.

Miller MT, Strömland K. Teratogen update: thalidomide: a review, with a focus on ocular findings and new potential uses. Teratology 1999; 60: 306–21.

Mishkin DS, Van Deinse W, Becker JM et al. Successful use of adalimumab for Crohn's disease in pregnancy. Inflamm Bowel Dis 2006; 12: 827–8.

Moskowitz DN, Bodian C, Chapman ML et al. The effect on the fetus of medications used to treat pregnant inflammatory bowel-disease patients. Am J Gastroenterol 2004; 99: 656–61.

Mubarak AAS, Kakil IR, Awidi A et al. Normal outcome of pregnancy in chronic myeloid leukemia treated with interferon-alpha in first trimester. Am J Hematol 2002; 69: 115–18.

Nagy S, Bush M, Berkowitz R et al. Pregnancy outcome in liver transplant recipients. Obstet Gynecol 2003; 102: 121–8.

2

Pregnancy

2.12 Immunomodulators

Nørgård B, Pedersen L, Fonager K et al. Azathioprine, mercaptopurine and birth outcome: a population-based cohort study. Aliment Pharmacol Ther 2003; 17: 827–34.

Nulman I, Sgro M, Barrera M et al. Neurodevelopment in children exposed in utero to cyclosporine and azathioprine following maternal renal transplant: preliminary results. Reprod Toxicol 2004; 18: 707–56.

Pergola PE, Kancharla A, Riley DJ. Kidney transplantation during the first trimester of pregnancy: immunosuppression with mycophenolate mofetil, tacrolimus, and prednisone. Transplantation 2001; 71: 994–7.

Polifka JE, Friedman JM. Teratogen uptake: azathioprine and 6-mercaptopurine. Teratology 2002; 65: 240–61.

Pons JC, Lebon P, Frydman R et al. Pharmacokinetics of interferon-alpha in pregnant women and fetoplacental passage. Fetal Diagn Ther 1995; 10: 7–10.

Rayes N, Neuhaus R, David M et al. Pregnancies following liver transplantation – how safe are they? A report of 19 cases under ciclosporine A and tacrolimus. Clin Transplant 1998; 12: 396–400.

Regierer AC, Schulz CO, Kuehnhardt D et al. Interferon-alpha therapy for chronic myeloid leukemia during pregnancy. Am J Hematol 2006; 81: 149–50.

Rieder MJ, McLean JL, Morrison C et al. Long-term follow-up of children with in utero exposure to immunosuppressives. Teratology 1997; 55: 37.

Roberts RM. Interferon-tau and pregnancy. J Interferon Cytokine Res 1996; 16: 271–3.

Roll C, Hans-Joachim L, Winter A et al. Hepatoblastoma in a 2-year-old child of a liver-transplanted mother. Lancet 1997; 349: 103.

Sandberg-Wollheim M, Frank D, Goodwin TM et al. Pregnancy outcomes during treatment with interferon beta-1a in patients with multiple sclerosis. Neurology 2005; 65: 802–6.

Sangalli MR, Peek M, McDonald A. Prophylactic granulocyte colony-stimulating factor treatment for aquired chronic severe neutropenia in pregnancy. Aust NZ J Obstet Gynaecol 2001; 41: 470–71.

Shaheen FAM, al Sulaiman MH, al Khader AA. Long-term nephrotoxicity after exposure to cyclosporine in utero. Transplantation 1993; 56: 224–5.

Sills ES, Perloe M, Tucker MJ et al. Successful ovulation induction, conception, and normal delivery after chronic therapy with etanercept: a recombinant fusion anticytokine treatment for rheumatoid arthritis. Am J Reprod Immunol 2001; 46: 366–8.

Stephens TD, Fillmore BJ. Hypothesis: thalidomide embryopathy-proposed mechanism of action. Teratology 2000; 61: 189–95.

Strömland K, Andersson-Grönlund M, Philipsson E. The children of the Swedes with thalidomide embryopathy {Abstract}. Teratology 2000; 61: 449.

Teratology Society. Public Affairs Committee. Position Paper, Thalidomide. Teratology 2000; 62: 172–3.

Vesga L, Terdiman JP, Madadevan U. Adalimumab use in pregnancy. Gut 2005; 54: 890.

Vilcek J. Adverse effects of interferon in virus infections, autoimmune diseases and acquired immunodeficiency. Progr Med Virol 1984; 30: 62–77.

Vyas S, Kumar A, Piecuch S et al. Outcome of twin pregnancy in a renal transplant recipient treated with tacrolimus. Transplantation 1999; 67: 490–92.

Wallace DJ, Weisman MH. The use of etanercept and other tumor necrosis factor-α blockers in infertility: it's time to get serious. J Rheumatol 2003; 30: 1897–9.

Wu A, Nashan B, Messner U et al. Outcome of 22 successful pregnancies after liver transplantation. Clin Transplant 1998; 12: 454–64.

Antineoplastic drugs

2.13

Corinna Weber-Schöndorfer and
Christof Schaefer

In practice, there arise two practical questions on this topic:

1. Does previous chemotherapy or radiotherapy, which has led to remission or cure, affect the course of future pregnancies?
2. What are the consequences resulting from a diagnosis of cancer and chemotherapy during pregnancy?

2.13.1   Cancer and pregnancy

▶ Pregnancy and previous chemotherapy

In a large number of patients, previous combination chemotherapy has not led to permanent infertility, to a significant increase in the rate of miscarriages, or to low birth weight babies in subsequent pregnancies (Falconer 2002). In addition to the duration, dosage, and type of cytotoxic drugs administered, the age of the woman undergoing chemotherapy can play an important role in future fertility (Minton 2002). A recent study investigated ovarian function after intensive chemotherapy for non-Hodgkin's lymphoma using cyclophosphamide, doxorubicin, and vincristin (Mega-CHOP). Only 1 of 13 patients, a woman of 40 (the oldest of the group) still had ovarian dysfunction 70 months after therapy was completed. Eight patients became pregnant and gave birth to a total of 12 children. Seven women – not including the 40-year-old, including five of the women who became pregnant – had undergone prophylactic monthly co-treatment with GnRH analog (Dann 2005).

Previous treatment with chemotherapy for cancer is not associated with a substantial risk of birth defects. Despite the mutagenic and cytotoxic potential of many antineoplastic agents, there has not been an increase in reports of clinically relevant chromosomal aberrations or genetic defects; there is therefore no need routinely to perform amniocenteses or chorionic biopsies. In a study of 2300 pregnancies where the father had undergone treatment for cancer, there was found a gender shift towards girls (Green 2003).

Likewise, radiotherapy dating back some time does not lead to persisting infertility in men or in women, unless the testes or ovaries have been irradiated specifically (Stovall 2004). Two studies reported that the probability of giving birth to children with restricted growth was higher if the pelvic area had been irradiated previously (Signorello 2006, Green 2002). The risk of being born preterm was also increased (Signorello 2006). In a multicenter study, Boice (2003) examined more than 6000 children of parents who had received radiotherapy in their own childhood; 46% of the parents had received a gonadal dose in excess of 100 mSv, and 16% had a dose in excess of 1000 mSv. There was no indication of a significant increase in genetic anomalies.

▶ **Cancer during pregnancy**

Cancer during pregnancy is rare, with an incidence of 0.2–1 per 1000 pregnancies. The most common cancers are lymphoma, leukemia, breast cancer, cervical and ovarian carcinoma, and melanoma, as well as thyroid and colon carcinoma. There is no substantial evidence that the pregnancy *per se* influences the outcome of the cancer. This also holds true for breast cancer (Merlob 2004), which is, however, frequently noticed only at a later stage of illness. Except for melanoma, there are no case reports regarding metastases in the placenta or fetus.

When a cancer is diagnosed during the first trimester, many couples opt to terminate the pregnancy in view of the potential teratogenic risk of the ensuing treatment; therefore, experience is limited. However, the cases that have been documented demonstrate that malformations are by no means mandatory. Depending upon the chemotherapy and the dose administered, multi-agent chemotherapy given during the second or third trimester may lead to fetal growth restriction and/or transient bone marrow depression, involving fetal anemia, leucopenia, and thrombocytopenia. Intrauterine fetal death has rarely been reported. Surprisingly, the fetus tolerates chemotherapy in most cases without persisting damage. So far, no impairment of intellectual development has been observed (Nulman 2001). Premature delivery is often discussed during the third trimester in order to have a "free hand" in the choice of therapy, and to avoid exposure of the fetus to potentially toxic substances.

As women in many countries are delaying childbearing, it seems probable that the incidence of *breast cancer* during pregnancy will increase. Compared to other malignant diseases, there is already a large amount of experience regarding breast cancer treatment which was indicated in the second or third trimester during pregnancy. A number of case reports and some studies provide evidence that neonatal related morbidity is low, including the following (see also various sections below):

- Giacalone (1999) reported on 20 pregnancies from a French national survey, where the most-used drugs in different chemotherapy regimens were fluorouracil (16 times), epirubicin (10 times) and cyclophosphamide (12 times)
- Ring (2005) reported on 28 women from five London teaching hospitals over 18 years; all had cyclophosphamide, together with doxorubicin ($n = 11$), or with epirubicin ($n = 5$), or with methotrexate and fluorouracil ($n = 12$)
- Hahn (2006) and Berry (1999) reported on 81 pregnant women treated after a standardized FAC protocol (5-fluorouracil, doxorubicin, cyclophosphamide).

The results of the largest study, by Hahn (2006), showed that the rate of cesarian sections was higher than usual; the mean gestational age at delivery was slightly earlier, as was the mean birth weight; 63% of neonates had no complications at all; 28% had breathing difficulties; and there was one subarachnoidal hemorrhage on day two in a child with neutropenia and thrombocytopenia, although the mother's complete blood count was normal and the last course of chemotherapy had been more than three weeks previously.

2

Pregnancy

2.13 Antineoplastic drugs

Recommendations. Following chemotherapy for cancer, a general waiting period is recommended, prior to conceiving, of 2 years for women and 6 months for men. However, there is no reason to terminate an intact and wanted pregnancy should conception occur earlier than this. Cancer during pregnancy is rare, and requires the largest possible interdisciplinary expert medical and psychosocial support.

A couple's decision regarding antineoplastic treatment when pregnant should be made after detailed information on the relevant risks, and with the support of the physician and the healthcare team. Each type of cancer during pregnancy requires individual consultation and treatment. Cancer and other malignant diseases are treated according to optimized therapy protocols which also apply to pregnancy, in order to ensure the best chances of survival for the pregnant woman. For this reason, this chapter does not contain suggestions for therapy from an embryo-toxicological perspective. Apart from careful gynecological monitoring, in any case of cancer therapy during pregnancy a detailed fetal ultrasound examination should be offered to evaluate morphological development.

There are no general recommendations concerning storing sperm or eggs before cancer therapy; the decision should be made on an individual basis.

2.13.2 Classification of the drugs used for chemotherapy

The agents used in cancer chemotherapy are divided into four groups.

1. *Cytostatics*, by far the largest group, are subdivided into six subgroups:
   - vinca alkaloids and their analogs
   - podophyllotoxin derivatives
   - alkylating agents (nitrogen mustards and analogs, and other alkylating agents)
   - antibiotics with antitumor properties
   - antimetabolites
   - other cytotoxic drugs.
2. *Other antineoplastics*, including:
   - platinum compounds
   - other agents
   - monoclonal antibodies.
3. *Endocrine antineoplastics*, including:
   - hormones
   - hormone antagonists
   - enzyme inhibitors.
4. *Phytocytostatics*.

Since cancer during pregnancy is fortunately rare, and antineo-plastic therapy is usually conducted as combination chemotherapy following established standard protocols, it is difficult to determine the teratogenic potential of individual cytostatic drugs in the human. Apparently, antimetabolites possess the strongest teratogenic potential after transretinoic acids such as tretinoin (see Chapter 2.17).

2.13.3   Vinca alkaloids and structural analogs

Vinblastine is an alkaloid derived from the periwinkle plant. Like the related vincristine, it inhibits cell division by interfering with the mitotic spindle. There are more than 15 case reports concerning the use of *vinblastine* during the first trimester, mostly in combination with other cytostatic drugs. In most cases, the course of pregnancy was apparently normal (Aviles 1991). However, there are also reports of children with malformations: a child with hydrocephalus after intrauterine exposure to vinblastine alone in week 3; a second with cleft palate whose mother had received vincristine and other cytostatic drugs from week 9 until delivery, following treatment with vinblastine until week 6; and a spontaneous miscarriage shortly after injection of vinblastine in week 6 (Mulvihill 1987). There is also a report of a spontaneous miscarriage of a male fetus with only four toes on each foot and syndactyly in week 24 of pregnancy (Garrett 1974), as well as a male infant delivered at 37 weeks weighing only 1900 g with a defect of the atrial septum who died of respiratory distress syndrome and whose mother had been treated with vincristine and vinblastine (Thomas 1976). The mothers of these latter four children had received vinblastine in combination with several other agents. There are some reports with normal outcome after exposure during the second and third trimesters (Doll 1989).

There are more than 20 case reports regarding apparently normal children following *vincristine* therapy during the first trimester (for an overview, see Schardein 2000 and www.motherisk.org). However, there are also reports of an aborted fetus with renal aplasia after combination therapy (Mennuti 1975); the newborn cited above (Thomas 1976) who had a defect an atrial septal defect and died of respiratory distress syndrome; a child with cleft palate after vincristine treatment until week 6 followed by vinblastine and other cytostatic drugs (Mulvihill 1987); and a woman receiving combination therapy for Hodgkin's disease during the first trimester whose hydrocephalic child died four hours after birth (Zemlicki 1992). Furthermore, there are reports about apparently normal pregnancies after exposure during the second and/or third trimesters, but also reports of neonatal pancytopenia (Pizzuto 1980) and intrauterine growth retardation.

Three children aged 2 and 3 years whose mothers were treated for breast cancer with *vinorelbine* plus 5-fluorouracil during the second and third trimesters developed normally (Cuvier 1997). Another pregnancy with vinorelbine and trastuzumab (see section 2.13.16) in the third trimester was complicated by an oligohydramnios, which was thought more likely to be a side effect of trastuzumab (Fanale 2005).

At present, there are no reports available on *vindesine*.

2.13.4   Podophyllotoxin derivatives

There are at least 13 case reports on *etoposide* (Han 2005, Rodriguez 1995, Arango 1994, Horbelt 1994, Brunet 1993), including two reports describing the delivery of healthy children after exposure during the first trimester (Aviles 1991). Development of these two children was normal up to the ages of 3 and 8, respectively.

Transient pancytopenia was reported in some children following exposure during the second/third trimester (Hsu 1995, Murray 1994). One case report describes a premature baby that developed cerebral atrophy with enlargement of the cerebral ventricles; its mother had been treated for an ovarian tumor and received $100\,mg/m^2$ etoposide for 5 days in week 26/27 in combination with bleomycin and cisplatin (Elit 1999). Another premature baby (gestational age 27 weeks) whose mother had received multi-agent chemotherapy with etoposide, bleomycin, and cisplatin in week 26, developed severe leukopenia and anemia postnatally on day 3. At the age of 10 days, the infant was noted to be losing her scalp hair and there was an associated rapid loss of lanugo. Hair growth recovered after 12 weeks. Re-examination after a year showed normal neurodevelopmental progress, but there was moderate sensorineural hearing loss bilaterally (Raffles 1989).

Teniposide is a semi-synthetic derivative of podophyllotoxin that inhibits topoisomerase, preventing DNA synthesis and cell entry into the prophase. An apparently healthy baby was born to a woman who received teniposide and other chemotherapeutic agents during the second half of pregnancy (Lowenthal 1982).

2.13.5   Nitrogen mustard agents

Streptozocin is a nitrosourea marketed for the treatment of metastatic islet cell carcinoma of the pancreas. Because of its diabetogenic effect in animals (Tuch 1993), concern was raised about human use of the drug. However, experimental animal diabetes induced by streptozocin seems not to occur in humans. Human fetal pancreatic islet cells appear to be resistant to streptozocin toxicity in comparison to rat fetal islet cells (Tuch 1989). There has been a single report of a human pregnancy in which streptozocin was used. No adverse effect was observed (Schapira 1984).

Carmustine is a nitrosourea that alkylates nucleic acids. One normal infant who had been exposed to this drug during early pregnancy was reported by Schardein (2000). No other reports are available.

Fotemustine, lomustine, nimustine, and *semustine* block DNA replication. No information is available about use of these drugs in pregnancy.

2.13.6   Nitrogen mustard analogs

Chlorambucil blocks the initiation of DNA replication. Two fetuses aborted after maternal treatment in the first trimester were found to have unilateral renal agenesis (Steege 1980, Shotton 1963). One of these was a twin pregnancy, where only one of the twins was affected. A third aborted fetus after intrauterine exposure in the first trimester showed retinal defects (Rugh 1965). Several normal pregnancies have also been reported (Jacobs 1981).

Cyclophosphamide is an alkylating agent used in cancer chemotherapy and as an immunosuppressant for the treatment of, for example, lupus erythematodes. Animal studies using rats, mice, rabbits, monkeys, and chicken showed malformations of the CNS, the craniofacial area and the skeleton (*cf.* Enns 1999).

Knowledge regarding the treatment of pregnant women with cyclophosphamide during the first trimester is based on a small cases series (Aviles 1991) and retrospective case reports. In total, there are reports on more than 30 women treated during the first trimester, including one twin pregnancy: 17 children were healthy or without congenital malformations (Férnandez 2006, Peres 2001, Aviles 1991, Pizzuto 1980), 11 fetuses and children had major or minor malformations (Paskulin 2005, Paladini 2004, Vaux 2003, Giannakopoulou 2000, Enns 1999, Mutchinick 1992, Kirshon 1988, Murray 1984, Toledo 1971, Greenberg 1964), two pregnancies ended in spontaneous miscarriage (Clowse 2005), and in two other pregnancies the fetuses died in weeks 25/26 (Peres 2001, Ba-Thike 1990). Furthermore, a boy who was born with multiple malformations developed thyroid cancer at 11 years of age and a neuroblastoma at age 14; at the age of 16 a metastasizing papillary thyroid carcinoma was diagnosed. His twin sister was healthy (Zemlickis 1993).

2

Pregnancy

2.13 Antineoplastic drugs

To date, in the TIS Berlin, five pregnancies with exposure during the first trimester have been prospectively analyzed; one ended in spontaneous abortion, one was terminated during the second trimester at the mother's request, despite apparently normal detailed ultrasound findings, and three children were born healthy.

Recently, a special cyclophosphamide embryopathy (Enns 1999) or cyclophosphamide–methotrexate–cytarabine embryopathy (Vaux 2003) has been proposed; characteristics include craniofacial abnormalities along with eye and ear malformations, limb defects, and growth retardation. Nine of the cases described above do at least partially follow this pattern, including those where the mothers had received cyclophosphamide as the only cytotoxic drug in connection with systemic lupus erythematosus.

Treatment with cyclophosphamide during the second and third trimesters may result in pancytopenia and reduced birth weight of newborns. There is also a higher incidence of premature births (Kerr 2005). Numerous case studies have reported an apparently normal outcome of the pregnancies, even in cases of malign illness (Hahn 2006, Ring 2005, Köseuglu 2001, Luisiri 1997, Oates 1990). In two patients with lupus who received cyclophosphamide during the second trimester due to the severity of the disease, the pregnancies ended in late abortion (Clowse 2005).

Ifosfamid and *trofosfamid* are structurally similar to cyclophosphamide. There is one case report of a healthy infant whose mother was treated with ifosfamid and other agents during the third trimester of pregnancy because of Ewing's sarcoma (Merimsky 1999).

Chromosomal abnormalities have been identified after treatment of humans with *melphalan*, often years after therapy has been completed (Mamuris 1989, Lambert 1984). This agent is believed to be associated with secondary malignancies. There is only one case report, describing a miscarriage that occurred in a woman who was treated with melphalan without other cancer chemotherapeutic agents during the first trimester of pregnancy (Zemlickis 1992).

There is one case report of a healthy child whose mother was treated with *bendamustin* in the first trimester of pregnancy (cited in Schardein 2000).

Pregnancies exposed to *estramustin* have not been described.

2.13.7 Other alkylating agents

Busulfan exerts its alkylating effect specifically on the bone marrow, and therefore is used in leukemia therapy and in preparation for bone marrow transplantation. At least 49 pregnancies, including 31 with application during the first trimester, have been published; six children or fetuses had various malformations without pattern (Briggs 2005).

Four of 12 pregnant women treated with *dacarbazine* had been exposed during the first trimester. All newborn babies appeared to be normal (di Paolo 1997, Aviles 1991).

In four of 12 case reports regarding therapy with *mechloretamine* during the first trimester (in conjunction with other cytotoxic substances), the following anomalies were described: oligodactyly, cerebral haemorrhage, hydrocephalus, and renal anomalies (Zemlickis 1992, Mennuti 1975). There were four cases of miscarriage and two induced abortions; the other pregnancies proceeded normally (Aviles 1991).

Procarbazine is a component of the combination therapy for Hodgkin's disease and other lymphomas. Only 3 of 10 newborn babies exposed during the first trimester were healthy (Aviles 1991, Schapira 1984). The malformations reported include multiple hemangiomas, anomalies of the kidneys and limbs, cleft palate, atrial septal defects, and intrauterine growth retardation. A woman who had accidentally ingested 50 mg daily for 30 days during the second trimester delivered a healthy child (Daw 1970). Since procarbazine is a weak monoamine oxidase inhibitor, hypertensive circulatory disorders may occur during simultaneous administration of synergistically acting drugs.

Thio-TEPA is the abbreviated name for triethylenethiophosphoramide; this agent is also known as *thiophosphamide*. There is one case report of a woman treated for leukemia during the early third trimester with thio-TEPA 30 mg/day. There were no drug-associated abnormalities in the child (Stevens 1965).

No information is available regarding the use of *chlormethin*, *temozolomid*, and *treosulfan* during pregnancy. The same applies for *pipobroman*, which is used for the treatment of polycythemia vera, and for *plicamycin*.

2.13.8   Cytotoxic anthracycline antibiotics

Daunorubicin interferes with DNA synthesis. The molecular size and relative hydrophilia of daunorubicin considerably restrict and delay its transfer to the placenta. According to Germann (2004), the concentrations in fetal tissues are between 100-fold and a 1000-fold lower than in adult and tumor tissues, respectively.

In his review, Briggs (2005) describes 29 pregnant women, of whom 4 had been exposed during the first trimester (Feliu 1988, Alegre 1982). The 22 children born alive did not show any malformations. In 2 of these children, transient neutropenia was observed at the age of 2 months. Re-examination of 13 children of this group when aged between 6 months and 9 years demonstrated that their development was normal. Zuazu (1991) describes two other pregnancies exposed during the first trimester; one ended in a spontaneous miscarriage 20 days after the end of multi-agent chemotherapy, and the other proceeded to delivery of a healthy premature baby in week 34. Artlich (1994) describes a patient who underwent treatment with daunorubicin and cytarabine at the time of conception, and received cytarabine and thioguanine 5 weeks later. The child had craniosynostosis and radial aplasia. When administered during the second/third trimester, daunorubicin may occasionally elicit myelosuppression.

Doxorubicin, also called *adriamycin*, has been described in numerous pregnancies, including at least 12 where it was administered during the first trimester (Garcia 1981, Blatt 1980, Hassenstein 1978). A child whose mother had received simultaneously cyclophosphamide and cobalt irradiation treatment of the left axilla and supraclavicular region, during weeks 8–13, showed anal atresia with rectovaginal fistula (Murray 1984). Kim (1996) describes a premature baby with blepharophimosis, microcephaly, hydrocephalus, and a balanced autosomal translocation inherited from the mother, who had received two cycles of cyclophosphamide, doxorubicin, and cisplatin during the first trimester. The other newborns did not show any anomalies.

In a review, Germann (2004) analyzed 160 case reports published between 1976 and 2001; 50 cases involved daunorubicin and 99 cases involved doxorubicin. Some of these have been quoted above. About 30 of the 160 patients received treatment during the first trimester and gave birth to 20 healthy children; 3 newborn infants showed malformations.

A case report (Nakajima 2004) showed again that cytotoxic therapy (doxorubicin and ifosfamide) during the second/third trimester may lead to healthy but growth-restricted children. This applies also to a study of 57 pregnant breast cancer patients who were treated with FAC (5-fluorouracil, doxorubicin, cyclophosphamide) (Hahn 2006). However, doxorubicin is known to have cardiotoxic side effects: there are three case reports of young pregnant women who had received doxorubicin treatment in their childhood or youth and, although their cardiac function appeared normal prior to pregnancy, they were decompensating at the end of pregnancy (Pan 2002).

There are at least 20 case reports on *epirubicin* in combination therapy, including two exposures during the first trimester which ended in spontaneous miscarriage. Regarding the other pregnancies, there was 1 abortion, 1 stillbirth and 1 child who died shortly after birth. Furthermore, there were cases of intrauterine growth restriction, premature births, and a transient leukopenia (Ring 2005, Gadducci 2003, Giacalone 1999, Müller 1996, Goldwasser 1995).

Placental transfer of epirubicin is low but slightly higher than that of doxorubicin (Gaillard 1995).

Five case reports describe combination therapy with *idarubicin* after the first trimester (Claahsen 1998, Reynoso 1994). In the first case, fetal death occurred after the beginning of the therapy, whereas the second report describes birth of a growth-restricted but otherwise healthy baby. The third child was born in week 28 and suffered from acute cardiac failure lasting for 3 days, which the authors attributed to idarubicin (Achtari 2000). Furthermore, transient dilated cardiomyopathy was reported in two other children (Niedermeier 2005, Siu 2002). One of these children also displayed a moderate-sized membranous ventricular septal defect, short digits and limbs, acrocyanosis, a shallow sacral dimple, and a prominent frontal skull with mild macrognathia which cannot be explained by exposure to idarubicin and cytarabine exclusively during the second and third trimesters (Niedermeier 2005). Although idarubicin is less cardiotoxic than traditional anthracyclines, its higher lipophilicity makes placental transfer easier. This could explain why the fetuses described in the few reports available frequently showed cardiac complications.

For *mitoxantrone*, four case reports are available. One of these describes a pregnancy with idarubicin exposure in combination with other drugs, which resulted in fetal death (Reynoso 1994). An apparently normal newborn was reported after intrauterine exposure to chemotherapy in weeks 24–34 (Azuno 1995). Giacalone (1999) reports a healthy child and a growth-restricted infant after therapy during the second trimester. Mitoxantrone has immunomodulatory properties, and is therefore used for certain forms of multiple sclerosis.

Nothing is known about the effects of the treatment of pregnant women with *aclarubicin* and *pirarubicin*.

2.13.9   Other cytotoxic antibiotics

Bleomycin is a glycopeptide antibiotic. These antineoplastic drugs appear to affect DNA binding, and act via radical formation. Isolated clinical reports are available on cases of Hodgkin's lymphoma, non-Hodgkin's lymphoma, and teratoma treated during the second and third trimesters of pregnancy. No fetal anomalies or chromosome changes were reported in these cases (Lowenthal 1982). Transient neonatal leukopenia and neutropenia were observed in a premature infant born to a woman who had been treated with bleomycin, etoposide, and cisplatin until 7–10 days prior to delivery (Raffles 1989; for a more detailed case description, see Chapters 2.13.4 and 2.13.14). Three infants who had been exposed to the same agents during the second/third trimester were apparently healthy (Han 2005) or with minor problems (Molegi 2007). Normal growth and development was found in a group of 22 children who were prenatally exposed to bleomycin. In 11 of them, maternal chemotherapy for cancer had begun in the first trimester (Aviles 1991).

Treatment with the cytotoxic antibiotic *dactinomycin* in early pregnancy has been reported in a few cases (overview by Briggs 2005), without any malformation described. Treatment after the first trimester has also been reported, without apparent adverse effects in three cases (Gililland 1983, Nicholson 1968).

No information is available about the use of *mitomycin D* in pregnancy, but it may have unwanted effects because of its folic acid antagonism.

2.13.10   Folate antagonistic antimetabolites

▶ Aminopterin

As early as the 1950s malformations were being described resulting from treatment with aminopterin, a substance related to methotrexate (Warkany 1959, Meltzer 1956, Thiersch 1952). There are reports about failed terminations of pregnancies using aminopterin, in which malformations such as the following have been described: CNS anomalies (meningo-encephalocele, hydrocephalus, brachycephaly, anencephaly); anomalies of the facial cranium (micrognathia, cheiloschisis, and cleft palate, craniostenosis, low-set ears, hypertelorism); malformations of the limbs; growth retardation; and mental retardation (see review by Briggs 2005). There are also some publications containing case reports with normal pregnancy outcome after exposure during the first trimester.

▶ Methotrexate (MTX)

Methotrexate (a methyl derivative of aminopterin, which is also called *amethopterin*) has a half-life of 12–24 hours, but approximately 5–35% is stored for several months as polyglutamate derivative in hepatocytes and erythrocytes (Hendel 1984). It is used for a wide range of indications – for example, to terminate ectopic or unwanted pregnancies, and for the treatment of autoimmune diseases, chronic inflammatory diseases, and neoplasias. Methotrexate carries a teratogenic risk, with a similar pattern of malformations to aminopterin (see above), so that sometimes reference is made to an aminopterin/methotrexate syndrome (Bawle 1998). However, in view of the close correspondence between the various malformations described for methotrexate, cyclophosphamide, and cytarabine (see section 2.13.6), the term aminopterin/methotrexate embryopathy does not seem justified. It is not clear whether these drugs have a common embryotoxic mechanism of action, as Vaux (2003) assumes. At present, it is not possible to say whether other antimetabolites cause similar malformations.

In children with characteristic malformations (skull ossification defects, facial dysmorphism, CNS anomalies with lower intelligence, and defects of the extremities) and intrauterine growth restriction, the latter seems to persist during postnatal development, resulting in short stature. During subsequent development, both normal intellectual development and mental retardation were observed.

In more than 30 published articles, there are over 200 cases of pregnant women treated during the first trimester. Since these were, in general, retrospective case reports and not a prospective study, statistical calculation of the malformation rate is not valid. Moreover, some of these publications do not contain details about dose and indication. For example, McElhatton (2000) describes 82 exposed fetuses, including 53 exposed during the first trimester; 12 (for which no exposure period is given) showed anomalies, including nine cranial anomalies and six other malformations of the skeleton. In the following paragraphs, only the more detailed case reports are presented.

Chemotherapy for cancer using MTX

Ten articles describe pregnant women who had received methotrexate as part of cancer therapy during the first trimester. It is noteworthy that 16 healthy children were born in this high-risk group (Zemlickis 1992, Aviles 1991, Feliu 1988, Dara 1981, Pizzuto 1980); 1 child had inguinal hernia (Giannakopoulou 2000), there was 1 spontaneous miscarriage (Giacalone 1999), and 1 stillbirth without malformations (Peres 2001). Only 1 child had characteristic malformations (Bawle 1998); this child's mother had been treated for breast cancer with a weekly dose of 80 mg MTX from weeks 8–29. Moreover, she had received irradiation treatment from weeks 16–25, with the fetal dose estimated at 14 rad.

When administered during the second and third trimesters, methotrexate may – like other cytostatic drugs – produce intrauterine growth restriction, myelosuppression in the fetus, and (albeit rarely) fetal death.

Abortion attempt using MTX

Eight publications contain case reports of unsuccessfully attempted terminations of pregnancy. All 11 children showed the malformations characteristic for MTX (see, for example, Seidahmed 2006, Milunsky

1968). The total dose was between 10 and 100 mg methotrexate. In seven of these pregnancies (eight children), misoprostol was administered additionally several days after methotrexate (Yedlinski 2005, Adam 2003, Wheeler 2002). In one instance, curettage had been performed beforehand but without success (Bawle 1998). Other reports discuss the anomalies of exposed fetuses which were diagnosed prenatally and led to termination of the pregnancy (Chapa 2003, Krähenmann 2002).

Antirheumatic therapy using MTX

Ten publications listing more than 110 pregnancies with exposure during the first trimester refer to the so-called "low-dose" therapy for rheumatic diseases. However, with the exception of a recently published small prospective study from France (Lewden 2004) and our own unpublished data, all listed cases represent retrospective reports or, at best, small prospective case studies describing a maximum of four pregnancies (Østensen 2000, Donnenfeld 1994).

There were a total of four children with characteristic malformations. Two of the mothers (Del Campo 1999, Powell 1971) had taken more MTX (one took 3×2.5 mg per week until week 10, and the other took 5 mg per day until week 8) than is usual for a "low-dose" therapy (i.e. maximally 25 mg per week). Another mother received 7.5 mg per day for 2 days in week 6 (Nguyen 2002), and the fourth woman received 12.5 mg per week until week 10 in combination with a daily dose of 1 mg folic acid (Buckley 1997).

In contrast to these publications, there are case reports of 14 healthy children whose mothers had a dosage of between 7.5 and 15 mg per week (Østensen 2000, Donnenfeld 1994, Feldkamp 1993, Kozlowski 1990), 4 spontaneous miscarriages (Østensen 2000, Kozlowski 1990), and 2 induced abortions without embryopathic background. Chakravarty (2003) describes 38 retrospective ascertained pregnancies with "low-dose" MTX therapy without giving details regarding the period of administration and the dose; 21 children were born healthy, 3 had malformations (no details given), there were 7 spontaneous miscarriages, and 8 pregnancies were electively terminated. A prospective French study (Lewden 2004) with 28 cases and a weekly median dose of 10.5 mg MTX reports 4 spontaneous miscarriages, 5 induced abortions, and 19 live births, none of which was a MTX embryopathy.

These findings are in agreement with those of the TIS Berlin: of the 22 prospectively ascertained pregnancies with exposure during the first trimester (with a weekly dose of 10–25 mg MTX), 3 pregnancies were terminated despite inconspicuous ultrasound findings, 5 resulted in spontaneous miscarriages, and 13 healthy children were born (1 premature infant at 36 weeks). One child whose mother additionally took phenprocoumon and other drugs weighed 1600 g at birth and was growth restricted, had an inguinal hernia, and was highly irritable for 14 days.

The dose ranges of MTX administered in combination chemotherapy, attempted abortions, and for rheumatic indications ("low-dose" treatment) overlap. Therefore, the conclusion is inadmissible that there are safe and risky indications for MTX. However, since there has been only one case with suspicious symptoms following 10 mg MTX per week, the hypothesis proposed by Feldkamp (1993) seems plausible: that MTX is teratogenic only at a weekly dose in excess of 10 mg. In addition, the author postulates a sensitive phase between weeks 8 and 10. However, the data available do not permit a definitive conclusion in this respect.

Recommendation. Developmental anomalies resulting from treatment with the teratogenic drug methotrexate have been observed in a number of pregnancies, essentially comprising growth restriction beginning at a prenatal stage, severe ossification defects of the calvaria, facial dysmorphisms, CNS anomalies with or without diminishing of intelligence, and defects of the extremities. A safe dose cannot be defined; however, at present there are no indications for teratogenic effects to occur below a weekly dose of 10 mg. Antirheumatic "low-dose" therapy which had been continued (inadvertently) during the first trimester seems to be associated at most with a slightly increased risk of malformations. In general, exposure during the first trimester does not necessarily lead to malformations, even when used to treat malignant diseases.

Although antirheumatic MTX treatment should be stopped before planning a pregnancy, the data available at present do not justify the advice to postpone pregnancy for at least 3 months after stopping methotrexate therapy. Pregnant women who have been (inadvertently) exposed to MTX during the first trimester should be offered a detailed ultrasound scan to obtain confirmation of the normal development of the fetus.

2.13.11   Purine-derived antimetabolites (purine antagonists)

6-Mercaptopurine is a purine analog, which acts as an inhibitor of nucleic acid synthesis (*cf.* azathioprine = AZA, a pro-drug of 6-MP). Until now, no specific malformation syndrome has been described. 6-MP is also used as an immunosuppressive, for example for chronic inflammatory bowel disease (IBD). The plasma half-lives of 6-MP and AZA of 1–3 hours are short, but the half-life of the cytostatic active metabolite, the thioguanine nucleotide, is 3–13 days. The mode of action and metabolic transformation of 6-MP vary

inter-individually, and involve the enzyme thiopurine-methyltransferase, TPMT, the activity of which is genetically determined. AZA
and 6-MP are able to cross the placenta (Polifka 2002).

In one report, more than 60 of over 100 pregnant women who
were exposed during the first trimester took 6-MP in connection with
IBD (Francella 2003), frequently in combination with prednisolone;
a small group took it continuously throughout the entire pregnancy.
The majority of the children of the pregnant women receiving 6-MP
described in this and other publications were born without anomalies (Moskowitz 2004, Polifka 2002, Aviles 1990, Dara 1981,
Pizzuto 1980). Some infants and fetuses showed malformations such
as polydactyly (Mulvihill 1987), hypospadia (Sosa Munoz 1983),
hydrocephalus (Francella 2003), hypoplasia of the lung, malformations of the urinary bladder and urethra (Nørgård 2003), cleft palate,
and facial dysmorphism (Tegay 2002). It is not possible to deduce a
significant teratogenic potential from these reports. There is overlap
between the therapeutic dose ranges of the two major indications for
treatment, IBD and leukemia. The indication in itself is therefore not
a distinguishing feature in terms of potential teratogenicity.

Thioguanine is a purine analog that produces single-strand
breaks in mammalian DNA. Schardein (2000) collected five cases
of thioguanine exposure during early pregnancy, of which none
resulted in a child with anomalies. In another case report, an infant
exposed to thioguanine and cytarabine during the sixth week postconception was born with craniosynostosis and radius aplasia, as
well as digital defects (Schafer 1981). Probably, cytarabine was the
substance causing the malformations. Artlich (1994) also reports
on a malformed child after intrauterine exposure during the first
trimester (see cytarbine; section 2.13.12). 6-Thioguanine is also
indicated for Crohn's disease. De Boer (2005) described two
patients with Crohn's disease treated with low-dose 6-thioguanine
throughout pregnancy who delivered healthy babies. Significantly
lower levels of 6-thioguaninenucleotides were found in the erythrocytes of the infants compared to the mother (ratio 1 : 12).

A woman with hairy cell leukemia diagnosed at 10 weeks' gestation who deferred therapy with *cladribine* until 6 months after giving birth, when she stopped nursing, had an uneventful pregnancy
outcome (Alothman 1994).

No information is available on use of *fludarabine* during pregnancy.

2.13.12 Pyrimidine-derived antimetabolites (pyrimidine antagonists)

The pyrimidine antagonist *cytarabine* (also called *cytosine arabinoside*
or *Ara C*) inhibits synthesis of DNA as well as RNA by displacement

of cytosine, from which it differs by its sugar component, arabinose. There have been 11 published reports on pregnancies following cytarabine exposure in the first trimester. Six children were healthy (Aviles 1991, 1990), and one spontaneous miscarriage occurred 20 days after the end of cytotoxic therapy (Zuazu 1991). There were two induced abortions, one of which was induced after 20 weeks with an apparently normally developed fetus (Zemlickis 1992, Lilleyman 1977). Three children had limb anomalies; one of them also had bilateral microtia and atresia of the exterior auditory canal (Wagner 1980). The mother had received cytarabine three times in connection with maintenance therapy for acute lymphatic leukemia: at the time of conception, in week 6/7, and in week 10. This is the only case report of a mono-drug therapy; all the other cases received multi-agent chemotherapy. The second anomalous child had radial aplasia on both sides and four fingers on each hand, with a hypoplastic thumb, a severe brachycephaly, hypoplasia of the basal skull and mid-face, as well as synostosis of the cranial sutures. The mother had been treated with cytarabine and other drugs at the time of conception and thereafter from day 35 or 37 onwards for acute myelocytic leukemia (Artlich 1994). The third case (Schafer 1981) is described above under thioguanine (see section 2.13.11). Regarding the specificity of the teratogenic damage caused by cytarabine, the reader is referred to Vaux (2003), who proposes an embryopathy induced by cyclophosphamide–methotrexate–cytarabine drugs (see section 2.13.6).

We have found approximately 30 published cases of exposure to cytarabine during the second/third trimester; further cases are mentioned in review articles. A large proportion of the children were healthy (Peres 2001, Veneri 1996, Requena 1995, Aviles 1991, 1990, Blatt 1980). There are also reports about late abortions and stillbirths (Greenlund 2001, citations in Zuazu 1991), and, furthermore, of three premature babies with severe but reversible pancytopenia (Hsu 1995, Murray 1994, Engert 1990). Reynoso (1987) reported on three healthy infants (one was premature at 34 weeks' gestation, the second had transient changes in the blood count, the third was a full-term baby) and one premature baby born at 29 weeks' gestation whose mother had received treatment for acute myeloid leukemia (AML) from week 25 of pregnancy onwards. At the age of 2 years, ophthalmologic evaluation revealed congenital adherence of the iris to the cornea of the left eye. Otherwise, the boy was still apparently developing normally at the age of 3 years.

5-Fluorouracil (5-FU) also interferes with DNA and RNA synthesis by displacing uracil. Five healthy children have been reported following local vaginal application of 5-fluorouracil during the first trimester (Kopelman 1990, Odom 1990). Case reports about treatment during the first trimester in conjunction with other therapeutic drugs describe four healthy children (Andreadis 2004, Peres 2001,

Pregnancy

2

2.13 Antineoplastic drugs

Zemlickis 1992), two spontaneous abortions (Giacalone 1999), and a complex deformity after exposure in weeks 11 and 12 (Stephens 1980). Paskulin (2005) describes a child who had been exposed *in utero* until week 16 to cyclophosphamide, fluorouracil, and doxorubicin, and who was born showing growth restriction, facial dysmorphism, and different malformations of the distal extremities. These anomalies were probably due to cyclophospamide.

The majority of more than 100 children with intrauterine exposure to 5-FU during the second and third trimesters were healthy (Ginopoulos 2004, Berry 1999). Intrauterine growth restriction was reported (Hahn 2006, Zemlickis 1992). Dreicer (1991) describes a boy who had been exposed to high doses of 5-FU during the second/third trimester (20 g in total), was born in week 38 of pregnancy weighing below average (2660 g); he was normally developed when 2 years old. Concerning the topical application of fluorouracil, refer to Chapter 2.17.

Regarding *gemcitabin* and *capecitabin*, there is no information available regarding drug tolerance during pregnancy.

2.13.13 Taxanes

Taxanes exert their antineoplastic effects by blocking the synthesis of the microtubuli. They are used for the treatment of breast cancer. There are no reports about application during the first trimester.

Six cases with exposure to *paclitaxel* in the second/third trimester reported healthy children (Gonzales-Angulo 2004, Cardonick 2004, Gadducci 2003, Mendez 2003, Sood 2001).

Docetaxel is a structural analog of paclitaxel. There are five case reports with exposure in the second/third trimester: four healthy infants (Nieto 2006, Potluri 2006, Gainford 2006, De Santis 2000) and one with hydrocephalus, which was diagnosed on ultrasound before docetaxel therapy (Potluri 2006).

2.13.14 Platin compounds

Cisplatin has been used in the treatment of a variety of solid tumors, including those of the urogenital system. As a result of poor placental transfer of cisplatin, the developing embryo may be protected from exposure to this agent, but toxic effects on the more developed fetus are possible (Kopf-Maier 1983).

At present, there is only one case report on multiple chemotherapy using cisplatin, cyclophosphamide, and doxorubicin in the first trimester (Kim 1996). A young pregnant woman received two cycles in weeks 7 and 12 respectively. In week 25, a boy was delivered by emergency cesarean section, weighing 1020 g; he showed blepharophimosis, microcephaly, and enlarged lateral ventricles on both sides. His mother and the baby were diagnosed with a balanced autosomal translocation. Ultrasound scans of the skull showed no alterations up to the thirtieth postnatal day. Jacobs (1980) describes an externally normal looking fetus following exposure to cisplatin after week 12 of pregnancy.

There are about 28 publications about treatment during the second and third trimesters, administered as mono-drug therapy as well as multi-agent chemotherapy. Han (2005) reports two cases with apparently normal outcome after therapy with cisplatin, etoposide, and bleomycin. Ferrandina (2005) describes a healthy male premature baby after prenatal exposure to six cycles of cisplatin. Tomlinson (1997) reports a normal pregnancy using cisplatin and cyclophosphamide, and gives a summary on nine further cases, including a premature birth with neutropenia and reversible hair loss from day 10 onwards which had been exposed to cisplatin, bleomycin, and etoposide until 6 days prior to birth. At the age of 1 year, the child was apparently normal except for a moderate sensineural hearing loss bilaterally (Raffles 1989; see also case description in section 2.13.4). One case report describes a premature infant that developed cerebral atrophy with enlargement of the cerebral ventricles; its mother had received 100 mg/m^2 etoposide for 5 days in week 26/27, in combination with bleomycin and cisplatin, to treat an ovarian tumor (Elit 1999). In a series of cases reported by Peres (2001), a stillbirth occurred at week 26 of pregnancy without malformations. The mother had received cisplatin and etoposide in week 22 as treatment for non-Hodgkin's lymphoma. All other children were healthy, but two had intrauterine growth restriction (Caluwaerts 2006, Ohara 2000, di Paolo 1997, Giacalone 1996, Hoffmann 1995, Henderson 1993).

One study found that animals prenatally exposed to cisplatin had an increased risk of tumor formation in various tissues. Although it is not known whether this finding has relevance for the use of cisplatin in the clinical setting, the authors recommend that infants exposed to this agent during gestation should be monitored for preneoplastic and neoplastic lesions in later life (Diwan 1993).

Carboplatin is related to cisplatin. In a case report involving fetal exposure to cisplatin between 20 and 30 weeks' gestation, and carboplatin between 31 and 36 weeks' gestation, no adverse effects on fetal development were detected (Henderson 1993). Another case report with carboplatin exposure between 17 and 33 weeks' gestation also describes a healthy infant (Mendez 2003).

There is no information on the use of *oxaliplatin* during pregnancy.

2.13.15   Other antineoplastic drugs

Hydroxycarbamide, also called *hydroxyurea*, reduces the synthesis of DNA. Currently, hydroxyurea is used in the management of chronic granulocytic leukemia, in polycythemia vera and thrombocythemia, and in cases of sickle cell anemia. To date, there are more than 25 reported cases of treatment with hydroxycarbamide during pregnancy. One apparently normal fetus was electively aborted in the midtrimester, and one woman delivered a stillborn male infant without gross abnormalities (Celiloglu 2000, Byrd 1999). There were no gross structural malformations among the live births whose mothers had predominantly been treated during the first trimester (Merlob 2005, Pata 2004, Thauvin-Robinet 2001, Wright 2001, Diav-Citrin 1999). There are case reports of successful therapy with hydroxyurea in the second or third trimester, when therapy of chronic granulocytic leukemia during pregnancy was necessary (Ault 2006).

Anagrelide is used for the treatment of essential thrombocythaemia. It inhibits phosphodiesterase III and acts during the postmitotic phase of megakaryocyte development. Thus, the number of thrombocytes is selectively reduced. It is not cytotoxic or mutagenic. The findings during pregnancy are limited to approximately ten reports, in which no teratogenic effects were noticed (al Kindi 2005A, Doubek 2004, TIS Berlin data).

Tretinoin or *all-trans-retinoic acid* (ATRA), is used orally as an antineoplastic in the treatment of acute promyelocytic leukemia. Most human reproductive studies on retinoids focus on the potent teratogenic effect of isotretinoin (an isomer of tretinoin), which is used in the oral therapy of cystic acne and is easily converted to tretinoin. Defects of the central nervous system, branchial arches, and cardiovascular system were observed. There are 22 case reports that include the use of systemic tretinoin ($45\,mg/m^2$ per day) for the treatment of acute promyelocytic leukemia during pregnancy. Only one of these exposures occurred during the first trimester (during the sixth week of gestation). No congenital abnormalities were observed in any of the exposed newborns. If problems in newborn babies arose, they were usually due to the premature birth and of a transient nature. There are also reports of growth restriction and fetal arrhythmia as well as cardiac arrest with successful recovery (Takitani 2005, Consoli 2004, Carradice 2002, Fadilah 2001, Terada 1997). A female full-term, who as a fetus had been exposed to ATRA and idarubicin from week 15 on, showed an atrial septal defect and a slight dilatative cardiomyopathy of the right ventricle, which regressed completely after 1–2 months. The hemodynamically insignificant atrial septal defect was still detectable (Siu 2002). For further details on retinoids, see Chapter 2.17.

There are no data available on the tolerance during pregnancy for *amsacrine* or *miltefosin*, which is also used against leishmaniosis.

The same is true for *pentostatin, mitoguazone*, and the topoisomerase inhibitors *irinotecan* and *topotecan*, for the photosensitizing agents *temoporfin* and *porfimer-sodium*, and for *bexaroten*, an agonist of the retinoid X receptor. Likewise, concerning *pemetrexed* (an inhibitor of thymidylate synthesis) and *mitotane*, there are no data available concerning the use during pregnancy.

Imatinib, a protein tyrosine kinase inhibitor, is used for the therapy of chronic granulocytic leukemia. There are only a few case reports about its use during pregnancy, and these prove neither its safety nor its teratogenicity. There were 11 pregnant patients on imatinib, of whom all but one took it until pregnancy was recognized: two had spontaneous abortions, one decided to have a therapeutic abortion, and eight pregnancies were carried to term, resulting in the birth of nine babies, of which one had a hypospadia that was surgically corrected (Ault 2006, Ali 2005). There are four case reports describing imatinib exposure throughout pregnancy. All babies were without congenital malformations, but two of them were small for gestational age (Al Kindi 2005B, Prabhasch 2005). Hensley (2003) described two healthy infants, a boy with hypospadia, and two induced abortions due to deformities (hydrocephalus, heart defect). Another case report with exposure to imatinib until week 7 concerns a girl with pyloric stenosis (Heartin 2004). Choudhary (2006) reported on a woman who inadvertently took imatinib until 6 weeks after gestation, and delivered a dead fetus with meningocele at the thirty-fourth week of pregnancy.

Erlotinib is a newly licensed cytotoxic drug for the treatment for non-small-cell lung cancer. *Altretamine* is an oral drug used to treat ovarian cancer, which was approved by the FDA in 1990. There are no data concerning the use during pregnancy.

2.13.16   Enzymes and antibodies exerting antineoplastic effects

Asparaginase is a bacterial enzyme that is typically used in combination with other antineoplastic agents, to interfere with the availability of the amino acid asparagine to rapidly growing cancer cells. There have been seven case reports of pregnant women exposed to asparaginase during the second trimester (Turchi 1988, Scheuning 1987, Awidi 1983, Karp 1983, Okun 1979, Khurshid 1978). In each case, asparaginase was administered in combination with a number of other chemotherapeutic agents in the treatment of acute leukemias. No birth defects were noted in the offspring of these women, but two infants had transient bone marrow hypoplasia. One child was found to have chromosomal gaps and a ring chromosome.

Because multiple chemotherapeutic agents were involved in each pregnancy, no direct association with asparaginase exposure can be made.

Alemtuzumab, ibritumomab-tiuxetan, cetuximab, edrecolomab, bortezomib, and *tositumomab* are monoclonal antibodies for which there are no data on tolerance during pregnancy.

There are four reports on *rituximab* with apparently normal pregnancy outcomes. Two treatments occurred inadvertently during the first trimester, the other from week 21 onwards (Ojeda-Uribe 2006, Kimby 2004, Herold 2001). The fourth patient, with a diffuse large B-cell lymphoma, was successfully treated with rituximab, cyclophosphamide, doxorubicin, vincristine, prednisolone, and *filgastrim* during the second trimester of pregnancy. At delivery of a premature but otherwise healthy girl the serum rituximab concentrations (half-life of 28 days) were similar in mother and child. The child's B cells were severely diminished at birth, but recovered faster than did those in the mother. Neither mother nor child developed any infections during the time of observation (Decker 2006).

Trastuzumab is a monoclonal antibody which blocks the "human epidermal growth factor 2" protein and has an estimated half-life of 12 days. Waterstone (2006) reported on an uneventful pregnancy and the delivery of a healthy girl whose mother conceived 3 days after her second cycle of trastuzumab. There is one case report of inadvertent exposure of a 28-year-old with breast cancer who was given the drug every 3 weeks until week 20 of her pregnancy. When, in week 23, the pregnancy was noticed, a lack of amniotic fluid prevailed with a healthy female fetus. Gradually, the amount of amniotic fluid recovered. In week 37, a healthy girl was delivered whose kidney function was normal at the age of 6 months and who showed no sign of pulmonary hypoplasia (Watson 2005). There is another report regarding the development of an oligohydramnios after trastuzumab therapy. Fanale (2005) described a case where therapy with trastuzumab and vinorelbine was started after week 27 because of metastatic breast cancer. Despite extra hydration, the amniotic fluid indexes were low so that delivery was induced in week 35. The male infant was healthy, and no immediate postpartum neonatal complications were noted.

Gefitinib is still in the testing stage for small-cell bronchial carcinoma, and there are not yet any data on pregnancy. The same is true of *lapatinib* and *bevacizumab*, which are administered together with 5-fluorouracil to treat metastasizing colon or rectal carcinomas.

Aldesleukin is produced by genetic engineering in *E. coli*, and is used for the treatment of metastasizing renal cell carcinoma. There are no data concerning its use during pregnancy. This is also the case with *lenalidomide*, as therapeutic approach for myelodysplastic syndrome. Lenalidomide is structurally similar to thalidomide;

however, they have different developmental effects in animal experiments. In contrast to thalidomide, lenalidomide does not produce limb malformations in rabbits, but deaths, abortions and total litter losses (Christian 2006).

The liposomal cancer vaccine *L-BLP25*, against non-small-cell bronchial carcinoma, is still being tested in clinical trials, as is *actinonin*, an antibiotic with proliferation-inhibiting properties. There are obviously no data concerning use during pregnancy.

2.13.17 Antineoplastic drugs with endocrine effects

The hormone antagonist *tamoxifen* is used for the treatment of breast cancer. Its effect on the endometrium might indirectly pose a risk to prenatal development. In 37 pregnancies collated by the manufacturer, 19 newborn babies were healthy and 2 children had craniofacial deformities. Two other case reports describe a child with anomalies resembling Goldenhar syndrome (Cullins 1994), and a newborn girl with indifferent genital development (Tewari 1997). An adenoma of the vagina was diagnosed in a girl aged 2 years whose mother had taken tamoxifen until the fourth month of pregnancy. There are also reports of apparently normal pregnancies (Andreadis 2004, Isaacs 2001, Lai 1994). Nine pregnancies following induction of ovulation with tamoxifen resulted in newborn babies that had no malformations (Ruiz-Velasco 1979). There is, however, insufficient data for a discriminative risk evaluation.

There is no information on *toremifene* and *fulvestrant*, an estrogen antagonist, during pregnancy. Enzyme inhibitors such as *aminoglutethimide* are also used for the therapy of Cushing's syndrome, with adrenocortical adenomas and carcinomas, and with ectopic ACTH syndrome. Some case reports with aminoglutethimide describe masculinization of female fetuses as well as normal development (overview in Schardein 2000).

The aromatase inhibitor *letrozole* is prescribed to postmenopausal women with hormone-dependent breast carcinoma. Recently, letrozole has also found application in the treatment of sterility, in order to stimulate ovulation – for example, as alternative to clomiphene. A recently published retrospective study on 911 newborns from women who conceived following clomiphene ($n = 397$) or letrozole ($n = 514$) treatment found no difference in the overall rates of major and minor congenital anomalies (Tulandi 2006).

There are no data on the use of the aromatase inhibitor *exemestane* during pregnancy.

Regarding *medroxyprogesterone, megestrol*, and *gosereline*, see Chapter 2.15.

2.13.18   Cytostatic drugs of plant origin

For mistletoe preparations (*Viscum album*), clinical observations in a few pregnancies do not indicate toxicity to the unborn. There were no cytotoxic or mutagenic effects in *in vitro* tests with amniotic fluid (Bussing 1995). However, because viscum album therapy may provoke fever and clinical data are insufficient to rule out prenatal toxicity, exposure should be avoided during pregnancy.

2.13.19   Occupational handling of cytostatic drugs

There has been some discussion about an increased risk of abortion for nurses who regularly handle cytostatic drugs during their pregnancy. However, according to the available information, a causal relationship can be neither proven nor eliminated (Stucker 1990).

> **Recommendation.** During pregnancy, regular professional handling of cytostatic drugs should be discontinued. However, if a nurse or pharmacist has been working in a relevant department before the pregnancy was known, there is no need to take any diagnostic measures and no justification for the termination of the pregnancy on the basis of an assumed risk.

References

Achtari C, Hohlfeld P. Cardiotoxic tranplacental effect of idarubicin administered during the second trimester of pregnancy. Am J Obstet Gynecol 2000; 183: 511–12.

Adam MP, Manning MA, Beck AE et al. Methotrexate/misoprostol embryopathy: report of four cases resulting from failed medical abortion. Am J Med Gen 2003; 123A: 72–8.

Alegre A, Chunchurreta R, Rodriguez-Alarcon J et al. Successful pregnancy in acute promyelocytic leukemia. Cancer 1982; 49: 152–3.

Ali R, Ozkalemkas F, Ozcelik T et al. Pregnancy under treatment of imatinib and successful labor in a patient with chronic myelogenous leukemia (CML). Outcome of discontinuation of imatinib therapy after achieving a molecular remission. Leuk Res 2005; 29: 971–3.

Al Kindi S (A), Dennison D, Pathate A. Successful outcome with anagrelide in pregnancy. Ann Hematol 2005; 84: 758–9.

Al Kindi S (B), Dennison D, Pathate A. Imatinib in pregnancy. Eur J Haematol 2005; 74: 535–7.

Alothman A, Sparling TG. Managing hairy cell leukemia in pregnancy. Ann Intern Med 1994; 120: 1048–9.

Andreadis CH, Charalampidou M, Diamantopoulos N et al. Combined chemotherapy and radiotherapy during conception and two trimesters of gestation in a woman with metastatic breast cancer. Gynecol Oncol 2004; 95: 252–5.

Arango HA, Deceeare SL, Lyman GH et al. Management of chemotherapy in a pregnancy complicated by a large neuroblastoma. Obstet Gynecol 1994; 84: 665–8.

Artlich A, Möller J, Tschakaloff A et al. Teratogenic effects in a case of maternal treatment for acute myelocytic leukaemia – neonatal und infantile course. Eur J Pediatr 1994; 153: 488–91.

Ault P, Kantarjian H, O'Brien S et al. Pregnancy among patients with chronic myeloid leukemia treated with imatinib. J Clin Oncol 2006; 24: 1204–8.

Aviles A, Diaz-Maqueo JC, Torras V et al. Non-Hodgkins lymphomas and pregnancy: presentation of 16 cases. Gynecol Oncol 1990; 37: 335–7.

Aviles A, Diaz Maqueo JC, Talavera A et al. Growth and development of children of mothers treated with chemotherapy during pregnancy: current status of 43 children. Am J Hematol 1991; 36: 243–8.

Awidi AS, Tarawneh MS, Shubair KS et al. Acute leukemia in pregnancy: report of five cases treated with a combination which included a low dose of adriamycin. Eur J Cancer Clin Oncol 1983; 19: 881–4.

Azuno Y, Kaku K, Fujita N. Mitoxantrone and etoposide in breast milk. Am J Hematol 1995; 48: 131–2.

Ba-Thike K, Oo N. Non-Hodgkin's lymphoma in pregnancy. Asia-Oceania J Obstet Gynaecol 1990; 16: 229–32.

Bawle EV, Conard JV, Weiss L. Adult and two children with fetal methotrexate syndrome. Teratology 1998; 57: 51–5.

Berry DL, Theirault RL, Holmes FA et al. Management of breast cancer during pregnancy using a standardized protocol. J Clin Oncol 1999; 17: 855–61.

Blatt J, Mulvihill JJ, Ziegler JL. Pregnancy outcome following cancer chemotherapy. Am J Med 1980; 69: 828–32.

Boice JD, Tawn EJ, Winther JF et al. Genetic effects of radiotherapy for childhood cancer. Health Physics 2003; 7: 65–80.

Briggs GG, Freeman RK, Yaffe SJ. Drugs in Pregnancy and Lactation, 7th edn. Baltimore, MD: Williams & Wilkins, 2005.

Brunet S, Sureda A, Mateu R et al. Full-term pregnancy in a patient diagnosed with acute leukemia treated with a protocol including VP-16. Med Clin (Barc) 1993; 100: 757–8.

Buckley LM, Bullaboy CA, Leichtman L et al. Multiple congenital anomalies associated with weekly low-dose methotrexate treatment of mother. Arthritis Rheum 1997; 40: 971–3.

Bussing A, Lehnert A, Schink M et al. Effect of Viscum album L. on rapidly proliferating amniotic fluid cells. Sister chromatid exchange frequency and proliferation index. Arzneimittelforsch 1995; 45: 81–3.

Byrd DC, Pitts SR, Alexander CK. Hydroxyurea in two pregnant women with sickle cell anemia. Pharmacotherapy 1999; 19: 1459–62.

Caluwaerts S, van Calsteren K, Mertens L et al. Neoadjuvant chemotherapy followed by radical hysterectomy for invasive cervical cancer diagnosed during pregnancy: report of a case and review of literature. Int J Gynecol Cancer 2006; 16: 905–8.

Cardonick E, Iacobucci A. Use of chemotherapy during human pregnancy. Lancet Oncol 2004; 5: 283–91.

Carradice D, Austin N, Bayston K et al. Successful treatment of acute promyelocytic leukaemia during pregnancy. Clin Lab Haem 2002; 24: 307–11.

Celiloglu M, Altunyurt S, Undar B. Hydroxyurea treatment for chronic myeloid leukemia during pregnancy. Acta Obstet Gynecol Scand 2000; 79: 803–4.

Chakravarty EF, Sanchez-Yamamoto D, Bush TM. The use of disease modifying antirheumatic drugs in women with rheumatoid arthritis of childbearing age: a survey of practice patterns and pregnancy outcomes. J Rheumatol 2003; 30: 241–6.

2

Pregnancy

2.13 Antineoplastic drugs

Chapa JB, Hibbard JU, Weber EM et al. Prenatal diagnosis of methotrexate embryopathy. Obstet Gynecol 2003; 101: 1104–7.

Choudhary DR, Mishra P, Kumar R et al. Pregnancy on imatinib: fatal outcome with meningocele. Ann Oncol 2006; 17: 178–9.

Christian MS, Teo S, Laskin O et al. Different pattern of developmental effects for structurally similar drugs, thalidomide and lenalidomide {Abstract}. Reprod Toxicol 2006; 22: 267–8.

Claahsen HL, Semmekrot BA, van Dongen PW et al. Successful fetal outcome after exposure to idarubicin and cytosine-arabinoside during the second trimester of pregnancy – a case report. Am J Perinatol 1998; 15: 295–7.

Clowse MEB, Magder L, Petri M. Cyclophosphamide for lupus during pregnancy. Lupus 2005; 14: 593–7.

Consoli U, Figuera A, Milone G et al. Acute promyelocytic leukemia during pregnancy: report of 3 cases. Int J Hemotol 2004; 79: 31–6.

Cullins SL, Pridjian G, Sutherland CM. Goldenhar's syndrome associated with tamoxifen given to the mother during gestation {Letter}. J Am Med Assoc 1994; 271: 1905–6.

Cuvier C, Espie M, Extra JM et al. Vinorelbin in pregnancy. Eur J Cancer 1997; 33: 168–9.

Dann EJ, Epelbaum R, Avivi I et al. Fertility and ovarian function are preserved in women treated with an intensified regimen of cyclophosphamide, adriamycin, vincristine and prednisone (Mega-CHOP) for non-Hodgkin lymphoma. Hum Reprod 2005; 20: 2247–9.

Dara P, Slater LM, Armentrout SA. Successful pregnancy during chemotherapy for acute leukemia. Cancer 1981; 47: 845–6.

Daw EG. Procarbazine in pregnancy. Lancet 1970; 2: 984.

De Boer NK, Elburg van RM, Wilhelm AJ. 6-Thioguanine for Crohn's disease during pregnancy: thiopurine metabolite measurements in both mother and child. Scand J Gastroenterol 2005; 40: 1374–7.

Decker M, Rothermundt C, Holländer G et al. Rituximab plus CHOP for treatment of diffuse large B-cell lymphoma during second trimester of pregnancy. Lancet Oncol 2006; 7: 693–4.

Del Campo M, Kosaki K, Bennett FC et al. Developmental delay in fetal aminopterin/methotrexate syndrome. Teratology 1999; 60: 10–12.

De Santis M, Lucchese A, de Carolis S et al. Metastatic breast cancer in pregnancy: first case of chemotherapy with docetaxel. Eur J Cancer 2000; 9: 235–7.

Diav-Citrin O, Hunnisett L, Sher GD et al. Hydroxyurea use during pregnancy: a case report in sickle cell disease and review of the literature. Am J Hematol 1999; 60: 148–50.

Di Paolo SR, Goodin S, Ratzell M et al. Chemotherapy for metastatic melanoma during pregnancy. Gynecol Oncol 1997; 66: 526–30.

Diwan BA, Anderson LM, Rehm S et al. Transplacental carcinogenicity of cisplatin: initiation of skin tumors and induction of other preneoplastic and neoplastic lesions in SENCAR mice. Cancer Res 1993; 53: 3874–6.

Doll DC, Ringenberg QS, Yarbro JW. Antineoplastic agents and pregnancy. Semin Oncol 1989; 16: 337–46.

Donnenfeld AE, Pasuszak A, Salkoff Noah J et al. Methotrexate exposure prior to and during pregnancy. Teratology 1994; 49: 79–81.

Doubek M, Brychtova Y, Doubek R et al. Anagrelide therapy in pregnancy: report of a case of essential thrombocythemia. Ann Hematol 2004; 83: 726–7.

Dreicer R, Love RR. High total dose 5-fluorouracil treatment during pregnancy. Wis Med J 1991; 90: 582–3.

2

Elit L, Bocking A, Kenyon C et al. An endodermal sinus tumor diagnosed in pregnancy: case report and review of the literature. Gynecol Oncol 1999; 72: 123–7.

Engert A, Lathan B, Cremer R et al. Non-Hodgkin lymphoma and pregnancy {in German}. Med Klin 1990; 85: 734–8.

Enns GM, Roeder E, Chan RT et al. Apparent cyclophosphamide (Cytoxan) embryopathy: a distinct phenotype? Am J Med Genet 1999; 86: 237–41.

Fadilah SA, Hatta AZ, Keng CS et al. Successful treatment of acute promyelocytic leukemia in pregnancy with all-trans retinoic acid. Leukemia 2001; 15: 1665–6.

Falconer AD, Fernis P. Pregnancy outcomes following treatment of cancer. J Obstet Gynaecol 2002; 22: 43–4.

Fanale MA, Uyei AR, Theirault RL et al. Treatment of metastatic breast cancer with trastuzumab and vinorelbine during pregnancy. Clin Breast Cancer 2005; 6: 354–6.

Feldkamp M, Carey JC. Clinical teratology counseling and consultation case report: low dose methotrexate exposure in the early weeks of pregnancy. Teratology 1993; 47: 533–9.

Feliu J, Juarez S, Ordonez A et al. Acute leukemia and pregnancy. Cancer 1988; 61: 580–84.

Férnandez M, Andrade R, Alarcón GS. Cyclophosphamide use and pregnancy in lupus. Lupus 2006, 15: 59.

Ferrandina G, Distefano M, Testa A et al. Management of an advanced ovarian cancer at 15 weeks of gestation: Case report and literature review. Gynecol Oncol 2005; 97: 693–6.

Francella A, Dyan A, Bodian C et al. The safety of 6-mercatopurine for childbearing patients with inflammatory bowel disease: a retrospective cohort study. Gastroenterology 2003; 124: 9–17.

Gadducci A, Cosio S, Fanucchi A et al. Chemotherapy with epirubicin and paclitaxel for breast cancer during pregnancy: case report and review of the literature. Anticancer Res 2003; 23: 5225–9.

Gaillard B, Leng JJ, Grellet J et al. Passage transplacentaire de l'épirubincine. J Gynecol Obstet Biol Reprod 1995; 24: 63–8.

Gainford MC, Clemons M. Breast cancer in pregnancy: Are taxanes safe? Clin Oncol (R Coll Radiol) 2006; 18: 159.

Garcia B, San Miguel J, Borrasca AL. Doxorubicin in the first trimester of pregnancy. Ann Intern Med 1981; 94: 547.

Garrett MJ. Teratogenic effects of combination chemotherapy. Ann Intern Med 1974; 80: 667.

Germann N, Goffinet F, Goldwasser F. Anthracyclines during pregnancy: embryofetal outcome in 160 patients. Ann Oncol 2004; 15: 146–50.

Giacalone PL, Benos P, Rousseau O et al. Cis-platinum neoadjuvant chemotherapy in a pregnant woman with invasive carcinoma of the uterine cervix. Br J Obstet Gynaecol 1996; 103: 932–4.

Giacalone PL, Laffargue F, Bénos P. Chemotherapy for breast carcinoma during pregnancy. Cancer 1999; 86: 2266–72.

Giannakopoulou C, Manoura A, Hatzidaki E et al. Multimodal cancer chemotherapy during the first and second trimester of pregnancy: a case report. Eur J Obstet Gynecol Reprod Biol 2000; 91: 95–7.

Gililland J, Weinstein L. The effects of cancer chemotherapeutic agents on the developing fetus. Obstet Gynecol Surv 1983; 38: 6–13.

Ginopoulos PV, Michail GD, Kourounis GS. Pregnancy associated breast cancer: a case report. Eur J Gynaecol Oncol 2004; 25: 261–3.

Goldwasser F, Pico JL, Cerrina J et al. Successful chemotherapy including epirubicin in a pregnant non-Hodgkin's lymphoma patient. Leuk Lymphoma 1995; 20: 173–6.

Gonzales-Angulo AM, Walters RS, Carpenter RJ et al. Paclitaxel chemotherapy in a pregnant patient with bilateral breast cancer. Clin Breast Cancer 2004; 5: 317–19.

Green DM, Whitton JA, Stovall M et al. Pregnancy outcome of female survivors of childhood cancer: a report from the childhood cancer survivor study. Am J Obstet Gynecol 2002; 187: 1070–80.

Green DM, Whitton JA, Stovall M et al. Pregnancy outcome of partners of male survivors of childhood cancer survivor study. J Clin Oncol 2003; 21: 716–21.

Greenberg LH, Tanaka KR. Congenital anomalies probably induced cyclophosphamide. J Am Med Assoc 1964; 4(188): 423–6.

Greenlund LJS, Letendre L, Tefferi A. Acute leukemia during pregnancy: a single institutional experience with 17 cases. Leuk Lymphoma 2001; 41: 571–7.

Hahn KME, Johnson PH, Gordon N et al. Treatment of pregnant breast cancer patients and outcomes of children exposed to chemotherapy in utero. Cancer 2006; 107: 1219–26.

Han J-Y, Nava-Ocampo AA, Kim T-J. Pregnancy outcome after prenatal exposure to bleomycin, etoposide and cisplatin for malignant ovarian germ cell tumors: report of 2 cases. Reprod Toxicol 2005; 19: 557–61.

Hassenstein E, Riedel H. Teratogenicity of adriamycin. A case report {in German}. Geburtshilfe Frauenheilkd 1978; 38: 131–3.

Heartin E, Walkinshaw S, Clark RE. Successful outcome of pregnancy in chronic myeloid leukaemia treated with imatinib. Leuk Lymphoma 2004; 45: 1307–8.

Hendel J, Nyfors A. Pharmakokinetics of methotrexate in erythrocytes in psoriasis. Eur J Clin Pharmacol 1984; 27: 607–10.

Henderson CE, Elia G, Garfinkel D et al. Platinum chemotherapy during pregnancy for serous cyst-adenocarcinoma of the ovary. Gynecol Oncol 1993; 49: 92–4.

Hensley ML, Ford JM. Imatinib treatment: specific issues related to safety, fertility, and pregnancy. Semin Hematol 2003; 40: 21–5.

Herold M, Schnohr S, Bittrich H. Efficacy and safety of a combined rituximab chemotherapy during pregnancy. J Clin Oncol 2001; 19: 3439.

Hoffmann M. Primary ovarian carcinoma during pregnancy. Clinical Cons Obstet Gynecol 1995; 7: 237–42.

Horbelt D, Delmore J, Meisel R et al. Mixed germ cell malignancy of the ovary concurrent with pregnancy. Obstet Gynecol 1994; 28: 662–4.

Hsu K-F, Chang Ch-H, Chou Ch-Y. Sinusoidal fetal heart rate pattern during chemotherapy in a pregnant woman with acute myelogenous leukemia. J Formos Med Assoc 1995; 94: 562–5.

Isaacs RJ, Hunter W, Clark K. Tamoxifen as systemic treatment of advanced breast cancer during pregnancy – case report and literature review. Gynecol Oncol 2001; 80: 405–8.

Jacobs AJ, Marchevski A, Gordon RE et al. Oat cell carcinoma of the uterine cervix in a pregnant woman treated with cis-diamminedichloroplatinum. Gynecol Oncol 1980; 9: 405–10.

Jacobs C, Donaldson SS, Rosenberg SA et al. Management of the pregnant patient with Hodgkin's disease. Ann Intern Med 1981; 95: 669–75.

Karp GI, Von Oeyen P, Valone F et al. Doxorubicin in pregnancy: possible transplacental passage. Cancer Treat Rep 1983; 67: 773–7.

Kerr JR. Neonatal effects of breast cancer chemotherapy administered during pregnancy. Pharmacotherapy 2005; 25: 438–41.

Khurshid M, Saleem M. Acute leukaemia in pregnancy. Lancet 1978; 2: 534–5.

Kim WY, Wehbe TW, Akerley W. A woman with a balanced autosomal translocation who received chemotherapy while pregnant. Med Health RI 1996; 79: 396–9.

Kimby E, Sverrisdottir A, Elinder G. Safety of rituximab therapy during the first trimester of pregnancy: a case history. Eur J Haematol 2004; 72: 292–5.

Kirshon B, Wasserstrum N, Willis R et al. Teratogenic effects of first-trimester cyclophosphamide therapy. Obstet Gynecol 1988; 72: 462–4.

Kopelman JN, Miyazawa K. Inadvertent 5-fluorouracil treatment in early pregnancy: a report of three cases. Reprod Toxicol 1990; 4: 233–5.

Kopf-Maier P. Stage of pregnancy-dependent transplacental passage of 195mPt after cis-platinum treatment. Eur J Cancer Clin Oncol 1983; 19: 533–6.

Köseoglu HK, Yücel AE, Künefeci G et al. Cyclophosphamide therapy in a serious case of lupus nephritis during pregnancy. Lupus 2001; 10: 818–20.

Kozlowski RD, Steinbrunner JV, MacKenzie AH et al. Outcome of first-trimester exposure to low-dose methotrexate in eight patients with rheumatic diesease. Am J Med 1990; 88: 589–92.

Krähenmann F, Østensen M, Stallmach Th et al. In utero first trimester exposure to low-dose methotrexate with increased fetal nuchal translucency and associated malformations. Prenatal Diagn 2002; 22: 487–500.

Lai CH, Hsueh S, Chao AS et al. Successful pregnancy after tamoxifen and megestrol acetate therapy for endometrial carcinoma. Br J Obstet Gynaecol 1994; 101: 547–9.

Lambert B, Holmberg K, Einhorn N. Persistence of chromosome rearrangements in peripheral lymphocytes from patients treated with melphalan for ovarian carcinoma. Hum Genet 1984; 67: 94–8.

Lewden B, Vial T, Eléfant E et al. Low dose methotrexate in the first trimester of pregnancy: result of a french collaborative study. J Rheumatol 2004; 31: 2360–65.

Lilleyman JS, Hill AS, Anderton KJ. Consequences of acute myelogenous leukemia in early pregnancy. Cancer 1977; 40: 1300–303.

Lowenthal RM, Funnell CF, Hope DM et al. Normal infant after combination chemotherapy including teniposide for Burkitt's lymphoma in pregnancy. Med Pediatr Oncol 1982; 10: 165–9.

Luisiri P, Lance NJ, Curran JJ. Wegener's granulomatosis in pregnancy. Arthritis Rheum 1997; 40: 1354–60.

Mamuris Z, Prieur M, Dutrillaux B et al. Specificity of melphalan-induced rearrangements and their transmission through cell divisions. Mutagenesis 1989; 4: 133–9.

McElhatton PR. A review of the reproductive toxicity of methotrexate in human pregnancy. Reprod Toxicol 2000; 14: 549.

Melzer HJ. Congenital anomalies due to attempted abortion with 4-amino pteroylglutamic acid. J Am Med Assoc 1956; 161: 1253.

Mendez LE, Mueller A, Salom E et al. Paclitaxel and carboplatin chemotherapy administered during pregnancy for advanced epithelial ovarian cancer. Obstet Gynecol 2003; 102: 1200–202.

Mennuti MT, Shepard TH, Mellman WJ. Fetal renal malformation following treatment of Hodgkin's disease during pregnancy. Obstet Gynecol 1975; 46: 194–6.

Merimsky O, le Chevalier T, Missenard G et al. Management of cancer in pregnancy: a case of Ewing's sarcoma of the pelvis in the third trimester. Ann Oncol 1999; 10: 345–50.

Merlob P. Infant or mother with malignant disease. Beltis Newsletter 2004; 12: 40–49.

Merlob P. Hydroxyurea in pregnant women with polycythemia vera. BELTIS Newsletter 2005; 13: 45–50.

Milunsky A, Graef JW, Gaynor MF. Methotrexate-induced congenital malformations. J Pediatr 1968; 72: 790–95.

2

Pregnancy

2.13 Antineoplastic drugs

Minton SE, Munster PN. Chemotherapy-induced amenorrhea and fertility in women undergoing adjuvant treatment for breast cancer. Cancer Control 2002; 9: 466–72.

Moskowitz DN, Bodian C, Chapman ML et al. The effect on the fetus of medications used to treat pregnant inflammatory bowel-disease patients. Am J Gastroenterol 2004; 99: 656–61.

Motegi M, Takakura S, Takano H et al. Adjuvant chemotherapy in a pregnant woman with endodermal sinus tumor of the ovary. Obstet Gynecol 2007; 109: 537–40.

Müller T, Hofmann J, Steck T. Eclampsia after polychemotherapy for nodal-positive breast cancer during pregnancy. Eur J Obstet Gynecol Reprod Biol 1996; 67: 197–8.

Mulvihill JJ, McKeen EA, Rosner F et al. Pregnancy outcome in cancer patients: experience in a large cooperative group. Cancer 1987; 60: 1143–50.

Murray CL, Reichert JA, Anderson J et al. Multimodal cancer therapy for breast cancer in first trimester of pregnancy. J Am Med Assoc 1984; 252: 2607–8.

Murray NA, Acolet D, Deane M et al. Fetal marrow suppression after maternal chemotherapy for leukaemia. Arch Dis Child 1994; 71: F209–10.

Mutchinick O, Aizpuru E, Grether P. The human teratogenic effect of cyclophosphamide. Teratology 1992; 45: 329.

Nakajima W, Ishida A, Takahashi M et al. Good outcome for infant of mother treated with chemotherapy for ewing sarcoma at 25 to 30 weeks gestation. J Pediatr Hematol Oncol 2004; 26: 308–11.

Nguyen Ch, Duhl AJ, Escallon C et al. Multiple anomalies in a fetus exposed to low-dose methotrexate in the first trimester. Obstet Gynecol 2002; 99: 599–602.

Nicholson HO. Cytotoxic drugs in pregnancy: review of reported cases. J Obstet Gynecol Br Commonw 1968; 75: 307–12.

Niedermeier DM, Frei-Lahr DA, Hall PD. Treatment of acute myeloid leukemia during the second and third trimesters of pregnancy. Pharmacotherapy 2005; 25: 1134–40.

Nieto Y, Santisteban M, Aramendía JM et al. Docetaxel administered during pregnancy for inflammatory breast carcinoma. Clin Breast Cancer 2006; 6: 533–4.

Nørgård B, Pedersen L, Fonager K et al. Azathioprine, mercaptopurine and birth outcome: a population-based cohort study. Aliment Pharmacol Ther 2003; 17: 827–34.

Nulman I, Laslo D, Fried S et al. Neurodevelopment of children exposed in utero to treatment of maternal malignancy. Br J Cancer 2001; 85: 1611–18.

Oates S. Non-Hodgkin's lymphoma in pregnancy. J Obstet Gynaecol 1990; 10: 531–2.

Odom LD, Plouffe l, Butler WJ. 5-Fluorouracil exposure during the period of conception: report on two cases. Am J Obstet Gynecol 1990; 163: 76–7.

Ohara N, Teramoto K. Successful treatment of an advanced cystadenocarcinoma in pregnancy with cisplatin, adriamycin and cyclophosphamid (CAP) regimen. Case report. Clin Exp Obstet Gynecol 2000; 2: 123–4.

Ojeda-Uribe M, Gillot C, Jung G et al. Administration of rituximab during the first trimester of pregnancy without consequences for the newborn. J Perinatol 2006; 26: 252–5.

Okun DB, Groncy PK, Sieger L et al. Acute leukemia in pregnancy: transient neonatal myelosuppression after combination chemotherapy in the mother. Med Pediatr Oncol 1979; 7: 315–19.

Østensen M, Hartmann H, Salvesen K. Low dose weekly methotrexate in early pregnancy. A case series and review of literature. J Rheumatol 2000; 27: 1872–5.

Paladini D, Vassallo M, d'Armiento MR et al. Prenatal detection of multiple fetal anomalies following inadvertent exposure to cyclophosphamide in the first trimester of pregnancy. Birth Def Res A 2004: 70: 99–100.

Pan PH, Moore CH. Doxorubicin-induced cardiomyopathy during pregnancy: three case reports of anesthetic management for cesarean and vaginal delivery in two kyphoscoliotic patients. Anesthesiology 2002; 97: 513–15.

Paskulin GA, Gazzola Zen PR, Camargo Pinto LL et al. Combined chemotherapy and teratogenicity. Birth Def Res A 2005; 73: 634–7.

Pata O, Tok CE, Yazici G et al. Polycythemia vera and pregnancy: a case report with the use of hydroxyurea in the first trimester. Am J Perinatol 2004; 21: 135–7.

Peres RM, Sanseverino MTV, Guimararaes JLM et al. Assessment of fetal risk associated with exposure to cancer chemotherapy during pregnancy: a multicenter study. Brazil J Med Biol Res 2001; 34: 1551–9.

Pizzuto J, Aviles A, Noriega L et al. Treatment of acute leukemia during pregnancy: presentation of nine cases. Cancer Treat Rep 1980; 64: 679–83.

Polifka JE, Friedman JM. Teratogen uptake: azathioprine and 6-mercaptopurine. Teratology 2002; 65: 240–61.

Potluri V, Lewis D, Burton GV. Chemotherapy with taxanes in breast cancer during pregnancy: case report and review of the literature. Clin Breast Cancer 2006; 7: 167–70.

Powell HR, Ekert H. Methotrexate-induced congenital malformations. Med J Aust 1971; 2: 1076–7.

Prabhash K, Sastry PS, Biswas G et al. Pregnancy outcome of two patients treated with imatinib. Ann Oncol 2005; 16: 1983–4.

Raffles A, Williams J, Costeloe K et al. Transplacental effects of maternal cancer chemotherapy. Case Report. Br J Obstet Gynaecol 1989; 96: 1099–100.

Requena A, Velasco JG, Pinilla J et al. Acute leukemia during pregnancy: obstetrics management nad perinatal outcome of two cases. Eur J Obstet Gynecol Reprod Biol 1995; 63: 139–41.

Reynoso EE, Huerta F. Acute leukemia and pregnancy – fatal fetal outcome after exposure to idarubicin during the second trimester. Acta Oncol 1994; 33: 703–16.

Reynoso EE, Shepherd FA, Messner HA et al. Acute leukemia during pregnancy: the Toronto leukemia study group experience with long-term follow-up of children exposed in utero to chemotherapeutic agents. J Clin Oncol 1987; 5: 1098–106.

Ring AE, Smith IA, Jones A et al. Chemotherapy for breast cancer during pregnancy: an 18-year experience from five London teaching hospitals. J Clin Oncol 2005; 23: 4192–7.

Rodriguez JM, Haggag M. VACOP-B chemotherapy for high grade non-Hodgkin's lymphoma in pregnancy. Clin Oncol (R Coll Radiol) 1995; 7: 319–20.

Rugh R, Skaredoff L. Radiation and radiomimetic chlorambucil and the fetal retina. Arch Ophthalmol 1965; 74: 382–93.

Ruiz-Velasco V, Rosas-Arceo J, Matute MM. Chemical inducers of ovulation: comparative results. Int J Fertil 1979; 24: 61–4.

Schafer AI. Teratogenic effects of antileukemic chemotherapy. Arch Intern Med 1981; 14: 514–15.

Schapira DV, Chudley AE. Successful pregnancy following continuous treatment with combination chemotherapy before conception and throughout pregnancy. Cancer 1984; 54: 800–803.

Schardein JL. Chemically Induced Birth Defects, 3rd edn. New York: Marcel Dekker, 2000.

Scheuning M, Clemm C. Chromosomal aberrations in a newborn whose mother received cytotoxic treatment during pregnancy. N Eng J Med 1987; 317: 1666–7.

Seidahmed MZ, Shaheed MM, Abdulbasit OB et al. A case of methotrexate embryopathy with holoprosencephaly, expanding the phenotype. Birth Def Res A 2006; 76: 138–42.

2

Pregnancy

2.13 Antineoplastic drugs

Shotton E, Monie IW. Possible teratogenic effect of chlorambucil on a human fetus. J Am Med Assoc 1963; 186: 180–81.

Signorello LB, Cohen SS, Bosetti C et al. Female survivors of childhood cancer: preterm birth and low birth weight among their children. J Natl Cancer Inst 2006; 98: 1453–61.

Siu BL, Alonzo MR, Vargo TA et al. Transient dilated cardiomyopathy in a newborn exposed to idarubicin and all-trans-retinoic acid (ATRA) early in the second trimester of pregnancy. Int J Gynecol Cancer 2002; 12: 399–402.

Sood AK, Shahin MS, Sorosky JI. Paclitaxel and platinum chemotherapy for ovarian carcinoma during pregnancy. Gynecol Oncol 2001; 83: 599–600.

Sosa Munoz JL, Perez Santana MT, Sosa Sanchez R et al. Acute leukemia and pregnancy. Rev Invest Clin 1983; 35: 55–8.

Steege JF, Caldwell DS. Renal agenesis after first trimester exposure to chlorambucil. South Med J 1980; 73: 1414–15.

Stephens TD, Golbus MS, Miller TR et al. Multiple congenital anomalies in a fetus exposed to 5-fluorouracil during the first trimester. Am J Obstet Gynecol 1980; 137: 747–9.

Stevens FRT, Fisher HM. Pregnancy in leukemia. Aust NZ J Obstet Gynaecol 1965; 5: 38–40.

Stovall M, Donaldson SS, Weathers RE et al. Genetic effects of radiotherapy for childhood cancer: gonadal dose reconstruction. J Radiat Oncol Biol Phys 2004; 60: 542–52.

Stucker I, Caillard JF, Collin R et al. Risk of spontaneous abortion among nurses handling antineoplastic drugs. Scand J Work Environ Health 1990; 16: 102–7.

Takitani K, Hino N, Terada Y et al. Plasma all-trans retinoic acid level in neonates of mothers with acute promyelocytic leukemia. Acta Haematol 2005; 114: 167–9.

Tegay DH, Tepper R, Willner JP. 6-Mercaptopurine teratogenicity. Postgrad Med J 2002; 78: 572.

Terada Y, Shindo T, Endoh A et al. Fetal arrhythmia during treatment of pregnancy-associated acute promyelocytic leukemia with all-trans retinoic acid and favorable outcome. Leukemia 1997; 11: 454–5.

Tewari K, Bonebrake RG, Asrat T et al. Ambiguous genitalia in infant exposed to tamoxifen in utero. Lancet 1997; 350: 183.

Thauvin-Robinet C, Maingueneau C, Robert E et al. Exposure to hydroxyurea during pregnancy: a case series. Leukemia 2001; 15: 1309–11.

Thiersch JB. Therapeutic abortion with a folic acid antagonist, 4-amino pteroylglutamic acid, administerd by the oral route. Am J Obstet Gynecol 1952; 63: 1298.

Thomas PRM, Peckham MJ. The investigation and management of Hodgkin's disease in the pregnant patient. Cancer 1976; 38: 1443–51.

Toledo TM, Harper RC, Moser RH. Fetal effects during cyclophosphamide and irradiation therapy. Ann Intern Med 1971; 74: 87–91.

Tomlinson MW, Treadwell MC, Deppe G. Platinum based chemotherapy to treat recurrent Sertoli-Leydig cell ovarian carcinoma during pregnancy. Eur J Gynaecol Oncol 1997; 18: 44–6.

Tuch BE, Turtle JR, Simeonovic CJ. Streptozotocin is not toxic to the human fetal B cell. Diabetologia 1989; 32: 678–84.

Tuch BE, Chen J. Resistance of the human fetal beta-cell to the toxic effect of multiple low-dose streptozotocin. Pancreas 1993; 8: 305–11.

Tulandi T, Martin J, al Fadhli R et al. Congenital malformation among 911 newborns conceived after infertility treatment with letrozole or clomiphene citrate. Fertil Steril 2006; 85: 1761–5.

2

Turchi JJ, Villasis C. Anthracyclines in the treatment of malignancy in pregnancy. Cancer 1988; 61: 435–40.

Vaux KK, Kahole NCO, Jones KL. Cyclophosphamide, methotrexate and cytarabine embryopathy: Is apotosis the common pathway? Birth Def Res A 2003; 67: 403–8.

Veneri D, Todeschini G, Pizzolo G et al. Acute leukemia and pregnancy. Clin Exp Obstet Gynecol 1996; 23: 112–15.

Wagner VM, Hill JS, Weaver D et al. Congenital abnormalities in baby born to cytarabine treated mother. Lancet 1980; 2: 98–9.

Warkany J, Beaudry PH, Hornstein S. Attempted abortion with aminopterin. Am J Dis Child 1959; 97: 274.

Waterstone AM, Graham J. Effect of adjuvant trastuzumab on pregnancy. J Clin Oncol 2006; 24: 321–2.

Watson WL. Herceptin (trastuzumab) therapy during pregnancy: association with reversible anhydramnios. Obstet Gynecol 2005; 105: 642–3.

Wheeler M, O'Meara P, Stanford M. Fetal methotrexate and misoprostol exposure: the past revisited. Teratology 2002; 66: 73–6.

Wright CA, Tefferi A. A single institutional experience with 43 pregnancies in essential thrombocythemia. Eur J Haematol 2001; 66: 152–9.

Yedlinski NT, Morgan FC, Whitecar PW. Anomalies associated with failed methotrexate and misoprostol termination. Obstet Gynecol 2005; 105: 1203–5.

Zemlickis D, Lishner M, Degendorfer P et al. Fetal outcome after in utero exposure to cancer chemotherapy. Arch Intern Med 1992; 152: 573–6.

Zemlickis D, Lisher M, Erlich R et al. Teratogenicity and carcinogenicity in a twin exposed in utero to cyclophosphamide. Teratogenesis Carcinog Mutagen 1993; 13: 139–43.

Zuazu J, Julia A, Sierra J et al. Pregnancy outcome in hematologic malignancies. Cancer 1991; 67: 703–9.

Pregnancy

2.13 Antineoplastic drugs

Uterine contraction agents, tocolytics, vaginal therapeutics, and local contraceptives

2.14

Herman van Geijn

2.14.1   Prostaglandins

Pharmacology and toxicology

Prostaglandins (PG) have a large number of biologic and reproductive functions. Of practical significance during pregnancy are the prostaglandins designated as PGE_2, $PGF_{2\alpha}$ and PGI_2 (prostacyclin).

Prostaglandins are synthesized from arachidonic acid by the enzyme phopholipase A_2. The half-life of naturally occurring prostaglandins, such as those produced in the uterus, is only a few minutes. The kidneys, liver, intestinal tract, and lungs contain enzymes that quickly destroy prostaglandins and limit their activity. The synthesis of prostaglandins in the genital tract is influenced by the hormones estradiol and progesterone, and by catecholamines.

PGE_2 causes so-called ripening of the cervix, characterized by connective tissue changes that facilitate softening, effacement, and dilatation of the cervix during uterine contractions. $PGF_{2\alpha}$ promotes contractions. PGI_2 is an arteriolar dilator. Deficiency of prostacyclin is associated with hypertensive disorders of pregnancy.

In practice, the following uses of prostaglandins can be distinguished:

- Preparation for labor induction by ripening the cervix with *dinoprostone*, a PGE_2 analog, applied in the form of intravaginal suppositories or as a gel intracervically, or with *misoprostol* (a PGE_2 analog) applied intravaginally
- Induction of birth or enhancement of contractions with dinoprostone, applied as intravaginal suppositories, as vaginal inserts, or as a gel intracervically or extra-amniotically
- Treatment of postpartum uterine atony with *dinoprost* or *sulprostone* application intravenously or into the myometrium, or transcervically into the uterus, or misoprostol orally
- Induction of abortion with dinoprostone (PGE_2) as an intracervical gel, with sulprostone cervically or in the myometrium, with dinoprostone extra-amniotically, and with *gemeprost*, intravaginally or misoprostol intravaginally or orally
- Sub-involution of the uterus after birth can be treated with oxytocin or ergotamine derivatives like methylergometrine.

With all contraction stimulants, overstimulation of the myometrium can occur. Because myometrial contractions are associated with a decrease in perfusion of the uterine vessels, a potential adverse effect of these agents is embryonic or fetal hypoxia. Disruption-type malformation due to reduced perfusion and, in extreme cases, fetal death might be the consequence (Bond 1994).

Failed abortion attempts with *misoprostol* have been associated with the occurrence of Moebius sequence (cranial nerve defects and limb defects) in the offspring. Other malformations, such as cranial bone defects, omphalocele, and gastroschizis, have also been observed. In these abortion attempts, misoprostol was used orally, often combined with vaginal administration as well. The most common total dose was 800 μg, with a range from 200 to 16 000 μg (4 tablets daily for 20 days). All cases were exposed in the first trimester, most commonly in the second month (Orioli 2000, Gonzalez 1998, Hofmeyr 1998, Castilla 1994, Schüler 1992). The medication history in the mothers of

94 children with Moebius sequence showed that nearly half had used misoprostol orally or vaginally.

A 200-μg dose of misoprostol has been associated with increased uterine artery resistance indices by Doppler ultrasound, suggesting that perfusion reduction could underlie the disruption-type malformations (Yip 2000).

In a prospective controlled study, on the contrary, no adverse effects on pregnancy or neonates were observed. However, the number of mothers exposed to misoprostol was only 86 (Schüler 1999). No increased risk for major malformations was again noted in a French collaborative study of 125 pregnancies exposed to misoprostol. No specific pattern of malformations was demonstrated; in particular, Moebius sequence or limb-reduction defects were not observed (Bellemin 1999). A recent systematic review and meta-analysis, including 4899 cases of congenital anomalies and 5742 controls, concluded, though, that misoprostol is associated with an increased risk of Moebius sequence (OR = 25; 95% CI 11–58) and terminal transverse limb defects (OR = 12; 95% CI 5–29) (Da Silva Dal Pizzol 2006).

In summary, an increased teratogenic risk after (accidental) exposure to misoprostol may exist. Among women with offspring with Moebius syndrome, the likelihood of exposure to misoprostol in the first trimester is high; however, the absolute risk is probably low following misoprostol exposure in the first trimester of pregnancy (Goldberg 2001).

Misoprostol is also increasingly used for the induction of an abortion or labor, and in the postpartum period, due to its simple oral administration and favorable costs. Titrating the misoprostol dose on the basis of the frequency and intensity of uterine contractions is frequently applied, particularly in developing countries. For labor induction after rupture of the membranes, it is the most effective drug that can be applied without an increased risk for infection. Overstimulation and pathologic fetal heart rate patterns in individual cases, however, are a reason to warn against indiscriminate use of misoprostol (Wing 2006). Misoprostol should not be used in term pregnancies with a uterine scar from a previous cesarean section or from major uterine surgery (ACOG opinion no 342, 2006).

Misoprostol is not approved for any indication in pregnancy, and administration of misoprostol for cervical ripening and/or labor induction currently is considered off-label (Wing 2006).

For misoprostol, see also Chapter 2.5 on ulcer therapeutics.

Recommendation. Prostaglandins may be used for cervical ripening and induction of labor. When pregnancy continues after a failed abortion attempt with prostaglandins, it is advised to perform detailed ultrasound scanning (at 12–14 and 18–20 weeks) to verify morphologic development of the fetus, on the grounds of possible embryotoxicity.

2.14.2   Oxytocin

Pharmacology and toxicology

Oxytocin is an octapeptide produced in the hypothalamus, stored in the posterior pituitary, and from there released into the blood. Inactivation occurs via a specific oxytocinase in the liver, spleen, and ovaries. During pregnancy, oxytocin is inactivated by another enzyme produced by the placenta, a cystinaminopeptidase. Oxytocin has a plasma half-life of only a few minutes.

The sites of oxytocin action are the uterine muscle and the myoepithelial cells surrounding the milk-producing units of the breast. The conditions for the action of oxytocin on a pregnant uterus are complex and are controlled by several factors. Among these factors are decreases in estrogen and progesterone concentrations in the blood, with a reduction in the α- and β-adrenergic activity in the uterine muscles. During pregnancy the concentration of oxytocin in the blood is slightly elevated, but towards the end of pregnancy both the concentration and the number of oxytocin receptors in the myometrium increase significantly. During the course of labor, a three- to four-fold increase in the plasma concentration of oxytocin is observed.

Because of its structural similarity to vasopressin, oxytocin has antidiuretic hormone activity, promoting the reabsorption of salt-free fluid in the distal renal tubules. High doses of oxytocin given with electrolyte-free solutions can lead to water intoxication, with cramps, coma and, rarely, death. Reduction of fluid intake and monitoring of electrolytes can eliminate the risk of water intoxication.

The oxytocin analog *pitocin* is used in low doses intravenously as a standard treatment for the induction or augmentation of labor. As with all contraction stimulants, overstimulation of the myometrium can occur. In that case, oxytocin increases the basal tone in the uterus, leading to a decrease in uteroplacental perfusion, with the possibility of fetal hypoxia and even fetal death occurring.

A second risk from overstimulation is uterine rupture, particularly in the presence of a scarred uterus; this may lead to substantial maternal blood loss, shock, loss of the uterus, and even maternal death. Uterine rupture, except when an emergency cesarean section can be performed, will inevitably lead to the death of the child. Oxytocin should be applied with extreme caution for induction or augmentation of labor, and only in combination with careful monitoring of maternal uterine contractions and the fetal heart rate (i.e. electronic fetal heart rate monitoring, cardiotocography).

> **Recommendation.** Oxytocin (pitocin) may be used when indicated for induction or augmentation of labor. It should be applied extremely carefully, and only in combination with monitoring of uterine activity and fetal heart rate.

2.14.3 Ergot alkaloids (see also Chapter 2.1)

Pharmacology and toxicology

Ergot alkaloids (ergotamine derivatives) are used to increase the strength of uterine contraction to limit postpartum bleeding and promote postpartum involution. Because ergot-associated contractions are tonic rather than rhythmic, these agents cannot be used during labor. Tonic contraction of the uterus during labor could result in fetal hypoxia and even death.

Pharmacologic agents in this group include *ergometrine* and *methylergometrine (methylergonovine)*.

> **Recommendation.** Ergot alkaloids are used only after birth for postpartum uterine hypotonia. They are contraindicated during pregnancy. Accidental use during the first trimester does not automatically require termination of the pregnancy. Detailed ultrasound scanning can exclude morphologic developmental disorders. For other ergotamine derivatives, see Chapters 2.1, 2.8 and 2.15.

2.14.4 Tocolytics in general

Tocolytic agents can stop uterine contractions and temporarily delay delivery. Critical analyses have demonstrated that most tocolytics are effective for prolongation of pregnancy for only 48–72 hours. This period allows for transport of the pregnant woman to a perinatal center, and for administration of glucocorticoids for lung maturation (Higby 1999, Katz 1999). No protocol of (long-term) tocolysis has unequivocally contributed to effective prevention of preterm birth or to improvement in neonatal outcome. When prescribing tocolytics, strict guidelines must be observed.

Among the most common agents used as tocolytics are calcium antagonists, β-adrenergic agents, oxytocin antagonists, prostaglandin antagonists, and magnesium sulfate.

2.14.5 β_2-sympathomimetics

Pharmacology and toxicology

β-adrenergic agents have for long been the most widely used contraction inhibitors (tocolytics), but are applied less frequently because of their pronounced side effects (Papatsonis 2003, Goldenberg 2002) and the short-acting effect (maximum of 48 hours) on the uterine musculature due to development of tachyphylaxis (Schiff 1993). *Ritodrine* and *fenoterol* are the most frequently used inhibitors of uterine contractions. *Clenbuterol, salbutamol, terbutaline*, and the less selective *isoxsuprine* are also used for tocolysis.

Maternal cardiovascular side effects, such as palpitations and pulmonary edema, are serious complications from intravenous application. A suspected cardioprotective effect of verapamil led for a time to combining both pharmaceutical agents (Weidinger 1973), until reports appeared of pulmonary edema following this combination (Grospietsch 1981).

The effectiveness of oral treatment with these agents has not been demonstrated. Oral administration may not produce blood levels adequate to maintain tocolysis, and effectiveness is limited by tachyphylaxis (Schiff 1993).

The use of fenoterol and other β-sympathomimetics, especially when combined with corticosteroids to enhance fetal lung maturity, can result in impaired carbohydrate tolerance, sometimes leading to an abrupt increase in insulin need in insulin-dependent diabetics. As in their mothers, β-sympathomimetics can cause fetal and neonatal cardiovascular side effects, as well as impaired carbohydrate tolerance in the neonate.

Transient alterations in neonatal behavior and hyperkinetic behavior have been observed (Thayer 1997).

> **Recommendation.** Use of tocolytics like β_2-sympathomimetics is difficult to justify at this time. Maternal, fetal, and neonatal cardiovascular side effects and impaired carbohydrate tolerance can occur.

2.14.6   Calcium antagonists

Pharmacology and toxicology

Calcium antagonists, such as *nifedipine* or *nicardipine*, are used for tocolysis. The oral use of slow-release preparations is considered an advantage over intravenous treatment schedules. Several studies have demonstrated that these agents are well-tolerated and effective compared with other tocolytics, such as β_2-sympathomimetics (Papatsonis 2000, 1997, El-Sayed 1998, Jannet 1997). Myocardial infarction and serious dyspnea with lung edema have been reported during tocolysis with calcium antagonists (Oei 2006, van Geijn 2005). Combined administration of calcium antagonists and magnesium may seriously potentiate the activity of magnesium, inducing hypotension and neuromuscular blockade, and thus endangering the mother and fetus.

Recommendation. Tocolysis with calcium antagonists is acceptable when clearly indicated and following a normal course of pregnancy. Caution is required regarding its use simultaneously with magnesium sulfate.

2.14.7   Magnesium sulfate

Pharmacology and toxicology

Magnesium sulfate, although not actually an antihypertensive, has proved valuable in the treatment of pre-eclampsia. Magnesium sulfate is the drug of choice for the prevention and treatment of seizures in eclampsia. Intravenous administration of the drug as an initial loading dose of 4–6 g, followed by an infusion of 2–3.5 g/h, was found not to be harmful. A significantly lower risk of repeated convulsions in eclampsia has been reported.

Magnesium sulfate also acts to inhibit contractions, but is ineffective as a tocolytic (Crowther 2002). Although it is still being used in the USA for tocolysis, there are better alternatives, such as atosiban or nifedipine. Grimes and colleagues present convincing arguments that intravenous magnesium sulfate tocolysis should stop (Grimes 2006). They consider its use as a tocolytic to be a North American anomaly.

Magnesium, when used in higher doses or when kidney function is limited, can cause marked muscle hypotonia in both mother and newborn. In extreme cases, especially when a calcium antagonist such as nifedipine enhances its effect, a dangerous drop in maternal blood pressure can occur, which may result in fetal hypoxia.

Recommendation. Magnesium sulfate can be used for appropriate indications such as pre-eclampsia and eclampsia. It is the drug of choice for treatment of seizures in eclampsia. Its use as a tocolytic is obsolete.

2.14.8 Oxytocin receptor antagonists

Pharmacology and toxicology

Atosiban is a new intravenously used compound registered for tocolysis. Global availability, however, is limited due to cost. Atosiban competes with oxytocin for binding to oxytocin receptors in the myometrium, thus preventing the increase of free calcium in the cell. In a worldwide double-blind randomized trial of atosiban versus b-agonists (Worldwide Atosiban versus β-agonists Study Group 2001), both compounds resulted in similar rates of delivery within 48 hours and 7 days after start of the therapy. Atosiban, though, resulted in far fewer and, particularly, less severe maternal side effects, and as a consequence substantially less discontinuations of therapy (Wing 2006). Atosiban is considered a safe drug in comparison with calcium antagonists and β-mimetics. However, atosiban was excluded and therefore not tested in the currently reported studies in patients with preeclampsia or eclampsia, suspected chorioamnionitis, abruptio placentae, undiagnosed vaginal bleeding, multiple gestation, intrauterine fetal distress, or fetal death.

> **Recommendation.** Atosiban appears to be safe when used properly, and can be considered for tocolysis.

2.14.9 Prostaglandin antagonists

Pharmacology and toxicology

Prostaglandin synthetase inhibitors such as *indomethacin* and *sulindac* are used as an adjunct in tocolysis (Higby 1999). These agents can produce premature closure of the ductus arteriosus and impairment of renal function, with subsequent oligohydramnios. In short-term tocolysis (maximum 48 hours) before the thirty-second week of pregnancy this is seldom problematic, although the magnitude of the risks is still a subject of debate (for further detail, see also Chapter 2.1).

> **Recommendation.** Additional use of prostaglandin synthetase inhibitor in tocolysis is controversial, and should be reserved for treatment in exceptional cases.

2.14.10 Other tocolytics

Nitroglycerin, administered as a patch and intravenously, is also effective and well-tolerated in tocolysis. However, documentation regarding safety, considering its potential effects on the neonatal circulation, is limited (see, for example, Black 1999, David 1998).

Ethyl alcohol has been used in the past for tocolysis, for its presumed inhibition of oxytocin release by the posterior pituitary gland. To be effective, substantial maternal serum levels are needed! The harmful effects of alcohol on the development of the child are well known, and thus alcohol is an obsolete tocolytic (see Chapter 2.21).

> **Recommendation.** Alcohol is contraindicated.

2.14.11   Vaginal therapeutics

Pharmacology and toxicology

In women with bacterial vaginosis, the normal vaginal flora is characterized by high concentrations of *Gardnerella vaginalis* and anaerobic bacteria, and a decrease in *Lactobacillus* species. Bacterial vaginosis in pregnancy has been associated with adverse outcomes of pregnancy, such as preterm labor, preterm birth, Preterm Premature Rupture of the Outer Membranes (PPROM), chorioamnionitis, and low birth weight of the infant, especially in women with at least one other factor known to be associated with preterm delivery – in particular, cervical incompetence.

Currently, treatment of bacterial vaginosis during pregnancy has not been proven unequivocally to be efficient in reducing the risk of preterm birth or PPROM. Results suggest that treatment of women at high risk for preterm delivery does decrease the rate of preterm birth, but this is not the case in low-risk women (Donders 1999). Oral therapy against possible subclinical upper genital tract infection appears more effective than intravaginal therapy (Donders 2000, Joesoef 1999).

Intravaginal *clindamycin* may lead to a transient increase in vaginal colonization by *E. coli*. In initial randomized trials, a trend towards increased preterm birth after treatment with vaginal clindamycin was noted (Joesoef 1999). In a randomized placebo-controlled trial, vaginal clindamycin given prophylactically to women at risk for preterm birth did not prevent preterm birth. The neonatal infectious morbidity in this group was significantly higher (Vermeulen 1999). In a recent study, however, clindamycin vaginal cream therapy was associated with a significant prolongation of pregnancy and reduced costs of neonatal care in women with bacterial vaginosis (Larsson 2006).

For local therapy of vaginal candida infection, see Chapter 2.6. Antimycotics of first choice for local therapy of vaginal candidiasis are nystatin, clotrimazole, and miconazole.

Vaginal douching with (povidone-) iodine solutions increases maternal serum iodine levels and transiently alters maternal and fetal thyroid function (from week 12 of gestation). Therefore, its use should be avoided during pregnancy (see Chapter 2.17).

To date, there is no indication that vaginally administered estrogens or disinfectants, such as *dequalium, hexetidine*, and *policresulenum*, have a teratogenic effect. However, it is good therapeutic practice to avoid obsolete and controversial agents.

> **Recommendation.** When treatment of bacterial vaginosis is indicated, oral antibiotics are the first choice (see details in Chapter 2.6). Vaginal administration of metronidazole or other antibiotics appears to be less effective.

2.14.12 Spermicide contraceptives

The "over-the-counter" (OTC) available spermicides, sold as cream, gel, tablets or foam, contain *nonoxinol-9*. This form of contraception had always been considered harmless. However, in one study of more than 700 children born to mothers who became pregnant in spite of the use of vaginal contraceptives, a slight increase in rate of malformations was observed (Jick 1981). A meta-analysis did not confirm this finding (Einarson 1990). Several publications suggest that by damaging the vaginal mucosa and disturbing the vaginal flora, the use of these spermicides may facilitate HIV infection (Rosenstein 1998, Stafford 1998).

> **Recommendation.** Conception using vaginal spermicidals containing nonoxinol-9 has not been associated with an identifiable risk of birth defects.

2.14.13 Intrauterine devices

In women who use a copper IUD as a contraceptive, the copper concentration in the fallopian tubes is elevated, but copper and ceruloplasmin levels in the serum are not changed (Wollen 1994). A number of reports suggest that pregnancy in association with copper IUDs results in an increased rate of spontaneous abortions and preterm birth in the group in which the IUD remained in the uterus, compared with the group in which the IUD was removed or expelled. No increase in the rate of birth defects was documented. This is also to be expected with *levonorgestrel*-containing "intrauterine systems".

> **Recommendation.** From the embryotoxicity point of view, an IUD remaining in utero is no indication for termination of pregnancy or invasive diagnostic procedures. However, increased spontaneous abortion has been reported with retained IUDs.

References

ACOG Committee Opinion No. 342. Induction of labor for vaginal birth after cesarean delivery. Obstet Gynaecol 2006; 108: 465–7.

Bellemin B, Carlier P, Vial T et al. Misoprostol exposure during pregnancy: a French collaborative study. Presentation at the 10th Annual Conference of the European Network of Teratology Information Services (ENTIS), Madrid, 1999.

Black RS, Lees C, Thompson C et al. Maternal and fetal cardiovascular effects of transdermal glyceryl trinitrate and intravenous ritodrine. Obstet Gynecol 1999; 94: 572–6.

Bond GR, Van Zee A. Overdosage of misoprostol in pregnancy. Am J Obstet Gynecol 1994; 71: 561–2.

Castilla EE, Orioli IM. Teratogenicity of misoprostol: data from the Latin-American collaborative study of congenital malformations (ECLAMC). Am J Med Genet 1994; 51: 161–2.

Crowther CA, Hiller JE, Doyle LW. Magnesium sulphate for preventing preterm birth in threatened preterm labour. Cochrane Database Syst Rev 2002; CD 001060.

Da Silva dal Pizzol T, Pozzobon Knop F, Serrate Mengue S. Prenatal exposure to misoprostol and congenital anomalies: systematic review and meta-analysis. Reproduct Toxicol 2006; 22: 666–71.

David M, Halle H, Lichtenegger W et al. Nitroglycerin to facilitate fetal extraction during cesarean delivery. Obstet Gynecol 1998; 91: 119–24.

Donders GG. Bacterial vaginosis during pregnancy: screen and treat? Eur J Obstet Gynecol Reprod Biol 1999; 83: 1–4.

Donders GG. Treatment of sexually transmitted bacterial diseases in pregnant women. Drugs 2000; 59: 477–85.

Einarson TR, Koren G, Mattice D et al. Maternal spermicide use and adverse reproductive outcome: a meta analysis. Am J Obstet Gynecol 1990; 162: 655–60.

El-Sayed Y, Holbrook RH Jr, Gibson R et al. Diltiazem for maintenance tocolysis of preterm labor: comparison to nifedipine in a randomized trial. J Matern Fetal Med 1998; 7: 217–21.

Goldberg AB, Greenberg MB, Darney PD. Misoprostol and pregnancy. N Engl J Med 2001; 344: 38–47.

Goldenberg RL. The management of preterm labor. Obstet Gynecol 2002; 100: 1020–37.

Gonzalez CH, Marques-Dias MJ, Kim CA et al. Congenital abnormalities in Brazilian children associated with misoprostol misuse in first trimester of pregnancy. Lancet 1998; 351: 1624–7.

Grimes DA, Nanda K. Magnesium sulfate tocolysis: time to quit. Obstet Gynecol 2006: 108: 986–9.

Grospietsch G, Fenske M, Kühn W. Pathophysiologie der Lungenödementstehung bei der tokolytischen Therapie mit Fenoterol. Arch Gynäkol 1981; 232: 504–12.

Higby K, Suiter CR. A risk–benefit assessment of therapies for premature labour. Drug Saf 1999; 21: 35–56.

Hofmeyr GJ, Milos D, Nikodem VC et al. Limb reduction anomaly after failed misoprostol abortion. S Afr Med J 1998: 88; 566–7.

Jannet D, Abankwa A, Guyard B et al. Nicardipine versus salbutamol in the treatment of premature labor. A prospective randomized study. Eur J Obstet Gynecol Reprod Biol 1997; 73: 11–16.

Jick H, Walker AM, Rothman KJ et al. Vaginal spermicides and congenital disorders. J Am Med Assoc 1981; 245: 1329–32.

Joesoef MR, Schmid GP, Hillier SL. Bacterial vaginosis: review of treatment options and potential clinical indications for therapy. Clin Infect Dis 1999; 28(Suppl 1): S57–65.

Katz VL, Farmer RM. Controversies in tocolytic therapy. Clin Obstet Gynecol 1999; 42(4): 802–19.

Larsson PG, Fahraeus L, Carlsson B et al. Late miscarriage and preterm birth after treatment with clindamycin: a randomised consent design study according to Zelen. Br J Obstet Gynaecol 2006; 113: 629–37.

Oei SG. Calcium channel blockers for tocolysis: a review of their role and safety following reports of serious adverse events. Eur J Obstet Gynecol 2006; 126: 137–45.

Orioli IM, Castilla EE. Epidemiological assessment of misoprostol teratogenicity. Br J Obstet Gynaecol 2000; 107: 519–23.

Papatsonis DN, van Geijn HP, Ader HJ et al. Nifedipine and ritodine in the management of preterm labor: a randomized multicenter trial. Obstet Gynecol 1997; 90: 230–34.

Papatsonis DN, Kok JH, van Geijn HP et al. Neonatal effects of nifedipine and ritodrine for preterm labor. Obstet Gynecol 2000; 95: 477–81.

Papatsonis DN, van Geijn HP, Beleker OP et al. Hemodynamic and metabolic effects after nifedipine and ritodrine tocolysis. Int J Gynaecol Obstet 2003; 82: 5–10.

Rosenstein IJ, Stafford MK, Kitchen VS et al. Effect on normal vaginal flora of three intravaginal microbicidal agents potentially active against human immunodeficiency virus type 1. J Infect Dis 1998; 177: 1386–90.

Schiff E, Sivan E, Terry S et al. Currently recommended oral regimens for ritodrine tocolysis result in extremely low plasma levels. Am J Obstet Gynecol 1993; 169: 1059–64.

Schüler L, Ashton PW, Sanseverino MT. Teratogenicity of misoprostol. Lancet 1992; 339: 437.

Schüler L, Pastuszak A, Sanseverino MTV et al. Pregnancy outcome after exposure to misoprostol in Brazil: a prospective, controlled study. Reprod Toxicol 1999; 13: 147–51.

Stafford MK, Ward H, Flanagan A et al. Safety study of nonoxynol-9 as a vaginal microbicide: evidence of adverse effects. J Acquir Immune Defic Syndr Hum Retrovirol 1998; 17: 327–31.

Thayer JS, Hupp SC. In utero exposure to terbutaline. Effects on infant behavior and maternal self esteem. J Obstet Gynecol Neonatal Nurs 1997; 27: 691–700.

van Geijn HP, Lenglet JE, Bolte AC. Nifedipine trials: effectiveness and safety aspects. Br J Obstet Gynaecol 2005: 112 (Suppl 1): 79–83.

Vermeulen GM, Bruinse HW. Prophylactic administration of clindamycin 2% vaginal cream to reduce the incidence of spontaneous preterm birth in women with an increased recurrence risk: a randomised placebo-controlled double-blind trial. Br J Obstet Gynaecol 1999; 106: 652–7.

Weidinger H, Wiest H. Die Behandlung des Spätabortes und der drohenden Frühgeburt mit Thll65a in Kombination mit Isoptin. Z Geburtsh Perinatol 1973; 177: 233–7.

Wing DA, Gaffaney CA. Vaginal misoprostol administration for cervical ripening and labor induction. Clin Obstet Gynecol 2006; 49: 627–41.

Wollen A-L, Sandvei R, Skare A et al. The localization and concentration of copper in the fallopian tube in women with or without an intrauterine contraceptive device. Acta Obstet Gynecol Scand 1994; 73: 195–9.

Worldwide Atosiban versus Beta-agonists Study Group. Effectiveness and safety of the oxytocin antagonist atosiban versus beta-adrenergic agonists in the treatment of preterm labour. The Worldwide Atosiban versus Beta-agonists Study Group. Br J Obstet Gynaecol 2001; 108: 133–42.

Yip S-K, Tse AO-K, Haines CJ et al. Misoprostol's effect on uterine arterial blood flow and fetal heart rate in early pregnancy. Obstet Gynecol 2000; 95: 232–5.

Hormones

2.15

Elvira Rodriguez-Pinilla and
Corinna Weber-Schöndorfer

Hormones are substances produced by organs of the body and that serve to induce and control physiologic processes in other organs. Many hormones are organized on three levels – the midbrain hypothalamic level (primary releasing function), the stimulator level in the anterior pituitary gland, and the glandular level in the body periphery. Hormonal secretion is controlled via feedback among the three levels.

When the mother is treated with hormones, there may also be effects on the fetus at the various levels of these regulatory mechanisms.

The classical hormones discussed in this chapter are distinguished from local tissue factors or mediators, which include, among others, the prostaglandins (see Chapter 2.14) and leukotrienes.

2.15.1   Hypothalamic releasing hormones

Pharmacology and toxicology

The hypothalamic control of anterior pituitary function is performed by a group of hormones referred to as releasing hormones. Because of their molecular size, hypothalamic releasing hormones can cross the placenta. The following hormones belong to this group.

Thyrotropin releasing hormone (TRH)

Synthetic analogs are protirelin and corticorelin. TRH controls thyroid function via the thyroid-stimulating hormone (TSH), and also stimulates prolactin secretion. There is evidence that TRH exerts a significant relaxant effect in human myometrium and in human umbilical vasculature. These effects could have clinical implications in treated pregnant women (Potter 2004). Some authors have suggested that TRH added to prenatal glucocorticoids in women at risk of preterm delivery could reduce pulmonary problems and neonatal lung disease. Nevertheless, some studies and an extensive review of the literature published on this topic, with over 4600 women analyzed, concluded that prenatal TRH in addition to corticosteroids did not reduce the risk of neonatal respiratory diseases, but can produce adverse effects in both women and their infants (Crowther 2004, 1997, Ballard 1998). Some authors described an association between maternal treatment with TRH and delay in mental development in antenatal exposed children (Briet 2002). Thus, there seems to be a general consensus that in preterm infants at risk for lung disease, antenatal administration of TRH and glucocorticoids is no more beneficial than glucocorticoids alone.

Gonadotropin releasing hormone (GnRH) or luteinizing hormone releasing hormone (LHRH)

Releasing hormones are responsible for regulating the synthesis and secretion of FSH and LH. Many synthetic human GnRH agonists are marketed, including *buserelin*, *gonadorelin*, *goserelin*, *leuprorelin*, *nafarelin*, and *triptorelin*. *Cetrorelix* and *ganirelix* are inhibitors of GnRH. In women, GnRH agonists have been used to treat estrogen-dependent breast cancer, endometriosis, hirsutism, and polycystic ovarian syndrome, but the widespread use of protocols using GnRH agonists/ antagonists in assisted reproductive technologies has led to an increasing number of pregnant women being exposed to these types of drugs. Most of the data concerning the safety of the GnRH analogs have not demonstrated serious side effects, such as increase in the incidence of miscarriage, birth defects, or fetal growth restriction, in human pregnancies exposed to GnRH (Tarlatzis 2004,

Ludwig 2001, Eléfant 1995, Wilshire 1993). Nevertheless, concern about its potential side effects on the CNS persists. In a controlled study, 6 pregnancies exposed to GnRH agonist and 20 unexposed controls were followed to a mean age of 8 years. Four of the antenatally exposed children showed neurological developmental disorders, including attention deficit hyperactivity disorder (three children), motor difficulties (three children), speech disturbances (one child) and epilepsy (one child). The authors suggested a possible toxic effect of GnRH analogs on development (Lahat 1999). More recently, another case of one 7-year-old child with attention deficit hyperactivity disorder exposed to GnRH agonist during pregnancy has been reported (Papanikolau 2005).

The available information concerning children exposed to GnRH antagonist is still rare. In a study carried out on the perinatal outcome of pregnancy in a total of 73 infants born to patients treated with the GnRH antagonist (ganirelix) during ovarian stimulation for *in vitro* fertilization (IVF) or intra-cytoplasmatic sperm injection (ICSI), the incidence of adverse obstetrical and neonatal outcome was comparable with reported incidences for IVF-embryo transfer pregnancies. Only one child was diagnosed with a major congenital malformation – a boy with Beckwith-Wiedemann syndrome (BWS). Five infants had minor anomalies (Olivennes 2001). Nevertheless, it is important to note that an association between imprinting disorder, such as BWS, and assisted reproductive technology (IVF and ICI) is suspected (Chang 2005, Shiota 2005, Maher 2003).

Growth hormone releasing hormone (GHRH)

Synthetic analogs are *sermorelin* and *somatorelin*. These hormones reduce blood flow to the uterus and inhibit endometrial proliferation. For these reasons, they are used preoperatively in treating uterine leiomyomata. In case of inadvertent use during pregnancy, miscarriage and fetal growth restriction are conceivable; however, these effects have not been reported to date.

Somatostatin inhibits the release of both growth hormone and TSH. In this respect, it is unique among the hypothalamic hormones. Therapeutically, it is used for carcinoids and to lower the growth hormone concentration in acromegaly. A synthetic octapeptide derivative of somatostatin, *octreotide*, is available for therapeutic use. In a few individual cases octreotide was used during a part of pregnancy or throughout pregnancy for treatment of acromegaly; no malformations or other adverse effects were reported (Cozzi 2006, Blackhurst 2002, Neal 2000, Takeuchi 1999, Colao 1997). It was reported that ultrasound monitoring of fetal parameters during octreotide long-acting repeatable treatment in a patient suggested the possibility of fetal growth retardation, prompting drug dosage decrease (Fassnacht 2001). However, experience with use of octreotide during pregnancy is insufficient for a well-grounded assessment of the teratogenic potential. There is no experience with exposure during pregnancy with *lanreotide*, an analog of somatostatin or with *pegvisomant*, a somatotropin receptor antagonist.

> **Recommendation.** There are only rare indications for using hypothalamic releasing hormones during pregnancy. Inadvertent use is not grounds for either termination of the pregnancy or invasive diagnostic procedures.

2.15.2   Anterior pituitary hormones

Pharmacology and toxicology

The hormones of the anterior lobe of the pituitary gland regulate hormone released by the peripheral hormone glands. The release of anterior pituitary hormones is controlled by the hypothalamic releasing hormones. Because of their high molecular weight, pituitary hormones do not cross the placenta. Therefore, a direct effect on the fetus is not to be expected. The following hormones are released from the anterior pituitary gland.

Growth hormone (GH, somatropin, STH)

This has effects on somatic growth and on metabolism. A hormone similar structurally and functionally to GH is produced in increasing quantities by the placenta in advanced pregnancy. It is referred to as human placental lactogen (HPL) or, less often, as human chorionic somatomammotropin (HCS). Functionally, this hormone is similar to prolactin.

Prolactin is a polypeptidic hormone whose main role consists of the stimulation of lactation in the postpartum period. A physiological increase in prolactin secretion occurs during pregnancy and lactation, but also in hypothalamic and pituitary diseases. Prolactin has no therapeutic use.

Follicle stimulating hormone (FSH, urofollitrophin, follitrophin-α, follitrophin-β)

This stimulates growth and maturation of the ovarian follicle, and granulosa cell release of estrogen. Luteinizing hormone (LH) stimulates ovulation. During pregnancy, human chorionic gonadotrophin (hCG), which is analogous to LH, is synthesized in the placenta, and is responsible for maintaining the corpus luteum of pregnancy. FSH and a mixture of FSH and LH have been used therapeutically. Human menopause gonadotrophins (hMG) and hCG are two of these mixtures (analogs are *menotropin* and *urogonadotropin*). These hormones are used for ovulation induction and for additional support of the corpus luteum. Inducing ovulation with gonadotrophins can lead to multiple pregnancies; of these, 5–6% involve triplets (Scialli 1986). Two publications report on a rare complex of multiple malformations and four cases of neuroblastoma in infants below 1 year, born of pregnancies involving exposure to gonadotrophins (Mandel 1994, Litwin 1991). These findings were not confirmed in other studies, nor were other pregnancy risks or abnormalities in early childhood and pubertal development associated with use of these agents for ovulation induction.

Thyroid stimulating hormone (thyrotropin, TSH)

This stimulates the synthesis and release of thyroxine.

Adrenocorticotropic hormone (ACTH, tetracosactid)

This stimulates the synthesis and release of the glucocorticoids and mineralocorticoids in the adrenal cortex.

Melatonin is secreted by the pineal gland. Melatonin secretion is regulated on the basis of photic stimuli; in the absence of photic stimuli (at night), melatonin secretion increases. Melatonin coordinates biological rhythms. It also stimulates progesterone secretion, inhibits prostaglandin synthesis, and has (experimentally) a tocolytic effect (Ayar 2001). The human fetal suprachiasmatic nucleus expresses melatonin-binding sites, and is therefore likely to be affected by both endogenous and exogenous melatonin, with consequences for the prenatal and postnatal expression and entrainment of circadian rhythms. The relevance of melatonin to the maintenance of pregnancy at the feto-maternal interface has been investigated, and results suggest that melatonin seems to regulate the human placental function in a paracrine/autocrine manner (Iwasaki 2005). There is insufficient experience with the therapeutic use of melatonin (for instance, for prevention of jetlag after intercontinental flights) in pregnancy.

> **Recommendation.** There are no indications for using anterior pituitary hormones during an already existing pregnancy. Inadvertent use is not grounds for pregnancy termination or for invasive diagnostic procedures.

2.15 Hormones

2.15.3   Prolactin antagonists

Pharmacology and toxicology

Infertility resulting from hyperprolactinemia is reversible after treatment with centrally acting dopamine agonists. Among these, *bromocriptine, cabergoline, lisuride, metergoline*, and *quinagolide* are the more frequently used in the clinic.

In a study of 2587 pregnancies in which *bromocriptine* was administered during the first weeks of pregnancy, there was a slight increase in the rate of early miscarriage but no increase in the rate of birth defects (Krupp 1987). Because most women stop therapy as soon as pregnancy is confirmed, this study also suggests that continuing hyperprolactinemia has no adverse effects on the fetus. A more recent report concerning 27 pregnancies also demonstrated effectiveness and apparent lack of adverse effect of continuing therapy for micro- or macroprolactinoma with bromocriptine or lisuride through early pregnancy. If, during the course of the pregnancy, ophthalmologic problems occur in connection with macroprolactinoma, restarting medication therapy is recommended (Ventz 1996). In individual cases, long-term therapy throughout pregnancy is sometimes indicated.

Cabergoline, which only needs to be taken once or twice a week because of its long-lasting effectiveness, gave no indication of increasing the risk of birth defects in more than 350 pregnancies, which occurred during this therapy. In a few of these pregnancies, treatment was continued throughout pregnancy (de Turris 2003, Ricci 2002, Liu 2001, Verhelst 1999, Ciccarelli 1997, Jones 1997, Robert 1996).

In nine pregnancies, women were treated with *quinagolide* because their prolactinomas were resistant to bromocriptine. No increase in abnormal outcomes was noted; in four cases treatment was continued throughout pregnancy (Morange 1996). The manufacturer is aware of 176 pregnancies in which quinagolide was continued for a median duration of 37 days. No increase was observed in the complication rate during pregnancy, and no indication for an increase in teratogenic risk was reported (Webster 1996).

Based on comparative studies, cabergoline and quinagolide seem to be more effective and better tolerated than bromocriptine in patients with hyperprolactinemia (Barlier 2006, Colao 2000, Schultz 2000, Biller 1999, Webster 1994, van der Heijden 1991).

Documented experience with the use of lisuride and metergoline during pregnancy is insufficient for a risk assessment, although in the scanty published information there is no evidence of risk (Falsetti 1982).

Recommendation. As a result of extensive testing, bromocriptine has been considered the dopamine agonist of choice for hyperprolactinemic amenorrhea. However, presently cabergoline and quinagolide could be considered good treatment options (especially in women with bromocriptine intolerance), given that they seem to be more effective and better tolerated than bromocriptine and have not been associated with any detrimental effect on pregnancy or birth defects. After conception, the medication should, as a rule, be discontinued. However, continuing treatment with it is not grounds for termination of pregnancy or for invasive diagnostic procedures. This recommendation regarding pregnancy exposure also applies to the use of lisuride and metergoline.

2.15.4   Posterior pituitary hormones

Pharmacology and toxicology

Oxytocin and *vasopressin* are released from the neurohypophysis, the posterior lobe of the pituitary. Structurally speaking, these octapeptide hormones are similar to the hypothalamic hormones.

Oxytocin produces contraction of the uterine muscle and the myoepithelial cells in the breast. During pregnancy, it is produced physiologically in increasing amounts; at the same time, it is inactivated by a similarly increased synthesis of the so-called pregnancy oxytocinase. A role for oxytocin in the natural initiation of labor has been suspected but not proven, but oxytocin is used clinically to induce or augment labor. Undesirable effects of administered oxytocin, such as fetal hypoxia, are associated with excessively strong uterine contractions or inadequate uterine relaxation between contractions (see also Chapter 2.14).

Vasopressin influences the transamniotic water transfer from the mother to the fetus. Vasopressin is inactivated by vasopressinase. During pregnancy, subclinical diabetes insipidus may be aggravated as a result of increased levels of placental vasopressinase. Vasopressin deficiency results in diabetes insipidus, for which vasopressin or its analogs have been used as therapy. The peripheral anomalies of the extremities that have been induced by vasopressin in animal experiments (Love 1973, Davies 1970, Jost 1951), apparently caused by vasoconstriction, have not, as yet, been observed in human beings. Among the natural and synthetic analogs are *argipressin, desmopressin* (*DDAVP*), *lypressin, ornipressin,* and *terlipressin. Desmopressin,* which is not inactivated by vasopressinase, has been most frequently described in connection with the treatment of pregnancy-related diabetes insipidus. DDAVP, at therapeutic maternal drug concentration, does not appear to cross the placenta within detectable limits using an *in vitro* human placental model (Ray 2004). The available experience from approximately 50 documented cases exposed to desmopressin is not sufficient for a well-grounded assessment of the teratogenic potential of these synthetic hormones (Brewster 2005, Lacassie 2005, Siristatidis 2004, El-Hennawy 2003, Ray 1998).

Because desmopressin can promote the release of clotting factors, this agent has been used in the management of mild hemophilia, von Willebrand's disease type I, and platelet dysfunction, such as after therapy with acetylsalicylic acid (ASS). It is usually administered only briefly peripartum (Castaman 2006, Gojnic 2005, Perez-Barrero 2003).

> **Recommendation.** Oxytocin may be used obstetrically for the induction or augmentation of labor. Clinically important vasopressin deficiency (diabetes insipidus) justifies the use of vasopressin or desmopressin during pregnancy. Careful control of circulatory and kidney function is essential. Von Willebrand's disease type I and platelet dysfunction can also be indications for the administration of desmopressin. The use of the other vasopressin analogs is not grounds for a termination of pregnancy or for invasive diagnostic procedures.

2.15.5   Thyroid function and iodine supply during pregnancy

During pregnancy, there are hormonal and metabolic changes that require an adaptation of thyroid function. A healthy pregnant woman can easily compensate for this change. The adaptation is an important prerequisite for normal embryonic and fetal development, and also for an uncomplicated pregnancy.

The fetal thyroid begins to function at the end of the third month of pregnancy (Burrow 1994). Before that, the embryo is exclusively dependent on the thyroid supply via the mother.

During pregnancy, the mother's need for *iodine* increases because the thyroid function of the fetus, as well as the mother, is dependent on a sufficient iodine supply.

In regions where iodine is in short supply, sufficient iodine should be assured even before pregnancy. In the case of severe iodine insufficiency, supplementation started after the second trimester may no longer counteract developmental abnormalities of the central nervous system (Xue-Yi 1994). Deficits in intellectual development are apparently correlated with maternal iodine-deficient hypothyroidism (Pharoah 1984).

The daily iodine requirement during pregnancy is 260 μg. When dietary iodine intake via iodized salt, iodized foods, and ocean fish is not reliable, supplementation in tablet form is necessary.

2.15.6 Hypothyroidism, triiodothyronine (T3), and thyroxine (T4)

Pregnant women with *hypothyroidism* have a higher risk of complications (Glinoer 1997), and hypothyroidism during pregnancy can impair the mental development of the child. In particular in relation to iodine deficiency, this has been understood for a long time.

According to a recent study on 60 hypothyroid women (whose disease was only diagnosed after 12 weeks of pregnancy), hypothyroidism impaired the mental and motor capacities of their children, who were tested at the age of 2 years compared to children of euthyroid or only discrete hypothyroid women during pregnancy (Pop 2003). Haddow (1999) draws similar conclusions from his study on 60 children aged 7–9 years. Their mothers only suffered from discrete hypothyroidism during pregnancy. Based on these results, hypofunction of the thyroid should be diagnosed and treated for the benefit of the developing unborn child. Regarding the risk of neonatal hypothyroidism after maternal thyrostatic therapy during pregnancy, see section 2.15.7.

Pharmacology and toxicology

Hormonally effective thyroid hormones are the L-forms of triiodothyronine (T3) and thyroxine (T4), which are only metabolically active in a free, non-protein-bound form. T3 is the biologically effective hormone with a short period of effectiveness, while T4 is a less effective prohormone or hormone depot that is deiodinated as needed to T3. Thyroid hormones are necessary for placental development. Placental transfer of thyroid hormones is limited (Burrow 1994). However, in the case of fetal thyroid agenesis, there is substantial transfer of maternal thyroxine because of the high concentration gradient.

L-thyroxine and *liothyronine* (T3) are available as medications. Correction of maternal thyroid deficiency with these medications is not associated with abnormal fetal outcome. The requirement for thyroid hormones increases during pregnancy. Therefore, hypothyroid women should increase their levothyroxine dose. Thereafter, serum thyrotropin levels should be monitored (Alexander 2004).

> **Recommendation.** When thyroid hormones are indicated, thyroxine preparations should be prescribed because the mother retains control over the actual hormonal activity due to the conversion to triiodothyronine. Iodine should be supplemented as necessary. As soon as pregnancy is confirmed, women with hypothyroidism should increase their levothyroxine dose by approximately 30%. A simple rule is to increase the dose by 25–50 μg at the beginning of pregnancy. During the second trimester a further dose increase is necessary, to an approximately 40–50% higher dose compared to the pre-pregnancy situation. Serum thyrotropin levels should be monitored in order to find the correct individual thyroxine dose. During thyrostatic therapy, thyroid hormones should not be given in addition because the need for placenta-permeable thyrostatics is increased as a result.

2.15.7   Hyperthyroidism and thyrostatics

An uncontrolled hyperthyroidism of a pregnant woman is a risk for the outcome of pregnancy and the fetus: fetal growth retardation, pre-eclampsia, prematurity, and intrauterine death or stillbirths occur more often (Glinoer 1997). In cases of Graves' disease or Hashimoto thyroiditis – the latter usually results in hypothyroidism – the maternal auto-antibodies should be tested at the beginning of pregnancy and early in the third trimester. A high concentration, especially of TSH-receptor antibodies (TRAb), is often correlated with a diaplacental transfer of these antibodies. It is estimated that 1–2% of pregnancies with Graves' disease result in a transient hyperthyroidism of the fetus or newborn, respectively (Carrol 2005). A recently published prospective study on 115 pregnant women reports a much higher rate of 12.6% of fetal/neonatal hyperthyroidism (Rosenfeld 2005).

Pharmacology and toxicology

Propylthiouracil (*PTU*), *carbimazole*, and *thiamazole* (*methimazole*) (an active metabolite of carbimazole) are drugs with antithyroid (thyrostatic) activity. They inhibit the synthesis of T3 and T4 by blocking the organification of iodine and the coupling of iodothyronine residues. All of these agents can reach the fetus.

Propylthiouracil has a higher protein-binding than the other thyrostatic substances, and presumably a lower placental transfer. However, no significant differences in neonatal thyroid function were found by several authors. With maternal daily doses up to 100 mg PTU or up to 10 mg methimazol, 21% and 14% respectively of the neonates had increased values of TSH (not significantly different) (Momotani 1997). In the study by Rosenfeld (2005) mentioned above,

9.5% of *in utero* PTU-exposed children developed hypothyroidism and 5.4% also developed goiter. Not all hypothyroid neonates demonstrated goiter directly after birth; some were noted only at the screening control 2 weeks later.

Individual case descriptions led to the hypothesis that methimazole could cause skin defects (aplasia cutis) in the fetus and other teratogenic effects like choanal atresia, esophagus atresia, tracheal esophageal fistula, hypoplastic nipples, facial dysmorphism, and psychomotoric developmental delay (Nakamura 2005, Barbero 2004, Karg 2004, Ferraris 2003, Karlsson 2002, Clementi 1999, Wilson 1998, Hall 1997, Johnsson 1997, Vogt 1995). Foulds (2005) reviewed all the published cases and concluded that there are 16 reports regarding infants or fetuses exposed to methimazol/thiamazol in first trimester, showing a similar pattern of malformations. He concluded that there exists a rare embryopathy.

However, multiple case collections have indicated neither morphologic developmental disturbances (Wing 1994) nor effects on the size or function of the thyroid or on the physical and intellectual development of children as a result of prenatal exposure to propylthiouracil or methimazole (Eisenstein 1992, Messer 1990). In a prospective multicenter case-control study on the outcome of 204 methimazole-exposed pregnancies, no significant total major malformation rate was reported. However, among the eight reported birth defects, there was one case of choanal atresia and one case of esophagus atresia (di Gianantonio 2001).

To date, thyrostatic drugs during pregnancy do not appear to induce a significant increase in the rate of major malformation. However, methimazole can cause a rare embryopathy with a frequency of 1:1000 to 1:10 000 exposed fetuses (Cooper 2002, Diav-Citrin 2002).

Carefully adjusted thyrostatic therapy with antithyroid medications is unlikely to lead to fetal goiter in pregnancy. Earlier goiter-caused obstructions of the airways and interference with the birth process were described as a result of therapy with thyrostatics, in combination, to some degree, with high levels of iodine or with thyroid hormones.

Perchlorate is indicated only in the rare case of excessive iodine intake. Used in pregnancy, it could impair iodine transfer to the fetus.

Recommendation. Hyperthyroidism has to be treated in pregnancy. Propylthiouracil is the thyrostatic drug of choice in pregnancy, especially in the first trimester. Thiamazole (methimazole) and carbimazole are to be considered second-choice drugs. The dose can be kept to a minimum by maintaining maternal thyroid status a little above normal. Thyrostatic therapy should not be combined with thyroxine supplementation, because this co-therapy increases the mother's thyrostatic needs. Fetal hypothyroidisms as a consequence of maternal antithyroid therapy as well as hyperthyroidism as a consequence of placental transfer of auto-antibodies in case of Graves' disease have been described. Therefore, the thyroid gland of the fetus should be monitored by ultrasound scan. The screening of thyroid parameters of the newborn is absolutely necessary, and this is compulsory in many countries. A second evaluation of the thyroid status should be performed 2 weeks after birth in the case of intrauterine exposure. Mild symptoms of hyperthyroidism with borderline laboratory parameters can be treated symptomatically without thyrostatics, for example with β-receptor blockers such as propranolol or metoprolol. If thiamazole (methimazole) or carbimazole has been used during organogenesis, a detailed anatomical ultrasound examination is recommended. In cases of severe thyrotoxicosis, thyroidectomy may be indicated – even during pregnancy.

For information regarding hyperthyroidism and radioiodine therapy, see Chapter 2.20.

2.15.8   Glucocorticoids

(See also Chapter 2.3.)

Pharmacology

The adrenal cortex synthesizes two classes of steroids: the corticosteroids (glucocorticoids and mineralocorticoids) and the androgens. Corticosteroids act on the carbohydrate, protein, and lipid metabolism; the maintenance of fluid and electrolyte balance; and the preservation of the normal function of the cardiovascular and immune systems, the kidneys, the skeletal muscle, and the endocrine and nervous systems. In addition, corticosteroids allow the organism to resist stressful circumstances such as noxious stimuli and environmental changes. The effects of glucocorticoids are mediated by genomic and non-genomic mechanisms (Czock 2005). Corticosteroids interact with specific receptor proteins in target tissues to regulate the expression of the corticosteroid-responsive genes, modifying the levels of proteins synthesized by these target tissues. The genomic mechanism includes activation of the cytosolic glucocorticoid receptors that lead to activation or repression of protein synthesis, including cytokines, chemokines, inflammatory enzymes, and adhesion molecules, which modify the inflammation and immune response mechanisms (Czock 2005). The therapeutic effects of glucocorticoids are predominantly mediated through the repression of genes encoding inflammatory mediators. However, inhibition of other transcription factors may account for the deleterious effects of glucocorticoids, such as adrenal suppression and osteoporosis (Roumestan 2004). In contrast with these genomic effects, some actions of corticosteroids can be immediate and mediated by membrane-bound receptors (Christ 1999). Pharmacokinetic parameters such as the elimination half-life, and pharmacodynamic parameters like the concentration producing the half-maximal effect, determine the duration and intensity of glucocorticoids' effects.

The corticosteroids are grouped according to their capacity for Na+ retention, their effects on carbohydrate metabolism, and their anti-inflammatory effects. Thus, glucocorticoids have pleiotropic effects and are used in clinical practice in (as well as replacement therapy in cases of adrenal insufficiency) treating diverse diseases such as inflammatory rheumatic disorders, asthma, autoimmune diseases (systemic lupus erythematosus and others), acute kidney transplant rejection, and allergic and skin diseases. In pregnant women at risk for preterm birth, corticosteroids are also used for the induction of lung maturity. High doses of daily glucocorticoids are usually required in patients with severe diseases involving major organs, whereas alternate-day regimens may be used in patients with less aggressive disease. Intravenous glucocorticoids (pulse therapy) are frequently used to initiate therapy in patients with rapidly progressive, inmunologically mediated diseases (Boumpas 1993).

All systemic glucocorticoids cross the placenta to some degree after administration to the mother (Levitz 1978), but the fetal serum concentrations can vary according to the glucocorticoid used. *Betamethasone* and *dexamethasone* cross the placenta well (this is the reason why they have been traditionally used by obstetricians to enhance fetal lung maturation), whereas *prednisone*, *methylprednisolone*, and *prednisolone* appear to cross the placenta only to a small extent, and may for this reason be preferred for the treatment of maternal illness.

Teratogenic effects

The maternal treatment with glucocorticosteroids during the first trimester of pregnancy does not seem to represent a major teratogenic risk in humans. In spite of children with congenital defects being described in several case reports of women treated during the first trimester of pregnancy for a wide variety of maternal diseases, there has been no consistent pattern of defects leading to the suggestion of a causal drug effect. Likewise, some prospective epidemiological studies have been published in which there was no evidence to suggest a significant increased risk of congenital malformations

(Gur 2004, Park-Wyllie 2000). Nevertheless, several epidemiological studies have associated maternal treatment with glucocorticoids with an increased risk of oral clefts (Källén 2003, Pradat 2003, Carmichael 1999, Rodríguez-Pinilla 1998). Moreover, in one prospective negative study the authors include a meta-analysis of the epidemiological studies published so far that concludes that therapeutic doses of corticosteroids in humans increase the risk of oral clefts by an order of 3.4-fold, which is consistent with existing animal studies (Park-Wyllie 2000).

The association between glucocorticoids and oral clefts has also been discussed following maternal use of topical corticosteroid during pregnancy (Edwards 2003, Czeizel 1997), although Czeizel discounted this finding because the mothers stopped the medication after the first month of gestation. The results of Edwards (2003) should be interpreted with caution because, although statistically significant, the confidence interval was extremely wide (1.67–586!) due to the small sample size.

Regarding the use of inhaled glucocorticoids (e.g. *budesonide* or *beclomethasone*) in pregnant women who have asthma or other allergic process (such a rhinitis), the available data show no evidence of an apparent fetal risk (Demoly 2003, Källén 1999; see also Chapter 2.3).

Thus, taking into consideration the existing data, it is reasonable to conclude that there is no evidence of a significant increase in the basal risk for congenital anomalies, although a possible association with clefts cannot be excluded.

Fetal toxicity

There is still concern regarding intrauterine glucocorticoid exposure as the origin of some adult diseases. Conditions that are suspected of having been programmed before birth include hypertension, diabetes, coronary heart disease, and stroke (Rennick 2006, Newnham 2001, Challis 1999). Thus, the long-term effects of fetal glucocorticoids (especially dexamethasone) in humans are unclear, and whether they have a role in programming the individual for adult degenerative diseases remains to be studied.

Some clinical studies have suggested a possible relationship between antenatal exposure to prednisone and other corticosteroids as a treatment for maternal diseases, and an increased incidence of fetal growth restriction. Nevertheless, the effect of the corticosteroids in these cases of intrauterine growth retardation is uncertain, and the underlying maternal disease (often autoimmunity diseases, renal transplantation, asthma) as well as the concomitance medications (such as immunosuppressant drugs) could be playing a predominant role.

Depending on dose and the treatment interval, adrenal cortical insufficiency in the newborn babies may occur.

2

Pregnancy

Fetal effects of betamethasone or dexamethasone for induction of lung maturity

The administration, between 24 and 34 weeks' gestation, of *betamethasone* (12 mg i.m. every 24 hours for two doses) or *dexamethasone* (6 mg i.m. every 12 hours for four doses) is a well-established intervention to promote fetal lung maturation and prevent neonatal respiratory distress syndrome, neonatal mortality, and ventricular hemorrhage. Antenatal exposure to betamethasone but not dexamethasone has been associated with a decreased risk of cystic periventricular leukomalacia among very premature infants (Baud 1999).

Nevertheless, multiple works have been published showing adverse effects on the fetus after the administration of two or more complete courses, such as decreased fetal growth (Thorp 2002), reduction in birth head circumference (Thorp 2002), transient hypertrophic cardiomyopathy (Yunis 1999), increased mortality (Banks 1999), prolonged adrenal suppression, increased risk of early-onset neonatal sepsis, and increased perinatal mortality. Also, adverse effects have been described in the pregnant woman exposed to multiple courses, such as a higher incidence of postpartum endometritis (Abbasi 2000).

Recently, a work has been published which analyzed a sample of 29 557 singleton live-born infants without congenital defects to study the effects on fetal growth of antenatal corticosteroid treatment used to promote fetal lung maturation (Rodríguez-Pinilla 2006). In this work, and controlling for potential confounder factors (year of birth, maternal age, gestational age, parity, maternal smoking and/or alcohol consumption, gestational diabetes, non-gestational diabetes, and other maternal chronic diseases), the exposure to more than one course of antenatal corticosteroids resulted in a significant reduction in birth weight, length, and head circumference in singleton preterm infants. The birth weight decreased by 22% ($p < 0.0001$), the length by 5% ($p = 0.002$), and the head circumference by 6% ($p = 0.0005$). Exposure to just one course of antenatal corticosteroids also significantly reduced the weight (by 17%; $p < 0.0001$) and the length (by 5%; $p = 0.0001$), but not the head circumference. This correlation between the administered dose and the weight of the newborn children had been previously proven in animal experiments (Ikegami 1997). In addition, the significant interaction found between the treatment and the gestational age at birth indicated that the effect of corticosteroids is enhanced in the most premature babies (Rodriguez-Pinilla 2006).

It is important to note the potential negative repercussions on the programming of the developing CNS of antenatal exposure to

2.15 Hormones

dexa/betamethasone. This has been demonstrated by comparing magnetic resonance indices of brain maturation in infants exposed to repeat antenatal glucocorticoid (GC) therapy and born at or close to term, with non-GC exposed control infants. GC-exposed infants had a significantly lower whole cortex convolution index (a measure of the complexity of cortical folding) and smaller surface area (Modi 2001). Nevertheless, at present there is no conclusive information to prove a significant decrease in the head circumference after the exposure to a single course of GC (Rodríguez-Pinilla 2006). Also, exposure to a single course has not been associated with later obvious adverse effects on growth, intellectual and motor development, school achievement, social-emotional functioning, and lung function in the 10–14-year-olds studied (Doyle 2000, Schmand 1990). Dalziel (2005) followed up, at age 30 years, 534 individuals whose mothers had participated in a double-blind, placebo-controlled, randomized trial of antenatal betamethasone for the prevention of neonatal respiratory distress syndrome. There were no differences between the two groups in body size, blood lipids, blood pressure, plasma cortisol, prevalence of diabetes, or history of cardiovascular disease. Only after a glucose tolerance test were the prenatally betamethasone-exposed identified as having higher plasma insulin concentrations. These facts, together with the evidence that the administration of a single course is effective to prevent the neonatal respiratory distress syndrome, justify its administration in the pregnant woman at risk of preterm delivery. Nevertheless, a recently published randomized controlled trial supported the use of repeat doses of corticosteroids (betamethasone), 7 or more days after the initial course, in women who remain at risk of very preterm birth (Crowther 2006). Beyond the thirty-fourth week of pregnancy, support of lung maturation is usually not necessary.

On the other hand, placebo-controlled studies with mice exposed to corticosteroids during pregnancy have shown that betamethasone has less detrimental effects than does dexamethasone on the neurobehavioral development of the offspring, and is more potent in accelerating fetal lung maturity (Christensen 1997, Rayburn 1997). These experimental results, together with clinical studies in premature infants, suggest that betamethasone must be the preferred corticosteroid for use in women at risk of preterm delivery (Groneck 2001, Baud 1999).

Recommendation. Replacement therapy can and should be conducted throughout pregnancy.

In maternal inflammatory diseases, the benefits of glucocorticoid therapy on the maternal health can be offset by the low risk to the fetus, as long as there is a sufficient indication for maternal treatment and no safer alternative is available. Beyond its use during the first trimester, a high-resolution echocardiography could be recommended, especially for the diagnosis of oral clefts.

In maternal asthma and allergic diseases, pregnancy is not considered to be a contraindication for the continuation of corticosteroids therapy. Severe asthma may compromise maternal and/or fetal oxygenation. Therefore, risk–benefit consideration still favors the use of oral or inhaled corticosteroids during pregnancy when indicated for the treatment for asthma.

In pregnant women at risk of preterm delivery, single course of GC treatment before preterm delivery is recommended until week 34. The use of betamethasone for this indication may be of advantage compared to dexamethasone.

For adrenal medulla hormones, see Chapter 2.3.

2.15.9   Diabetes mellitus and pregnancy

Diabetes mellitus is the collective name for heterogeneous disturbances of metabolism which all are characterized by chronic hyperglycemia. In essence, there are three different types. While type I is caused by a disturbed secretion of insulin, type II and gestational diabetes are characterized by a disturbed action of insulin. Both causes can also occur simultaneously.

A poor glycemic control in pregestational diabetes, as measured by glycosylated hemoglobin (HbA1c > 6.5%), is correlated with an increased risk of major congenital malformations. HbA1c is a parameter for the blood glucose concentration of the last 120 days, the survival time of erythrocytes; it can also be referred to as the "blood sugar memory". The higher the concentration of HbA1c, the higher the statistically confirmed rate of malformations: an HbA1c of 8.5% is correlated with a malformation rate of 4%; an HbA1c of 10.5% has a risk for abnormalities of 6%. The most common birth defects are anomalies of the spine and extremities, of the heart and circulatory system, and neural tube defects. Urogenital defects, gastrointestinal fistulas, and atresias are seen more seldom (for an overview, see Briggs 2005, Loffredo 2001).

During pregnancy, women with all types of diabetes, as well as their infants, are at increased risk for a number of different complications: the miscarriage rate is increased, the perinatal morbidity is above average, and the rate of prematurity is almost 20% (Arbeitsgemeinschaft 2004, Gamson 2004). Characteristics of neonatal morbidity include macrosomia (an extremely large newborn) with immature organ functions or hypotrophy, and postpartum metabolic derangements of the newborn – especially hypoglycemia.

Pre-existing diabetes may be associated with vascular disease, leading to uteroplacental insufficiency and hypertensive disorders, resulting, for example, in pre-eclampsia.

The vast majority of type II or gestational diabetes occurs within the bounds of metabolic syndrome X (obesity, hyperlipidemia, hypertension, impaired glucose tolerance). In the beginning, there is insulin resistance of the insulin-dependent tissues. Therefore, an elevated insulin concentration is necessary for utilization of glucose. Hyperinsulinemia again intensifies the feeling of being hungry, which results in eating more and more, which leads to further weight gain, and so on – a vicious circle. Weight reduction results in lower insulin levels, and an increasing sensibility and amount of insulin receptors. Ideally, a body mass index of 27 kg/m^2 and below should be achieved prior to pregnancy! Regarding the risk of pre-existing obesity for a pregnancy, see Chapter 2.5.

Achieving and maintaining euglycemia throughout gestation is the aim of diabetes therapy, because diabetic fetopathy appears to be due to fetal hyperglycemia and hyperinsulinemia, secondary to maternal hyperglycemia. Fetal hyperinsulinemia leads to hyperplasia and hypertrophy of islet cells, and increases the risk of respiratory distress syndrome (RDS). Children of mothers with insufficient blood sugar control during pregnancy have an increased risk of becoming obese during puberty or in early adulthood, or of developing diabetes or an imbalanced glucose tolerance.

Being overweight and gestational diabetes are steadily increasing in industrial countries: it is estimated that approximately 20% of pregnancies in overweight women are complicated by gestational diabetes. Therefore, the recommendation is to have a glucose tolerance test at least once in every pregnancy.

Insulin action changes during the course of pregnancy. At 10–14 weeks' gestation, insulin sensitivity is slightly increased; however, it then declines for the rest of the pregnancy, with insulin resistance being highest late in the third trimester. Insulin sensitivity rebounds with the delivery of the placenta. In cases of pre-existing diabetes, these changes contribute to a degree of hypoglycemia in the first trimester and increased insulin requirements during later pregnancy, and reinstitution of the pre-pregnancy insulin requirement after delivery.

Recommendation. Maintaining euglycemia throughout pregnancy is the best prerequisite for an uncomplicated course of pre- and postnatal development of the child, and for minimal maternal morbidity. This aim should ideally be achieved prior to pregnancy. Pregnant women with diabetes – no matter what type – should consult a specialist, if possible, and deliver in a perinatal center. All pregnant women should be screened for a diabetic metabolic disorder, especially if they are obese. An anatomical ultrasound and α-fetoprotein screening should be considered, especially for patients who are not euglycemic.

2.15.10   Insulin

Pharmacology and toxicology

The endocrine part of the pancreas produces and secretes insulin, glucagons, and somatostatin. Insulin is necessary for storage of metabolic substrates such as glucose, fatty acids, and amino acids. Glucagon is important for the reverse regulation in hypoglycemia.

Human insulin does not cross the placenta, contrary to oral antidiabetic drugs. An intensified insulin dose regimen with at least three daily injections of regular insulin preprandially, perhaps added by an intermediate insulin dose at night-time, improves pregnancy outcome.

Extensive experience with human insulin substitution therapy in pregnancy does not indicate any embryotoxic potential.

In order to be used during pregnancy, ideally insulin or insulin analogs should mimic natural pancreatic insulin secretion; improve maternal glycemic control, be non-immunogenic, not cross the placenta; not increase the risk for maternal-fetal morbidity, and have minimal IGF-I- activity, thus not aggravating pre-existing diabetic retinopathy. Usually the therapy of diabetic pregnant women is with regular human insulin or delayed insulin.

The development of rapid-acting insulin analogs designed to control meal-related glycemic excursions began in 1996, first with the release of *insulin lispro*, followed by *insulin aspart* and *insulin glulisin*. Long-acting insulin analogs are *insulin glargine* and *insulin detemir*.

Among insulin analogs, there is most information regarding the use of *insulin lispro* during pregnancy. There are small retrospective and prospective studies with approximately 500 exposed pregnancies (Wyatt 2005, Cypryk 2004, Garg 2003, Masson 2003, Person 2002, Scherbaum 2002, Bhattacharyya 2001). To date, there has been no increased rate of congenital malformations when using insulin lispro; achievement of glucose control is comparable to that with human insulin, and the serum glucose concentration 1 hour postprandially is even lower on insulin lispro (Mecacci 2003). However, it cannot be concluded that the outcome of newborns of mothers who were on insulin lispro during pregnancy is favorable compared to those on

2.15 Hormones

2 Pregnancy

human insulin. A Dutch study involving 289 pregnant women with diabetes mellitus type I analyzed their offspring and compared two groups; infants with normal birth weight, and macrosomic newborns. Mothers of macrosomic infants took insulin lispro in 15% and regular human insulin in 8% of cases, a difference which is significant (Evers 2002). Aggravation of retinopathy during pregnancy on insulin lispro has not been reported yet, but experience is still limited (Loukovaara 2003, Buchbinder 2000). Gamson (2004) describes immunogenic effects as being comparably low on human insulin and on insulin lispro.

There is less information on the use of *insulin aspart* during pregnancy. A multinational European study compared the maternal and fetal complications of type I diabetic pregnant women on regular insulin (Actrapid®) ($n = 165$) and on insulin aspart ($n = 157$). Similar numbers of live births, fetal losses, and congenital anomalies were reported in both groups, as well as similar rates of neonatal hypoglycemia and infant birth characteristics. Overall glycemic control was similar, as well as the maternal and obstetric complications during pregnancy (Hod 2006).

The other insulin analogs, insulin glulisin, insulin detemir, and insulin glargine, have rarely been used in pregnancies to date. The long-acting *insulin glargine* might worsen a retinopathy (overview see Gamson 2004), as indicated in case reports. Therefore, the long-acting insulin analogs should not be used during pregnancy, or the mother should be switched to regular insulin as soon as pregnancy is confirmed. A few case reports regarding the use of insulin glargine during embryogenesis or throughout pregnancy have not shown adverse fetal effects (al Shaikh 2006, di Cianni 2005, Woolderink 2005, Holstein 2003). Single cases have reported severe hypoglycemia at night on regular insulin, which no longer occurred after a change of therapy to insulin glargine (Devlin 2002).

The rapid-acting inhaled insulin *pramlintid* is currently under investigation.

Recommendation. A type I diabetic woman should have good glycemic control before becoming pregnant. The drug of choice is regular insulin. If there is excellent glycemic control on insulin lispro, it is not compulsory to change to regular insulin if the patient is pregnant. Long-acting insulin analogs should be avoided during pregnancy.

Pregnant women with type II diabetes or gestational diabetes should have regular insulin, if diet alone is insufficient for control. If blood sugar levels are only at a critical threshold and if there is accompanying fetal macrosomia, therapy with insulin should be initiated.

Insulin of animal origin is contraindicated during pregnancy. The insulin requirements in pregnant women on insulin can increase. As well as serum glucose levels and HbA1c values, which are vital for control, ultrasound biometry of the growing fetus should be performed. Because glucocorticoids and some tocolytic medications decrease the mother's carbohydrate tolerance, the monitoring of metabolic factors is recommended when these medications are used.

2.15.11 Oral antidiabetics

Oral antidiabetics are not hormones and do not work in the way that insulin does; they are not substitutes. The most commonly used sulfonylurea derivatives merely stimulate those β-cells in the pancreas that still have the ability to function. Among these medications are the second-generation sulfonylureas *glibenclamide* (*glyburide*), *glibornuride*, *gliclazide*, *glimepiride*, *glipizide*, *gliquidone*, and *glisoxepide*. First-generation sulfonylureas are *acetohexamide*, *chlorpropamide*, *tolazamide*, and *tolbutamide*.

In contrast, the biguanide derivatives, *metformin* and *phenformin*, decrease glucose synthesis in the liver, delay glucose resorption from the gut, and increase glucose utilization in the muscular system.

Acarbose and *miglitol*, as glucosidase inhibitors, inhibit carbohydrate absorption in the intestine – a controversial therapy for diabetes. *Nateglinide* and *repaglinide* regulate postprandial blood sugar by a short increase in insulin secretion from the β-cells. *Pioglitazone* and *rosiglitazone* increase the sensitivity to insulin. *Muraglitazar* belongs to the same group, but results of studies have shown an increased risk for serious cardiovascular adverse effects, so there is no approval by the FDA for the USA. *Sitagliptin* and *vildagliptin* mimic incretin hormones, which naturally work in the gut and increase insulin production, dependent on meal supply. In diabetics, less incretin hormones than normal are produced. Both substances are still being tested in clinical trials.

These drugs have in common the fact that there is no evidence so far of effective prevention of diabetic late complications. Insulin, metformin, and sulfonylureas are the only antidiabetic substances where evidence-based data have shown positive effects on the late diabetic complications, such as neuropathy, nephropathy, etc., or coronary sclerosis and others.

Because oral antidiabetics have not been shown to regulate blood sugar as reliably as insulin, they are not considered suitable for treating diabetes during pregnancy. Studies on use during pregnancy only exist for glyburide and metformin.

▶ **Glyburide/glibenclamide**

Hypoglycemia of the newborn may be noted if treatment has been continued until delivery. In older studies, an increased risk for congenital malformations was described (Piacquadio 1991), which at first was taken as a suggestion that oral antidiabetics might have a teratogenic risk (Towner 1995). Currently, the results are interpreted differently: other studies did not confirm such an association, but stated that inadequately treated hyperglycemia and associated metabolic disruption lead to an increase in birth defects (Gutzin 2001). More recently published case reports do not report an increased rate of malformations, but they do not allow a differentiated risk assessment either. Therefore, substance-specific differences in placental permeability (e.g. tolbutamide is more placenta permeable than glipizide) are of less relevance. Recently published results of perfusion studies examine why the transplacental transfer of glyburide is low, and what might influence it (Kraemer 2006, Nanovskaya 2006).

Randomized studies have compared several hundred women with gestational diabetes on glyburide to those on insulin therapy, and have not found any differences concerning the course of pregnancy and the well-being of the newborns. Therapy was started after embryogenesis. Glyburide was not detected in umbilical cord blood samples, and there was no significant difference concerning the number of hypoglycemic newborn infants or birth weight (Jacobson 2005, Langer 2005, Kremer 2004). Jacobson (2005) reported an increased need for neonatal phototherapy and a higher rate of pre-eclampsia on glyburide. This latter finding is of particular concern in light of recent findings by Crowther (2005) that pre-eclampsia is more prevalent among patients with untreated gestational diabetes. It is doubtful whether the positive results are yet sufficient to question the current recommendation, regarding therapy of gestational diabetes, in favor of insulin (Rand 2006, Greene 2000).

▶ **Metformin**

In contrast to glibenclamide, metformin does not stimulate insulin secretion and thus does not lead to hypoglycemia of the pregnant woman or newborn. In overweight patients, diabetic therapy with metformin, which raises insulin sensitivity and decreases the insulin requirement, is more logical than therapy with glyburide.

Metformin is not only indicated for diabetes type II, but also for women with polycystic ovary syndrome (PCOS) in order to improve poor conception rates and decrease high pregnancy loss rates during first trimester. Gestational diabetes is also a frequent symptom of PCOS, which might be another indication for metformin. No teratogenic risk was reported in a study on 179 retrospectively ascertained pregnancies (Thatcher 2006) and in a case series of 50 pregnancies (Turner 2006). A meta-analysis of eight studies (five with retrospective and three with prospective data collection) published until 2004, and including 172 pregnancies, arrived at the same result (Gilbert 2006). A retrospective case-control study compared the neonatal outcome of 33 women with PCOS, treated with metformin in the first trimester, with 66 normal healthy women. There was a slight but statistically significant lower mean birth weight in the former (Kovo 2006). Some studies reported a decrease in the rate of miscarriage in women with PCOS on metformin (Thatcher 2006, Palomba 2005, Jakubowicz 2002). There is a debate concerning the duration of therapy in cases of PCOS: how long should metformin be maintained in order to "stabilize a pregnancy"? There is no evidence that therapy after gestational weeks 6–8 is correlated with a better pregnancy outcome. Glueck (2004), who has collected data on 126 intrauterine metformin-exposed infants of mothers with PCOS (of whom some are included in the above-mentioned meta-analysis), postulated that metformin, if taken throughout pregnancy, has a preventive effect concerning the occurrence of gestational diabetes, but this could not be confirmed by a randomized prospective study (Vanky 2004). The results from a recent study indicate that metformin freely passes the placenta and that the fetus is exposed to therapeutic concentrations, but it does not seem to influence pH levels in umbilical artery blood (Vanky 2005). Further research is necessary.

There are only a few case reports concerning the use of *rosiglitazone* and *acarbose* in pregnancy (Kalyoncu 2005, Yaris 2004). No data are available concerning the other oral antidiabetics.

Recommendation. As in type I diabetes, type II diabetics should be controlled with insulin therapy before a planned pregnancy. Nevertheless, when therapy with oral antidiabetics has been carried out during pregnancy, this is not an indication to terminate the pregnancy. A detailed ultrasound examination to verify normal morphologic development of the fetus is recommended. Whether the sulfonylureas glyburide (glibenclamide) or metformin are alternatives for insulin in gestational diabetes after the first trimester should be evaluated with reserve. Regular insulin is still the substance of choice. If metformin was taken to stabilize a pregnancy in cases of PCOS, therapy should be stopped by gestational weeks 6–8.

2.15.12 Estrogens

Pharmacology and toxicology

It is only during pregnancy that, in addition to estrone and estradiol, estriol (which otherwise only appears as a metabolite) and estetrol are synthesized to a large extent.

Physiologically as well as pharmacologically, estrogens act as a stimulus to uterine and fallopian tube growth and, most particularly, to the growth of the endometrium. In addition, estrogens produce thickening of the vaginal epithelium, an increase in cervical mucus production, and widening of the cervical canal. The earlier (sometimes routine) use of estrogens to improve contractions has been superseded by more effective pharmaceuticals.

Therapeutically, estrogens are used in oral contraceptives, as replacement therapy during the menopause, and for treatment of some malignancies. Among the available substances are estradiol and its derivatives, *ethinylestradiol* (the estrogen in most of the estrogen-containing birth control pills), *mestranol*, *estrone*, *conjugated equine estrogens*, *polyestradiol*, *estriol*, *fosfestrole*, *chlorotrianisen*, and *epimestrol*.

The relatively low-dosage preparations for hormonal contraception (preparations of combined estrogen and gestagen), including emergency contraception (the "morning-after pill"), have been quite well-studied because of their frequent accidental use during pregnancy. They do not involve detectable risk as far as is known today (Ahn 2005, Raman-Wilms 1995, Källén 1991, Harlap 1985A), and do not produce disturbances of gender differentiation when treatment is given during the sensitive phase from the eighth week of pregnancy. However, it should be mentioned that after the early reported association (based on case reports from the 1970s) between use of hormonal medications and heart defects, VACTERL (or VATER) syndrome, etc., newer publications citing increased rates of (urinary tract) anomalies have appeared (see Li 1995).

Several studies have analyzed the relationship between oral contraceptives and Down syndrome, some of them with negative results (Källén 1989, Harlap 1985B, Ericson 1983), but others have suggested that women who take oral contraceptives during the month just before conception (Mikkelsen 1991) or who fall pregnant following oral contraceptive failure (Harlap 1980) have an increased risk for Down syndrome. A more recent case-control study has demonstrated an increased risk of 2.8-fold for infants with Down syndrome in women younger than 35 years of age if the mother became pregnant while she was taking oral contraceptives (Martínez-Frias 2001).

The effects on later fertility have been hypothesized but not confirmed by controlled studies. An older publication reported deviant

2

psychosexual development in boys whose diabetic mothers were treated with estradiol and progesterone (Yalom 1973). There are no indications that these developmental disturbances occur in connection with currently used estrogenic medications. Likewise, there is no strong epidemiological evidence to indicate that prenatal exposure to estrogens increases the risk to abnormal development of the male reproductive organs (Storgaard 2006).

There is insufficient experience with high-dosage use of estrogen in, for example, malignancies. Experimental animal studies suggest that high doses of many different estrogens can produce histologic changes in the genital tract of the offspring similar to those after exposure to diethylstilbestrol. A human estrogen-exposure syndrome analogous to that occurring after diethylstilbestrol has not been described with regard to other estrogens.

Recommendation. During pregnancy there is no indication for estrogen treatment. The (accidental) use of oral contraceptives in early pregnancy does not require either a termination of the pregnancy or additional diagnostic studies. This statement also applies to emergency contraception (the "morning-after pill") and amenorrhea treatment with ethinylestradiol and norethisterone acetate (see progestins) or other oral contraceptive preparations. The accidental administration of high-dose preparations for other indications has no risk-based reason for a termination of pregnancy either. In cases of repeated high-dose administration, at least, a detailed ultrasound examination could verify a normal morphologic development of the fetus.

2.15.13 Progestins (gestagens)

Pharmacology and toxicology

Progesterone is manufactured by the theca and lutein cells in the ovary; during pregnancy, it is also produced in larger quantities by the placenta. Progesterone is metabolized by the fetus and placenta. The placenta is able to oxidize individual metabolites enzymatically to progesterone again. Progesterone is excreted as pregnandiol and decomposed in part to pregnantriol. Although progesterone is available as a pharmaceutical preparation, it is not well-absorbed orally. Alteration of the progesterone molecule produces progestins such as *medroxyprogesterone acetate*, which are better absorbed but differ from progesterone in some of their pharmacologic activities. Progestins are also obtained from modification of testosterone, with removal of one carbon to decrease the androgenicity of these preparations.

The following substances are available as pharmaceuticals: *chlormadinon, desogestrel, drospirenon, dydrogestone, ethynodiol diacetate, gestonorone, gestodene, hydroxyprogesterone, levonorgestrel, lynestrenol, medrogestone, medroxyprogesterone, megestrol, norethisterone (norethindrone)* and its acetate, *norethynodrel, norgestimate,* and *norgestrel.*

For about 40 years, progesterone and its partially or completely synthesized derivatives (i.e. *17-hydroxyprogesterone*) have been used to treat threatened or habitual miscarriage, although there is still no proof of the effectiveness of this therapy. A WHO Symposium on Drug Treatment during Pregnancy established the ineffectiveness of this sort of therapeutic effort, which was widespread in Germany, France and Italy, but not in Scandinavia (WHO Report 1984). The only indication for hormonal prevention of miscarriage which is currently discussed is hCG therapy for the rare corpus luteum insufficiency. However, therapy with progestins continues to be recommended, nowadays mostly with natural progesterone. In addition, it is common to use a progestin to support corpus luteum function after *in vitro* fertilization and embryo transfer.

Recently, randomized controlled trials have shown that treatment with progesterone started in the second trimester of pregnancy reduces the risk of delivery before 37 weeks' gestation, among pregnant women at increased risk of spontaneous preterm birth. However, as the authors of a recent meta-analysis emphasize, the effect on neonatal morbidity is still uncertain (Mackenzie 2006).

A possible association between hormone therapy and hypospadias has been previously debated (Källén 1992). More recently, a statistically significant risk for hypospadias in the newborn of mothers exposed to progestins for the purpose of becoming pregnant or preventing pregnancy loss (from 4 weeks before conception until the end of the first trimester) has been observed in a retrospective case-control study (OR = 3.7; CI 2.3–6.0), whereas progestin intake for the purpose of oral contraception was not associated with an increased risk for hypospadias (Carmichael 2005). Wogelius (2006) could not confirm this association with a case-control study on oral contraceptive use during early pregnancy. Nevertheless, more controlled studies are necessary to conclude a relationship between progestins and hypospadias. There are no epidemiological studies that support a significant relationship between progestational drugs and congenital malformations (Brent 2005, Martínez-Frias 1998).

Disturbances of gender differentiation have not been observed with use of progestins in contraceptive doses when given during the sensitive phase from the eighth week of pregnancy. However, when higher doses of the 19-nor-ethinyl-testosterone derived progestins are used in this sensitive phase, a transient clitoris hypertrophy may occur due to the androgenic properties of these agents. Effects on later fertility have been hypothesized but not confirmed by controlled studies. An older publication reported deviant psychosexual development in children whose diabetic mothers were treated with estradiol and progesterone or high-dosage norethisterone derivatives (e.g. Yalom 1973). There are no indications that these developmental disturbances occur in connection with currently-used progestin medications. Development through adolescence appears age-appropriate according to large long-term studies on medroxyprogesterone-depot preparations (Pardthaisong 1992).

The use of emergency contraception (postcoital contraception, the "morning-after pill") is presently increasing, especially the new regimen consisting of only levonorgestrel. To date, there appears to be no increased risk for congenital birth defects among pill users who become pregnant; however, the suspicion exists for a potential risk for ectopic pregnancy following emergency levonorgestrel contraception (Basu 2005, Gainer 2004, Harrison-Woolrych 2003, Fabunmi 2002). Nevertheless, the risk for ectopic pregnancy would probably be very small.

There is insufficient documented experience with administration of high-dose progestins, such as used in therapy for malignancies, in pregnancy.

Tibolone is a progestin-like agent that has been used with or without estrogen for the treatment of menopausal symptoms. There is no information concerning pregnancy outcome after exposure to this agent, which is used in postmenopausal women.

Recommendation. During pregnancy, there is no valid indication for the therapy with progestins. Use of progestins to prevent miscarriage is not indicated. Contraceptives taken by accident in early pregnancy are not grounds for termination of pregnancy or for additional diagnostic procedures. This statement applies to the contraceptive preparations that are in use today and to emergency contraception (the "morning-after pill") as well as to treatment for amenorrhea with norethisterone acetate and ethinylestradiol, or other oral contraceptive preparations, or miscarriage prophylaxis with progesterone derivatives. Since emergency contraception is not 100% effective, pill users should be warned about the small risk of ectopic pregnancy in cases of method failure. The accidental administration of high-dose preparations for other indications has no risk-based reason for a termination of pregnancy either. A detailed ultrasound examination could verify a normal morphologic development of the fetus.

2.15.14   Diethylstilbestrol

Pharmacology and toxicology

Diethylstilbestrol (DES) is a synthetic nonsteroidal estrogenic drug that was used therapeutically in the USA in the 1970s for threatened miscarriage and for maternal diabetes mellitus. The discovery of increased rates of vaginal clear-cell adenocarcinoma in adolescence among daughters whose mothers had received DES during pregnancy produced an international sensation (Herbst 1975). This drug provides the only proven example in human beings of prenatally-caused cancer (transplacental carcinogenesis). At least 25% of those young women who had prenatal exposure in the first trimester were born with vaginal, uterine, or fallopian tube anomalies. With male offspring, there appears to be an increased risk for cryptorchidism, testicular hypoplasia, and abnormal semen cell morphology (Bibbo 1981).

Recently, the possibility of a transgenerational effect of DES has been under discussion. Some studies have found an increased risk of hypospadias in the sons of women exposed to DES *in utero* (Pons 2005, Klip 2002), but the results of an ongoing study of DES-exposed persons, with data from 3916 exposed and 1746 unexposed women, do not support this potential transgenerational effect (Palmer 2005). Likewise, following intrauterine exposure to DES there have been three cases of newborns with limb-reduction defects reported, and two cases with deafness in the second generation after intrauterine exposure to DES (Stoll 2003). Several mechanisms could be involved in this possible transgenerational effect, such as a genotoxic effect of DES upon the germ cells, or imprinting, or genetic or epigenetic changes in the primordial oocytes, among others. Nevertheless, more studies should be conducted to confirm this potential effect.

> **Recommendation.** Diethylstilbestrol use during pregnancy is contraindicated.

2.15.15   Androgens and anabolics

Pharmacology and toxicology

Among the androgens available in drug form are *mesterolone*, *testolactone*, and *testosterone*. There is no indication for using this class of drugs during pregnancy. All of the earlier common reasons (i.e. psychosexual) for giving androgens to premenopausal women are considered outdated. Use of androgens to inhibit lactation also reflects outmoded practice.

Among anabolics on the market are *closterol, metenolone*, and *nandrolone*. There is no indication for treatment with this class of drugs during pregnancy. However, imported "black market" preparations used in connection with sports involving strength have been continued "accidentally" during pregnancy. Practical experience in human pregnancy with these agents is insufficient for a differentiated risk assessment, also with regard to masculinization.

> **Recommendation.** Androgens and anabolics are absolutely contraindicated in pregnancy. However, accidental use does not require a risk-based termination of the pregnancy. After repeated exposure, a detailed ultrasound examination is recommended to verify a normal morphologic development of the fetus.

2.15.16   Antiestrogens, antiandrogens, and danazol

Pharmacology and toxicology

Bicalutamide, cyproterone, and *flutamide* belong to the group of antiandrogens. *Aminoglutethimide, anastrozole, formestan, raloxifene,* and *tamoxifen* are antiestrogen drugs. *Danazol* is a gonadotropin inhibitor with androgenic activity. (For aminoglutethimide and tamoxifen, see Chapter 2.13.)

Cyproterone acetate is the antiandrogen most commonly used during the reproductive years. It is available in combination with *ethinylestradiol*. This preparation is frequently prescribed as "the pill", especially when acne is also present. The German Institute for Drugs and Medical Products restricted the therapeutic usage of this preparation because it was suspected of causing liver tumors. It may only be prescribed for symptoms of androgenization and acne with scarring.

The antiandrogenous effect of cyproterone acetate could potentially lead to the feminization of male fetuses. To date this effect has not been observed, even in the case of accidental continuation of 2 mg daily treatment during the sensitive phase from the eighth week of pregnancy (Bye 1986, Statham 1985). The manufacturer reported 44 human male fetuses unintentionally exposed to cyproterone during pregnancy. Of these, 38 were exposed during part of genital organogenesis, and 23 throughout genital organogenesis, to 2 mg/d; 5 were exposed to high doses (25–100 mg/d) during genital organogenesis. In all cases, normal boys were born (Jahn 1996). There is no indication of teratogenic effects in human beings as yet with this medication (unpublished experiences of the European Network of Teratology Information Services); however, the number of evaluated pregnancy outcomes is insufficient for a profound risk evaluation.

Danazol, a synthetically modified androgen, is derived from *ethisterone* and is also classified as an antiestrogen. Danazol is used in treating endometriosis, mastalgia, and hereditary angioneurotic edema, and was in the past used as a contraceptive. Publications on over 100 women exposed in pregnancy have revealed a risk of masculinization in female fetuses, at least when the mothers were treated with 200 mg or more daily and after the eighth week of pregnancy (when the androgen receptors begin to function) (Kingsbury 1985, Rosa 1984). Despite normal internal genitalia, over 50% of the girls exposed prenatally had, to some extent, an enlarged clitoris or a fully developed female pseudohermaphroditism. In as much as later development was observed, there was nothing further of note with respect to virilization or sexual behavior (Money 1982). The increased rate of spontaneous abortion associated with danazol could also have been caused by the endometriosis – the indication for therapy itself.

There is no experience with exposure during pregnancy to the other antiandrogens and antiestrogens mentioned in this chapter; this makes a differentiated risk assessment impossible.

> **Recommendation.** Antiestrogens, antiandrogens, and danazol are absolutely contraindicated in pregnancy. Accidental use is not necessarily grounds for termination of a pregnancy. Development abnormalities of the external genitalia of female fetuses after repeated high-dose exposure might be detectable by antenatal high-resolution ultrasound.

2.15.17   Mifepristone (RU486)

Pharmacology and toxicology

Mifepristone is a progesterone and glucocorticoid antagonist. It has been the subject of intense study and health policy discussion as an "abortion pill", and it has been approved as an abortifacient in several countries. A dose of 600 mg is required for the interruption of early pregnancy; however, in combination with a prostaglandin preparation (e.g. *misoprostol*) 200 mg is just as effective (Peyron 1993).

Among the pharmacologic effects of mifepristone are a lowering of luteinizing hormone (LH) secretion, more rapid corpus luteum regression, and an increased contractility of the uterine muscles. Effects on the placental production of progesterone, chorionic gonadotrophin (hCG), and lactogen (hPL) have also been observed (Das 1987).

As a result of its progesterone antagonism, mifepristone has also been tried as an "interceptive" medication to be taken monthly. In contrast to a contraceptive, it is effective after conception. However, mifepristone is unreliable for interception and for medical treatment of ectopic pregnancy. Mifepristone administration for ripening of the cervix and labor induction, as well as for endometriosis and uterus myomatosis, is also a topic of discussion (Mazouni 2006, Sitruk-Ware 2006, Fedele 2004, Jiang 2001).

Mifepristone crosses the placenta but, according to animal experiments, does not influence the concentrations of fetal progesterone, estradiol or cortisol. Only aldosterone concentration seems to increase.

Case reports have mainly cited normal babies born after treatment with mifepristone in early pregnancy (Pons 1991, Lim 1990). In a series of 71 pregnancies that continued after a failed attempt at early termination with mifepristone alone or in combination with a prostaglandin, 8 fetuses or infants with different anomalies were observed; among these were four with talipes equinovarus (Sitruk-Ware 1998). There is no controlled experience with which to predict the magnitude of developmental risk.

> **Recommendation.** If a pregnancy is continued after the accidental use of mifepristone, a detailed ultrasound diagnosis can be used to assess fetal development.

2.15.18   Clomiphene

Pharmacology and toxicology

Clomiphene has been in use for many years for ovulation induction. Among the undesirable side effects are increased rates of twinning, and ovarian hyperstimulation. The mechanism of ovulation induction is based on competitive inhibition of the estrogen receptor in the pituitary and hypothalamus, which in turn leads to increased follicle stimulating hormone (FSH) secretion. Clomiphene has a half-life of about 5 days, although its metabolites have been found in feces up to 6 weeks after administration. That is why fetal exposure cannot be totally eliminated in mothers treated with this drug before pregnancy.

The suspicion that ovulation induction with clomiphene increases the risk of birth defects such as neural tube defects (NTD) continues (van Loon 1992). A large population-based study found no increased risk of NTD after fertility treatments, where clomiphene citrate was the most commonly used drug (Whiteman 2000). One case report of iniencephaly, a rare type of NTD, has been described from a mother exposed to clomiphene for two consecutive cycles (Bhambhani 2004). Nevertheless, a cause–effect relationship can not be established.

Hypospadias has been also investigated in relation to clomiphene exposure. A population-based case-control study on a sample of 319 cases of hypospadias showed no increased risk of this defect in women exposed to clomiphene during the first trimester and 90 days before conception (Sorensen 2005). Nevertheless, a retrospective case-control study found a significantly increased risk for penoscrotal hypospadias (OR = 6.08; 95% CI 1.40–26.33), but not for the mild or moderate forms of this defect. The authors stress the importance of a detailed clinical definition in birth-defect studies (Meijer 2006). More studies are necessary to confirm the relationship between clomiphene and hypospadias. Moreover, a relationship between craniosynostosis and fertility treatments (specifically clomiphene citrate) has been described (OR = 3.8; 95% CI 1.1–12.3) in a small study covering 20 pregnant women; this also needs to be confirmed in further studies (Reefhuis 2003). One case report, referring to ocular effects in women, described a child with persistent hyperplastic primary vitreous whose mother took 100 mg clomiphene up to approximately week 6 of pregnancy (Bishai 1999).

If there are any teratogenic effects at all, they are slight. In Japan, 1034 pregnancies following clomiphene-induced ovulation were observed over 5 years. Of the 935 live-born children, 2.3% had identifiable birth defects. This was not significantly different from a control group (30 000 births with a 1.7% birth-defect rate) (Kurachi 1983). Cases collected by one manufacturer indicated 58 birth defects (2.4%) among 2379 clomiphene patients. In 158 women, clomiphene was also taken after conception. In this group, 8 children (5.1%) had birth defects.

Recommendation. Clomiphene may be prescribed to induce ovulation in patients who have been informed about the still not fully dismissed suspicion of organ-developmental disorders, and who accept the significantly increased incidence of multiple pregnancies. It is also important to note that a woman who is going to undergo fertility treatment should be informed about the possibility of an increased risk of congenital disorders because of her inherent fertility problem. Before starting treatment with clomiphene, any already existing pregnancy should be excluded.

References

Abbasi S, Hirsch D, Davis J et al. Effect of single versus multiple courses of antenatal corticosteroids on maternal and neonatal outcome. Am J Obstet Gynecol 2000; 182: 1243–9.

2

Pregnancy

Ahn HK, Choi JS, Han JY et al. Fetal outcome after exposure to oral contraceptives during the periconceptional period {Abstract}. Birth Def Res A 2005; 73: 350.

Alexander EK, Marqusee E, Lawrence J et al. Timing and magnitude of increases in levothyroxine requirements during pregnancy in women with hypothyroidism. N Engl J Med 2004; 351: 241–9.

al Shaikh AA. Pregnant women with type 1 diabetes mellitus treated by glargine insulin. Saudi Med J 2006; 27: 563–5.

Arbeitsgemeinschaft der Wissenschaftlichen Medizinischen Fachgesellschaften (AWMF-Leitlinien-Register; Nr. 015/020) "Die ärztliche Betreuung der schwangeren Diabetikerin", Stand 3/2004 unter "www.uni-duesseldorf.de/WWW/AWMF/ll/015-020.htm".

Ayar A, Kutlu S, Yilmaz B et al. Melatonin inhibits spontaneous and oxytocin-induced contractions of rat myometrium in vitro. Neuro Endocrinol Lett 2001; 22: 199–207.

Banks BA, Cnaan A, Morgan MA et al. Multiple courses of antenatal corticosteroides and outcome of premature neonates. North American Thyrotropin-Releasing Hormone Study Group. Am J Obstet Gynecol 1999; 181: 709–17.

Ballard RA, Ballard PL, Cnaan A et al. Antenatal thyrotropin-releasing hormone to prevent lung disease in preterm infants. North American Thyrotropin-Releasing Hormone Study Group. N Engl J Med 1998; 338: 493–8.

Barbero P, Ricagni C, Mercado G et al. Choanal atresia associated with prenatal methimazole exposure: three new patients. Am J Med Gen 2004; 129: 83–6.

Barlier A, Jaquet P. Quinagolide – a valuable treatment option for hyperprolactinaemia. European Journal of Endocrinology 2006; 154: 187–95.

Basu A, Candelier C. Ectopic pregnancy with postcoital contraception – a case report. Eur J Contracept Reprod Health Care 2005; 10: 6–8.

Baud O, Foix-l'Helias L, Kaminski M et al. Antenatal glucocorticoid treatment and cystic periventricular leucomalacia in very premature infants. N Eng J Med 1999; 341: 1190–6.

Bhambhani V, George S. Association of clomiphene with iniencephaly. Indian Pediatrics 2004; 41: 517.

Bhattacharyya A, Brown S, Hughes S et al. Insulin lispro and regular insulin in pregnancy. Q J Med 2001; 94: 255–60.

Bibbo N, Gill WB. Screening of adolescents exposed to diethylstilbestrol in utero. Pediatr Clin North Am 1981; 28: 379–88.

Biller BM, Luciano A, Crosignani P et al. Guidelines for the diagnosis and treatment of hyperprolactinemia. J Reprod Med 1999; 44: 1075–84.

Bishai R, Arbour L, Lyons C et al. Intrauterine exposure to clomiphene and neonatal persistent hyperplastic primary vitreous. Teratology 1999; 60: 143–5.

Blackhurst G, Strachan MW, Collie D et al. The treatment of a thyrotropin-secreting pituitary macroadenoma with octreotide in twin pregnancy. Clin Endocrinol (Oxf) 2002; 57: 401–4.

Boumpas DT, Chrousos GP, Wilder RL et al. Glucocorticoid therapy for immune-mediated diseases: basic and clinical correlates. Ann Intern Med 1993; 119: 1198–208.

Brent RL. Nongenital malformations following exposure to progestational drugs: the last chapter of an erroneous allegation. Birth Def Res A 2005; 73: 906–18.

Brewster UC, Hayslett JP. Diabetes insipidus in the third trimester of pregnancy. Obstet Gynecol 2005; 105: 1171–2.

Briet JM, van Sonderen L, Buimer M et al. Neurodevelopmental outcome of children treated with antenatal thyrotropin-releasing hormone. Pediatrics 2002; 110: 249–53.

2.15 Hormones

Briggs GG, Freeman RK, Yaffe SJ. Drugs in Pregnancy and Lactation, 7th edn. Baltimore, MD: Williams & Wilkins, 2005.

Buchbinder A, Miodovnik M, McElvy S et al. Is insulin lispro associated with the development or progression of diabetic retinopathy during pregnancy? Am J Obstet Gynecol 2000; 183: 1162–5.

Burrow GN, Fisher DA, Larsen PR. Maternal and fetal thyroid function. N Engl J Med 1994; 331: 1072–8.

Bye P. Comments on "Conception during 'Diane' therapy a successful outcome" {letter}. Br J Dermatol 1986; 114: 516.

Carmichael SL, Shaw GM. Maternal corticosteroid use and risk of selected congenital anomalies. Am J Med Genet 1999; 86: 242–4.

Carmichael SL, Shaw GM, Laurent C et al. Maternal progestin intake and risk of hypospadias. Arch Pediatr Adolesc Med 2005; 159: 957–62.

Carroll DN, Kamath P, Stewart L. Congenital viral infection? Lancet 2005; 365: 1110.

Castaman G, Federichi AB, Bernardi M et al. Factor VIII and von Willebrand factor changes after desmopressin and during pregnancy in type 2M von Willebrand disease Vicenza: a prospective study comparing patients with single (R1205H) and double (R1205H-M740I) defect. J Thromb Haemost 2006; 4: 357–60.

Challis JRG, Cox DB, Sloboda DM. Regulation of corticosteroids in the fetus: Control of birth and influence on adult disease. Semin Neonatol 1999; 4: 96–7.

Chang AS, Moley KH, Wangler M et al. Association between Beckwith–Wiedemann syndrome and assisted reproductive technology: a case series of 19 patients. Fertil Steril 2005; 83: 349–54.

Christ M, Haseroth K, Falkenstein E et al. Nongenomic steroids actions: fact or fantasy? Vitam Horm 1999; 57: 325–73.

Christensen HD, Sienko AE, Rayburn WF et al. A placebo-controlled, blinded comparison between betamethasone and dexamethasone to enhance lung maturation in fetal mouse. J Soc Gynecol Investig 1997; 4: 130–34.

Ciccarelli E, Grottoli S, Razzore P et al. Long-term treatment with cabergoline, a new long-lasting ergoline derivate, in idiopathic or tumorous hyperprolactinaemia and outcome of drug-induced pregnancy. J Endocrinol Invest 1997; 20: 547–51.

Clementi M, Di Gianantonio E, Pelo E et al. Methimazole embryopathy: delineation of the phenotype. Am J Med Genet 1999; 83: 436.

Colao A, Merola B, Ferone D et al. Acromegaly. J Clin Endocrinol Metabol 1997; 82: 2777–81.

Colao A, Lombardi G, Annunziato L. Cabergoline. Expert Opin Pharmacother 2000; 1: 555–74.

Cooper DS, Mandel S. Author's response: severe embryopathy and exposure to methimazole in early pregnancy. J Clin Endocrinol Metab 2002; 87: 948–9.

Cozzi R, Attanasio R, Barausse M. Pregnancy in acromegaly: a one-center experience. Eur J Endocrinol 2006; 155: 279–84.

Crowther CA, Hiller JE, Haslam RR et al. Australian Collaborative Trial of Antenatal Thyrotropin-releasing hormone: adverse effects at 12-month follow-up. ACTOBAT Study Group. Pediatrics 1997; 99: 311–17.

Crowther CA, Alfirevic Z, Haslam RR. Thyrotropin-releasing hormone added to corticosteroids for women at risk of preterm birth for preventing neonatal respiratory disease. Cochrane Database Syst Rev. 2004; CD000019.

Crowther CA, Hiller JE, Moss JR et al. Effect of treatment of gestational diabetes mellitus on pregnancy outcomes. N Engl J Med 2005; 352: 2477–86.

Crowther CA, Haslam RR, Hiller JE et al. Australian Collaborative Trial of Repeat Doses of Steroids (ACTORDS) Study Group. Neonatal respiratory distress syndrome after repeat exposure to antenatal corticosteroids: a randomised controlled trial. Lancet 2006; 367: 1913–19.

Cypryk K, Sobczak M, Pertynska-Marczewska M et al. Pregnancy complications and perinatal outcome in diabetic woman treated with Humalog (insulin lispro) or regular human insulin during pregnancy. Med Sci Monit 2004; 10: 129–32.

Czeizel AE, Rockenbauer M. Population-based case-control study of teratogenic potential of corticosteroids. Teratology 1997; 56: 335–40.

Czock D, Keller F, Rasche FM et al. Pharmacokinetics and pharmacodynamics of systemically administered glucocorticoids. Clin Pharmacokinet 2005; 44: 61–98.

Dalziel SR, Walker NK, Parag V et al. Cardiovascular risk factors after antenatal exposure to betamethasone: 30-year follow-up of a randomised controlled study. Lancet 2005; 365; 1856–62.

Das C, Catt KJ. Antifertility actions of the progesterone antagonist RU 486 include direct inhibition of placental hormone secretion. Lancet 1987; 2(8559): 599–601.

Davies J, Robson JM. Effects of vasopressin, adrenalin and noradrenaline on the mouse fetus. Br J Pharmacol 1970; 38: 446.

Demoly P, Piette V, Daures JP. Treatment of allergic rhinitis during pregnancy. Drugs 2003; 63: 1813–20.

de Turris P, Venuti L, Zuppa AA. Long-term treatment with cabergoline in pregnancy and neonatal outcome: report of a clinical case. Pediatr Med Chir 2003; 25: 178–80.

Devlin J, Hothersall L, Wilkis JL. Use of insulin glargine during pregnancy in a type 1 diabetic woman {Letter}. Diabetes Care 2002; 25: 1095–6.

Diav-Citrin O, Ornoy A. Teratogen update: Antithyroid drugs – methimazole, carbimazole and propylthiouracil. Teratology 2002; 65: 38–44.

di Cianni G, Volpe L, Lencioni C et al. Use of insulin glargine during the first weeks of pregnancy in five cases. Diabetes Care 2005; 28: 982–3.

di Gianantonio E, Schaefer C, Mastroiacovo PP et al. Adverse effects of prenatal methimazole exposure. Teratology 2001; 64: 262–6.

Doyle LW, Ford GW, Rickards AL et al. Antenatal corticosteroids and outcome at 14 years of age in children with birth weight less than 1501 grams. Pediatrics 2000; 106: E2.

Edwards MJ, Agho K, Attia J et al. Case-control study of cleft lip or palate after maternal use of topical corticosteroids during pregnancy. Am J Med Genet A 2003; 120: 459–63.

Eisenstein Z, Weiss M, Katz Y et al. Intellectual capacity of subjects exposed to methimazole or propylthiouracil in utero. Eur J Pediatr 1992; 151: 558–9.

Eléfant E, Biour B, Blumberg-Tick J et al. Administration of a gonadotropin-releasing hormone agonist during pregnancy, follow-up of 28 pregnancies exposed to triptorelin. Fertil Steril 1995; 63: 1111–13.

El-Hennawy AS, Bassi T, Koradia N et al. Transient gestational diabetes insipidus: report of two cases and review of pathophysiology and treatment. J Matern Fetal Neonatal Med 2003; 14: 349–52.

Ericson A, Källén B, Lindsten J. Lack of correlation between contraceptive pills and Down's syndrome. Acta Obstet Gynecol Scand 1983; 62: 511–14.

Evers IM, de Valk HW, Mol BWJ et al. Macrosomia despite good glycaemic control in type I diabetic pregnancy; results of a nationwide study in The Netherlands. Diabetologia 2002; 45: 1484–9.

Fabunmi L, Perks N. Caesarean section scar ectopic pregnancy following post-coital contraception. J Fam Plan Reprod Health Care 2002; 28: 155–6.

Falsetti L, Voltolini AM, Crosignani PG et al. Metergoline in the management of hyperprolactinemic amenorrhea and anovulation. Gynecol Obstet Invest 1982; 13: 108–16.

Fassnacht M, Capeller B, Arit W et al. Octreotide LAR treatment throughout pregnancy in a acromegalic woman. Clin Endocrinol (Oxf) 2001; 55: 411–15.

Fedele L, Berlanga N. Emerging drugs for endometriosis. Expert Opin Emerg Drugs 2004; 9: 167–77.

Ferraris S, Valenzise M, Lerone M et al. Malformations following methimazole exposure in utero: an open issue. Birth Def Res A 2003; 67: 989–92.

Foulds N, Walpole I, Elmslie F et al. Carbimazole embryopathy: an emerging phenotype. Am J Med Gen 2005; 132: 130–35.

Gainer E, Méry C, Ulmann A. Ectopic pregnancies following emergency levonorgestrel contraception. Contraception 2004; 69: 83–4.

Gamson K, Chia S, Jovanovic L. The safety and efficacy of insulin analogs in pregnancy. J Matern Fetal Med 2004; 15: 26–34.

Garg SK, Frias JP, Anil S et al. Insulin lispro therapy in pregnancies complicated by type 1 diabetes: glycemic control and maternal and fetal outcomes. Endocrin Pract 2003; 9: 187–93.

Gilbert C, Valois M, Koren G. Pregnancy outcome after first-trimester exposure to metformin; a meta-analysis. Fertil Steril 2006; 86: 658–63.

Glinoer D. The regulation of thyroid function in pregnancy: pathways of endocrine adaptation from physiology to pathology. Endocrin Rev 1997; 18: 404–33.

Glueck C J, Goldenberg N, Pranikoff J et al. Height, weight, and motor-social development during first 18 months of life in 126 infants born to 109 mothers with polycystic ovary syndrome who conceived on and continued metformin through pregnancy. Hum Reprod 2004; 19: 1323–30.

Gojnic M, Fazlagic A, Likic I et al. New approach of the treatment of von Willebrand's disease during pregnancy. Arch Gynecol Obstet 2005; 273: 35–8.

Greene MF. Oral hypoglycemic drugs for gestational diabetes (editorial). N Engl J Med 2000; 343: 1178–9.

Groneck P. Perinatal glucocorticosteroid therapy: time for reconsideration. Z Geburtshilfe Neonatol 2001; 205: 231–5.

Gur C, Diav-Citrin O, Shechtman S et al. Pregnancy outcome after first trimester exposure to corticosteroids: a prospective controlled study. Reprod Toxicol 2004; 18: 93–101.

Gutzin S, Kozer E, Magee L et al. The safety of oral hypoglycemic agents in the first trimester of pregnancy: a meta-analysis. Teratology 2001; 63: 268.

Haddow JE, Palomaki GE, Allan WC et al. Maternal thyroid deficiency during pregnancy and subsequent neuropsychological development of the child. N Engl J Med 1999; 341: 549–55.

Hall BD. Methimazole as a teratogenic etiology of choanal tresia/multiple congenital anomaly syndrome. Am J Hum Genet 1997; 61: A100.

Harlap S, Eldor J. Births following oral contraceptive failure. Obstet Gynecol 1980; 55: 447–52.

Harlap S (A), Shiono PH, Ramcharan S. Congenital abnormalities in the offspring of women who used oral and other contraceptives around the time of conception. Int J Fertil 1985; 30: 39–47.

Harlap S (B), Shiono PH, Ramcharan S et al. Chromosomal abnormalities in the Kaiser-Permanente Birth Defects Study, with special reference to contraceptive use around the time of conception. Teratology 1985; 31: 381–7.

Harrison-Woolrych ML. Progestogen-only emergency contraception and ectopic pregnancy. J Fam Plan Reprod Health Care 2003; 29: 5–6.

Herbst AL, Poskanzer DC, Robboy SJ et al. Prenatal exposure to stilbestrol. N Engl J Med 1975; 292: 334–9.

Hod M, Visser G, Damm P et al. Safety and perinatal outcome in pregnancy: a randomized trial comparing insulin aspart with human insulin in 322 subjects with type 1 diabetes. Diabetes 2006, June Supplement: Poster number: 1805-P.

Holstein A, Plaschke A, Egberts EH. Use of insulin glargine during embryogenesis in a pregnant woman with type 1 diabetes. Daibet Med 2003; 20: 777–80.

Ikegami M, Jobe AH, Newnham J et al. Repetitive prenatal glucocorticoids improve lung function and decrease growth in preterm lambs. Am J Respir Crit Care Med 1997; 156: 178–84.

Iwasaki S, Nakazawa K, Sakai J et al. Melatonin as a local regulator of human placental function. J Pineal Res 2005; 39: 261–5.

Jacobson GF, Ramos GA, Ching JY et al. Comparison of glyburide and insulin for the management of gestational diabetes in a large managed care organization. Am J Obstet Gynecol 2005; 193: 118–24.

Jahn A, Blode H, Schützel H et al. Developmental toxicology data of cyproterone acetate – their relevance for clinical safety assessment. Teratology 1996; 53: 31A.

Jakubowicz DJ, Iuorno MJ, Jakubowicz S et al. Effects of metformin on early pregnancy loss in the polycystic ovary syndrome. J Clin Endocrinol Metab 2002; 87: 524–9.

Jiang J, Lu J, Wu R. Mifepristone following conservative surgery in the treatment of endometriosis. Zhonghua Fu Chan Ke Za Zhi 2001; 36: 717–20.

Johnsson E, Larsson G, Ljunggren M. Severe malformations in infant born to hyperthyroid woman on methimazole. Lancet 1997; 350: 1520.

Jones J, Bashir T, Olney J et al. Cabergoline treatment for a large macroprolactinoma throughout pregnancy. J Obstet Gynaecol 1997; 17: 375–6.

Jost A. Role of vasopressin and corticostimuline (ACTH) in experimental production of lesions of the fetal extremities (hemorrhages, necroses, congenital amputations). C R Soc Biol 1951; 145: 1805–9.

Källén B. Maternal use of oral contraceptives and Down syndrome. Contraception 1989; 39: 503–6.

Källén B, Mastroiacovo P, Lancaster PAL et al. Oral contraceptives in the etiology of isolated hypospadias. Contraception 1991; 44: 173–82.

Källén B, Martinez-Frias EE, Castilla E et al. Hormone therapy during pregnancy and isolated hypospadias: an international case-control study. Intl J Risk Saf Med 1992; 3: 183–98.

Källén B, Rydhstroem H, Aberg A. Congenital malformations after the use of inhaled budesonide in early pregnancy. Obstet Gynecol 1999; 93: 392–5.

Källén B. Maternal drug use and infant cleft lip/palate with special reference to corticoids. Cleft Palate Craniofac J 2003; 40: 624–8.

Kalyoncu NI, Yaris F, Ulku C et al. A case of rosiglitazone exposure in the second trimester of pregnancy. Reprod Toxicol 2005; 19: 563–4.

Karg E, Bereg E, Gaspar L et al. Aplasia cutis congenita after methimazole exposure in utero. Pediatr Dermatol 2004; 21: 491–4.

Karlsson FA, Axelsson O, Melhus H. Severe embryopathy and exposure to methimazole in early pregnancy. J Clin Endocrinol Metab 2002; 87: 946–51.

Kingsbury AC. Danazol and fetal masculinization: a warning. Med J Aust 1985; 143: 410–11.

Klip H, Verloop J, van Gool JD et al. OMEGA Project Group. Hypospadias in sons of women esposed to diethylstilbestrol in utero: a cohort study. Lancet 2002; 359: 1102–7.

Kovo M, Weissman A, Gur D et al. Neonatal outcome in polycystic ovarian syndrome patients treated with metformin during pregnancy. J Matern Fetal Neonatal Med 2006; 19: 415–19.

2

Pregnancy

2.15 Hormones

Kraemer J, Klein J, Lubetsky A et al. Perfusion studies of glyburide transfer across the human placenta: Implications for fetal safety. Obstet Gynecol 2006; 195: 270–4.

Kremer CJ, Duff P. Glyburide for the treatment of gestational diabetes. Am J Obstet Gynecol 2004; 190: 1438–9.

Krupp P, Monka C. Bromocriptine in pregnancy: safety aspects {in German}. Klin Wochenschr 1987; 65: 823–7.

Lacassie HJ, Muir HA, Millar S et al. Perioperative anesthetic management for Cesarean section of a parturient with gestational diabetes insipidus. Can J Anaesth 2005; 52: 733–6.

Lahat E, Raziel A, Friedler S et al. Long-term follow-up of children born after inadvertent administration of a gonadotrophin-releasing hormone agonist in early pregnancy. Hum Reprod 1999; 14: 2656–60.

Langer O, Yogev Y, Xenakis EMJ et al. Insulin and glyburide therapy: dosage, severity level of gestational diabetes, and pregnancy outcome. Am J Obstet Gynecol 2005; 192: 134–9.

Levitz M, Jansen V, Dancis J. The transfer and metabolism of corticosteroids in the perfused human placenta. Am J Obstet Gynecol 1978; 132: 362–6.

Li DK, Daling JR, Mueller BA et al. Oral contraceptive use after conception in relation to the risk of congenital urinary tract anomalies. Teratology 1995; 51: 30–6.

Lim BH, Lees DA, Bjornsson S et al. Normal development after exposure to mifepristone in early pregnancy. Lancet 1990; 336: 257–8.

Litwin A, Amodai I, Fisch B et al. Limb–body wall complex with complete absence of external genitalia after in vitro fertilization. Fertil Steril 1991; 55: 634–6.

Liu C, Tyrrell JB. Successful treatment of a large macroprolactinoma with cabergoline during pregnancy. Pituitary 2001; 4: 179–85.

Loffredo CA, Wilson PD, Ferencz CH. Maternal diabetes: An independent risk factor for major malformations with increased mortality of affected infants. Teratology 2001; 64: 98–106.

Loukovaara S, Immonen I, Teramo KA et al. Progression of retinopathy during pregnancy in type 1 diabetic women treated with insulin lispro. Diabetes Care 2003; 26: 1193–8.

Love AM, Vickers TH. Vasopressin induced dysmelia in rats and its relation to amniocentesis dysmelia. Br J Exp Pathol 1973; 54: 291–7.

Ludwig M, Riethmuller-Winzen H, Felberbaun RE et al. Health of 227 children born after controlled ovarian stimulation for in vitro fertilization using the luteinizing hormone-releasing antagonist cetrorelix. Fertil Steril 2001; 75: 18–22.

Mackenzie R, Walker M, Armson A et al. Progesterone for the prevention of preterm birth among women at increased risk: a systematic review and meta-analysis of randomized controlled trials. Am J Obstet Gynecol 2006; 194: 1234–42.

Maher ER, Brueton LA, Bowdin SC et al. Beckwith–Wiedemann syndrome and assisted reproduction technology (ART). J Med Genet 2003; 40: 62–4.

Mandel M, Toren A, Rechavi G et al. Hormonal treatment in pregnancy: a possible risk factor for neuroblastoma. Med Pediatr Oncol 1994; 23: 133–5.

Martínez-Frias M-L, Rodriguez-Pinilla E, Bermejo E et al. Prenatal exposure to sex hormones: a case-control study. Teratology 1998; 57: 8–12.

Martínez-Frias M-L, Bermejo E, Rodriguez-Pinilla E et al. Periconceptional exposure to contraceptive pills and risk for Down syndrome. J Perinatol 2001; 21: 288–92.

Masson EA, Patmore JE, Brash PD et al. Pregnancy outcome in type 1 diabetes mellitus treated with insulin lispro (Humalog). Diab Med 2003; 20: 46–50.

Mazouni C, Provensal M, Porcu G et al. Termination of pregnancy in patients with previous cesarean section. Contraception 2006; 73: 244–8.

Mecacci F, Carignani L, Cioni R et al. Maternal metabolic control and perinatal outcome in women with gestational diabetes treated with regular or lispro insulin: comparison with non-diabetic pregnant women. Eur J Obstet Gynecol Repro Biol 2003, 111: 19–24.

Meijer WM, de Jong-van den Berg LT, van den Berg MD et al. Clomiphene and hypospadias on a detailed level: signal or chance? Birth Def Res A 2006; 76: 249–52.

Messer PM, Hauffa BP, Olbricht T. Antithyroid drug treatment of Graves' disease in pregnancy: long term effects on somatic growth, intellectual development and thyroid function of the offspring. Acta Endocrinol (Copenh) 1990; 123: 311–16.

Mikkelsen M. Epidemiology of trisomy 21: population, peri- and antenatal data. Hum Genet 1981; 2: 211–26.

Modi N, Lewis H, Al-Naqeeb N et al. The effects of repeated antenatal glucocorticoid therapy on the developing brain. Pediatr Res 2001; 50: 581–5.

Momotani N, Noh JY, Ishikawa N et al. Effects of propylthiouracil and methimazole on fetal thyroid status in mothers with Graves' hyperthyroidism. J Clin Endocrinol Metab 1997; 82: 3633–6.

Money J, Mathews D. Prenatal exposure to virilizing progestins: an adult follow-up study of twelve women. Arch Sex Behav 1982; 11: 73–83.

Morange I, Barlier A, Pellegrini I et al. Prolactinomas resistant to bromocriptine: long-term efficacy of quinagolide and outcome of pregnancy. Europ J Endocrinol 1996; 135: 413–20.

Nakamura S, Nishikawa T, Isaji M et al. Aplasia cutis congenita and skull defects after exposure to methimazole in utero. Intern Med 2005; 44: 1202–3.

Nanovskaya TN, Nekhayeva I, Hankins GDV et al. Effect of human serum albumin on transplacental transfer of glyburide. Biochem Pharmacol 2006; 72: 632–9.

Neal JM. Successful pregnancy in a woman with acromegaly treated with octreotide. Endocrin Pract 2000; 6: 148–50.

Newnham JP. Is prenatal glucocorticoid administration another origin of adult disease? Clin Exp Pharmacol Physiol 2001; 28: 957–61.

Olivennes F, Mannaerts B, Struijs M et al. Perinatal outcome of pregnancy after GnRH antagonist (ganirelix) treatment during ovarian stimulation for conventional IVF or ICSI: a preliminary report. Hum Reprod 2001; 16: 1588–91.

Palmer JR, Wise LA, Robboy SJ et al. Hypospadias in sons of women exposed to diethylstilbestrol in utero. Epidemiology 2005; 16: 583–6.

Palomba S, Orio F, Falbo A et al. Prospective parallel randomized, double-blind, double-dummy controlled clinical trial comparing clomiphene citrate and metformin as the first-line treatment for ovulation induction in nonobese anovulatory women with polycystic ovary syndrome. J Clin Endocrinol Metab 2005; 90: 4068–74.

Papanikolaou EG, Platteau P, Albano C et al. Achievement of pregnancy three times in the same patient during luteal GnRH agonist administration. Reprod Biomed Online 2005; 10: 347–9.

Pardthaisong T, Yenchit C, Gray R. The long-term growth and development of children exposed to Depo-Provera during pregnancy and lactation. Contraception 1992; 45: 313–24.

Park-Wyllie L, Mazzotta P, Pastuszak A et al. Birth defects after maternal exposure to corticosteroids: Prospective cohort study and meta-analysis of epidemiological studies. Teratology 2000; 62: 385–92.

Perez-Barrero P, Gil L, Martinez C et al. Treatment with desmopressin before epidural anesthesia in a patient with type I von Willebrand disease. Rev Esp Anestesiol Reanim 2003; 50: 526–9.

2

Pregnancy

2.15 Hormones

Persson B, Swahn M-L, Hjertberg R et al. Insulin lispro therapy in pregnancies complicated by type 1 diabetes mellitus. Diab Res Clin Pract 2002; 58: 115–21.

Peyron R, Aubeny E, Targosz V et al. Early termination of pregnancy with mifepristone (RU 486) and the orally active prostaglandin misoprostol. N Engl J Med 1993; 328: 1509–13.

Pharoah POD, Connolly KJ, Ekins RP et al. Maternal thyroid hormone levels in pregnancy and the subsequent cognitive and motor performance of the children. Clin Endocrinol 1984; 21: 265–70.

Piacquadio K, Hollingsworth DR, Murphy H. Effects of in-utero exposure to oral hypoglycemic drugs. Lancet 1991; 338: 866–9.

Pons JC, Imber MC, Eléfant E et al. Development after exposure to mifepristone in early pregnancy. Lancet 1991; 338: 763.

Pons JC, Papiernik E, Billon A et al. Hypospadias in sons of women exposed to diethylstilbestrol in utero. Prenat Diagn 2005; 25: 417–28.

Pop VJ, Brouwers EP, Vader HL et al. Maternal hypothyroxinaemia during early pregnancy and subsequent child development: a 3-year follow-up study. Clin Endocrinol (Oxf) 2003; 59: 282–8.

Potter SM, Astbury K, Morrison JJ. Effects of thyrotropin-releasing hormone on human myometrium and umbilical vasculature in vitro. Am J Obstet Gynecol 2004; 190: 246–51.

Pradat P, Robert-Gnansia E, Di Tanna GL et al. First trimester exposure to corticosteroids and oral clefts. Birth Def Res A 2003; 67: 968–70.

Raman-Wilms L, Tseng AL, Wighardt S et al. Fetal genital effects of first-trimester sex hormone exposure: a meta-analysis. Obstet Gynecol 1995; 85: 141–9.

Rand L. Comparison of glyburide and insulin for the management of gestational diabetes in a large managed care organization. Am J Obstet Gynecol 2006; 195: 628–9.

Ray JG. DDAVP use during pregnancy: an analysis of its safety for mother and child. Obstet Gynecol Survey 1998; 53: 450–55.

Ray JG, Boskovic R, Knie B et al. In vitro analysis of human transplacental transport of desmopressin. Clin Biochem 2004; 37: 10–13.

Rayburn WF, Christensen HD, Gonzalez CL. A placebo-controlled comparison between betamethasone and dexamethasone for fetal maturation: differences in neurobehavioral development of mice offspring. Am J Obstet Gynecol 1997; 176: 842–50.

Reefhuis J, Honein MA, Shaw GM et al. Fertility treatments and craniosynostosis: California, Georgia, and Iowa, 1993–1997. Pediatrics 2003; 111: 1163–6.

Rennick GJ. Use of systemic glucocorticoids in pregnancy: be alert but not alarmed. Australas J Dermatol 2006; 47: 34–6.

Ricci E, Parazzini F, Motta T et al. Pregnancy outcome after cabergoline treatment in early weeks of gestation. Reprod Toxicol 2002; 16: 791–3.

Robert E, Musatti L, Piscitelli B et al. Pregnancy outcome after treatment with the ergot derivative, cabergoline. Reprod Toxicol 1996; 10: 333–7.

Rodríguez-Pinilla E, Martinez-Frias ML. Corticosteroids during pregnancy and oral defects. A case-control study. Teratology 1998; 58: 2–5.

Rodríguez-Pinilla E, Prieto-Merino D, Dequino G et al. Grupo del ECEMC. Exposición prenatal a glucocorticoides para maduración pulmonar fetal y su repercusión sobre el peso, talla y perímetro cefálico del recién nacido. Med Clin (Barc) 2006; 127(10): 361–7.

Rosa FW. Virilization of the female fetus with maternal danazol exposure. Am J Obstet Gynecol 1984; 149: 99–100.

Rosenfeld H, Diav-Citrin O, Arnon J et al. Impaired thyroid function in offspring of propylthiouracil treated women: a prospective controlled study on 115 pregnancies. Reprod Toxicol 2005; 20: 480.

Roumestan C, Cougat C, Jaffuel D et al. Glucocorticoids and their receptor: mechanisms of action and clinical implications. Rev Med Intere 2004; 25: 636–47.

Scherbaum WA, Lankisch MR, Pawlowski B et al. Insulin lispro in pregnancy – retrospective analysis of 33 cases and matched controls. Exp Clin Endocrinol Diabetes 2002; 110: 6–9.

Schmand B, Neuvel J, Smolders-de Haas H et al. Psychological development of children who were treated antenatally with corticosteroids to prevent respiratory distress syndrome. Pediatrics 1990; 86: 58–64.

Schultz PN, Ginsberg L, McCutcheon IE et al. Quinagolide in the management of prolactinoma. Pituitary 2000; 3: 239–49.

Scialli, A. The reproductive toxicity of ovulation induction. Fertil Steril 1986; 45: 315–23.

Shiota K, Yamada S. Assisted reproductive technologies and birth defects. Congenit Anom (Kyoto) 2005; 45: 39–43.

Siristatidis C, Salamalekis E, Iakovidou H et al. Three cases of diabetes insipidus complicating pregnancy. J Matern Fetal Neonatal Med 2004; 16: 61–3.

Sitruk-Ware R, Davey A, Sakiz E. Fetal malformations and failed medical termination of pregnancy. Lancet 1998; 352: 323.

Sitruk-Ware R. Mifepristone and misoprosol sequential regimen side effects, complications and safety. Contraception 2006; 74: 48–55.

Sorensen HT, Pedersen L, Skriver MV et al. Use of clomifene during early pregnancy and risk of hypospadias: a population based case–control study. Br Med J 2005; 330: 126–7.

Statham BN, Cunliffe WJ, Clayton JK. "Conception during 'Diane' therapy a successful outcome" {Letter}. Br J Dermatol 1985; 113: 374.

Stoll C, Alembik Y, Dott B. Limb reduction defects in the first generation and deafness in the second generation of intrauterine exposed fetuses to diethylstilbestrol. Anales de Génétique 2003; 46: 459–65.

Storgaard L, Bonde JP, Olsen J. Male reproductive disorders in humans and prenatal indicators of estrogen exposure. A review of published epidemiological studies. Reprod Toxicol 2006; 21: 4–15.

Takeuchi K, Funakoshi T, Oomori S et al. Successful pregnancy in an acromegalic woman treated with octreotide. Obstet Gynecol 1999; 93: 848.

Tarlatzis BC, Bili H. Safety of GnRH agonist and antagonist. Expert Opin Drug Saf 2004; 3: 39–46.

Thatcher SS, Jackson EM. Pregnancy outcome in infertile patients with polycystic ovary syndrome who were treated with metformin. Fertil Steril 2006; 85: 1002–9.

Thorp JA, Jones FG, Knox E et al. Does antenatal costicosteriod therapy affect birth weight and head cercunference? Obstet Gynecol 2002; 99(1): 101–8.

Towner D, Kjos SL, Leung B et al. Congenital malformations in pregnancies complicated by NIDDM. Diabetes Care 1995; 18: 1446–51.

Turner MJ, Walsh J, Byrne KM et al. Outcome of clinical pregnancies after ovulation induction using metformin. J Obstet Gynaecol 2006; 26: 233–5.

van der Heijden PF, de Wit W, Brownell J et al. CV 205-502, a new dopamine agonist, versus bromocriptine in the treatment of hyperprolactinaemia. Eur J Obstet Gynecol Reprod Biol 1991; 40: 111–18.

Vanky E, Salvesen KA, Heimstad R et al. Metformin reduces pregnancy complications without affecting androgen levels in pregnant polycystic ovary syndrome women: results of a randomized study. Hum Reprod 2004; 19: 1734–40.

Vanky E, Zahlsen K, Spigset O et al. Placental passage of metformin in women with polycystic ovary syndrome. Fertil Steril 2005; 83: 1575–8.

van Loon K, Besseghir K, Eshkol A. Neural tube defects after infertility treatment: a review. Fertil Steril 1992; 58: 875–84.

2

Pregnancy

2.15 Hormones

Ventz M, Puhlmann B, Knappe G et al. Schwangerschaften bei hyperprolaktinämischen Patientinnen. Zentralbl Gynäkol 1996; 118: 610–15.

Verhelst J, Abs R, Maiter D et al. Cabergoline in the treatment of hyperprolactinemia: a study in 455 patients. J Clin Endocrinol Metab 1999; 84: 2518–22.

Vogt T, Stolz W, Landthaler M. Aplasia cutis congenita after exposure to methimazole: a causal relationship? Br J Dermatol 1995; 1333: 994–6.

Webster J. A comparative review of the tolerability profiles of dopamine agonists in the treatment of hyperprolactinaemia and inhibition of pregnancy. Drug Saf 1996; 14: 228–38.

Whiteman D, Murphy M, Hey K et al. Reproductive factors, subfertility, and risk of neural tube defects: a case-control study based on the Oxford Record Linkage Study Register. Am J Epidemiol 2000; 152: 823–8.

Wilshire GB, Emmi AM, Gagliardi CC et al. Gonadotropin-releasing hormone agonist administration in early human pregnancy is associated with normal outcomes. Fertil Steril 1993; 60: 980–83.

Wilson LC, Kerr BA, Wilkinson R et al. Choanal atresia and hypothelia following methimazole exposure in utero: a second report. Am J Med Genet 1998; 75: 220–22.

Wing DA, Millar LK, Koonings PP et al. Comparison of propylthiouracil versus methimazole in the treatment of hyperthyroidism in pregnancy. Am J Obstet Gynecol 1994; 170: 90–95.

Wogelius P, Horvath-Puho E, Pedersen L et al. Maternal use of oral contraceptives and risk of hypospadias – a population-based case-control study. Eur J Epidemiol 2006; Nov 1 {Epub ahead of print}.

Woolderink JM, van Loon AJ, Storms F et al. Use of insulin glargine during pregnancy in seven type 1 diabetic women. Diabetes Care 2005; 28: 2594.

Wyatt JW, Frais JL, Hoyme HE et al. Congenital anomaly rate in offspring of mothers with diabetes treated with insulin lispro during pregnancy. Diabet Med 2005; 22: 803–7.

Xue-Yi C, Xin-Min J, Zhi-Hong D et al. Timing of vulnerability of the brain to iodine deficiency in endemic cretinism. N Engl J Med 1994; 331: 1739–44.

Yalom ID, Green R, Fisk N. Prenatal exposure to female hormones. Effect of psychosexual development in boys. Arch Gen Psychiatry 1973; 28: 554–61.

Yaris F, Yaris E, Kadioglu M et al. Normal pregnancy outcome following inadvertent exposure to rosiglitazone, gliclazide, and atorvastatin in a diabetic and hypertensive woman. Reprod Toxicol 2004; 18: 619–21.

Yunis KA, Bitar FF, Havek P, et al. Transient hypertrophic cardiomyopathy in the newborn following multiple doses of antenatal corticosteroids. Am J Perinatol 1999; 16(1): 17–21.

General and local anesthetics and muscle relaxants

2.16

Asher Ornoy

Due to their lipid solubility, general anesthetic agents rapidly cross the placenta. They also rapidly cross the blood–brain barrier – hence their instantaneous effects on the brain. Since general anesthetics have a suppressive effect on the breathing center, there is concern if maternal hypoxia occurs; however, it is of course the role of the anesthesiologist to avoid such hypoxia. These agents, when used for delivery – i.e. for cesarean sections – might result in the suppression of the newborn's respiration. Local anesthetics are either injected or sprayed, but they often spread to the maternal circulation and hence to the fetus. This can be minimized by vasoconstrictors that decrease their absorption in the circulation in order to sustain and improve their local effects (Johnston 1976).

Muscle relaxants, often used as adjuncts to most surgical procedures performed under general anesthesia, can also reach the fetus. Local disinfectants are generally poorly absorbed through the skin, depending on its integrity, and hence, these disinfectants do not usually reach the fetus.

In spite of the fact that there have been very few epidemiological studies on specific and individual anesthetic agents, there have been several relatively large-scale studies looking at the effects of surgery (including anesthesia) in pregnancy, often using a combination of different anesthetic agents. As a general rule, none of these studies has demonstrated significant damaging effects on the outcome of pregnancy (Ebi 1994, Mazze 1989, Duncan 1986). An increased rate of spontaneous abortions was demonstrated in some reports (Brodsky 1980), but it is difficult to attribute that to the direct effects of the anesthetic agents. Therefore, we can conclude from the current state of knowledge that none of the commonly used anesthetics produces an increase in congenital malformations. However, anesthetic complications involving compromise of the mother's breathing or circulation (i.e. pulmonary hypertension) or anesthetic-associated malignant hyperthermia have been described, and might have adverse consequences for the fetus (Bonnin 2005). The various anesthetic agents in use will be described individually. We should also remember that in surgery a mixture of anesthetics is often used, and the data on the outcome of "surgery in pregnancy" may be more valid than the data on individual anesthetics. Indeed, most studies report pregnancy outcome following anesthesia in pregnancy, rather than looking into the effects of individual anesthetic agents (Cohen-Kerem 2005).

Animal studies will be cited in the chapter, especially because few specific human data are available. However, these studies, often performed with repeated and high doses, cannot substitute for human epidemiologic studies, and the safety of these agents during human pregnancies cannot be deduced from them.

Long-term occupational exposure to anesthetic agents, such as may occur in operating-theater personnel, deserves special consideration, and this will be dealt with (Ratzon 2004).

2.16.1 Halogenated inhalation agents for general anesthesia

Halothane, *fluothane*, *isoflurane*, *desflurane*, *enflurane*, and *sevoflurane* are halogenated inhalation agents with similar clinical effects. They transit the placental barrier, and are also secreted in small concentrations into mother's milk, see also Chapter 4.11.10.

▶ **Halothane**

This fluorinated hydrocarbon was the first one in this group used for general anesthesia. There are few studies regarding its possible effects on the human fetus (Mazze 1989), but there are more animal studies.

Skeletal and other fetal anomalies, fetal growth retardation, and death have been found in some animal studies, as well as behavioral abnormalities in the offspring (Baeder 1990, Levin 1990, Koëter 1986). In these studies rodents were repeatedly exposed to high doses of halothane, making these studies irrelevant to the human situation, where exposures are to lower doses and usually only once or twice in pregnancy. Indeed, no increase in anomalies were observed in the offspring of women undergoing general anesthesia in pregnancy, and, from the few studies published, there is no indication that halothane anesthesia in pregnancy imposes an increased risk to the fetus (Kuczkowski 2006, Cohen-Kerem 2005, Heinonen 1977).

When halothane is administered to women at delivery (i.e. cesarean section), there is a uterine relaxant effect, which can lead to diminished contractions and a suppressive effect on breathing; however, this seems to be rare, and the use of halothane in labor is considered safe (Hood 1990).

Among the halogenated inhalation anesthetics, halothane is thought to have the strongest circulatory depressant effect. High doses may lead to cardiac arrhythmias and cardiac arrest when α-sympathomimetic tocolytics are given at the same time. Liver damage as a result of toxic metabolites has been described following repeated use. Depressive effects on the circulatory system and liver toxicity have led to a preference for enflurane and isoflurane. However, the rapid action and excretion from the circulatory system are favorable characteristics for ambulatory anesthesia.

Isoflurane

Although human studies related to the use of isoflurane in pregnancy are few, they have not demonstrated any deleterious effect on the human fetus. Beilin (1999) found no reduction in the implantation rate in women anesthetized by isoflurane (or other anesthetic agents) for ova transfer. The use of isoflurane for cesarean sections does not seem to cause any damage to the fetus, except for a possible increase in bilirubin blood levels (de Amivi 2001). Although animal studies have demonstrated increased rate of various congenital anomalies, fetal growth restriction, and neonatal behavioral changes in mice but not in rats, the animals were repeatedly anesthetized in pregnancy by large doses of isoflurane, and hence there is no relevance to the human situation (Rice 1994, 1986).

Enflurane

No epidemiological studies in women having surgery during pregnancy with enflurane anesthesia have been found. Its use as an

2

Pregnancy

2.16 General and local anesthetics and muscle relaxants

anesthetic agent for cesarean section has not been associated with problems in the fetus (Tunstall 1989, Abboud 1985). Most animal studies regarding the teratogenicity of enflurane are negative, although a few demonstrated, after repeated administration of high doses in pregnancy, an increase in limb and other defects in rabbits, rats, and mice (Natsume 1990, Mazze 1986, Wharton 1981).

▶ **Desflurane and sevoflurane**

There seem to be no studies on human exposure in pregnancy to desflurane or sevoflurane, or on the use of these agents for cesarean sections. Two cases of fetal complications using sevoflurane anesthesia have been reported (Ong 2003, Schwartz 2001), and two of malignant hyperthermia following desflurane anesthesia (Allen 1998, Fu 1996), but it is impossible to be sure about such causal relations from these case reports. Animal studies are also few and inconclusive.

> **Recommendation.** Halogenated anesthetics are among the standard agents used in obstetrics, during either pregnancy or labor (mainly for cesarean sections). They can be used at any time during the pregnancy. When used during labor, there is a need for careful monitoring, and the newborn should be observed for possible respiratory or circulatory effects, and perhaps hyperbilirubinemia.

2.16.2   Ether (diethyl ether)

Ether is a fluid with a boiling point of 35°C, which is rarely used now; this is mainly because of its undesirable characteristics and complications, such as post-anesthesia vomiting and excitability. Ether crosses the placenta and reaches the fetus within a few minutes, achieving a steady-state concentration. The extent of the newborn respiratory depression is dependent on the length and depth of the anesthesia. There seem to be no human epidemiologic studies regarding the possible effects of ether in pregnancy. In experimental studies in rats and mice, repeated use of ether anesthesia caused increased skeletal anomalies and decreased head growth (Schwetz 1970); again, these studies have little relevance for man.

> **Recommendation.** Ether anesthesia is not indicated during pregnancy and labor, as other anesthetic agents are in use that have fewer side effects. However, it does not seem to be teratogenic, and hence increased damage to the fetus, if indeed it exists, seems to be negligible.

2.16.3   Nitrous oxide

Nitrous oxide (laughing gas) is a slow-acting gas with good analgesic and limited anesthetic effects, so it must be combined with other anesthetics and/or muscle relaxants to obtain complete anesthesia. It is more often used in dentistry for analgesia and partial anesthesia.

Compared to halogenated inhalation anesthetics, nitrous oxide is a well-tolerated anesthetic with no negative effects on the circulatory system or on the uterus. By inhalation of a nitrous oxide–oxygen mixture during labor, the quickest and most simple analgesic effect can be achieved, which can be controlled very well. In rare cases, nitrous oxide can be associated with neonatal respiratory depression requiring resuscitation (Langanke 1987).

There are several epidemiologic studies in pregnant women (altogether over 1000 exposures) administered nitrous oxide during pregnancy, reporting that its use during pregnancy has not been associated with an increase in congenital malformations (Crawford 1986, Heinonen 1977). On the other hand, there are studies demonstrating several deleterious effects on the newborn infant following the use of nitrous oxide during delivery. Taylor (1993) found a higher use of nitrous oxide during delivery in children with developmental delay, and Polvi (1996) found alterations in fetal cerebral vascular resistance. These studies have been criticized, as there are possible confounding factors that are not well-delineated. Occupational exposure to nitrous oxide has been associated with an increased rate of spontaneous abortions and reduced fertility whenever scavenging devices for the reduction in nitrous oxide concentrations have not been used (Rowland 1995, 1992). Animal studies have demonstrated an increase in the rate of congenital anomalies, resorptions, decreased growth, and behavioral changes in rats (Rice 1994, Rodier 1986) but not in hamsters. These studies, however, usually use prolonged exposure to high doses, and their relevance to man is questionable.

> **Recommendation.** Nitrous oxide is an acceptable inhalation agent for use during pregnancy and labor. When used during labor, the newborn should be evaluated for respiratory depression.

2.16.4   Injectable anesthetics

Etomidate, *ketamine*, *methohexital*, *propofol*, and *thiopentone* (*thiopental*) are among the injectable anesthetics. If administered intravenously, injectable anesthetics reach their maximum concentrations immediately. The concentration in plasma falls rapidly due to rapid redistribution and excretion. After use in labor, the longer the time between the injection of the anesthetic and the infant's birth, the lower the concentration in the newborn, and the less the possible transient effects of these agents. As a rule, they can all be used in pregnancy. The main drugs will be discussed individually.

▶ **Etomidate**

This non-barbiturate imidazole derivative is inactivated by non-specific esterases. It is an inhibitor of steroid biosynthesis, and has been found to reduce serum cortisol concentrations in neonates following the use of etomidate during delivery without any long-term consequences (Reddy 1988). Etomidate does not have cardio-depressive characteristics. Its half-life is very short, being in the serum for about 3 minutes. The brief duration of the effect, like that of barbiturates, is dependent on redistribution from the brain, with its large blood supply, to tissues such as muscle and fat, which are less well-vascularized. There are no epidemiologic studies on the adminis-tration of etomidate in pregnancy, and there has been no long-term follow-up. Animal studies regarding congenital anomalies are incon-clusive, and even high doses were not teratogenic in rats (USP DI 2003, Doenicke 1977).

> **Recommendation.** Etomidate may be used in pregnancy, but if it is used in labor then the baby should be observed for possible respiratory depressant effects.

▶ **Ketamine**

Ketamine (*Ketalar*) is a fast-acting anesthetic agent that has a good analgesic effect and little effect on respiration. There are no epi-demiologic studies in man evaluating its possible effects on fetal development. Due to its enhancement of sympathomimetic sensi-tivity, ketamine administration can be associated with marked car-diovascular effects such as increased heart rate and blood pressure. Ketamine increases the uterine tone and the frequency of uterine contractions in a dose-related fashion (Krissel 1994). High doses may depress fetal functions and hence distort fetal monitoring dur-ing parturition (Baraka 1990, Reich 1989). Use of ketamine during cesarean section has in several cases led to clinically important panic disorders, which restricts its use during birth. In addition, neonatal behavioral alterations, including reduction in sucking, have also been described in infants whose mothers were given ketamine for cesarean section (Hodgkinson 1978). In a study on 20 women who received ketamine for cesarean section, no neonatal depression was observed if the induction-to-delivery and incision-to-delivery times were short, but complications occurred if these intervals were longer than 10 and 1.5 minutes respectively (Baraka 1990). Most animal studies regarding congenital anomalies are negative (Abdel-Rahman 2000) even with doses 10–25 times the human dose. On microscopic evaluation, however, several tissues have shown degenerative changes in the offspring of rats treated in pregnancy with ketamine (Kochar 1986).

> **Recommendation.** It seems preferable not to use ketamine during pregnancy. As ketamine can increase blood pressure, it is especially contraindicated in cases of hypertension or pre-eclampsia in pregnancy, and with uterine hyperactivity or suspicion of fetal hypoxia during labor.

Propofol

Propofol is a general anesthetic administered intravenously. It crosses the human placenta with cord blood levels at term approximately 70% those of maternal blood (Dailland 1990). Similar findings have also been reported for samples taken during gestational weeks 12–18 (Jauniaux 1998). All studies except one on pregnancy rates in ova collection for *in vitro* fertilization following propofol anesthesia demonstrated no adverse effects on the rate of pregnancy (Beilin 1999, Christiaens 1998).

There are several reports which conclude that propofol used during delivery has no adverse effects on neonatal well-being (d'Alessio 1998, Moore 1989). These either have no controls or are compared to infants exposed to thiopental, and in most cases the conclusions are based on Apgar scores or the lack of need for ventilatory assistance. One of these reports, using the early neonatal neurobehavioral scale (ENNS), found newborns exposed to propofol for cesarean section to have a decrement in some areas of neurobehavioral status when compared with children exposed to thiopental (Celleno 1989, d'Alessio 1998). These effects were always transitory. In another study by Gin (1993), propofol was found to be superior to thiopental when used for anesthesia in women undergoing cesarean section. Animal studies reported by the manufacturer appear negative in the doses used for anesthesia.

2 Pregnancy

2.16 General and local anesthetics and muscle relaxants

> **Recommendation.** Propofol may be used in obstetrics to initiate anesthesia for operations during pregnancy and labor, or for ova transfer and IVF. Newborns should be observed for a depressive effect on the breathing if used in labor.

▶ **Sodium thiopentone (thiopental) and methohexital (sodium brevital)**

Sodium thiopentone is a thiobarbiturate characterized by its rapid action. Thiopentone accumulates in the brain, owing to this organ's large blood supply, where it acts rapidly. Subsequent redistribution to muscle and fat causes the concentration in the brain to fall rapidly below the threshold of anesthetic effectiveness, enabling rapid awakening. There seems to be only one epidemiologic human study showing that this drug, when serving for anesthesia in 152 women, did not increase the rate of congenital anomalies (Heinonen 1977).

Thiobarbiturates can be detected in fetal blood as rapidly as 1 minute after injection, at a concentration only slightly less than that in the mother's blood, but its concentrations in the fetal brain are low as it is rapidly taken up by the fetal liver. With low doses (i.v. up to 5 mg/kg) during labor, no fetal impairment is expected. With higher doses, neonatal respiratory depression may occur (Langanke 1987).

Methohexital (*sodium brevital, barbital*) is also a short-acting barbiturate, administered intravenously as an adjunct anesthetic during surgical procedures, including cesarean section. No human data regarding the safety of this drug in pregnancy are available, but it is widely used without any reported deleterious effects on pregnancy outcome (Cohen 1971). It readily crosses the placenta in both directions, thus fetal concentrations are similar to those in the mother (Herman 2000).

In animal studies, both drugs did not seem to increase the rate of congenital anomalies among the offspring of mice, rats or rabbits treated with this drug during pregnancy (Persaud 1965).

> **Recommendation.** Short-acting barbiturates like sodium thiopentone may be used to initiate anesthesia for operations during pregnancy. When given during labor, newborns should be observed for a depressive effect on breathing.

2.16.5   Local anesthetics

Local anesthetics, if absorbed, may stimulate the central nervous system and inhibit electrical stimulation of the heart. *Noradrenaline* (*norepinephrine*) or *adrenaline* (*epinephrine*) are often added to produce vasoconstriction, limiting local anesthetic uptake by the circulatory system. Local anesthetics are either esters, which are quickly deactivated in tissue by non-specific esterases, or amides, which are more slowly deactivated by amidases. Generally, these local anesthetics are well-tolerated in all phases of pregnancy, and they seem to have no effect on the neurophysiologic state of the newborn. Local anesthetics, whether injected into various organs, the epidural space or the cerebrospinal fluid, can also reach the fetus. Following epidural anesthesia, cord blood levels were about half the maternal blood levels (Guay 1992, Sakuma 1985). In pudendal nerve block, the levels in cord blood are much lower (Sakuma 1985). No specific teratogenic effects have been described in human beings after treatment with local anesthetics in pregnancy.

▶ Lidocaine

This widely used local anesthetic is able to cross the placenta, but it does not seem to have any adverse effect on pregnancy outcome. In prospective studies of more than 1200 pregnant women, there was no increase in major or minor anomalies (Heinonen 1977).

Lidocaine is also used for epidural analgesia in labor, to alleviate the pain without affecting uterine contractions. However, lidocaine is transferred to the fetus (Guay 1992, Sakuma 1985), and several adverse effects have been demonstrated, albeit rarely. They include transient alterations of fetal cardiopulmonary adaptation (Bozynski 1987), alterations in brain-stem evoked potential (Bozynski 1989, Diaz 1988), and possible loss of fetal thermoregulatory control (Macaulay 1992). Although epidural anesthesia has been associated in some studies with abnormalities of neurobehavioral testing in the neonate, more recent studies have shown that such abnormalities are rare and, if occurring, they are mild or transient (Decocq 1997, Fernando 1997, Guay 1992). Just as rare are the reported loss of thermoregulatory control and possible fetal hyperthermia after epidural anesthesia during prolonged labor (Macaulay 1992). Animal studies have shown transient alterations of neonatal behavior in rat offspring (Smith 1989, 1986). The relevance to humans is unknown.

▶ Bupivacaine and ropivacaine

These agents are often used in epidural and spinal anesthesia for pain relief, as they are believed to have reduced cardiovascular effects. They are transferred through the placenta, with fetal blood levels being about one-third the maternal levels (Kuhnert 1987). Ropivacaine, with its lower cardiovascular toxicity and less intense motor blockade, may have advantages over bupivacaine in epidural pain relief during labor. In a meta-analysis of six studies, significantly lower rates of instrumental deliveries and higher neurological and adaptive capacity scores in neonates at 24 hours postpartum were noted after epidural pain relief with ropivacaine during labor, compared with bupivacaine (Cederholm 1997).

▶ Ethyl chloride (chloroethane)

This is a refrigerant and topical anesthetic agent. There seem to be no data in man, but, owing to its local use and relatively low absorbance, it would appear to be safe during pregnancy. Ethyl chloride has been given by inhalation to pregnant mice without any teratogenic or toxic effects on the offspring (Hanley 1987).

> **Recommendation.** Local anesthetics may be used during pregnancy for infiltration (as in dentistry) and conduction anesthesia. The co-administration of adrenalin or noradrenalin to limit vascular absorption is acceptable, as it reduces absorption into the blood. Older members of this group are often preferred when they offer features such as rapid deactivation, or limited placental transfer due to extensive protein binding (e.g. bupivacaine or etidocaine).

2.16.6 Epidural and spinal analgesia/anesthesia in pregnancy

These methods (epidural anesthesia, spinal anesthesia, or a combination of both methods) are commonly used for pain relief during labor or for cesarean deliveries because they are immediately effective, the failure and complication rates are low, ambulation is possible, and they do not seem to interfere with the progress of labor (Mattingly 2003, Albright 2000). Among the many anesthetics used are *lidocaine*, *bupivacaine*, *ropivacaine*, and *fentanyl*. These agents have already been discussed individually (see above). Most studies looking at the effects of this type of anesthesia on the newborn infant showed some slight and transitory effects, with clearing of symptoms and elimination of the drugs from the infant's circulation within 24 hours. There seem to be no studies on the possible long-term effects of epidural/spinal analgesia on the development of the children.

2.16.7   Muscle relaxants

Muscle relaxants are usually used in surgical anesthesia because most anesthetics alone do not produce sufficient relaxation of the skeletal muscles. In contrast to general and local anesthetics, muscle relaxants cross the blood–brain barrier and the placenta only in limited amounts due to their high degree of ionization and limited lipid solubility. Thus, in fetal tissue these agents achieve only 5–10% of the concentration measured in the maternal blood (Demetriou 1982, Abouleish 1980). Hence, under regular anesthesia, it is presumed that the concentrations of these agents in fetal blood are well below the effective dose for production of fetal muscle relaxation. Indeed, no effects were observed in the fetuses of 25 women treated with tubocurarine in the second or third trimester of pregnancy (Moise 1987). On the other hand, there is one case report of an infant born with multiple congenital joint contractures whose mother was treated with multiple doses of tubocurarine (Jago 1970). Even if this case is indeed a result of tubocurarine injection, it has no resemblance to the doses and mode of administration in surgery. Of the different muscle relaxants in use, *alcuronium, atracurium, cisatracurium, mivacurium, pancuronium, rocuronium*, and *vecuronium* seem to be used to the same extent as tubocurarine. They are all known to block, completely and reversibly, the neuromuscular junctions. Umbilical serum concentrations at term are 10–20% of maternal serum concentrations, which means that transfer to the fetus, although reduced, does take place. However, their use during labor is well tolerated.

▶ **Pancuronium**

There are no human studies on pancuronium in pregnancy. This agent is particularly useful during childbirth. After a maternal dose of 0.03 mg/kg, no side effects were observed in newborns in 800 deliveries (Langanke 1987). It was also used to directly induce fetal paralysis for intrauterine fetal transfusion by injections to the fetus (Moise 1987). Repeated use in rats may result in joint contractures; single daily injections in rats and rabbits seem to have no effect. As stated, this has little relevance to man.

▶ **Atracurium**

Atracurium's use as a fetal muscle relaxant to arrest fetal activity during intrauterine intravascular transfusions has also been described in a small number of cases. One group of investigators concluded that atracurium was superior to pancuronium for this purpose (Mouw 1999).

▶ **Vecuronium**

Some investigators point out the advantage of vecuronium for cesarean sections over other muscle relaxants, as it seems to have negligible residual effects on the fetal heart function and on the newborn (Watson 1996, Das 1993).

▶ **Suxamethonium**

Suxamethonium (succinylcholine) is a depolarizing muscle relaxant. No anomalies were observed in 26 infants born to mothers treated with succinylcholine during pregnancy (Heinonen 1977). Transient respiratory depression has been described after succinylcholine use during labor, but this complication is apparently rare. If the plasma cholinesterase activity is low (as found in 3–4% of the population), the muscle relaxant effect of this agent may be prolonged and can result in apnea in the newborn infant (Cherala 1989). Proper care should be taken to avoid these complications, and hence the lowest effective doses should be administered.

> **Recommendation.** The common muscle relaxants may be used as part of anesthetic regimens during pregnancy and labor, as well as for the purpose of relaxation of fetal muscles. Use of multiple recurrent doses (i.e. for the treatment of tetanus) may cause some harm, but in this indication, the benefit seems to outweigh the possible hazard to the fetus. Use of low doses may reduce the likelihood of fetal side effects.

2.16.8   Occupational exposure to inhalation anesthetics

Pregnant women employed in operating rooms (ORs) may be chronically exposed to physical work load as well as to low doses of waste anesthetic gases. Volatile and gaseous inhalation anesthetics are administered as mixtures in different combinations, and can be delivered to the patient through an endotracheal tube or via a face-mask. Until several years ago, ventilation systems were apparently not efficient enough in preventing exposure to relatively high levels of anesthetics. Modern ORs are usually equipped with scavenging systems which significantly reduce the exposure of the OR staff to the gases. Nevertheless, measurements indicate that the staff may still be exposed to significant levels of waste anesthetic gases, since there is no hermetic way to avoid leakage of these gases into the workspace. The effectiveness of the preventive measures varies from one place to another, and proper maintenance is critical. Workers in dentistry often use nitrous oxide that is not administered via endotracheal tubes. The fact that common anesthetic gases easily cross the placenta means that they may pose a higher risk for the fetus and the mother (Herman 2000, Cordier 1992).

From the occupational safety perspective, different countries have set limits on the operating room air concentrations of anesthetic agents. For example, a maximum concentration of 25 ppm of nitrous oxide in the operating room is recommended in the USA. In Germany, a maximum workplace concentration of 100 ppm is considered harmless. However, it is often difficult to impose these rules, and therefore routine monitoring is advisable.

Over the past three decades, research exploring the effects of inhalation anesthetics on pregnancy has focused on fertility problems and the rate of congenital anomalies. Research findings regarding the effects of anesthetics on the developing fetus have been inconclusive (Tannenbaum 1985, Pharoah 1977). An increased rate of spontaneous abortion has been reported among OR personnel exposed in the course of their work, which has been attributed to chronic exposure to inhalation anesthetics, particularly nitrous oxide (Hemminki 1985, Vessey 1980). In a retrospective study by Rowland (1995), female dental assistants who worked more than 3 hours a week with nitrous oxide, and not using scavenging equipment, had a higher rate of spontaneous abortion. It is, however, difficult to eliminate the possibility that these effects may be a result of confounding factors such as stress, coffee consumption, smoking, and body position, as well as a tendency to miscarriage (Rowland 1995, 1992). Moreover, similar findings have not been confirmed in other epidemiologic studies.

Only a few studies have looked into the effects of maternal occupational exposure to anesthetics on the newborn. Several studies have identified outcomes of low birth weight and shortened gestational age at delivery (Ericson 1979, Rosenberg 1978, Pharoah 1977, Cohen 1971) in occupationally exposed groups. There are very few studies on the long-term development of children born to women occupationally exposed to anesthetic agents. One such study was performed recently (Ratzon 2004). The study population included 40 children (aged 5–13 years) born to female anesthesiologists and nurses working in ORs, who were thus exposed to waste anesthetic gases, and 40 children born to female nurses and physicians who worked in hospitals during their pregnancy but did not work in ORs. No differences were noted, regarding developmental milestones, in the exposed group as newborns or at the ages of 5–13 years. However, the mean score of gross motor ability was significantly lower in the exposed versus the unexposed group, and their scores on the DSM-III-R Parent–Teacher Questionnaire (PTQ), which measures inattention/hyperactivity, was higher in the exposed group, implying a higher rate of inattention. The level of exposure was significantly and negatively correlated with fine motor ability and the IQ score. However, these groups of children are too small to be conclusive.

Occupational exposure to injectable anesthetics does not impose any specific problem in pregnancy.

> **Recommendation.** It is safe to work in modern operating rooms with most volatile anesthetics because of the state-of-the-art scavenging systems in place, but it is important to monitor the concentrations in the air. Levels of anesthetics should not exceed the maximal allowable concentrations (Threshold Limit Value, TLV) for each agent. The data on congenital anomalies are reassuring, while the data on spontaneous abortions and developmental delay need further corroboration. Work with nitrous oxide in rooms without scavenging systems should be reduced in pregnancy, whenever possible.

References

Abboud TK, Kim SH, Henriksen EH et al. Comparative maternal and neonatal effects of halothane and enflurane for cesarean section. Acta Anaesthesiol Scand 1985; 29: 663–8.

Abdel-Rahman MS, Ismail EE. Teratogenic effect of ketamine and cocaine in CF-1 mice. Teratology 2000; 61: 291–6.

Abouleish E, Wingard LB Jr, de la Vega S et al. Pancuronium in cesarean section and its placental transfer. Br J Anaesth 1980; 52: 531–6.

Albright GA, Forster RM. The safety and efficacy of combined spinal and epidural analgesia/anesthesia (6,002 blocks) in a community hospital. Reg Anest Pain Med 1999; 24: 117–25.

Allen GC, Brubaker CL. Human malignant hyperthermia associated with desflurane anesthesia. Anesth Analg 1998; 86: 1328–31.

Baeder CH, Albrecht M. Embryotoxic/teratogenic potential of halothane. Intl Arch Occup Environ Health 1990; 62: 263–71.

Baraka A, Louis F, Dalleh R. Maternal awareness and neonatal outcome after ketamine induction for anesthesia for Cesarean section. Can J Anaesth 1990; 37: 641–4.

Beilin Y, Bodian CA, Mukerjee T et al. The use of propofol, nitrous oxide or isoflurane does not affect the reproductive success rate following gamete intrafalopian transfer (GIFT). Anesthesiology 1999; 90: 36–41.

Bonnin M, Mercier FJ, Sitbon O et al. Severe pulmonary hypertension during pregnancy: mode of delivery and anesthetic management of 15 consecutive cases. Anesthesiology 2005; 102: 1133–7.

Bozynski MEA, Rubarth LB, Patel JA. Lidocaine toxicity after maternal pudendal anesthesia in a term infant with fetal distress. Am J Perinatol 1987; 4: 164–6.

Bozynski MEA, Schumacher RE, Deschener LS et al. Effect of prenatal lignocaine on auditory brain stem evoked response. Arch Dis Child 1989; 64: 934–8.

Brodsky JB, Cohen EN, Brown BW Jr et al. Surgery during pregnancy and fetal outcome. Am J Obstet Gynecol 1980; 138: 1165–7.

Cederholm I. Preliminary risk-benefit analysis of ropivacaine in labour and following surgery. Drug Saf 1997; 16: 391–402.

Celleno D, Capogna G, Thomasseti M et al. Neurobehavioural effects of propofol on the neonate following elective caesarean section. Br J Anaesth 1989; 62: 649–54.

Cherala SR, Eddie DN, Sechzer PH. Placental transfer of succinylcholine causing transient respiratory depression in the newborn. Anaesth Intensive Care 1989; 17: 202–4.

Christiaens F, Janssenswillen C, van Steirteghem AC et al. Comparison of assisted reproductive technology performance after oocyte retrieval under general anaesthesia (propofol) versus paracervical local anaesthetic block. A case controlled study. Hum Reprod 1998; 13: 2456–60.

Cohen EN, Bellville JW, Brown BW Jr. Anaesthesia, pregnancy, and miscarriage: a study of operating room nurses and anaesthetists. Anesthesiology 1971; 35: 343–7.

Cohen-Kerem R, Railton C, Oren D et al. Pregnancy outcome following non-obstetric surgical intervention. Am J Surg 2005; 190: 467–73.

Cordier S, Ha MC, Ayme S et al. Maternal occupational exposure and congenital malformations. Scand J Work Environm Health 1992; 18: 11–17.

Crawford JS, Lewis M. Nitrous oxide in early human pregnancy. Anaesthesia 1986; 41: 900–905.

Dailland P, Cockshott ID, Lirzin JD et al. Intravenous propofol during cesarean section: placental transfer, concentrations in breast milk, and neonatal effects. A preliminary study. Anesthesiology 1989; 71: 827–34.

d'Alessio JG, Ramanathan J. Effects of maternal anesthesia in the neonate. Semin Perinatol 1998; 22: 350–62.

Das S, Bhattacharjee M, Maitra S. Study of neonatal status after use of vecuronium as a muscle relaxant in cesarean section. J Indian Med Assoc 1993; 91: 54–6.

de Amivi D, Delmonte P, Martinnoti L et al. Can anesthesiologic strategies for cesarean section influence newborn jaundice? A retrospective and prospective study. Biol Neonate 2001; 79: 97–102.

Decocq G, Brazier M, Hary L. Serum bupivacaine concentrations and transplacental transfer following repeated epidural administrations in term parturients during labour. Fundam Clin Pharmacol 1997; 11: 365–70.

Demetriou M, Depoix JP, Diakite B et al. Placental transfer of org nc 45 in women undergoing cesarean section. Br J Anaesth 1982; 54: 643–5.

Diaz M, Graff M, Hiatt IM et al. Prenatal lidocaine and the auditory evoked responses in term infants. Am J Dis Child 1988; 142: 160–61.

Doenicke A, Haehl M. Teratogenicity of etomidate. Anaesthesiol Resuscitation 1977; 106: 23–4.

Duncan PG, Pope WD, Cohen MM et al. The safety of anesthesia and surgery during pregnancy. Anesthesiology 1986; 64: 790–94.

Ebi KL, Rice SA. Reproductive and developmental toxicity of anesthetics in humans. In: SA Rice, KA Fish (eds), Anesthetic Toxicity. New York: Raven Press Ltd, 1994, pp. 175–98.

Ericson HA, Källén AJB. Survey of infants born in 1973 or 1975 to Swedish women working in operating rooms during their pregnancy. Anesth Analg 1979; 58: 302–5.

Fernando R, Bonello E, Gill P et al. Neonatal welfare and placental transfer of fentanyl and bupivacaine during ambulatory combined spinal epidural analgesia for labour. Anaesthesia 1997; 52: 517–24.

Fu ES, Scharf JE, Mangar D et al. Malignant hyperthermia involving the administration of desflurane. Can J Anesth 1996; 43: 687–90.

Gin T, O'Meara ME, Kan AF et al. Plasma catecholamines and neonatal condition after induction of anaesthesia with propofol or thiopentone at caesarean section. Br J Anaesth 1993; 70: 311–16.

Guay J, Gaudreault P, Boulanger A et al. Lidocaine hydrocarbonate and lidocaine hydrochloride for cesarean section: transplacental passage and neonatal effects. Acta Anaesthesiol Scand 1992; 36: 722–7.

Hanley TR, Scortichini BH, Johnson KA et al. Effects of inhaled ethyl chloride on fetal development in CF-1 mice. Toxicologist 1987; 7: 189.

Heinonen OP, Slone D, Shapiro S. Birth defects and drugs in pregnancy. Littleton, MA: John Wright-PSG, 1977.

Hemminki K, Vineis P. Extrapolation of the evidence on teratogenicity of chemicals between humans and experimental animals: chemicals other than drugs. Teratogen Carcinogen Mutagen 1985; 5: 251–318.

Herman NL, Li AT, van Decar TK et al. Transfer of methohexital across the perfused human placenta. J Clin Anesth 2000; 12: 25–30.

Hodgkinson R, Bhatt M, Kim SS et al. Neonatal neurobehavioral tests following cesarean section under general and spinal anesthesia. Am J Obstet Gynecol 1978; 132: 670–74.

Hood DD, Holubac DM. Elective repeat cesarean section. Effects of anesthesia type on blood loss. J Reprod Med 1990; 35: 368–72.

Jago RH. Arthrogryposis following treatment of maternal tetanus with muscle relaxants. Arch Dis Child 1970; 45: 277–9.

Jauniaux E, Gulbis B, Shannon C et al. Placental propofol transfer and fetal sedaton during maternal general anaesthesia in early pregnancy. Lancet 1998; 352: 290–91.

Johnston RR, Eger EI, Wilson C. A comparative interaction of epinephrine with enflurane, isoflurane and halothane in man. Anesth Analg 1976; 55: 709–12.

Kochhar MM, Aykac I, Davidson PP et al. Teratologic effects of d 1-2-(o-chlorophenyl)-2-(methylamino) cyclohexanone hydrochloride (ketamine hydrochloride) in rats. Res Commun Chem Pathol Pharmacol 1986; 54: 413–16.

Koëter HBWM, Rodier PM. Behavioral effects in mice exposed to nitrous oxide or halothane: prenatal vs. postnatal exposure. Neurobehav Toxicol Teratol 1986; 8: 189–94.

Krissel J, Kick WF, Leyser KH et al. Thiopentone, thiopentane/ketamine, and ketamine for induction of anaesthesia ceasarean section. Eur J Anaesthosial 1994: 11: 115–22.

Kuczkowski KM. The safety of anaesthetics in pregnant women. Expert Opin Drug Saf 2006; 5: 251–64.

Kuhnert BR, Zuspan KJ, Kuhnert PM et al. Bupivacaine disposition in mother, fetus and neonate after spinal anesthesia for cesarean section. Anesth Analg 1987; 66: 407–12.

Langanke D, Jährig K. Narkotika, Muskelrelaxantien und Lokalanästhetika. In: H Hüller, D Jährig, G Göretzlehner, A Träger A (eds) Arzneimittelanwendung in Schwangerschaft und Stillperiode. Berlin: Volk und Gesundheit, 1987, pp. 105–17.

Levin ED, de Luna R, Uemura E et al. Long term effects of developmental halothane exposure on radial arm maze performance in rats. Behav Brain Res 1990; 36: 147–54.

Macaulay JH, Bond K, Steer PJ. Epidural analgesia in labor and fetal hyperthermia. Obstet Gynecol 1992; 80: 665–8.

Mattingly JE, d'Alessio J, Ramanathan J. Effects of obstetric analgesics and anesthetics on the neonate: a review. Paediatr Drugs 2003; 5: 615–27.

Mazze RI, Fujinaga M, Rice SA et al. Reproductive and teratogenic affects of nitrous oxide, halothane, isoflurane and enflurane in Sprague-Dawley rats. Anesthesiology 1986; 64: 339–44.

Mazze RI, Källén B. Reproductive outcome after anesthesia and operation during pregnancy. A registry study of 5405 cases. Am J Obstet Gynecol 1989; 161: 1178–85.

Moise KR Jr, Carpenter RJ Jr, Kirshon B et al. The use of fetal neuromuscular blockade during intrauterine procedures. Am J Obstet Gynecol 1987; 157: 874–9.

Moore J, Bill KM, Flynn RJ. A comparison between propofol and thiopentone as induction agents in obstetric anesthesia. Anaesthesia 1989; 44: 758–62.

Mouw RJ, Klumper F, Hermans J et al. Effect of atracurium or pancuronium on the anemic fetus during and directly after intravascular intrauterine transfusion. A double blind randomized study. Acta Obstet Gynecol Scand 1999; 78: 763–7.

Natsume N, Miura S, Sugimoto S et al. Teratogenicity caused by halothane, enflurane and sevoflurane and changes depending on O_2 concentrations. Teratology 1990; 42: 30A.

Ong BY, Baron K, Stearns EL et al. Severe fetal cradycardia in a pregnant surgical patient despite normal oxygenation and blood pressure. Canad J Anaest 2003; 50: 922–5.

Persaud TVN. Animal experimental studies on the problem of the teratogenic effect of barbiturates. Acta Biol Med Ger 1965; 14: 89–90.

Pharoah PO, Alberman E, Doyle P. Outcome of pregnancy among women in anesthetic practice. Lancet 1977; 1: 34–6.

Polvi HJ, Pirhonen JP, Erkkola RU. Nitrous oxide inhalation: effects on maternal and fetal circulation at term. Obstet Gynecol 1996; 87: 1045–8.

Ratzon NZ, Ornoy A, Pardo A et al. Developmental evaluation of children born to mothers occupationally exposed to waste anesthetic gases. Birth Def Res A 2004; 70: 476–82.

Reddy BK, Pizer B, Bull PT. Neonatal serum cortisol suppression by etidomate compared with thiopentone for elective caesarean section. Eur J Anaesthesiol 1988; 5: 171–6.

Reich DL, Silvay G. Ketamine: an update on the first twenty-five years of clinical experience. Can J Anaesth 1989; 36: 186–97.

Rice SA. Behavioral effects of in utero isoflurane exposure in young SW mice. Teratology 1986; 33: C100–101.

Rice SA. Reproductive and development toxicity of anesthetics in animals. In: SA Rice, FK Fish (eds), Anesthetic Toxicity. New York: Raven Press, 1994, pp. 157–74.

Rodier PM, Koëter HBWM. General activity from weaning to maturity in mice exposed to halothane or nitrous oxide. Neurobehav Toxicol Teratol 1986; 8: 195–9.

2

Pregnancy

2.16 General and local anesthetics and muscle relaxants

Rosenberg PH, Vanttinen H. Occupational hazards to reproduction and health in anaesthetists and pediatricians. Intl J Epidemiol 1978; 11: 250–56.

Rowland AS, Baird DD, Weinberg CR et al. Reduced fertility among women employed as dental assistants exposed to high levels of nitrous oxide. N Engl J Med 1992; 327: 993–7.

Rowland AS, Baird DD, Shore DL et al. Nitrous oxide and spontaneous abortion in female dental assistants. Am J Epidemiol 1995; 141: 531–8.

Sakuma S, Oka T, Okuno A et al. Placental transfer of lidocaine and elimination from newborns following obstetrical epidural and pudendal anesthesia. Pediatr Pharmacol 1985; 5: 107–15.

Schwartz DA, Moriarty KP, Tasjian DB et al. Anesthetic management of the EXIT (ex utero intrapartum treatment) procedure. J Clin Anesth 2001; 13: 387–91.

Schwetz BA, Becker BA. Embryotoxicity and fetal malformations of rats and mice due to maternally administered ether. Toxicol Appl Pharmacol 1970; 17: 275.

Smith RF, Wharton GG, Kurtz SL et al. Behavioral effects of mid-pregnancy administration of lidocaine and mepivacaine in the rat. Neurobehav Toxicol Teratol 1986; 8: 61–8.

Smith RF, Kuurkjian MF, Mattran KM et al. Behavioral effects of prenatal exposure to lidocaine in the rat: effects of dosage and of gestational age at administration. Neurotoxicol Teratol 1989; 11: 395–403.

Tannenbaum TN, Goldberg RJ. Exposure to anesthetic gases and reproductive outcome. J Occup Med 1985; 27: 659–68.

Taylor DJ, Nelson J, Howie PW. Neurodevelopmental disability: a sibling-control study. Dev Med Child Neurol 1993; 35: 957–64.

Tunstall ME, Sheikh A. Comparison of 1.5% enflurane with 1.25% isoflurane in oxygen for caesarean section: avoidance of awareness without nitrous oxide. Br J Anaesth 1989; 62: 138–43.

USP DI: Etomidate. In: USP Dissensing information, Vol I. Drug Information for the Health Care Professional, 23rd edn. Greenwood Village, CO: Thomson Micromedex, 2003, p. 1285.

Vessey MP, Nunn JF. Occupational hazards of anesthesia. Br Med J 1980; 281: 696–8.

Watson WJ, Atchison SR, Harlass FE. Comparison of pancuronium and vecuronium for fetal neuro-muscular blockade during invasive procedures. J Matern Fetal Med 1996; 5: 151–4.

Wharton RS, Mazze RI, Wilson AI. Reproduction and fetal development in mice chronically exposed to enflurane. Anesthesiology 1981; 54: 505–10.

Dermatological medications and local therapeutics

2.17

Paul Peters and Christof Schaefer

In this chapter, the most important dermatological medications as well as other frequently used local therapies will be discussed. More extensive information on many medications can be found under the substance headings in other chapters. Vaginal therapeutics are discussed in Chapter 2.14.

2.17.1 Typical skin changes during pregnancy

The adaptation of the organism during pregnancy leads to typical morphological and functional changes in the skin. These are completely normal and do not need treatment. They include the following:

- *Pigmentation.* Spotty hyperpigmentation (melasma) may appear on the face, and usually disappears spontaneously after birth.

This is intensified by exposure to UV light (i.e. to direct sunlight), and using sun block can minimize it. Additionally, pigmentation of the nipples and the areola, the area around the navel, the armpits, and the genital and anal regions is intensified. In general, sensitivity to light is increased in pregnancy.

- *Striae.* During the second half of pregnancy, striae distensae appear relatively often on the stomach, the hips, the thighs and the breasts. As body size increases, these become wider and more plentiful. The skin in the area around the striae is thin, flabby, and inelastic. There is no known physical measure or drug that is effective as prophylaxis.
- *Fibroma.* Soft fibromata appear more frequently during pregnancy, especially in the neck and axillary regions.
- *Blood vessel changes.* Blood circulation in the skin is increased; it feels warm, and the vasomotor excitability of the vessels in the face increases. This can lead to quick blushing and blanching, and to increased dermatographism. In addition, the veins in the breast and stomach skin are much more visible, and varicosities in the legs and the vulva, as well as hemorrhoids, may appear.
- *Skin glands, hair and nails.* Especially in early pregnancy, the secretion of the sebaceous glands can increase significantly. Acne frequently improves. On the other hand, an acute pregnancy acne (acne gravidarum) can occur during the third month. This disappears during the postpartum period. The growth of hair on the head and of nails is generally enhanced during pregnancy. After birth, hair loss often seems quite threatening; however, this synchronal transition from anagen to telogen hair is fully physiologic, and usually returns to normal over the next few months postpartum. It does not require therapy.

Topically applied substances are absorbed in greater quantities during pregnancy. This applies especially to skin that has been altered by infection, and to sore areas; this can lead to increased exposure to the system and thus to the fetus.

2.17.2   Anti-infective agents

▶ **Local antibiotics**

Pharmacology and toxicology

Fusidin acid is an antibiotic used almost exclusively topically, for which, despite it having been introduced to the market quite some time ago, there are no systematic studies on its tolerability during pregnancy. It has only a narrow effectiveness spectrum against gram-positive bacteria (staphylococci), and for this reason is not recommended for non-specific treatment. Basically, every external antibiotic therapy must be critically examined from the perspective of whether there is a bacterial infection that might possibly be more effectively treated systemically. In addition, sensibilization and the development of bacteriological resistance need to be considered with topical antibiotic treatment. With acne therapy, the bacteriostatic *sodium sulfacetamide*, mostly in combination with sulfur preparations, is topically applied. The skin resorption is approximately 4%, according to Akhavan (2003). There are no safety data for the application of sodiumsulfacetamide and *silversulfadiazine* during pregnancy; the latter is used as prophylaxis against infected burns. Twelve pregnant women topically treated with *neomycin* (seven exposures in the first trimester) were reported. Follow-up did not mention developmental disorders (Akhavan 2003).

No data are available related to the specific locally-used antibiotics *framycetine, meclocycline, mupirocine, nadifloxacine*, and *tyrothricine*.

There has been no suspicion of teratogenic effects with any topically used anti-infectives. Antibiotics that can be used systematically can be used topically (see Chapter 2.6).

► Local antimycotics

See Chapter 2.6.

► Local antivirals

No risk during pregnancy has been identified for the virostatic *acyclovir* (see also extensive experience with sytemic use during pregnancy, Chapter 2.6) or for local treatment for condylomata acuminata (venereal warts) with *podophyllotoxin*, a plant-based mitosis inhibitor (Robert 1994, Bargman 1988, Karol 1980).

There are reports on eight pregnant women with condylomata acuminata who were treated with *imiquimode*, an immune modulator and virostatic for topical application. Two were exposed during the first trimester; all newborn were healthy (Einarson 2006, Maw 2004).

There is insufficient experience available using the virustatics *sodium foscarnet, idoxuridine, penciclovir, tromantadine*, and *vidarabine*. For further information concerning individual anti-infectives, see Chapter 2.6.

Recommendation. Anti-infectives may be used on the skin, the mucosa, and even in the eye and ear for the appropriate indications during pregnancy. For theoretical reasons, the best-tested substances should also be the first choice for topical usage; however, *chloramphenicol* should not be used. For usage over wide skin areas, preparations should be viewed as critically as systemic usage because of the danger of absorbing larger amounts of the agent. For *condylomata acuminata* during pregnancy, cryotherapy or *trichloroacetic acid* are the treatments of choice.

2.17.3   Antiseptics and disinfectants

Disinfectants should have a strong bactericidal or bacteriostatic action, and skin, mucosa, and wounds should tolerate them well. In addition, they should not cause systemic toxic effects when they are absorbed.

▶ **Alcohol**

Pharmacology and toxicology

No toxic effects have been observed, as yet, from the local topical use of alcohols during pregnancy. *Ethanol* and *isopropyl alcohol (isopropanol)* are the primary alcohols used.

Recommendation. Alcohols may be used topically as disinfectants during pregnancy.

▶ **Benzoyl peroxide**

Pharmacology and toxicology

Benzoyl peroxide is used, in particular, for external treatment of acne. Approximately 5% is absorbed. It is converted to benzoic acid in the skin. Concurrent topical therapy with retinoids increases the absorption of these agents. Benzoyl peroxide is also used in the food and plastics industries. There are insufficient experimental or epidemiological data for a risk assessment; however, there are also no case reports indicating teratogenic effects.

Recommendation. Benzoyl peroxide in therapeutic concentrations may be used topically on a limited area (i.e. the face) to treat acne.

Povidone iodine

Pharmacology and toxicology

When *povidone iodine* is used as a local disinfectant on intact skin, on wounds and on the mucosa as well as in body cavities, iodine transfer to the fetus must be assumed. This can lead to functional disturbances in the fetal thyroid gland. The intake of iodine from a vaginal douche during labor can lead to a temporary TSH-increase in the newborn's blood – a sign of transient hypothyroidism (Weber 1998). This should be considered in the interest of the undisturbed thyroid status necessary for central nervous system differentiation. Retrospective evaluation of children born to mothers who applied iodine vaginal douching did not show indications of teratogenic effects (Czeizel 2004). However, this study did not identify the time of exposure or usage during pregnancy.

> **Recommendation.** Iodine-containing disinfectants may only be used during pregnancy on small areas for a few days. Body cavities should not be cleaned with iodine-containing solutions. However, its use is not connected to any irreversible damage.

Phenol derivatives

Pharmacology and toxicology

Phenol derivatives are used primarily in over-the-counter preparations for rinsing the mouth, disinfecting the skin, and treating perianal infections. Solutions of phenol derivatives, such as *cresol* and *thymol*, as well as the chlorinated phenol derivatives (i.e. *4-chlorocresol* and *triclosan*) are viewed as relatively safe during pregnancy (see, for example, Bhargava 1996). They should not be used in a concentration stronger than 2%, and should only be used on intact skin. With higher concentrations, incremental absorption must be assumed.

Chlorhexidine is appropriate for pregnant women to disinfect the skin and mucosa. It is effective as a disinfectant of the vagina and vulva before birth, and for the abdomen before cesarean section (Briggs 2005).

In contrast, caution should be exercised during pregnancy with the neurotoxic phenol derivative *hexachlorophene*, because when larger areas are treated with concentrations of more than 3%, poisoning, with central nervous system symptoms, has been observed in treated patients (Lockhart 1972). In some animal studies, hexachlorophene has been shown to be teratogenic (Kimmel 1972). In many publications over the last decades, workplace contact with hexachlorophene has been controversially discussed with respect to fetotoxic effects. A Swedish study of medical staff, involving about 3000 pregnant women who were occupationally exposed and 1653 control pregnancies, did not report an increase in perinatal death or congenital malformations (Baltzar 1979). A further retrospective study associated mental retardation in 306 children from women with, among others, hexachlorophene exposure in the last trimester (Roeleveld 1993).

> **Recommendation.** Hexachlorophene should be avoided during pregnancy. However, accidental use requires no action. Pregnant women should use the other phenol derivatives mentioned, such as chlorhexidine, for disinfecting the skin and mucosa.

▶ Mercury compounds

Pharmacology and toxicology

Mercury can be substantially absorbed from external use, and is a potential developmental toxicant (Lauwerys 1987; see also Chapters 2.23 and 4.18).

> **Recommendation.** Mercury-containing disinfectants are contraindicated. However, their accidental limited application does not justify either a pregnancy interruption or additional diagnostic procedures.

▶ Other antiseptics

Pharmacology and toxicology

Quinoline sulfate has been discussed with respect to mutagenic properties (Andersen 2006). *Clioquinol* is one of the iodine-containing antiseptics. *Gentian violet* or *crystal violet* has been in widespread use for many years. In animal studies, there are indications of a carcinogenic activity, and contradictory data on teratogenicity (Aidoo 1990, Au 1978). Neither of these has been confirmed as yet in humans. There have also been no adverse effects described for *pyoktanin* as a result of use in pregnancy. However, there are no systematic studies on prenatal toxicity for these substances. The same can be said about *ethacridine*, used for purulent skin infections.

> **Recommendation.** Short-term topical use of the substances mentioned, over limited areas, is acceptable for relevant indications.

Glucocorticoids and nonsteroid anti-inflammatory drugs

Pharmacology and toxicology

When glucocorticoids (see also Chapter 2.15) or nonsteroid anti-inflammatory drugs such as *bufexamac* are applied regularly over larger areas of skin, absorption through the skin and transfer to the fetus must be assumed.

Mygind (2002) found no greater risk for developmental disorders, or difference in birth data, in 363 children born to mothers who had used topical glucocorticoids (170 during the first trimester) (see also Chapter 2.15).

There are no systematic studies for *bufexamac*, which is used widely in dermatology. Furthermore, there are no studies on other topically applied nonsteroid anti-inflammatory substances such as *levomenol* and *benzydamine*. NSAIDs for systemic treatment have not, as yet, shown any teratogenic effects (see Chapter 2.1).

> **Recommendation.** There is no objection to topical therapy with glucocorticoids or bufexamac, as long as treatment time is brief and the area covered is moderately sized. Because of their prostaglandin antagonism, nonsteroid anti-inflammatory drugs should be limited to small areas after the thirtieth week of gestation.

2.17.4   Astringents

Pharmacology and toxicology

In mucosa and in wounds, astringents lead (via protein precipitation) to sealing and shriveling of the surface layers of tissue. They are used for local treatment of inflamed mucosa and wounds. Two groups are used therapeutically – tannin-containing preparations, and dilute solutions of metal salts e.g. aluminum aceticum and zinc salts.

> **Recommendation.** There is no problem in treatment with astringents during pregnancy, as their absorption is not likely.

2.17.5   Polidocanol

Pharmacology and toxicology

Polidocanol is used externally in cases of itching. In addition, it is used intravenously to obliterate varicose veins, for lesions of the mouth mucosa, in vaginal spermicides, and in cosmetics. Polidocanol in combination with *benzethonium* and *carbamide* (*urea*) has been applied in wound therapeutics. No teratogenic action has been observed to date, in either animal or human studies, for this widely used substance. However, there have been no systematic studies published.

> **Recommendation.** Pregnant women may use polidocanol in cases of itching.

2.17.6   Camphor and menthol

Pharmacology and toxicology

A small amount of *camphor* applied to the skin has a cooling and local anesthetic effect. Rubbing it in vigorously enhances the circulation to the skin. Because of these effects, camphor and other essential oils are included in a large number of hyperemia-causing dermatological products.

Menthol is used topically for itching. No teratogenic action has, as yet, been observed in either animal or human studies for topical application.

> **Recommendation.** Camphor and other essential oils may be used topically during pregnancy.

2.17.7   Coal tar and slate oil preparations

Pharmacology and toxicology

Coal tar as treatment for neurodermatitis has not been suspected of having a teratogenic effect. A retrospective study of 23 exposed women revealed nothing notable (Franssen 1999). Experimentally, coal tar products have, to some extent, demonstrated mutagenic or carcinogenic properties, but there has not yet been any indication of this in the longstanding and well-tried use of the group of substances employed therapeutically in humans.

The slate oil extracts *ammonium bitumen sulfonate* and *sodium bitumen sulfonate* are used topically for chronically inflamed dermatitis and other indications. There are no systematic studies on prenatal toxicity, but also no indications of teratogenic effects in humans.

> **Recommendation.** Coal tar preparations should ideally not be used in pregnancy; however, accidental use does not require any action. The use of slate oil extracts is acceptable.

2.17.8   Local immunomodulators and neurodermatitis therapy

Pharmacology and toxicology

Tacrolimus and *pimecrolimus* are used as local treatment for neurodermatitis. Although there are no studies regarding topical use, these exist for systemic use of tacrolimus in transplant medicine (see Chapter 2.12).

The results do not indicate a risk of developmental disorders. Obviously, serum levels after local treatment with tacrolimus are much lower than in transplant patients. Therefore, this substance can be used topically when there are no acceptable alternatives. There are no data related to pimecrolimus.

> **Recommendation.** When no alternatives exist, topical use on small surfaces is permissible. The use of pimecrolimus is not advised, but if it is used then no invasive prenatal diagnostics are indicated and certainly there is no reason for termination of pregnancy.

2.17.9   Keratolytics

▶ Salicylate and carbamide preparations

Pharmacology and toxicology

Keratolytics are used to soften the keratin layer and for loosening scales. *Salicylates* are used as keratolytics in 2–10% solutions, or in 30–50% solutions in petroleum jelly for treatment of warts.

Carbamide preparations are used in 10% solutions. Systemic effects would not be expected, even in pregnancy, when used for the appropriate indications.

> **Recommendation.** Topical use of the keratolytics mentioned above is no cause for concern with pregnant women when the medications are used on limited areas for limited periods of time.

▶ Calcipotriol and dithranol

Pharmacology and toxicology

Calcipotriol is a vitamin D_3 derivative. Generally, D-hypervitaminosis should be avoided during pregnancy. However, use in the recommended dosage range ($\leqslant 100\,g$/week of a 0.005% solution) does not lead to a disturbance in calcium homeostasis.

Systematic studies on prenatal toxicity in humans are lacking here, as they are with *dithranol*. As an antimitotic substance, it is theoretically suspect for pregnant women, though substantial absorption of the preparation (usually 1–3%) is not likely. There is no information on the topical use of the vitamin D derivative *tacalcitrol* during pregnancy. It is comparable to calcipotriol.

> **Recommendation.** The above-mentioned substances should not be used over large areas, especially in the presence of inflammatory changes in the skin that make absorption more likely.

▶ Selenium disulfide

Pharmacology and toxicology

Selenium disulfide is used as a topical antifungal in the treatment of tinea vesicolor, as a topical keratolytic, and is applied topically to the scalp to control seborrheic dermatitis and dandruff. There are no systematic data implicating teratogenicity.

> **Recommendation.** Local application in small areas and for a limited period is acceptable.

Azelaic acid

Pharmacology and toxicology

Azelaic acid (nonanedioic acid) is an oxidation product of oleic acid occurring in rancid fats. It has anti-inflammatory, antibacterial, and keratolytic effects. It is also used in acne therapy. About 4–8% of the topically applied substance is absorbed systemically. Animal experiments have not shown teratogenicity (Akhavan 2003). Epidemiologic studies are lacking.

Recommendation. Azelaic acid is only to be used in pregnancy when absolutely necessary, on small skin surfaces, and preferably not during the first trimester. When used in pregnancy, there is no justification for invasive prenatal diagnostics or termination of pregnancy.

Precipitated sulfur

Pharmacology and toxicology

Sulfur (milk of sulfur) is present (at 2–10%) in lotions, creams, and powders, and is used as a mild keratolytic and bacteriostatic treatment. The bioavailability of topical sulfur is about 1% (Akhavan 2003). There are no data on its use during pregnancy.

Recommendation. When there is an indication for sulfur, it can be used on small skin areas in pregnancy. Systemic activity is unlikely.

Resorcin

Pharmacology and toxicology

Resorcin is an aromatic alcohol that is used in local acne therapy and in the treatment of other dermatoses as a bactericidal, fungicidal, keratolytic, exfoliative, and antipruritic agent, and for seborrheic dermatitis and psoriasis. It is also to be found in cosmetics and hair dye. There are no indications for teratogenicity. Systematic epidemiological research is lacking.

Recommendation. Topical treatment on a small area with resorcin, when indicated, is acceptable during pregnancy.

2

Pregnancy

2.17 Dermatological medications and local therapeutics

2.17.10   Retinoids for acne and psoriasis therapy

Pharmacology

Isotretinoin (*13-cis-retinoic acid*) and *tretinoin* (all-trans-retinoic acid) are natural derivatives of vitamin A (retinol). In synthetic derivate form, they have been used with great success for over 20 years, both externally and systemically, to treat cystic acne. Tretinoin is also licensed as a systemic preparation for treating promyelocytic leukemia. As far as we know today, tretinoin is identical to the body's own growth factor, which is in all cells and is bound to specific retinoid receptors (Committee on Developmental Toxicology 2000). Retinoic acid has a very important role during the embryonic phase because it controls, among other things, the development of the brain, face, thymus, heart, and spinal cord.

Retinoids also stimulate the proliferation of epidermal cells. In the skin, they loosen the keratin layer and in this way ease the scaling process. Isotretinoin also causes the sebaceous glands to atrophy. This explains its effectiveness in acne therapy. The half-lives of isotretinoin and of its metabolite, *4-oxo-isotretinoin*, are, on average, 29 hours and 22 hours respectively. In extreme cases the half-lives can be up to a week (Nulman 1998).

Acitretin and *etretinate* (which is now no longer sold) have proved themselves in the treatment of psoriasis. Both lead to prolonged high concentrations of retinoids in the body. Acitretin is metabolized to etretinate, which has a half-life of 80–175 days. A correlation has been established between alcohol consumption and increasing etretinate serum levels (Larsen 2000).

Adapalene belongs to the synthetic, polyaromatic, receptor-selective retinoids. These are indicated for the treatment of severe acne vulgaris, and *tazarotine* is indicated for the treatment of psoriasis. Topical treatment of AIDS-associated Kaposi sarcoma can be carried out using the 0.1% gel *alitretinoine*. By activating retinoid receptors, tumor growth will be blocked.

Toxicology

The marked teratogenic properties of retinoids have long been known from experimental animal embryo/fetotoxicology. Today, retinoids should be considered to be the most teratogenic medications since thalidomide. Their use in pregnancy increases the risk for spontaneous abortion, and leads to the characteristic retinoid embryopathy: anomalies of the ears (including agenesis or stenosis of the auditory canal), facial and palatine defects, micrognathia, cardiovascular (conotruncal) defects, and developmental defects of the thymus (with possible immunological consequences) and the central nervous system (ranging from neurological damage to the eyes and inner ear, to hydrocephalus) (Lammer 1988, 1985). Intelligence deficits have also been described to some extent in children without recognizable birth defects (Adams 1991).

Prospective epidemiological studies on maternal intake of isotretinoin showed 40% spontaneous abortions, an increased rate of premature births, and up to 35% major birth defects. Follow-up studies with intrauterine retinoid-exposed children at the age of 5–10 years showed high rates of mental retardation and, specifically, weaknesses in visual-spatial orientation and in behavior. In 25% of the children, no major malformations were diagnosed (Adams 2004).

Even though the scientific community – for example, the Teratology Society (1991) in the USA – has given forceful warnings of the teratogenic risk, children with birth defects due to isotretinoin have continued to be born in North America. Apparently, in many cases the required explanation of the risks is still not effective today (Robertson 2005, Honein 2000). The pharmaceutical companies and the U.S. FDA have received notification of more than 150 cases of children with developmental disorders after intrauterine exposure to isotretinoin.

In a retrospective study in California, 5 of 14 pregnancies where the mothers had isotretinoin therapy were voluntarily terminated, 4 aborted spontaneously, and there were 5 live births, of which only one showed the characteristic malformations (Honein 2001). The fetopathological results from two voluntarily aborted fetuses did not show gross malformations, but there were middle and internal ear anomalies (Moerike 2002). Three casuistic publications (Barbero 2004, de Die-Smulders 1995, Geiger 1994) have described the classical acitretin embryopathy (microcephaly, facial dysmorphology, atrioseptal defect, and bilateral sensorineural deafness). At 18 months, this child showed a persistent microcephaly and retarded neurological development. The mother had taken 10 mg of acitretin daily till the tenth gestational week (Barbero 2004).

From post-marketing studies, 13 acitretin-treated fathers were found (9 retrospective and 4 prospective); 11 fathers had been treated with acitretin until conception, and 2 stopped the therapy between 6 months and 4 weeks before conception. Of the latter, the pregnancy from the last-mentioned treated father ended in a spontaneous abortion, and the other with termination of pregnancy because of unspecified developmental disorders. The outcomes for the 11 fathers treated at least up until conception were 5 healthy children, 5 spontaneous abortions, and 1 termination of pregnancy (Geiger 2002). Furthermore, Geiger (1994) describes 75 pregnancies where the mother was exposed to acitretin either during (8 cases) or before (67 cases) pregnancy. In the group of 8 cases exposed during pregnancy, 4 aborted spontaneously and 2 were electively terminated. There was one typical malformation in a fetus after induced abortion (microtia, and malformations of the face and extremities); the mother had received 50 mg of acitretin daily for the first 19 weeks of pregnancy. In one of the 2 live-born infants, a high-frequency hearing disorder was diagnosed. Of the group of 67 women exposed to acitretin before pregnancy (mean, 5 months before conception), no typical malformations were found where information on the fetus was available.

In the same publication, Geiger (1994) reports on 75 women who underwent etretinate treatment during pregnancy. Of 29 neonates, 6 had typical malformations and 3 had non-typical abnormalities. There were 5 spontaneous abortions, and of the 41 induced abortions for which there was information, 5 fetuses had the typical malformations. Another group of 173 women who underwent etrenitate therapy before pregnancy delivered 88 newborns, of which 5 showed typical malformations and 13 showed non-typical abnormalities (not specified). Thirteen pregnancies ended in induced abortions for which fetal information is available; this shows that three of these fetuses had typical malformations and one had non-typical malformations. The rate of spontaneous abortions was lower when exposure was only before pregnancy. It was concluded that no threshold dose could be established in human therapy, based on these data.

External use

Five case descriptions in the last few years have raised the suspicion that typical retinoid birth defects cannot be absolutely ruled out after topical use of tretinoin (Selcen 2000, Colley 1998, Navarre-Belhassen 1998, Lipson 1993, Camera 1992). Two controlled studies involving a total of 300 pregnant women gave no indication of a teratogenic effect (Shapiro 1997, Jick 1993). However, the larger of these studies was based on prescription protocols from which it cannot be definitively determined that the medication was, in fact, used. In addition, the design and number of cases in this study do not allow the assumption that tretinoin is harmless (Martínez-Frias 1999). A prospective study of 106 tretinoin topically-treated women during the first trimester did not indicate either a higher spontaneous abortion rate or an increased risk of malformations (Loureiro 2005).

Pharmacologically, an average absorption rate of 2% with a maximum of about 6% (van Hoogdalem 1998), the usual concentration of 0.05% in topical retinoid preparations, and evidence that a noteworthy rise in endogenous retinoid concentration in the plasma $(2–5 \, \mu g/1)$ does not occur after external use indicate that a teratogenic effect is unlikely if the treated area and thus the resorption is not very large. Normal circulating levels in women are within that range, while teratogenic levels are much higher (Miller 1998).

The usual daily dosage is a maximum of 2 g of ointment with 1 mg of the active ingredient (0.05%). However, it must be kept in mind that with severely inflamed skin or additional (disinfectant) use (i.e. benzoyl peroxide – see section 2.17.3), the absorption rate may be increased. External use of isotretinoin has to be judged in a similar way to that of tretinoin.

A case report on *adapalene* used until week 13 of pregnancy mentions a terminated pregnancy based upon ultrasonographic diagnosis of cerebral and ocular disorders that are not judged to be typical for retinoids (Autret 1997). A prospective epidemiological study included 94 pregnancies exposed to topical retinoid (tretinoin, isotretinoid or adapalene); no indications for increased spontaneous abortion or higher risk of developmental disorders were found (Carlier 1998). The publication is, however, rather poor in details regarding the time and type of treatment, and dysmorphological criteria.

Topical use of *tazarotene* gives 6% resorption of the application. It has been found to have a half-life of 18 hours. The hydrophilic properties of the metabolites prevent fat storage. General remarks (without details) refer to healthy children being born to mothers who had local application of tazarotene during pregnancy (Menter 2000).

There is no experience with topical treatment with *alitretinoin* during pregnancy.

Recommendation. Systemic therapy with the retinoids, acitretin, etretinate, isotretinoin, and tretinoin, is absolutely contraindicated during pregnancy. For women of childbearing age, treatment is only permitted when other therapeutic measures have not been effective, when there is sufficient contraceptive protection with two separate effective forms of birth control at the same time (Food and Drug Administration 2004), and after ruling out a pregnancy. Reliable contraception must be used for 2 years after stopping acitretin and etretinate, and for a month after ending treatment with isotretinoin. When considerably less time has passed, especially when there has been treatment in early pregnancy, severe damage to embryonic development, including spontaneous abortion, is possible. Diagnostic ultrasonography is indicated in such cases. Hence, in some instances, interruption of the pregnancy must be discussed. For additional information about pregnancy prevention, see www.ipledgeprogram.com.

Topical use of retinoids is also contraindicated during pregnancy. In cases of such therapy in early pregnancy, interruption of pregnancy is unnecessary because of the apparently limited teratogenic risk – if, indeed, there exists any risk at all. However, a detailed fetal ultrasound diagnosis should be planned. There is insufficient experience available concerning the synthetic, polyaromatic receptor selective retinoids adapalene, tzarotine, and alitretinoin.

2.17.11 Photochemotherapy and fumaric acid

Pharmacology and toxicology

Photochemotherapy (PUVA therapy) for extremely severe psoriasis is given either orally or – as preferred today – by external application of *8-methoxypsoralen* followed by long-wave UVA irradiation. The psoralen is activated chemically through the UV light, binds more strongly to the DNA, and damages the cells. The cytotoxic effect of PUVA treatment is minimal because of the limited depth of penetration. The European Network of Teratology Information Services (ENTIS) analyzed 41 pregnancies in which systemic PUVA therapy with 8-methoxypsoralen was administered (Garbis 1993). In this study, in which the PUVA therapy was limited to the first trimester, and in a Scandinavian study (Gunnarskog 1993), no indications of embryotoxic effects were reported.

Fumaric acid is used as an antioxidant, in small amounts, in the food industry. With increasing dosages, it is prescribed as therapy in cases of psoriasis (several hundred milligrams daily); leukopenia and lymphopenia may occur as adverse reactions. There is no information about effects on the unborn. However, one of the current authors (C.S.) has documented data on 15 pregnancies treated during the first trimester for psoriasis with numeric acid. No embryotoxic or teratogenic effects were found (there was one spontaneous abortion and one stillbirth).

> **Recommendation.** Photochemotherapy with 8-methoxypsoralen and UVA irradiation is not recommended during pregnancy because of possible mutagenic effects. However, if there has been treatment it does not justify either an interruption of pregnancy or invasive diagnostic procedures. Because of the topical application and the limited area of application, it is unlikely that these agents have substantial risk of developmental toxicity.

2.17.12 Sex hormones and cyproterone acetate

See also Chapter 2.15.

Pharmacology and toxicology

Androgens, such as testosterone, act directly on hair growth and the sebaceous glands; this explains juvenile acne during puberty. Because of their anti-androgenic properties, a great many sex hormones, such as many progestins/gestagens and estrogens and, in particular, the inhibiting substance *cyproterone acetate*, have an anti-acne action. This effect is used therapeutically. Most widely used is the combination of *ethinylestradiol* and cyproterone acetate in oral contraceptives (see also Chapter 2.15).

> **Recommendation.** Acne therapy with sex hormones and their inhibiting substances is contraindicated during pregnancy. However, inadvertent exposure does not justify either an interruption of pregnancy or invasive diagnostic procedures.

2.17.13   5-Fluorouracil

See also Chapter 2.13.

Pharmacology and toxicology

The cytostatic, *5-fluorouracil*, was not found to cause any embryotoxic effects when used in early pregnancy for local treatment of vaginal condylomata (Koepelman 1990, Odom 1990).

> **Recommendation.** Dermal treatment with 5-fluorouracil is contraindicated in pregnancy, apart from for the treatment of an individual wart. Treatment of vaginal warts should be postponed until after the birth, or other treatments (such as cryotherapy) used instead. Local use of the cytostatic is, however, not an indication for interruption of pregnancy or for invasive diagnostic procedures.

2.17.14   Lithium

Pharmacology and toxicology

Lithium is not only used orally in cases of bipolar disorders (see Chapter 2.11), but also for local treatment of seborrheic dermatitis. Lithium has an anti-inflammatory activity, and the percutaneous resorption is small. Therefore, the plasma concentration is much lower than with oral treatment (Sparsa 2004).

> **Recommendation.** Dermal treatment with lithium is not advisable because of insufficient data. Use of lithium in pregnancy does not justify termination of a wanted pregnancy, or invasive diagnostic measures. Cryotherapy should be used instead. However, (inadvertent) use is not an indication for an interruption of the pregnancy or for invasive diagnostic procedures.

2.17 Dermatological medications and local therapeutics   Pregnancy   2

2.17.15   Scabies and lice medications

Pharmacology and toxicology

Benzyl benzoate, lindane, and the pyrethroid *allethrin* are available for external use in treating scabies. *Ivermectin* is indicated for oral usage. For lice, coconut oil, pyrethrum extract, the pyrethroids *allethrin* and *pyrethrin*, and lindane are used. *Crotamiton* and the pyrithroid *permethrin* are used for both scabies and lice infestations.

Benzyl benzoate was banned in the USA because its metabolite, *benzyl alcohol*, was associated with neonatal fatal intoxication (the "gasping syndrome", with encephalopathy, severe metabolic acidosis, bone marrow depression, and multiple organ failure). However, intoxication occurred only when benzyl alcohol itself was used to rinse central vein catheters. Apart from local skin irritation, there has to date been no substantial toxicity observed after topical application of benzyl benzoate (Fölster-Holst 2000). A prospective study of 113 pregnant women using permethrine shampoo during pregnancy, 31 of them during the first trimester, did not reveal prenatal toxicity (Kennedy 2005, 2003).

Approximately 10% of *lindane* is absorbed through the skin (see also Chapter 4.12). Lindane is potentially neurotoxic. Animal experience has demonstrated that it is stored in fat tissue and in the testes. Damage of Leydig cells has been observed (Suwalsky 2000). According to European environmental guidelines, its use is not permitted after 2007.

The synthetic pyrethroids, *allethrin, permethrin*, and *pyrethrin*, have longer half-lives than the "natural" *pyrethrum*. About 2% of permethrin is absorbed after topical application (Fölster-Holst 2000).

Less than 1% of *crotamiton* is absorbed after dermal application.

No teratogenic effects have been observed with any of the substances mentioned after normal usage.

> **Recommendation.** Scabies should be treated with benzyl benzoate or crotamiton, and lice infestation with coconut oil or pyrethrum extract. Synthetic pyrethroids are the drugs of second choice during pregnancy. Lindane should be avoided; however, if there has been acute topical treatment, no action need be taken.

2.17.16   Diethyltoluamide and icaridin

Pharmacology and toxicology

Mosquito repellents, such as *diethyltoluamide* (*DEET*), are rubbed into or sprayed on the skin. Absorption through the skin is about

8–17% (Sudakin 2003). A mother in Africa who gave birth to a mentally retarded child had not only been using malarial prophylaxis (chloroquine), but also rubbing her arms and legs daily with a 25% DEET lotion (Schaefer 1992). Since DEET has neurotoxic properties and is absorbed through the skin, the authors cannot entirely eliminate a causal connection. However, there are no further reports on toxic effects on prenatal development.

A randomized prospective study covering 449 pregnant women with an average topical application of 1.7 g daily of DEET during the second and third trimesters could not demonstrate any difference in the newborn and the development of the infants up to the age of 1 year compared to the control group. However, DEET was found in 8% of the cord blood specimens (McGready 2001).

There is insufficient documented experience on DEET during the first trimester.

Icaridin is less toxic in general than DEET. There are no studies on its use during pregnancy.

> **Recommendation.** Pregnant women should be advised against using insect repellents of the DEET type on large areas of their bodies for a long time unless there is a strong indication. In areas where the risk of malaria is high (which should only be visited during pregnancy when there are compelling grounds to do so), the risk for both mother and child associated with the use of DEET is still clearly less than the risk of a malarial infection. However, apart from non-chemical protection (covering the skin, etc.), less toxic repellents (including icaridin) should be chosen. The use of DEET in the first trimester justifies neither an interruption of the pregnancy nor invasive diagnostic procedures.

2.17.17   Eye, nose, and ear drops

Eye, nose, and ear drops may generally be used during pregnancy for the appropriate indications. However, medication should be chosen carefully, and questionable combination preparations as well as (pseudo)-innovations should be avoided during pregnancy. Where there is some doubt, the recommendations on systemic therapy in the appropriate chapters can serve as guidance.

Eye drops and glaucoma therapy

With eye drops, quantitative absorption of the medication via the conjunctiva should be considered. For this reason, the possibility that, for example, atropine-like substances and β-receptor blockers

2

Pregnancy

2.17 Dermatological medications and local therapeutics

in the eye drops might reach the fetus and increase or decrease its heart rate cannot be eliminated – and has, in fact, been observed to some extent (e.g. Wagenvoort 1998). However, at-risk situations would not be expected with the doses used in drops for diagnosing long-distance vision or for glaucoma treatment.

The carbonic anhydrase inhibitors *brinzolamide, dorzolamide*, and for systemic application, *acetazolamide*, which are used for glaucoma therapy, have not been systematically studied. A newborn of 34 weeks' gestation was tachypnoic, and a combined respiratory-metabolic acidosis, hypoglycemia, and hypokalemia was diagnosed. Its mother had been treated with 750 mg *azetazolamide* daily during the 3 days prior to delivery. There was 2.9 µg/ml in the blood of the newborn when this was measured 5 hours after birth – almost a therapeutic concentration (3–10 µg/ml). There was no substance detectable on day 11. Further development of the child was uneventful (Ozawa 2001). There were no birth defects or postnatal disorders observed in the newborn of 12 women using, on average, 500 mg azetazolamide daily for idiopathic increased intracranial pressure. Nine of them were exposed during the first trimester (Lee 2005).

De Santis (2004) reported on 10 prospectively recorded pregnancies where the women used *latanoprost* eye drops during the first trimester. One spontaneous abortion occurred, while nine pregnancies resulted in healthy term newborns. Another publication observed normal outcome in two cases after first-trimester exposure (one throughout pregnancy; Johnson 2001).

There is no published experience on *bimatoprost* and *travoprost*.

In general, there has not as yet been any indication for lasting negative effects on the fetus – at least not with the preparations that have been in use for a long time. This also applies to *brimonidine*, and cholinergics such as *pilocarpin* and *clonidine* preparations.

> **Recommendation.** Eye drops may generally be used during pregnancy for the appropriate indications. Since prostaglandins increase uterine tone and can cause reduced perfusion to the fetus, general caution is advised. However, if there are compelling treatment indications in a case of severe glaucoma, they should not be withheld. The dosage should be kept as low as therapeutically possible.

▶ **Nasal decongestants**

There are no systematic studies on the embryotoxicity of nasal decongestant drops or sprays. However, these *xylometazoline* and *oxymetazoline* preparations, which are very frequently used during pregnancy, have not as yet been shown to be a risk for the fetus, although theoretically they could (in high doses) cause reduced circulation to the fetus as a result of systemic vasoconstriction (see also section 2.3.12). However, there is no reason for concern about this with the usual dosages. Many women (including pregnant women) take nasal decongestants for months instead of the recommended period of a few days. In the interest of their own nasal mucosa, which can be damaged by the medication, a "withdrawal" strategy is recommended.

There is no specific information on the use of *indanazoline, naphazoline, tetryzoline*, and *tramazoline* during pregnancy.

> **Recommendation.** If nasal decongestant drops or sprays are needed during pregnancy, xylometazoline or oxymetazoline are preferred. The dosage and treatment interval should be kept as low as possible. Physiological sodium chloride solution or steam inhalation may be considered as alternatives.

▶ Other eye, nose, and ear preparations

Glucocorticoids, cromoglicic acid, antihistamines, antibiotics, and *acyclovir*, as well as "artificial tears" such as, for instance, *povidone*, may be used for the appropriate indications. The antibiotic *chloramphenicol* should not be used (see Chapter 2.6). Nasal or inhalative application of *budesonide* (Källén 2003) or nasal *fluticason* (Ellegard 2001) has not been associated with developmental disorders in the newborn. There is no specific experience yet with loteprednol during pregnancy.

2.17.18 Hemorrhoid medications

Pharmacology and toxicology

Hemorrhoid medications (salves and suppositories) are local therapeutics which, for the most part, contain local anesthetics, glucocorticoids, antibiotics, and disinfectants, either as individual substances or in combination. These preparations are also used following surgical procedures in the rectal–anal area. Substantial absorption is not to be expected. There are no reports on fetal toxicity of the usual hemorrhoid medications.

> **Recommendation.** The usual hemorrhoid medications have proved to be safe during pregnancy.

2.17.19 Vein therapeutics

Aescin preparations (horse chestnut extract) for vein complaints during pregnancy do not appear to be a problem for pregnant women or their fetuses; however, they have not been sufficiently studied.

Sclerotherapy for varicosities, as with *polidocanol*, may be used during pregnancy if urgently needed.

2.17.20 Antihidrotica

Pharmacology and teratology

Methinamine salve is a topical therapeutic used in cases of excessive sweating. There have been no systematic studies regarding the safety of this substance during pregnancy. The resorption from local application is low. There is no documented experience with intracutaneous application of *C. botulinum toxin* (botox) preparations. However, the risk for systemic toxicity is remote (see also section 2.22.8).

> **Recommendation.** Methinamide can be used in pregnancy when it is applied on a small skin area. *C. botulinum* toxin must not be used in pregnancy. However, inadvertent exposure does not justify either interruption of pregnancy or invasive diagnostic procedures.

2.17.21 Minoxidil

Pharmacology and teratology

Minoxidil is used orally as a systemic antihypertensive drug with vasodilatory activity. Topically, it is used in cases of androgenetic alopecia and other types of baldness. The ingredient is lipophylic, and the resorption rate is 2–3%. The concentrations in the serum are far below therapeutic levels in adults. In a prospective study, 17 pregnant women were treated with minoxidil. Of 15 newborns, 1 had an unspecified developmental disorder of the heart (Shapiro 2003). A case report (Smorlesi 2003) describes a woman who applied minoxidil to her scalp at least twice daily during pregnancy. Fetal pathology revealed an enlarged heart with distal stenosis of the aorta, an enlarged sigmoid colon and mesentery, and enlarged cerebral ventricles with brain hemorrhages. The placenta had numerous ischemic and indurative areas, and a discrepancy between gestational age and villi maturation. Another publication reveals a developmental sacral disorder and malformation of the lower extremities, lower vertebral aplasia, agenesis of both kidneys, and an atresic esophagus in a severely hypertrophic fetus born to a mother who had used minodil for years (Rojanski 2002).

There is no experience with *eflornithin* for hirsutism during pregnancy.

2

Pregnancy

> **Recommendation.** Since there are no conclusive studies, neither oral nor topical treatment with minoxidil is acceptable during pregnancy. However, inadvertent exposure does not justify either interruption of pregnancy or invasive diagnostic procedures. The same holds for eflornithin.

2.17.22   Cosmetics

Cosmetics and hair products, including those for coloring and permanent waves, may be used in usual quantities – especially if this makes the pregnant woman happier! However, labels should be checked for ingredients, and products from ethical manufacturers should be used. Contamination of products with environmental contaminants, such as lead, have been reported in products from lesser-known manufacturers.

References

Adams J, Lammer EJ. Relationship between dysmorphology and neuropsychological functions in children exposed to isotretinoin (in utero). In: T. Fujii, GJ Boer (eds), Functional Neuroteratology of Short Term Exposure to Drugs. Tokyo: Teiko University Press, 1991, pp. 159–68.

Adams J. The adverse effect profile of neurobehavioral teratogens: retinoic acid. Birth Def Res A 2004; 70: 344.

Aidoo A, Gao N, Neft RE et al. Evaluation of the genotoxicity of gentian violet in bacterial and mammalian cell systems. Teratogen Carcinogen Mutagen 1990; 10: 449–62.

Akhavan A, Bershad S. Topical acne drugs. Am J Clin Dermatol 2003; 4: 473–92.

Andersen A. Final amended report on the safety assessment of oxyquinoline and oxyquinoline sulfate as used in cosmetics. Intl J Toxicol 2006; 25 (Suppl 1): 1–9.

Au W, Pathak S, Collie CJ et al. Cytogenetic toxicity of gentian violet and crystal violet on mammalian cells *in vitro*. Mutat Res 1978; 58: 269–76.

Autret E, Berjot M, Jonville-Bera AP et al. Anophthalmia and agenesis of optic chiasma associated with adapalene gel in early pregnancy. Lancet 1997; 350: 339.

2.17   Dermatological medications and local therapeutics

Baltzar B, Ericson A, Källén B et al. Delivery outcome in women employed in medical occupations in Sweden. J Occup Med 1979; 21: 543–8.

Barbero P, Lotersztein V, Bronberg R et al. Acitretin embryopathy: a case report. Birth Def Res A 2004; 70: 831–3.

Bargman H. Is podophyllin a safe drug to use and can it be used in pregnancy? Arch Dermatol 1988; 124: 1718–20.

Bhargava HN, Leonard PA. Triclosan: applications and safety. Am J Infect Control 1996; 24: 209–18.

Briggs GG, Freeman RK, Yaffe SJ. Drugs in Pregnancy and Lactation, 7th edn. Baltimore, MD: Williams & Wilkins, 2005.

Camera G, Pregliasco P. Ear malformation in baby born to mother using tretinoin cream {Letter}. Lancet 1992; 339: 687.

Carlier P, Choulika S, Dally S. Topical retinoids exposure in pregnancy. Cooperative Study from January 1992 to April 1997: 132 cases and 94 with known pregnancy outcome. Thérapie 1998; 53: 180.

Colley S, Walepole I, Fabian VA et al. Topical tretinoin and fetal malformations. Med J Aust 1998; 168: 467.

Committee on Developmental Toxicology NAS/NRC. Scientific Frontiers in Developmental Toxicology and Risk Assessment. National Research Council, Washington DC, 2000.

Czeizel AE, Kazy Z, Vargha P. Vaginal treatment with povidone-iodine suppositories during pregnancy. Intl J Gynaecol Obstet 2004; 84: 83–5.

de Die-Smulders CEM, Sturkenboom MCJM, Veraart J et al. Severe limb defects and craniofacial abnormalities in fetus conceived during acitretine therapy. Teratology 1995; 52: 215–19.

de Santis M, Lucchese A, Carducci B et al. Latanoprost exposure in pregnancy. Am J Ophthalmol 2004; 138: 305–6.

Einarson A, Costei A, Kalra S et al. The use of topical 5% imiquimod during pregnancy: a case series. Reprod Toxicol 2006; 21: 1–2.

Ellegard EK, Hellgren M, Karlsson NG. Fluticasone propionate aqueous nasal spray in pregnancy rhinitis. Clin Otolaryngol 2001; 26: 394–400.

Fölster-Holst R, Rufli T, Christophers E. Treatment of scabies with special consideration of the approach in infancy, pregnancy and while nursing {in German}. Hautarzt 2000; 51: 7–13.

Food and Drug Administration. New measures to manage risks associated with accutane. J Am Med Assoc 2001; 283: 1146.

Franssen ME, van der Wilt GJ, de Jong PC et al. A retrospective study of the teratogenicity of dermatological coal tar products {Letter}. Acta Derm Venereol 1999; 79: 390–91.

Garbis H, Eléfant E, Bertolotti E et al. Pregnancy outcome after periconceptional and first trimester exposure to methoxsalen photochemotherapy. Arch Dermatol 1993; 131: 492–3.

Geiger JM, Baudin M, Saurat JH. Teratogenic risk with etretinate and acitretine treatment. Dermatology 1994; 189: 109–16.

Geiger JM, Walker M. Is there a reproductive safety risk in male patients treated with acitretine? Dermatology 2002; 205: 105–7.

Gunnarskog JG, Källén B, Lindelof BG et al. Psoralen photochemotherapy (PUVA) and pregnancy. Arch Dermatol 1993; 129: 320–23.

Honein MA, Paulozzi LJ. Accutane®-exposed pregnancies. Teratology 2000; 61: 442.

Honein MA, Paulozzi LJ, Erickson JD. Continued occurrence of accutane®-exposed pregnancies. Teratology 2001; 64: 142–7.

2

Pregnancy

Jick SS, Terris BZ, Jick H. First trimester topical tretinoin. Lancet 1993; 341: 1181–2.

Johnson SM, Martinez M, Freedman S. Management of glaucoma in pregnancy and lactation. Survey Ophthalmol 2001; 45: 449–54.

Källén BAJ, Otterblad Olaussen P. Maternal drug use in early pregnancy and infant cardiovascular defect. Reprod Toxicol 2003; 17: 255–61.

Karol MD, Conner CS, Watanabe AS et al. Podophyllum: suspected teratogenicity from topical application. Clin Toxicol 1980; 16: 283–6.

Kennedy D, Hurst V, Konradsdottir E et al. Outcome of pregnancy following exposure to permethrin head lice shampoo. Birth Def Res B 2003; 68: 294–5.

Kennedy D, Hurst V, Konradsdottir E et al. Pregnanc outcome following exposure to permethrin and use of teratogen information. Am J Perinatol 2005; 22: 87–90.

Kimmel CA, Moore W, Stara JF. Hexachlorophene teratogenicity in rats. Lancet 1972; 2: 765.

Koepelman JN, Miyazawa K. Inadvertent 5-fluorouracil treatment in early pregnancy: a report of three cases. Reprod Toxicol 1990; 4: 233–5.

Lammer EJ, Chen DT, Hoar RM et al. Retinoic acid embryopathy. N Engl J Med 1985; 313: 837–41.

Lammer EJ, Hayes AM, Schunior A et al. Unusually high risk for adverse outcomes of pregnancy following fetal isotretinoin exposure. Am J Hum Genet 1988; 43: A58.

Larsen FG, Steinkjer B, Jakobsen P et al. Acitretin is converted to etretinate only during concomitant alcohol intake. Br J Dermatol 2000; 143: 1164–9.

Lauwerys R, Bonnier C, Eurard P et al. Prenatal and early postnatal intoxication by inorganic mercury resulting from maternal use of mercury containing soap. Hum Toxicol 1987; 6: 253–6.

Lee AG, Pless M, Falardeau J et al. The use of acetazolamide in idiopathic intracranial hypertension during pregnancy. Am J Ophthalmol 2005; 139: 855–9.

Lipson AH, Collins F, Webster WS. Multiple congenital defects associated with maternal use of topical tretinoin. Lancet 1993; 341: 1352–3.

Lockhart JD. How toxic is hexachlorophene? Pediatrics 1972; 50: 220–35.

Loureiro KD, Kao KK, Jones KL et al. Minor malformations characteristic of the retinoic acid embryopathy and other birth outcomes in children of women exposed to topical tretinoin during early pregnancy. Am J Med Genet 2005; 136A: 117–21.

Martínez-Frias ML, Rodriguez-Pinilla E. First-trimester exposure to topical tretinoin: its safety is not warranted {Letter}. Teratology 1999; 60: 5.

Maw RD. Treatment of external genital warts with 5% imiquiod cream during pregnancy: a case report. Br J Obstet Gynaecol 2004; 111: 1475.

McGready R, Hamilton KA, Simpson JA et al. Safety of the insect repelent n,n,-diethyl-m-toluamide (DEET) in pregnancy. Am J Trop Med 2001; 65: 285–9.

Menter A. Pharmacokinetics and safety of tazarotene. J Am Acad Dermatol 2000; 43: 31–5.

Miller RK, Hendrickx AG, Millls JL et al. Periconceptional vitamin A use: how much is teratogenic? Reprod Toxicol 1998; 12: 75–88.

Moerike S, Pantzar JT, De Sa D. Temporal bone pathology in fetuses exposed to isotretinoin. Pediatr Dev Pathol 2002; 5: 405–9.

Mygind H, Thulstrup AM, Pedersen L et al. Risk of intrauterine growth retardation, malformations and other birth outcomes in children after topical use of corticosteroid in pregnancy. Acta Obstet Gynaecol Scand 2002; 81: 234–9.

Navarre-Belhassen C, Blancehet P, Hillaire-Buys D et al. Multiple congenital malformations associated with topical tretinoin. Ann Pharmacother 1998; 32: 505–6.

2.17 Dermatological medications and local therapeutics

Nulman I, Berkovitch M, Klein J et al. Steady-state pharmacokinetics of isotretinoin and ist 4-oxo metabolite: implications for fetal safety. J Clin Pharmacol 1998; 38: 926–30.

Odom LD, Plouffe J, Butler WJ. 5-fluorouracil exposure during the period of conception: a report of two cases. Am J Obstet Gynecol 1990; 163: 76–7.

Ozawa H, Azuma E, Shindo K et al. Transient renal tubular acidosis in a neonate following transplacental acetazolamide. Eur J Pediatr 2001; 160: 321–2.

Robert E, Scialli AR. Topical medications during pregnancy. Reprod Toxicol 1994; 8: 197–202.

Robertson J, Polifka JE, Avner M et al. A survey of pregnant women using isotretinoin. Birth Def Res A 2005; 73: 881–7.

Roeleveld N, Zielhuis GA, Gabreels F. Mental retardation and parental occupation: a study on the applicability of job exposure matrices. Br J Indust Med 1993; 50: 945–54.

Rojansky N, Fasouliotis SJ, Ariel I et al. Extreme caudal agenesis. J Reprod Med 2002; 47: 241–5.

Schaefer C, Peters PWJ. Intrauterine diethyltoluamide exposure and fetal outcome. Reprod Toxicol 1992; 6: 175–6.

Selcen D, Seidman S, Nigro MA. Otocerebral anomalies associated with topical tretinoin use. Brain Dev 2000; 22: 218–20.

Shapiro J. Safety of topical minoxidil solution: a one-year, prospective, observational study. J Cutan Med Surg 2003; 7: 322–9.

Shapiro L, Pastuszak A, Cutro G et al. Safety of first-trimester exposure to topical tretinoin: prospective cohort study. Lancet 1997; 350: 1143–4.

Smorlesi C, Caldarella A, Caramelli L et al. Topically applied minoxidil may cause fetal malformation: a case report. Birth Def Res A 2003; 67: 997–1001.

Sparsa A, Bonnetblanc JM. Lithium. Ann Dermatol Venereol 2004; 131: 255–61.

Sudakin DL, Trevathan WR. DEET: a review and update of safety and risk in the general population. J Toxicol Clin Toxicol 2003; 41: 831–9.

Suwalsky M, Villena F, Marcus D et al . Plasma absorption and ultrastructural changes of rat testicular cells induced by lindane. Hum Exp Toxicol 2000; 19: 529–33.

Swan SH, Main KM, Liu F et al. Decrease in anogenital distance among male infants with prenatal phthalate exposure. Environ Health Perspect 2005; 113: 1056–61.

Teratology Society. Recommendations for isotretinoin use in women of child bearing potential. Teratology 1991; 44: 1–6.

Van Hoogdalem EJ. Transdermal absorption of topical anti-acne agents in man; review of clinical pharmacokinetic data. J Eur Acad Dermatol Venereol 1998; 11: S13–19, S28–9.

Wagenvoort AM, van Vugt JMG, Sobotka M et al. Topical timolol therapy in pregnancy: is it safe for the fetus? Teratology 1998; 58: 258–62.

Weber G, Vigone MC, Rapa A et al. Neonatal transient hypothyroidism: etiological study. Italian collaborative study on transient hypothyroidism. Arch Dis Childhood Fet Neonat Ed 1998; 79: F70–2.

Vitamins, minerals, and trace elements

2.18

Paul Peters and Christof Schaefer

Vitamins and minerals are organic food substances found only in plants and animals, and are essential to the normal functioning of the body. However, the actual meaning of the term "essential" does not hold for all vitamins. Vitamin imbalances can be divided into three categories:

1. Hypovitaminosis – shortage of one or more vitamins
2. Avitaminosis – depletion of one or more vitamins
3. Hypervitaminosis – excess of certain vitamins by overdose, and hence intoxication.

Altered maternal metabolism, the growth of the fetus, and additional storage of some vitamins in the yolk sac and placenta, in particular vitamins A, B_1, B_2, B_3, B_6, B_{12}, C, and folic acid, increase vitamin requirements during pregnancy. A varied and balanced composition of the daily diet is the preferred basis of the vitamin supply. Folic acid might be the only vitamin that has to be supplemented before and during pregnancy. Vitamins A and D are the only vitamins that might, in cases of hypervitaminosis, cause toxicity for the unborn.

2.18.1 Vitamin A (retinol)

Pharmacology

Vitamin A is a fat-soluble vitamin that occurs in two forms in nature. It is found in food derived from animals, such as fish oils and liver. The body readily uses this form. Vitamin A values are expressed in different ways.

The nutrient was originally measured in IU (international units), but in 1974 the United States began using a measurement called Retinol Equivalents (REs), where 1 RE = 1 μg of retinol, or 6 μg of β-carotene, or 3.333 IU of vitamin A. The recommended daily allowance for pregnant women is 700 RE.

Vitamin A can also be found in vegetables in the form of β-carotene or provitamin A. This form is found in plants, and is the precursor of the actual vitamin. Vitamin A is the basic substance needed for rhodopsin (visual purple). In addition, epithelial cells need vitamin A for growth and functional maintenance. Vitamin A, like vitamin C, accumulates in the embryo. The endogenous concentration of vitamin A metabolites in the serum is reduced in pregnant women during the first trimester, and amounts to between 0.26 and 7.7 μg/l. Even after 3 weeks of supplementation with 30 000 IU vitamin A per day, the peak values of the metabolites *retinoic acid* and *isotretinoin* are, at most, slightly above the concentrations measured previously (Wiegand 1998). During the second half of pregnancy, the endogenous concentration increases to about 150% of the level in nonpregnant women (Malone 1975).

Toxicology

The teratogenic action on humans of vitamin A derivatives such as the retinoids isotretinoin and *acitretin*, which are used as therapy for severe forms of acne and psoriasis, is discussed in Chapter 2.17. Retinoids are absolutely contraindicated during pregnancy.

About three decades ago, the possibility was first discussed that vitamin A preparations in doses over 25 000 IU daily might have a teratogenic action on humans similar to that of retinoids, and could cause characteristic "retinoid effects" (Rosa 1986). At the end of the 1980s, manufacturers of multivitamin preparations in many countries changed the composition of their products, following the opinions of the Teratology Society and at the insistence of regulatory authorities, so that a daily dose did not contain more than 6000 IU (Teratology Society 1987). The safety of such doses has been confirmed repeatedly in many studies, among them the Dudas (1992) study on pregnant women in Hungary. Amazingly, a later study from the European Network of Teratology Information Services (ENTIS) gave no indication of a teratogenic effect, even with higher vitamin A doses (10 000–300 000, mean 50 000 IU per day), taken in the first trimester. In particular, the observations in another study that high doses (i.e. over 15 000 IU daily) cause neural crest anomalies (Rothman 1995) could not be confirmed (Miller 1998). The ENTIS study of 423 pregnant women is the largest vitamin A study to date (Mastroiacovo 1999). There was no increase in the rate of birth defects either among the 311 live-born children, or within the high-dose group of 120 children whose mothers took 50 000 IU daily. Nevertheless, looking at these case numbers statistically, they only allow a relative risk above 2.8 to be ruled out.

A retrospective study discussed a higher risk for transposition of the great vessels with maternal vitamin A intake >10 000 IU daily during the 12 months prior to conception (Botto 2003). However, the number of affected children was low, and these results are not confirmed by other studies. Another retrospective study found no association between oral clefts and the (normal) vitamin A levels of women taking supplementation or consuming liver (Mitchell 2003).

There is a general warning against eating liver, because a portion (100 g) may contain up to 400 000 IU; however, there is no clear indication yet of teratogenic effects from liver consumption. According to a pharmacokinetic study by Buss (1994), the peak value of vitamin A or of the ultimate teratogen, all-trans-retinoic acid, in the serum after eating liver is only 1/20 of that measured after taking vitamin A tablets. However, the three- to five-fold observed increase in plasma concentrations and the dose-dependent increase in exposure to 13-cis and 13-cis-4-oxo retinoic acid support the current safety recommendation: that women should be cautious regarding their consumption of liver-containing meals during pregnancy (Hartmann 2005).

β-carotene, also called *pro-vitamin A*, is converted as needed by the organism to vitamin A (retinol). Even high doses of β-carotene do not increase the retinol concentration in the serum and do not pose any teratogenic risk (Miller 1998; Polifka 1996).

> **Recommendation.** A pregnant woman should not take more than 6000 IU of vitamin A as retinyl esters, retinal or retinol per day. Basically, there is no reason to take a vitamin A supplement, particularly when nutrition is reasonably well balanced. Exceptions are, of course, illnesses where there is a proven deficiency – for example, as a result of limited intestinal absorption. If, however, a dosage of more than 25 000 IU per day has been given by accident, interruption of the pregnancy is in no way indicated. An individual risk assessment should be made using detailed fetal ultrasound. Potentially pregnant women should not eat liver. However, single liver meals do not require any action. β-carotene is safe during pregnancy.

2.18.2   Vitamin B$_1$ (thiamine)

Pharmacology and toxicology

Thiamine is important as a co-enzyme in carbohydrate metabolism. The need for vitamin B$_1$ (1–1.2 mg daily) only increases slightly during pregnancy, and there is a higher concentration in the fetal blood than in that of the mother. Thiamine deficiency can induce clinical symptoms within 1 week. Severe polyneuropathy can occur in chronic hyperemesis in pregnancy, and needs to be treated.

> **Recommendation.** Supplementation with vitamin B$_1$ during pregnancy is, as a rule, unnecessary. There are no data suggesting teratogenicity with overdoses of thiamine.

2.18.3   Vitamin B$_2$ (riboflavin)

Pharmacology and toxicology

Riboflavin is an important co-enzyme in energy metabolism. In newborns whose mothers had clinical or laboratory signs of riboflavin deficiency, no developmental disorders could be shown (Heller 1974). The same study showed that the *vitamin B$_2$* concentration in the cord blood was four times as high as in the maternal blood. It would appear that an active transplacental transport of vitamin B$_2$ prevents deficiency in the fetus. A suggestion has been made that riboflavin hypovitaminosis might be an additional risk factor for pre-eclampsia (Wacker 2000).

2

> **Recommendation.** Supplementation with vitamin B2 during pregnancy is, as a rule, unnecessary. Embryo- or fetotoxicity with an overdose of riboflavin has not been reported.

2.18.4   Vitamin B$_3$ (nicotinamide)

Pharmacology and toxicology

Nicotinamide is an ingredient in many important enzymes. Deficiencies in pregnancy have not been reported.

> **Recommendation.** Supplementation with vitamin B$_3$ during pregnancy is, as a rule, unnecessary. No adverse reactions are known.

2.18.5   Vitamin B$_6$ (pyridoxine)

Pharmacology and toxicology

Pyridoxine is the co-enzyme of some amino acid decarboxylases and transaminases. *Vitamin B$_6$* is used in North America in combination with doxylamine as therapy for excessive vomiting in pregnancy (hyperemesis) (see Chapter 2.4). The vitamin B$_6$ concentration in the mother's blood is reduced throughout the entire pregnancy. By contrast, the concentrations in the fetal blood are about three times as high (Cleary 1975). There is no indication as yet for teratogenicity (see Chapter 2.4).

> **Recommendation.** Supplementation with vitamin B$_6$ is only necessary in exceptional cases, for example during tuberculostatic treatment with *isoniazid* (see Chapter 2.6). For treatment of nausea and vomiting in pregnancy, see Chapter 2.4.

2.18.6   Vitamin B$_{12}$ (cyanocobalamin)

Pharmacology and toxicology

Vitamin B$_{12}$ (cyanocobalamin) is a factor in animal proteins necessary for the maturation of the erythroblasts. Its absence leads to megaloblastic (pernicious) anemia, with neurological consequences. Although the concentration of vitamin B$_{12}$ in the maternal serum drops slightly during the pregnancy, there is no reduction in the vitamin B$_{12}$ stored in the mother's liver (about 3000 μg). The newborn's need for about 50 μg of stored vitamin B$_{12}$ is comparatively modest.

Diets in Western Europe commonly include 5–15 µg vitamin B_{12} per day. The daily requirement for vitamin B_{12} is 2 µg for non-pregnant women; during pregnancy this rises to 3 µg per day. Low vitamin B_{12} levels have been discussed as a risk factor for early recurrent abortion (Reznikoff-Etiévant 2002). Another genetic problem is transcobalamin II deficiency, which reduces the transfer of vitamin B_{12} into the cell.

> **Recommendation.** Because vitamin B_{12} deficiency is not caused by pregnancy, supplementation with vitamin B_{12} is not routinely necessary. At most, it might be indicated with an unbalanced vegetarian or vegan diet. Anemia in the pregnancy caused by a vitamin B_{12} deficiency should, of course, be treated.

2.18.7   Folic acid

Pharmacology and toxicology

Folic acid, a pteridine derivate, is a B vitamin that is essential for nucleoprotein synthesis in general, and especially for growing tissues – i.e. for blood synthesis, embryonic and fetal development. It also keeps homocysteine levels low. The organism metabolizes folic acid in its biologically effective form, folinic acid. With a balanced diet, the effects on the maternal blood production caused by a deficiency should not be of any concern. However, with the rare, marked, folic acid deficiency, macrocytic anemia can develop.

As with all vitamin and nutritional standards, committees of experts set folate requirement. This explains the differences between countries and at various times. For example, in 1970 the US Food and Nutrition Board (FNB 1970) set the recommended *folate* intake for pregnant women at 0.4 mg per day. This was reduced to 0.270 mg per day in 1989, mainly because of data showing that healthy folate-replete adults ingested this amount. The recommendation was increased to 0.450 mg per day in 1999 by the same authority, in order to maintain adequate folate status in pregnant women (Tamura 2006). In the UK, the recommended daily intake of folic acid for pregnant women is set at 0.6 mg/day in 2006.

In the UK in 1965, an association between a relative folic acid deficiency in the mother and a high rate for neural tube defects (NTDs), especially open spina bifida and anencephaly, was suggested for the first time (Hubbard 1965). In 1980, the first studies seemed to indicate that these serious birth defects could be prevented by giving multivitamin preparations (Smithells 1980), or by supplementation with folic acid (Laurence 1981) in pregnancies with a recurrent risk (Teratology Society 1994, Rosenberg 1992, MRC 1991). Since there are no clinical studies that indicate prevention of NTDs in a recurrent risk situation with less than 4 mg folic acid per day, it is ethically and practically not common to use lower daily doses in such a situation.

Comprehensive studies in the USA (Mulinare 1988), Australia (Bower 1989), Cuba (Vergel 1990), England (MRC 1991), Hungary (Czeizel 1992), and China (Berry 1999) have suggested a possible protective action of folic acid supplementation for NTDs in cases where there is no recurrent risk. However, in the Hungarian study there was probably a selection bias in the control group, since the risk of NTDs in that control group was higher than in the general Hungarian population (Anonymous 1991). Apart from NTDs, there have been studies that found a protective effect with respect to other birth defects (Bailey 2005, Czeizel 2004), such as cardiac defects (Czeizel 2004, Botto 2003), anal atresia (Myers 2001), and miscarriage (Gindler 2001, Nelen 2000).

The association between folic acid and open neural tube defects has not yet been fully established, and epidemiological studies have, to date, indicated but not completely confirmed the protective effects of folic acid supplementation. A biological plausibility is not yet demonstrated. It has to be stressed that folding of the neural walls and closure of the neural tube (neural tube formation) takes place between about 22 and 28 days post-conception – i.e. before the pregnant woman is about 14 days "overdue", and before she is 42 days pregnant (counting from the first day of the last menstruation). Thus, if folic acid supplementation is effective in preventing neural tube defects, such supplementation must take place from at least some time before conception and during the first 2 months of pregnancy. The issue of placental transfer of folic acid is of less interest because during the important part of neural tube morphogenesis, the placenta is not yet formed or will only just start functioning. Therefore, neural tube closure is more dependent on the functioning of the yolk sac (Garbis-Berkvens 1987). Shaw (1997) and others have discussed the relation of methionine and folic acid with respect to neural tube formation – for example, they observed that a higher dietary intake of methionine was associated with a reduction in NTD risk irrespective of maternal folate intake.

Based on current experience, a tablet dose of folic acid of up to 5 mg daily is not dangerous for embryonic development. The possible masking of a rare vitamin B_{12} deficiency anemia, repeatedly mentioned as a risk of taking folic acid, is possible, but in light of the recommended temporary supplementation this is not relevant.

In the USA, the Food and Drug Administration (FDA) has required folic acid enrichment of foods (grain-based products) with 1.4 mg/kg since January 1988. This ruling is also true in Canada (0.15 mg per 100 g flour), in Chile (2.2 mg per kg flour) and Costa Rica. In the UK, enrichment has been assessed at 0.240 mg folic acid per 100 g flour, and a final consultation on mandatory fortification of flour with folic acid will be held in 2007. Food fortification was introduced in

Hungary, but was not successful because of the higher price of the enriched bread and flour (Czeizel 2006). The issue of food fortification is still being discussed in other European countries, since only a small number of pregnant women actually take the supplementary tablets, and the average diet contains only 0.2 mg per day. Occasionally there has been discussion regarding whether or not a balanced diet would provide sufficient folic acid anyway. Moreover, the decrease of NTD prevalence observed in line with the implementation of food fortification with folic acid might well also be correlated with the genetic and/or nutritional characteristics of the population involved. For example, Ireland, Wales, and North China were, in the past, high risk areas for NTDs, and it may be that changing nutritional habits in those countries explains a lowering of NTDs (Rosano 1999).

Finally, it should not remain unsaid that, after critical evaluation of all the available data, doubts are still expressed today about the protective action of folic acid supplementation (Kalter 2000). We agree with the statement of Källén (2002) that folic acid should not be promoted as a teratologic panacea, and certainly that a woman with a spina bifida child should not feel any guilt for not having taken enough folic acid tablets before and during her pregnancy.

Concomitant use of the high dosage of 5 mg folic acid supplementation compromises the efficacy of *sulfadoxine-pyrimethamine* for the treatment of uncomplicated malaria in pregnant women. Countries that use this medication for treatment or prevention of malaria in pregnancy need to evaluate their antenatal policy on the timing or dosage of folic acid supplementation (Ouma 2006) (see also Chapter 2.6).

Recommendation. For the protective action of folic acid against open neural tube defects to be effective, supplementation with 0.4–0.8 mg folic acid per day should begin as early as possible when a pregnancy is planned, and be continued throughout the first 8 weeks of pregnancy. Pregnant women should also be encouraged to consume foods high in folate, such as green leafy vegetables, and fruit. If the mother has already given birth to a child with a neural tube defect (i.e. has a recurrent risk), the supplementary dosage should be 4–5 mg per day. This is also suggested in connection with the intake of certain medications with a folic acid antagonist action. Folic acid deficiency anemia should be treated in the usual way during pregnancy.

2.18.8   Vitamin C (ascorbic acid)

Pharmacology and toxicology

Vitamin C is important in cellular metabolism for the maintenance of oxidation–reduction balance. The daily requirement is set at 100 mg.

Vitamin C deficiency leads to scurvy, with disturbances in the collagen metabolism, and to a tendency to bleed. Vitamin C concentration in the fetal blood is three times as high as in the maternal blood because vitamin C accumulates in the fetus after the placental transfer of dehydroascorbic acid (Malone 1975). It is not known whether giving vitamin C affects the fetal reduction–oxidation balance. Recently, the association of vitamin C deficiency with gestational diabetes has been discussed (Zhang 2004A, 2004B), as has vitamin C supplementation during second and third trimesters to prevent premature rupture of membranes (Casanueve 2005, Tejero 2003).

2

Pregnancy

> **Recommendation.** Vitamin C supplementation is not necessary during pregnancy if the diet is balanced.

2.18.9   Vitamin D group

Pharmacology and toxicology

Several fat-soluble vitamins with a central role in calcium metabolism are referred to collectively as *vitamin D*. Vitamin D promotes the resorption of calcium and phosphate from the intestines. The daily requirement for vitamin D is 5 μg calciferol (1 μg × 40 iu; 1 iu × 0.025 μg). Vitamin D deficiency causes a disturbance in bone growth and development, which manifests itself as rickets in children and as osteomalacia in adults. Vitamin D_2 (*ergocalciferol*) and vitamin D_3 (*colecalciferol*), are found in milk, cod-liver oil, and butter. Colecalciferol and ergocalciferol are transformed into the active form of vitamin D under the influence of UV rays. In the fetus, the active form of vitamin D is related to the maternal concentration – i.e., it is normally about 70–90% of this concentration, but increases significantly to over 100% when the maternal vitamin D concentration is deficient (Pitkin 1975).

A longitudinal study up to the age of 9 years, covering 198 mother–child pairs, indicated that vitamin D deficiency in late pregnancy may lead to significantly reduced ossification of the whole skeleton, and in particular of the lower spine. A lower than normal calcium concentration in the cord blood may also predict poorer ossification (Javaid 2006).

Other derivatives of vitamin D are *alfacalcidol* and *calcitriol*.

Dihydrotachysterol is a vitamin D analog for the treatment of hypoparathyroidism. There have been no studies on its use during pregnancy. However, dihydrotachysterol dosages are adjusted to maintain physiological conditions. Therefore, developmental toxicity is unlikely.

2.18 Vitamins, minerals, and trace elements

Paricalcitol is a synthetic vitamin D derivative used for the prevention and treatment of secondary hyperparathyroidism and osteoporosis. There is no experience with treatment during pregnancy.

> **Recommendation.** During pregnancy, very high doses of vitamin D are contraindicated because they can lead to hypercalcaemia in both the mother and the newborn. For healthy women, the need for vitamin D does not increase in pregnancy. When the diet is balanced, there is no need for supplementation. However, if there is a documented deficiency, supplementation, vitamin D may – or even must – be given until the maternal plasma concentrations are normal. This also applies to high doses for inherited dominant X-chromosomal vitamin D-resistant rickets needing treatment. In this case, it seems that a genetically healthy fetus is not damaged even with daily doses as high as 20 000 IU. Where there is phosphate diabetes, interruption of the vitamin D therapy should be discussed if the maternal symptoms allow this. Generally speaking, with these diseases the calcium and phosphate concentrations in the blood of both mother and newborn should be measured regularly.

2.18.10 Vitamin E (tocopherol)

Pharmacology and toxicology

Vitamin E is not essential for human beings, and deficiencies are unknown. The usual requirement for vitamin E is provided by a normal diet (10–20 IU). There have not, as yet, been any observations of vitamin E deficiency during pregnancy.

Among 82 prospectively ascertained pregnancies exposed to high doses of vitamin E during the first trimester (400–1200 IU daily), the birth weight was significantly lower than among non-exposed controls. However, it was not clear whether the authors adjusted for gestational age at birth. There were no increased rates of prematurity, miscarriage, or birth defects (Boskovic 2004A, 2004B).

> **Recommendation.** Routine supplementation with vitamin E is not necessary.

2.18.11 Vitamin K

See Chapter 2.9.

2.18.12   Multivitamin preparations

Pharmacology and toxicology

Multivitamin preparations are frequently prescribed during pregnancy, or are taken by patients without a doctor's prescription. There is a controversy over whether or not supplementation of additional vitamins might prevent birth defects (Groenen 2004, Krapels 2004, Shaw 2000). However, there is no proven indication as yet for using multivitamins, either as supplements or as a preventive measure, with the exception of folic acid supplementation. Despite the lack of scientific justification, it has become common practice to prescribe certain vitamin (and mineral) combinations.

> **Recommendation.** Prophylactic administration of multivitamin preparations to healthy pregnant women is controversial, because a balanced diet is sufficient, and vitamins A and D may be toxic for the embryo in higher doses (when preparations are used inappropriately). However, most multivitamins include a combination of beta-carotene and a retinyl ester for vitamin A to reduce risk. See section 2.18.7 on the need for folic acid prophylaxis.

2.18.13   Iron

The total amount of *iron* in the human body is 4–5 g. Of this, about 70% is bound to hemoglobin (Hb). With the help of a protein, ferritin, iron is actively absorbed from the intestine. In the blood, iron is bound to the transport protein, transferrin, and reaches the unborn in this form through the placenta. During pregnancy, the need for iron increases due to the increase in the maternal blood volume as well as the increased need of the fetus and the placenta. The maternal plasma volume increases more than the number of erythrocytes (hemodilution), and this in turn leads to a relative decline in the hemoglobin value. The need of the embryo (and later the fetus) for iron increases during pregnancy, from 4 mg to 6.6 mg per day. Keeping in mind that the daily rate of excretion of iron is 1.5 mg, a pregnant woman needs about 5 mg of iron per day. The increased need for iron in pregnancy is not sufficiently covered by food. For this reason, stored iron is mobilized from the mother's broken-down hemoglobin. Over the course of the pregnancy, the hemoglobin level drops by 20 g/l, primarily because of the increase in blood volume. With uncomplicated labor and normalization of the blood volume, the hemoglobin value returns to a normal level by the end of the postpartum period.

2 Pregnancy

2.18 Vitamins, minerals, and trace elements

Pharmacology

Iron (II) salts are well-absorbed after oral intake, and are suitable for supplementation during pregnancy. The addition of vitamins and trace elements to oral iron (II) preparations has no proven value. Combination preparations with folic acid cannot be recommended, because iron absorption with these preparations is reduced by up to 60%. About 15–20% of the patients who take iron (II) preparations complain of gastrointestinal problems, which may force a change to another preparation or even cessation of iron supplementation, especially in the presence of morning sickness. Parenteral administration of iron preparations (Singh 2000) such as iron (III)-gluconate complex is only indicated with marked anemia, for instance, and, in combination with other anti-anemics, eliminates, for the most part, the need for transfusions in pregnancy.

Toxicology

The suspicion that the birth defect rate could increase slightly with routine iron supplementation in pregnancy has not been confirmed by comprehensive prospective studies (Royal College of General Practitioners 1975). For iron overdose, see Chapter 2.22.

> **Recommendation.** Iron supplementation during pregnancy is indicated if the hemoglobin level is = 100 g/l. It should be given orally, using an iron (II) preparation. If for some reason parenteral iron supplementation is necessary, this should be given intravenously with an iron (III) preparation. For iron overdose, see Chapter 2.22.

2.18.14   Calcium

Pharmacology and toxicology

Nearly all the *calcium* in the body, totaling about 1100–1200 g, is found in the bones, bound in complexes with phosphate and hydroxyapatite. The daily calcium requirement is 800–1000 mg. Calcium metabolism and fetal bone development are dependent on the maternal vitamin D metabolism and pregnancy-related changes in the activity of different hormones (parathormone, calcitonin, cortisteroids, estrogens). Calcium is actively transported through the placenta to the fetus. In the last trimester, bone development is enhanced as a result of low parathormone concentrations and high calcitonin concentrations in the fetus. Over the course of the pregnancy, the fetus takes in about 30 g of calcium. This amount is normally mobilized during pregnancy from maternal storage, without additional administration of calcium salts. However, it is generally advised that a supplement of about 500 mg per day be taken to ensure the daily requirement is met. Calcium should not be given as a phosphate salt because of leg muscle cramps. Organic salts, such as *calcium citrate, calcium aspartate, calcium globionate* and *calcium gluconate*, are more appropriate for calcium supplementation.

> **Recommendation.** It makes sense to take 500 mg of calcium per day orally, or to drink a liter of milk. The milk has the advantage that it supplies not only the calcium but also the daily vitamin D requirement.

2.18.15   Fluoride

Pharmacology and toxicology

Whether a *fluoride* supplement during pregnancy of about 1 mg/day in tablet form (equivalent to about 2 mg sodium fluoride), or ingested via fluoridated drinking water (about 1 mg/l), actually reduces the incidence of caries in the baby is somewhat controversial. However, such fluoride prophylaxis does not appear to harm the fetus. Earlier suspicions regarding the possible toxic effect of regular fluoride on reproduction – for example, an increased rate of Down syndrome – is biologically implausible. Even high fluoride doses as a result of environmentally contaminated drinking water (above 10 mg/1) do not apparently cause any increase in birth defects. Prenatally induced fluorosis of the teeth and bones in the second half of pregnancy is theoretically possible, and has been described in individual cases after extreme continuous exposure, but would not be expected after (as has occasionally happened) accidental intake of an osteoporosis preparation containing about 25 mg of fluoride.

> **Recommendation.** Fluoride supplementation of about 1 mg per day can be given during pregnancy without risk. Calcium (including milk products) and fluoride must not be taken together because of the formation of insoluble calcium fluoride, which cannot be absorbed. High-dose fluoride therapy for osteoporosis is contraindicated. However, accidental intake of higher doses does not justify either interruption of the pregnancy or additional diagnostic procedures.

2.18.16   Strontium

Pharmacology and toxicology

Strontium is prescribed in cases of postmenopausal osteoporosis. There are insufficient data concerning the use of strontium in pregnancy. Experimental data on bone marrow cells have given indications for clastogenic effects. Strontium also has an effect on capacitation, both in humans and animals (Sharma 1989), and on the activation of oocytes in rodents (Fraser 1987).

> **Recommendation.** Indications for treatment with strontium are outside the scope of this book. Therefore, and because of the possible mutagenic activity, the use of strontium is not indicated in pregnancy. In cases of unintended strontium use, invasive diagnostics or interruption of pregnancy is not justified.

2.18.17   Biphosphonates and other osteoporosis drugs

Pharmacology and toxicology

Alendronatic acid, clodronic acid, etidronic acid, ibandronic acid, pamidronic acid, risedronic acid, tiludronic acid and *zoledronic acid* are among the osteolysis inhibitors. They are used for Morbus Paget, postmenopausal osteoporosis, and other osteolytic processes. There are no systematic studies on their use during pregnancy. Animal experiments suggest a possible placental transfer and effect on fetal skeletal development (Ornoy 1998).

In one study, there was no major congenital anomaly among 24 pregnancies with pre-pregnancy or early pregnancy exposure to alendronate (Ornoy 2006). Another case report describes a healthy newborn, with normal bone structure and uneventful development until the age of 1 year, who was exposed to 10 mg per day throughout pregnancy (Rutgers-Verhage 2003). Another report was on a woman receiving zoledronic acid during the second and third trimesters, after chemotherapy for breast cancer during the first trimester. The child was born at 35 weeks' gestation, and was followed until the age of 1 year, during which time development was normal (Andreadis 2004).

A prospective study covering 15 pregnancies where the mothers underwent biphosphonate treatment (alendronatic acid, 7; etidronic acid, 5; pamidronic acid, 1; risedronic acid, 2), and where 9 of the mothers were being treated during the first trimester, resulted in 14 live births and 1 spontaneous abortion. There was no indication of developmental toxicity (Levy 2004).

There are insufficient data on the use of calcitonin, cinacalet, and raloxifen during pregnancy.

> **Recommendation.** Biphosphonates and the other osteoporosis drugs are not indicated during pregnancy. Accidental acute use of individual doses in the first trimester does not justify either interruption of the pregnancy or additional diagnostic procedures.

2.18.18 Iodide

See Chapter 2.15.

2.18.19 Trace elements

Pharmacology and toxicology

Trace elements such as chromium, copper, selenium, or zinc are not normally supplemented in pregnancy. However, *zinc* is used therapeutically in cases of Wilson's disease. In a prospective study of 26 pregnancies (in 19 women) with this condition, the mothers received 25–50 mg zinc three times daily. All the pregnancies resulted in live-born children; one child had a cardiac disorder and another had microcephaly (Brewer 2000). Teratogenicity cannot be concluded, based on these findings.

Chromium is, according to some investigators, associated with glucose intolerance which commonly develops during late pregnancy (Saner 1981). This theory has been criticized as poorly supported by available data (Knopp 1982).

Selenium (see also Chapter 2.17) is an essential trace element. Selenium poisoning can be caused by high concentrations in drinking water. In this respect, it has been associated with miscarriages (Robertson 1970). No definitive data are available – certainly not to evaluate the use of selenium as an antioxidant.

> **Recommendation.** Supplementation with trace elements such as chromium, copper, and zinc is not necessary during pregnancy, apart from those instances when there is a documented deficiency or particular treatment indication (e.g. Wilson's disease). "Detoxification treatment" with selenium should not be undertaken either. However, the accidental use of these trace elements does not require any action.

References

Andreadis C, Charalampidou M, Diamantopoulos N et al. Combined chemotherapy and radiotherapy during conception and first two trimesters of gestation in a women with metastatic breast cancer. Gynecol Oncol 2004; 95: 252–5.

Anonymous. Congenital Malformations Worldwide, A Report from the International Clearinghouse for Birth Defects Monitoring Systems. Amsterdam: Elsevier, 1991.

Bailey LB, Berry RJ. Folic acid supplementation and the occurrence of congenital heart defects, orofacial clefts, multiple births, and miscarriage. Am J Clin Nutr 2005; 81: 1213–17.

Berry RJ, Li Z, Erickson JD et al. Prevention of neural-tube defects with folic acid in China. China–US Collaborative Project for Neural Tube Defect Prevention. N Engl J Med 1999; 341: 1485–90.

Boskovic R (A), Cargaun L, Dulus J et al. High doses of vitamin E and pregnancy outcome. Reprod Toxicol 2004; 18: 722.

Boskovic R (B), Cargaun L, Oren D et al. Pregnancy outcome following high doses of vitamin E supplementation; a prospective controlled study. Birth Def Res A 2004; 70: 358.

Botto LD, Mulinare J, Erickson JD. Do multivitamin or folic acid supplements reduce the risk for congenital heart defects? Evidence and gaps. Am J Med Genet 2003; 121A: 95–101.

Bower C, Stanley FJ. Dietary folate as a risk factor for neural-tube defects: evidence from a case-control study in Western Australia. Med J Aust 1989; 150: 613–19.

Brewer GJ, Johnson VD, Dick RD et al. Treatment of Wilson's disease with zinc. XVII: Treatment during pregnancy. Hepatology 2000; 31: 364–70.

Buss NE, Tembe EA, Prendergast BD et al. The teratogenic metabolites of vitamin A in women following supplements and liver. Hum Exp Toxicol 1994; 13: 33–43.

Casanueva E, Ripoll C, Tolentino M et al. Vitmin C supplementation to prevent premature rupture of the chorioamniotic. Am J Clin Nutr 2005; 81: 859–63.

Cleary RE, Lumeng L, Li T. Maternal and fetal plasma levels of pyridoxal phosphate at term: adequacy of vitamin B_6 supplementation during pregnancy. Am J Obstet Gynecol 1975; 121: 25–8.

Czeizel AE, Dudas I. Prevention of the first occurrence of neural-tube defects by periconceptional vitamin supplementation. N Engl J Med 1992; 327: 1832–5.

Czeizel AE, Dobo M, Varga P. Hungarian cohort control trial of periconceptional multivitamin supplementation shows a reduction in certain congenital abnormalities. Birth Def Res A 2004; 70: 853–61.

Czeizel AE. Folic acid: a public health challenge. Lancet 2006; 367: 2056.

Dudas I, Czeizel AE. Use of 6,000 IU vitamin A during early pregnancy without teratogenic effect. Teratology 1992; 45: 335–6.

FNB, NRC. Maternal nutrition and the course of pregnancy. Washington, DC: NAS, 1970.

Fraser LR. Strontium supports capacitation and the acrosome reaction in mouse sperm and rapidly activates mouse eggs. Gamete Res 1987; 18: 363–74.

Garbis-Berkvens JM, Peters PWJ. Comparative morphology and physiology of embryonic and fetal membranes. In: H Nau, WJ Scott (eds), Pharmacokinetics in Teratogenesis, Vol. I. Boca Raton, FL: CRC Press, 1987, pp. 13–44.

Gindler J, Li Z, Berry RJ et al. Folic acid supplements during pregnancy and the risk of miscarriage. Lancet 2001; 358: 796–800.

Groenen PM, van Rooij IA, Peer PG et al. Low maternal dietary intake of iron, magnesium, and niacin are associated with spina bifida in the offspring. J Nutr 2004; 134: 1516–22.

Hartmann S, Brors O, Bock J et al. Exposure to retinoic acids in non-pregnant women following high vitamin A intake with a liver meal. Intl J Vit Nutr Res 2005; 75: 187–94.

Heller SP, Salkeld RM, Korner WE. Riboflavin status in pregnancy. Am J Clin Nutr 1974; 27: 1225–39.

Hubbard ED, Smithells RW. Folic acid metabolism and human embryopathy. Lancet 1965; 1: 1254.

Javaid MK, Crozier SR, Harvey NC et al. Maternal vitamin D status during pregnancy and childhood bone mass at age 9 years: a longitudinal study. Lancet 2006; 367: 36–43.

Källén BAJ, Otterblad Olausson P. Use of folic acid and delivery outcome: a prospective registry study. Reprod Toxicol 2002; 16: 327–32.

Kalter H. Folic acid and human malformation: a summary and evaluation. Reprod Toxicol 2000; 14: 463–76.

Krapels IP, van Rooij IA, Ocke MC et al. Maternal nutritional status and the risk for orofacial cleft in humans. J Nutr 2004; 134: 3106–13.

Laurence KM, James N, Miller MH et al. Double-blind randomised controlled trial of folate treatment before conception to prevent recurrence of neural-tube defects. Br Med J 1981; 282: 1509–11.

Levy S, Fayez I, Han JY et al. Fetal outcome after intrauterine exposure to biphosphonates. Birth Def Res A 2004; 70: 359–60.

Malone JM. Vitamin passage across the placenta. Clin Perinatol 1975; 2: 295–307.

Mastroiacovo P, Mazzone T, Addis A et al. High vitamin A intake in early pregnancy and major malformations: a multicenter prospective controlled study. Teratology 1999; 59: 7–11.

Miller RK, Hendrickx AG, Millls JL. Periconceptional Vitamin A use: how much is teratogenic? Reprod Toxicol 1998; 12: 75–88.

Mitchell LE, Murray JC, O'Brien S et al. Retinoic acid receptor alpha gene variants, multivitamin use, and liver intake as risk factors for oral clefts: a population-based case-control study in Denmark, 1991–1994. Am J Epidemiol 2003; 158: 69–76.

MRC (Medical Research Council) Vitamin Study Research Group. Prevention of neural tube defects: results of the MRC vitamin study. Lancet 1991; 338: 131–7.

Mulinare J, Cordero JF, Erickson JD et al. Periconceptional use of multivitamins and the occurrence of neural tube defetcts. J Am Med Assoc 1988; 260: 3141–5.

Myers MF, Li S, Correa-Villasenor A et al. Folic acid supplementation and risk for imperforate anus in China. Am J Epidemiol 2001; 154: 1051–6.

Nelen WLDM, Blom HJ, Steegers EAP et al. Homocysteine and folate levels as risk factors for recurrent early pregnancy loss. Obstet Gynecol 2000; 95: 519–24.

Ornoy A, Patlas N, Pinto T et al. The transplacental effects of alendronate on the fetal skeleton in rats. Teratology 1998; 57: 242.

Ornoy A, Wajnberg R, Diav-Citrin O. The outcome of pregnancy following pre-pregnancy or early pregnancy alendronate treatment. Reprod Toxicol 2006; 22: 578–9.

Ouma P, Parise ME, Hamel MJ et al. A randomized controlled trial of folate supplementation when treating malaria in pregnancy with sulfadoxine-pyrimethamine. PLoS Clin Trials 2006; 6: 20–21.

Pitkin RM. Vitamins and minerals in pregnancy. Clin Perinatol 1975; 2: 221–32.

Polifka JE, Donlan CR, Donlan MA et al. Clinical teratology counseling and consultation report: high-dose β-carotene use during early pregnancy. Teratology 1996; 54: 103–7.

Reznikoff-Etiévant MC, Zittoun J, Vaylet C et al. Low vitamin B_{12} level as a risk factor for early recurrent abortion. Eur J Obstet Gynecol 2002; 104: 156–9.

Robertson DSF. Selenium a possible teratogen? Lancet 1970; 1: 518–19.

Rosa EW, Wilk AL, Kelsey EO. Vitamin A congeners. Teratology 1986; 33: 355–64.

Rosano A, Smithells D, Cacciani L et al. Time trends in neural tube defects prevalence in relation to preventive strategies: an international study. J Epidemiol Community Health 1999; 53: 630–35.

Rosenberg IH. Folic acid and neural-tube defects time for action? N Engl J Med 1992; 327: 1875–7.

Rothman KJ, Moore LL, Singer MR et al. A. Teratogenicity of high vitamin A intake N Engl J Med 1995; 333: 1369–73.

2

Pregnancy

2.18 Vitamins, minerals, and trace elements

Royal College of General Practitioners. Morbidity and drugs in pregnancy. J R Coll Gen Pract 1975; 25: 631–5.

Rutgers-Verhage AR, de Vries TW. No effects of biphosphonates on the human fetus. Birth Def Res A 2003; 67: 203–4.

Saner G. Urinary chromium excretion during pregnancy and its relationship with intravenous glucose loading. Am J Clin Nutr 1981; 34: 1676–9.

Sharma A, Talukder G. Effects of metals on chromosomes of higher organisms. Environ Mut 1989; 9: 191–226.

Shaw GM, Velie EM, Schaffer DM. Is dietary intake of methionine associated with a reduction in risk for neural tube defect-affected pregnancies? Teratology 1997; 56: 295–9.

Shaw GM, Croen LA, Todoroff K et al. Periconceptional intake of vitamin supplements and risk of multiple congenital anomalies. Am J Med Genet 2000; 93: 188–93.

Singh K, Fong YF. Letter to the editor: Intravenous iron polymaltose complex for treatment of iron deficiency anaemia in pregnancy resistant to oral iron therapy. Eur J Haematol 2000; 64: 272–4.

Smithells RW, Sheppard S, Schorah CJ et al. Possible prevention of neutral-tube defects by periconceptional vitamin supplementation. Lancet 1980; 1: 339–400.

Tamura T, Picciano F. Folate and human reproduction. Am J Clin Nutr 2006; 83: 993–1016.

Tejero E, Perichart O, Pfeffer F et al. Collagen snthesis during pregnancy, vitamin C availability, and risk of premature rupture of fetal membranes. Intl J Gynaecol Obstet 2003; 81: 29–34.

Teratology Society. Position Paper: Recommendations for Vitamin A use During Pregnancy. Teratology 1987; 35: 269–75.

Teratology Society. Summary of the 1993 Teratology Society Public Affairs Committee Symposium: folic acid prevention of neural tube defects – public policy issues. Teratology 1994; 49: 239–41.

Vergel RG, Sanchez LR, Heredero BL et al. Primary prevention of neural tube defects with folic acid supplementation: Cuban experience. Prenatal Diagn 1990; 10: 149–52.

Wacker J, Fruhauf J, Schulz M et al. Riboflavin deficiency and pre-eclampsia. Obstet Gynecol 2000; 96: 38–44.

Wiegand UW, Hartmann S, Hummler H. Safety of vitamin A: recent results. Intl J Vit Nutr Res 1998; 68: 411–16.

Zhang C (A), Williams MA, Sorensen TK et al. Maternal plasma ascorbic acid (vitamin C) and risk of gestational diabetes mellitus. Epidemiol 2004; 15: 597–604.

Zhang C (B), Williams MA, Frederick IO et al. Vitamin C and the risk of gestational diabetes mellitus: a case-control study. J Reprod Med 2004; 49: 257–66.

Herbs during pregnancy

2.19

Henry M. Hess and Richard K. Miller

Plants and plant extracts have been used for medicinal purposes since before recorded time. Many pharmaceutical agents have their origins in plant-based compounds. In a trend towards returning to the "natural", and believing that such agents are safer, patients worldwide are more and more frequently consulting natural therapists and taking herbs to enhance their nutrition, stay healthy, and treat their illnesses. Women taking herbs can and do get pregnant. They take herbal therapies to ensure that they are healthy prior to and during their pregnancy, and also to treat medical conditions during their pregnancy. A 2003 study of 578 pregnant women in the United States showed that 45 percent of respondents used herbal medicines (Glover 2003).

2.19.1 The safety of herbs during pregnancy

The difficulties in evaluating the safety and risk of *herbal therapies* are known, and are faced by everyone who takes or is considering taking herbs. These concerns are enhanced in pregnant women, and risks are even more difficult to evaluate. The problems of determining the safety of herbs in this context are as follows:

- There are few published clinical trials or investigations of these substances establishing the efficacy and/or toxicity of the preparations at specific doses.
- There are limited standards for the preparation and for the established amounts of specific ingredients in the products marketed, and there are few regulating bodies that certify the products sold or doses used (for example, the US Food and Drug Administration (FDA), the European Medicines Agency (EMEA) and the European Evaluation Food Safety Authority (EFSA)). The German Commission E does provide some oversight on selected herbal products (Blumenthal 2003, 1998).
- There are differing health claims made by the agencies in Europe, the United States, and other countries around the world.
- Some of the products available worldwide may contain (and in some instances have been shown to contain) unknown contaminants such as lead and/or arsenic from the agricultural or manufacturing processes. These could have devastating effects on the pregnant woman.
- It is always important to know the potential side effects of anything we take, and this is even more significant during pregnancy. The fetus is growing rapidly, and is vulnerable to substances that affect cellular growth and division. In addition, certain herbs and natural substances can affect the muscle tone and circulation of the uterus, and some can act as uterine stimulants, abortifacients or teratogens (Low Dog 2005).

2.19.2   Counseling a pregnant woman about herbs

For the above reasons, it is difficult even for an experienced healthcare provider to counsel a pregnant woman on the use of herbal preparations. As providers, evidence-based medicine is expected. However, few herbs and natural therapies even have good scientific evidence, never mind the evidence-based medicine that people expect today. Rather, herbal therapies use more traditional evidence as their proof of safety. This is evidence passed down by culture and tradition, and is often only oral. There is almost no solid scientific evidence regarding the benefits or the risks of herbs in pregnancy to the mother or fetus. It is difficult to reassure patients under these circumstances.

There is some good news, though. There is a considerable body of traditional evidence that can be used as a basis for a discussion with patients. This is traditional evidence – a different kind of evidence-based medicine. It can be very helpful to patients, when put in the proper perspective and used with appropriate understanding. This chapter presents the latest and best evidence that is available, to help counsel pregnant patients, and is organized to optimize the thinking and approach to understanding the most up-to-date knowledge regarding the safety of herbs during pregnancy.

Following a general discussion of herbs during pregnancy, descriptions of some of the frequently used herbs during pregnancy are presented here, along with the best evidence available regarding their safety and risk assessment during pregnancy. Next, there is a description of some common herbs where there is controversy over their use during pregnancy. Again, there is a description and discussion of the latest known evidence for these herbs. Finally, there is a list of herbs thought to be contraindicated during pregnancy. These are organized into groups according to how they might negatively affect a pregnant woman. This can be helpful in terms of counseling a patient.

The chapter focuses on herbal preparations for the pregnant woman. It does not include information on *ayruvedic* preparations, Chinese herbs and/or medicines, or *homeopathy*, where evidenced-based safety data for the pregnant woman are even more limited.

Sections and tables are presented identifying herbs where there is some evidence supporting the safety of their use during pregnancy, but only at the doses and in the preparations mentioned. It should be emphasized that any product can have potential adverse effects, based upon the quantity or doses used. Since manufacturing standards have not been established, it is impossible to be certain of the dosage in many products produced around the world. While manufacturers in developed countries have tried to establish more defined preparations, this still remains an area of concern. In addition, the stability of products and possible contamination of the plant or product grown in other parts of the world may still be an issue because of the lack of regulatory standards. Therefore, it is a requirement for any consumers of these products, and the provider counseling them, to evaluate carefully the stated preparation of each product used, focusing upon the reported concentrations of the ingredients, the country of origin, the manufacturer and its reputation, and any reported incidents of contamination for that type of product. For pregnant or lactating women, or any woman of reproductive age, further caution is necessary because of the potential for enhanced effects of these substances on the mother, the embryo/fetus, and the breastfed baby. With regard to purity and the safety of specific products, there is a valuable and important resource. Consumer Labs (ConsumerLab.com) is an independent laboratory for the testing of herbal, vitamin, and mineral supplements. A subscription service at

ConsumerLab.com is a valuable resource for any provider who counsels patients, including pregnant women, about the purity of specific brands of natural substances.

2.19.3   General concepts regarding the use of herbs during pregnancy

There are a few points that are important for consideration of the use of herbs in pregnancy:

1. Herbs should only be recommended by a competent and qualified provider caring for the pregnant woman, and one who is comfortable with and knowledgeable about the efficacy and risk assessment of herbs in pregnancy. It is well worth becoming familiar with Blumenthal (2003), Rotblatt (2002), and ConsumerLab.com.
2. Herbs are extracts of plants or plant roots, and they contain numerous compounds. Different forms of the herbal preparations will have different compounds in the herbal preparations, as well as differing concentrations. How the herb is prepared is very important to the effect and safety of the pregnant woman and fetus. Herbal preparations come in the following forms:
   - teas or infusions (infusions are hot-water extracts of dried herbs)
   - capsules
   - dried extracts
   - tinctures (tinctures are alcohol extracts of dried herbs).

   The most commonly used herbs in pregnancy are teas or infusions (which are similar to teas). These usually have the lowest concentrations and contain the least amount of the compounds. Capsules and dried extracts are less commonly used; examples include ginger and echinacea. Tinctures should be avoided in pregnancy because of their higher concentrations as well as the use of alcohol as a carrier.
3. The effects and safety of herbs will depend on the trimester. One of the most important concepts is that herbs – just like pharmaceuticals – should be used with caution in the first trimester. In general, there is no pharmaceutical or herb that is absolutely safe in the first trimester, based upon our current knowledge. It is important to be aware that the rapid cellular development in organogenesis can be altered by any compound, and that some herbs may increase uterine tone, increasing the risk of pregnancy loss.

4. The pregnant woman has an altered physiological state. Drugs and herbs may therefore behave differently in the pregnant woman's body compared to in a non-pregnant woman.

(See Low Dog 2005, Blumenthal 2003.)

2.19.4   Herbs used as foods

The safest herbs in pregnancy are, in general, those considered to be food. Herbs commonly used as food or food additives are usually safe for use during pregnancy, and can be used daily (at the levels generally used as food ingredients) without affecting the pregnant woman or fetus. (See Low Dog 2005, Fleming 2004, Blumenthal 2003, Weed 1986.)

2.19.5   Essential oils that are safe during pregnancy

Some essential oils can be safely used as aromatherapy during pregnancy, based on traditional and historic use. There are no evidenced-based studies that will assure their safety. They should always be used carefully, in a well-diluted form, and should not be ingested. They should be used in an aromatherapy diffuser. Such oils, and their uses, are listed in Table 2.19.1. (See Low Dog 2005, Fleming 2004, Blumenthal 2003, Weed 1986.)

Table 2.19.1 Essential oils considered to be safe during pregnancy

Essential oil	Common usage
Chamomile	Respiratory tract disorders
Tangerine	Antispasmodic, decongestant, general relaxant
Grapefruit	Stimulant, antidepressant
Geranium	Dermatitis, hormone imbalances, PMS, menstrual problems, viral infections
Rose	Astringent, used for mild inflammation of the oral and pharyngeal mucosa
Jasmine	Stimulant, antidepressant, anxiety
Ylang-ylang	Antispasmodic, cardiac arrhythmias, anxiety, antidepressant, hair loss, intestinal problems
Lavender	Loss of appetite, nervousness, and insomnia

2.19.6   Herbs frequently used during pregnancy

Herbs are frequently used as teas or infusions. Although there are no clinical trials available, and there is no evidence-based proof in terms of Western medical standards, some herbal teas/infusions have been used for many years without adverse effects, and are considered to be safe. The evidence of their safety comes from their traditional use and from traditional evidence passed down through history by traditional users. Although there are no data to suggest how much is "safe", it is suggested that consumption of herbal teas be limited to two cups per day during pregnancy. This is similar to the safety data regarding coffee in pregnancy. Their safety is unknown when used at higher levels, so the use of herbs above these amounts is not recommended. If the quantities consumed are above these recommended levels, no special action is required except stopping usage at high doses. (See Low Dog 2005, Blumenthal 2003, Weed 1986.).

Table 2.19.2 lists those herbs that are frequently used during pregnancy.

Table 2.19.2 Herbs frequently used during pregnancy

Herb	Usage	Form
1. Red raspberry leaf	Relief of nausea, increase in milk production, increase in uterine tone, and ease of labor pains; there is some controversy over its use in the first trimester, primarily because of concern of stimulating uterine tone and causing miscarriage (McFarland 1999, Parsons 1999, 2001, Brinker 1997)	Tea or infusion
2. Peppermint	Nausea, flatulence	Tea or infusion is the most common; enteric-coated tablets (187 mg) three times a day (maximum), are also used; peppermint may cause gastroesophageal reflux
3. Chamomile (German)	Gastrointestinal irritation, insomnia, and joint irritation	Tea or infusion
4. Dandelion	A mild diuretic, and to nourish the liver; dandelion is known for high amounts of vitamins A and C, and elements of iron, calcium, and potassium, as well as trace elements	Tea or infusion

(Continued)

Table 2.19.2 *(Continued)*

Herb	Usage	Form
5. Alfalfa	General pregnancy tonic; a source of high levels of vitamins A, D, E, and K, minerals, and digestive enzymes; thought to reduce the risk of postpartum hemorrhage in late pregnancy	Tea or infusion
6. Oat and oat straw	Sources of calcium and magnesium; helps to relieve anxiety, restlessness, insomnia, and irritable skin	Tea or infusion
7. Nettle leaf	All-around pregnancy tonic; sources of high amounts of vitamins A, C, K, and calcium, potassium; and iron. **NB**: Nettle root (different from nettle leaf) is used for inducing abortions and is not safe in pregnancy; nettle-leaf tea is a traditional tea in pregnancy and lactation	Tea or infusion
8. Slippery elm bark	Nausea, heartburn, and vaginal irritations	Tea or infusion

2.19.7   Herbs controversially used during pregnancy

More controversial herbs are listed in Table 2.19.3.

2.19.8   Herbs contraindicated during pregnancy

There are numerous herbs that are thought to be contraindicated during pregnancy, or that traditional herbalists consider potentially contraindicated during pregnancy. Studies are minimal, however. (See Low Dog 2005, Blumenthal, 2003, 1998, Weed 1986.) These herbs can be classified into five subgroups for an understanding of their potential effect on a pregnant woman:

1. *Herbs used traditionally to stimulate menstruation* (Table 2.19.4). Herbs that may stimulate the smooth muscle of the uterus may be risky during pregnancy, as they may cause a pregnancy loss.
2. *Alkaloid-containing herbs* (Table 2.19.5). Alkaloids are a diverse group of chemical plant constituents that have a wide range of pharmacological impacts on the body. Some alkaloids have been shown to be hepatotoxic and potentially carcinogenic. In some instances these compounds can be very potent, and they

Table 2.19.3 Herbs controversially used during pregnancy

Herb	Usage	Form and dosage	Safety
1. Ginger	Nausea and vomiting, or morning sickness	250 mg four times a day maximum; ginger is also frequently used as a tea or infusion	Ginger is the only herb with reasonable evidence-based data regarding its benefit and safety during pregnancy. In several studies, it is estimated to be safe when used at doses of 250 mg four times a day or less (Blumenthal 2003, Low Dog 2005).
			Three published placebo-controlled trials have addressed the safety and efficacy of ginger for morning sickness. In 1990, Fischer-Rasmussen reported 30 pregnant women, randomly assigned, who were admitted to the hospital before 20 weeks' gestation, and received either 250 mg of powdered ginger capsules or placebo four times a day over a 4-day period. No adverse effects on the pregnancy and outcome were noted.
			Vutyavanich (2001) conducted a randomized double-blind placebo-controlled study of 70 women with nausea of pregnancy with or without vomiting before the seventeenth week. Again, either 250 mg powdered ginger capsules or placebo four times a day was used. Good efficacy was reported, and no adverse effects were noted on pregnancy outcomes. A study in 2003 by Willetts, in a double-blind placebo-controlled trial, randomly assigned 120 women before the twentieth week of gestation who had experienced morning sickness daily for at least a week. These patients received either 125 mg of ginger extract or placebo four times a day. Again, the efficacy was excellent, and outcomes were normal. Follow-up of the pregnancies revealed normal ranges of birth weight, gestational age, Apgar scores, and frequencies of congenital abnormalities when the study group infants were compared to the general population of infants born that year.
			Surprisingly, the German Commission E (Blumenthal 1998) and the American Herbal Products Association (McGaffin 1997) contraindicate the use of ginger during pregnancy. This is definitely not supported by the popular data, popular

experience, or traditional-based evidence. Their advice appears to be based on two concerns. The first is that inhibition of thromboxane synthetase may affect testosterone binding in the fetus, although this usually happens at much higher doses than those practically used or used in the studies (Backon 1991). The second concern is *in vitro* evidence that gingerol and shogoal, isolated components of ginger, exhibit mutagenic activity in certain salmonella strains (Nagabhushan 1987). However, researchers have also found potential antimutagenic compounds in ginger (Fudler 1991). In that regard, however, a study of rats failed to find malformations in the offspring of animals administered 20 g/l or 50 g/l of ginger tea in their drinking water in early pregnancy.

Researchers at the Hospital For Sick Children in Toronto, Canada, studied 187 pregnant women who used some form of ginger in the first trimester (Portnoi 2003). In this small study, there were no increased risks in babies with congenital malformations compared to a control group.

With the vast number of women taking ginger during pregnancy, it is reasonable to assume that it is safe for women to use small amounts (up to 250 mg four times a day) of ginger during pregnancy. However, it is prudent to use ginger in moderation (Low Dog 2005, Blumenthal 2003, Muller 1991, Fudler 1991).

2. Cranberry	Prevention and treatment of urinary tract infection (Low Dog 2005, Blumenthal 2003)	300–400 mg three times daily

Although there is a long history of the safe use of cranberry during pregnancy there are no studies confirming this.

3. Evening primrose oil	Mastalgia, mood swings (Hibbeln 2002)	500 mg daily

There are no known restrictions on the use of evening primrose oil during pregnancy (Chen 1999, Brown 1996, Harrobin 1992, 1991). No teratogenic effects have been seen, based on animal studies. According to The World

(Continued)

2

Pregnancy

2.19 Herbs during pregnancy

Table 2.19.3 (Continued)

Herb	Usage	Form and dosage	Safety
			Health Organization, pregnant and lactating women should obtain 5 percent of their total daily caloric intake from EFA (essential fatty acids).
4. Aloe vera gel	Topical use (only), for burns (Low Dog 2005, Blumenthal 2003)	Gel	Although there is a long history of safe topical use during pregnancy, there are no studies showing its safety
5. Echinacea	Prevention and treatment of upper respiratory tract infections, vaginitis, and herpes simplex virus (Gallo 2000, Blumenthal 1998, McGaffin 1997, Mengs 1991)	900 mg of dried root (or equivalent) three times daily	Although there is a long history of safe use during pregnancy, there are very few studies (Gallo 2000, Mengs 1991) showing its safety. Early animal studies have failed to demonstrate evidence of mutagenicity or carcinogenicity after 4 weeks of ingestion of the expressed use of Echinacea at doses that far exceed normal human consumption. A prospective study of 206 pregnant women found no increased risk for fetal malformations when Echinacea was ingested during pregnancy, even during the first trimester (Gallo 2000). The authors of these studies suggest that gestational use of Echinacea during organogenesis is not associated with a detectable increased risk of malformations, but these studies did not have the statistical power or sufficient scientific rigor to assure this. *The British Herbal Compendium*, *The German Commission E Monograph* (Blumenthal 1998), and The American Herbal Products Association (McGaffin 1997) have listed the use of Echinacea as not contraindicated during pregnancy.
6. St John's wort	Mild to moderate depression (Low Dog 2005, Blumenthal 2003)	300 mg three times daily, of a standardized extract	Although its safety in pregnancy has not been scientifically evaluated, the German Commission E (Blumenthal 2003, 1998) and the American Herbal Products Association (Blumenthal 2003, McGaffin 1997) state that St John's wort is not contraindicated. Its use in pregnant women is commonly reported. However, there have not been any adequate clinical trials using evidence-based

2

Pregnancy

		principles that can absolutely reassure of safety of St John's wort for the pregnant or lactating woman. In one study in mice (Fudler 1991), maternal administration of 180 mg/kg of hypericum before and throughout gestation did not affect the long-term growth or physical maturation of exposed mouse offspring. In another study, no adverse effects were noted in the offspring of animals given 1.5 g/kg per day of hypericum. No chromosomal abberations have been found on *in vitro* or animal testing. In one published case report, low levels of hyperforin were found in the breast milk of a woman who had been taking 300 mg three times a day of a standard extract of St John's wort while nursing (a standard dose). However, hyperforin and hypericin, compounds in St. John's wort, were undetectable in the baby's plasma. No adverse effects were noted in the mother or the infant (Rayburn 2001, Mills 2000, Okpanyi 1991). It should be noted that St John's wort induces CYP 3A4 and P-glycoprotein, which can result in decreased action of many drugs. Photosensitization has also been reported.
7. Valerian root	Anxiety, insomnia (Low Dog 2005, Blumenthal 2003)	Tea/capsule – 2–3 g of crude herb at bedtime	No contraindications have been found in the literature, including the German Commission E (Blumenthal 2003, McGaffin1997) and the *Botanical Safety Handbook* (McGaffin 1997). Several articles and books support the use of valerian during pregnancy, and generally conclude that occasional use, for insomnia, is safe. Traditional clinical use supports its safety, and therapists use it for pregnant and lactating women. The World Health Organization (WHO) (Low Dog 2005), on the other hand, contraindicates the use of valerian during pregnancy and lactation as a general precaution, because its safety has not been established clinically – i.e. there are no clinical trials available using evidence-based medicine to prove its safety. In one study, *valepotriates*, the key constituent in valerian, was given orally for 30 days to pregnant rats, and there were no adverse findings in the pregnant rats or in their offspring. To date, there have been no studies of human pregnancies (Low Dog 1005, Blumenthal 1998, Tufik 1994).

2.19 Herbs during pregnancy

Table 2.19.4 Herbs used traditionally to stimulate menstruation (not recommended during pregnancy)

Herb	Usage
Angelica	Diuretic and diaphoretic
Celandine	Loss of appetite; liver and gallbladder complaints
Goldenseal	Dyspepsia, gastritis, diarrhea, menorrhagia
Shepherd's purse	Arrhythmia, hypertension, hypotension, nosebleeds, PMS
Barberry	Constipation, loss of appetite, heartburn
Dong Quai	Hormone imbalance, PMS, menopause
Motherwort	Arrhythmia, hyperthyroid, flatulence, PMS
Southernwood	Anxiety, depression
Black Cohosh	Menstrual irregularity, PMS, menopause
Ephedra	Bronchospasms (bronchodilator), nasal congestion, weight loss
Mugwort	Gastrointestinal complaints, sedative
Tansy	Migraines, antihelminthic, neuralgia, rheumatism, loss of appetite
Blue Cohosh*	Gynecologic disorders, dysmenorrhea, dyspareunia, menorrhagia, labor induction, antispasmatic symptoms during labor
Feverfew	Migraines; nausea and vomiting associated with migraines
Rue	Menstrual disorders, contraception, abortifacient, anti-inflammatory
Yarrow	Loss of appetite, dyspepsia, liver and gallbladder complaints
Nettle root	Urinary tract infections, kidney and bladder stones, rheumatism
Baldo	Depression, stimulant
Andrographis	Anxiety, gastritis

*Blue Cohosh has been used by some medical providers to induce labor at the end of a pregnancy (Weed 1986)

have been isolated as medications or as the active ingredients in many pharmaceuticals and herbs.

3. *Essential oils* (Table 2.19.6). Essential oils are frequently used by patients in many situations. Some essential oils are potentially very dangerous during pregnancy when ingested. All essential oils

2

Table 2.19.5 Alkaloid-containing herbs (contraindicated during pregnancy)

Herb	Usage
Autumn crocus	Digestion stimulation
Broom	Hypertension, edema, menorrhagia, postpartum hemorrhage
Comfrey	Gastritis, gastrointestinal ulcers, external bruises, and blunt injuries
Mandrake (podophyllin)*	One of the oldest medicinal plants; stomach ulcers, colic, hay fever
Barberry	Constipation, loss of appetite, heartburn
Coffee**	Stimulation, increased performance, migraines, diarrhea, inflammation of the mouth/pharynx, weight loss
Goldenseal	Dyspepsia, gastritis, diarrhea, and menorrhagia
Tansy	Migraines, antihelminthic, neuralgia, rheumatism, loss of appetite
Blood root	Expectorant, antiplaque agent, mouthwash
Colt's foot	Treatment and prevention of diseases of the respiratory tract

*Animal studies have suggested risks of reproductive and developmental toxicity (Joneja 1974, Dwornik 1967, Thiersch 1963).
**More than two cups per day of freshly brewed coffee (Christian 2001, Mills et al. 1993).

Table 2.19.6 Essential oils (contraindicated during pregnancy when taken orally)

Herb	Usage
Arbor vitae	Liver cleanse, loss of appetite, anxiety
Juniper	Acne, liver problems, urinary tract infections, fluid retention
Pennyroyal	Digestive disorders, colds, increased micturition
Nutmeg	Stomach complaints
Catnip	Colds, colic, migraines, nervous disorders, gynecologic disorders
Rosemary	Loss of appetite, blood pressure problems, liver and gallbladder complaints, rheumatism
Baldo	Depression, stimulant

should be appropriately diluted when used, and none should be taken internally. In some instances, especially with external use, essential oils may be safe, but in general – especially during pregnancy – they are contraindicated.

4. *Anthraquinone laxatives* (Table 2.19.7). Anthraquinones are very potent compounds which can stimulate bowel peristalsis. They are frequently used as potential laxative agents. In pregnancy, overstimulation of the bowel or bladder has the potential to irritate/stimulate the uterus in some women, and may cause premature labor.
5. *Herbs thought to have an effect on the hormonal system* (Table 2.19.8). Herbs that may have an effect on the hormonal system, and that have potential estrogen-like properties, give scientists cause for concern regarding the possible effects on the fetus.

Table 2.19.7 Anthraquinone laxatives (not recommended during pregnancy)

Herb	Usage
Alder buckthorn	Constipation, anal fissures, hemorrhoids, diuretic
Cascara	Constipation, anal fissures, hemorrhoids
Purging buckthorn	Constipation, anal fissures, hemorrhoids
Senna	Constipation, anal fissures, hemorrhoids

Table 2.19.8 Herbs with potential hormonal action (not recommended during pregnancy)

Herb	Usage
Ginseng	Adaptogen, general tonic, fatigue
Licorice	Gastric disorders, upper respiratory disorders, menorrhagia, menopause
Chasteberry (Vitex)*	Menstrual disorders
Saw palmetto	Benign prostatic hyperplasia, menopause
Passion flower	Nervousness and insomnia
Isoflavones	PMS, menstrual disorders, menopause
Red clover	Coughs, respiratory conditions, PMS, menopause
Flaxseed	Hyperlipidemia, atherosclerosis, breast cancer, constipation, IBS, diverticulitis, gastritis
Hops	Anxiety, insomnia

*Chasteberry is sometimes used by experienced practitioners to treat and/or prevent postpartum bleeding.

> **Recommendation.** It is important to remember, and to remind patients, that it is critical to know the safety issues regarding particular herbs during pregnancy, and also critical to know the doses, stability, and purity of the product. ConsumerLab.com is an extremely helpful resource in this regard.

2

Pregnancy

References

Backon J, Fischer-Rasmussen W. Ginger in preventing nausea and vomiting of pregnancy; a caveat do to its thromboxane synthetase activity and effect on testosterone binding. Eur J Obstet Gynecol Reprod Biol 1991; 42: 163–4.

Blumenthal M, Gruenwald J, Hall C et al. EDS, The Complete German Commission E Monographs: Therapeutic Guide To Herbal Medicine. Boston, MA: Integrative Medicine Communications, 1998.

Blumenthal M. (ed.) The ABC Clinical Guide To Herbs. New York: Thieme Medical Publishing, 2003.

Brinker F. Herb Contraindications And Drug Interactions. Sandy, OR: Eclectic Institute, 1997.

Brown D. Herbal Prescriptions for Better Health. Rockland, CA: Prima Publishing, 1996, pp. 79–89.

Chen J. Evening Primrose Oil – Continuing Education Module. Bolder, CO: University of Southern California School of Pharmacy, 1999.

Christian MS, Brent RL. Teratogen update: evaluation of the reproductive and developmental risks of caffeine. Teratology 2001; 64: 51–78.

Dwornik JJ, Moore KL. Congenital anomalies produced in the rat by podophyllin. Anat Rec 1967; 157: 237.

Fischer-Rasmussen W. Ginger treatment of hyperemesis gravidarum. Eur J Obstet Gynecol Reprod Biol 1990; 38: 19–24.

Fleming T. (ed.) PDR For Herbal Medicines, 3rd edn. Montvale, NJ: Medical Economics Company, 2004.

Fudler S, Tenne M. Ginger as an anti-nausea remedy in pregnancy; the issue of safety. Herbalgram 1991; 38: 47–50.

Gallo M, Sarkarm M, Au W. Pregnancy outcome following gestational exposure to Echinacea: a prospective controlled study. Arch Intern Med 2000; 160: 3141–3.

Glover DG, Amonkar M, Rybeck BF. Prescription, over-the-counter, and herbal medicine use in a rural, obstetric population. Am J Obstet Gynecol 2003; 88: 1039–45.

Harrobin N, Alice K, Morris-Fisher The effects of evening primrose oil, safflower oil and paraffin on plasma fatty acid levels in humans: choice of an appropriate placebo for clinical studies on primrose oil. Prostagland Leukot Essent Fatty Acids 1991; 42: 245–9.

Harrobin N. Nutritional and medical importance of gamma-linolenic acid. Progn Lipid Reis 1992; 31: 163–94.

Hibbeln JR. Seafood consumption, the DHA content of mother's milk and prevalence rates of postpartum depression: a cross-national, ecological analysis. J Affect Disord 2002; 69(1–3): 15–29.

Joneja MG, LeLiever WC. Effects of vinblastine and podophyllin on DBA on mouse fetuses. Toxicol Appl Pharmacol 1974; 27: 408–14.

2.19 Herbs during pregnancy

Low Dog T, Micozzi MS. Women's Health in Complementary and Integrative Medicine: A Clinical Guide. Oxford: Elsevier, 2005.

McFarland BC, Gilson MH, O'Rear J et al. A national survey of herbal preparation use by nurse midwives for labor stimulation. Review of the literature and recommendations for practice. J Nurse Midwif 1999; 44: 205–16.

McGaffin M, Hobb C, Upton R et al. American Herbal Products Association's Botanical Safety Handbook. Boca Raton, FL: CRC Press, 1997.

Mengs U, Clare CB, Poiley JA. Toxicity of *Echinacea purpurea*. Acute, subacute and genotoxicity studies. Arzneim-Forsch Drug Res 1991; 41: 1976–81.

Mills JL, Holmes LB, Aarons JH et al. Moderate caffeine use and the risk of spontaneous abortion and intrauterine growth retardation. J Am Med Assoc 1993; 269: 593–7.

Mills S, Bone K. Principles and Practice of Phytotherapy. London: Churchill Livingstone, 2000, pp. 548–9.

Muller J, Clauson KA. Pharmaceutical considerations of common herbal medicine. Am J Managed Care 1997; 3: 1753–70.

Nagabhushan M. Mutagenicity of gingerol and shogoal and antimutagenicity of zingerone, in Parsons Salmonella/microsome assay. Cancer Lett 1987; 36: 221–3.

Okpanyi SN, Lidzba H, Scholl BC. Genotoxicity of standardized Hypericum extract. Arzneimettl-Forsch 1991; 40(8 Pt 2): 851–5.

Parsons M, Simpson M, Ponton TJ. Raspberry leaf and its effect on labour: safety and efficacy. Aust Coll Midwives 1999; 12: 20–25.

Portnoi G, Chng LA, Karimi-Tabesh L et al. Prospective comparative study of the safety and effectiveness of ginger for the treatment of nausea and vomiting in pregnancy. Am J Obstet Gynecol 2003; 189: 1374–7.

Rayburn WF, Gonzalez CL, Christense HB. Effect of prenatally administered hypericum (St John's wort) on growth and physical maturation of mouse offspring. Am J Obstet Gynecol 2001; 184: 191–5.

Rotblatt M, Zimint I. Evidence-Based Herbal Medicine. Philadelphia, PA: Lippincott Williams & Wilkins, 2002.

Simpson M, Parsons M, Greenwood J. Raspberry leaf in pregnancy: its safety and efficacy in labor. J Midwifery Women's Health 2001; 46: 151–9.

Thiersch JB. Effect of podophyllin and podophyllotoxine on the rat litter in utero. Proc Soc Exper Biol 1903; 113: 124–7.

Tufik S, Fujita K, Seabra M de L. Effects of a prolonged administration of valepotriates in rats on the mothers and their offspring. J Ethnophamacol 1994; 41: 39–44.

Vutyavanich T, Kraisarint T. Ginger for nausea and vomiting in pregnancy: randomized, double-masked, placebo-controlled trial. Ruangsrira Obstet Gynecol 2001; 97: 577–82.

Weed S. Wise Woman Herbal For The Childbearing Year. Woodstock, NY: Ash Tree Publishing, 1986.

Willetts KE, Ekangahi A, Eden JA. Effect of a ginger extract on pregnancy-induced nausea: a randomised controlled trial. Aust NZ J Obstet Gynaecol 2003; 43: 139–44.

▶ **Useful websites**

American Botanical Council (www.herbalgram.org).

CAM On Pubmed (www.nlm.nih.gov/nccam/camonpubmed.hlml, and www.pubmed.gov).

HerbMed (www.herbmed.org).

International Bibliographic Information On Dietary Supplements (IBIDS) Database (http://ods.od.nih.gov/health_information/ibids.aspx).

Natural Medicines Comprehensive Data Base (www.naturaldatabase.com).

Natural Standard (www.naturalstandard.com).

United States Pharmacopeia Dietary Supplement Verification Program (www. uspverified.org).

www.ConsumerLab.com (for evaluating preparations).

Diagnostic agents

2.20

Elisabeth Robert-Gnansia

2.20.1   X-ray examinations

X-rays are ionizing radiation, and doses are expressed in rad or in Gray (Gy), where 1 Gray = 100 rads = 100 000 mrad. Only the radiation dose that reaches the organ in question – in this case, the uterus, ovaries or the fetus – is relevant. In the target organism, i.e. the embryo, the actually determined dose is expressed in rem or Sievert (Sv), where 1 Sievert = 100 rem = 100 000 mrem. Assuming that the emitted dose to the organ corresponds to the dose delivered to the embryo, 1 Sv corresponds to 1 Gy.

The cardinal manifestations of intrauterine radiation effects in humans are growth retardation and defects of the central nervous system (CNS) – mainly microcephaly with mental retardation, and eye malformations. These effects are a function of the dose administered and of the stage of development of the embryo. Embryo/fetal death may also occur during the first 5 days after conception (i.e. in the "all-or-none period"); the lowest lethal dose is 10 rads (0.1 Gy). During embryogenesis, the lowest lethal dose for the embryo increases to 25–50 rads and later to more than 100 rads (1 Gy) (Brent 1999). Severe CNS malformations are to be expected with exposures above 20 rads during early gestation (18–36 days after conception). Microcephaly and mental retardation were observed only after exposures above 20 rads between weeks 8 and 15 after conception. The conclusion from most studies is that for doses lower than 0.05 Gy (i.e. 5 rads) there is no significant increase of the malformation rate in humans, and the risk clearly is increased above 20–50 rads (Brent 1999, Sternberg 1973). A common and important finding is the absence of visceral, limb or other malformations unless there is growth retardation, microcephaly or congenital malformation of the brain, or visible eye malformations such as microphthalmia, optic atrophy, or cataract. De Santis (2005A) and Brent (1999) reviewed the literature and concluded that inadvertent exposure to ionizing radiations due to diagnostic procedures during pregnancy doesn't increase the background risk of congenital anomalies. It has nevertheless been suggested by different authors that pregnancy exposure to ionizing radiations increases the risk of low birth weight (Hamilton 1984). Hujoel (2004) performed a case-control study and concluded that dental X-rays during pregnancy were a risk factor for low birth weight. They suggest as an interpretation that an alteration of the maternal hypothalamus–hypophysis–thyroid axis might affect birth weight, with a threshold dose-effect of 0.4 mGy at the thyroid. De Santis (2005B) studied the pregnancy outcome of 224 women who underwent thyroid irradiation as a diagnostic procedure during the first trimester, and also found a moderate reduction in the birth weight with a dose threshold of 0.4–0.8 mGy at the thyroid level. These studies concerning the thyroid are considered to be inconsistent, because hypothyroidism cannot be produced with 0.4 mGy (Brent 2005, Boice 2004).

The mutagenic or transplacental carcinogenetic risk of ionizing radiation is more difficult to evaluate than the teratogenic risk. Mutagenic effects are stochastic events, and no threshold can be established for this kind of risk. Point mutations often occur spontaneously. Estimations have been made that a dose of 100–200 rads may induce a doubling of the point mutation rate (Brent 1999, Neel 1999). On the one hand, a doubling of the mutation rate of a given gene does not mean a doubling of the disease frequency; on the other hand, insufficient knowledge regarding the possible effects on later generations prevents definition of safety limit values of exposures for a population (Brent 1999). The dose capable of increasing

2

Pregnancy

2.20 Diagnostic agents

the cancer risk, especially the risk of childhood leukemia following prenatal exposure, is also not well established. In a case-control study on neuroblastoma, Patton (2004) found no consistent exposure – response gradient based upon the number of maternal or paternal medical radiation examinations. In a study of twin pregnancies conducted by Harvey (1985), it was concluded that a prenatal dose of 0.01 Sv (1 rem) might multiply the risk of childhood leukemia by a factor of 2.4. Wakeford (2003) concluded, from the Oxford Survey of Childhood Cancers, that doses to the fetus *in utero* of the order of 10 mSv discernibly increases the risk of childhood cancer.

However, uncertainties in risk estimates are such that it is difficult to conclude reliably from these epidemiological data what the level of risk at these low doses might be, beyond the inference that the risk is not zero or grossly underestimated. Other authors assume that there is no increased risk for the embryo with exposures of 0.02–0.05 Sv (Boice 1999) because the increased lifetime risk would be very small – the current risk is 18 per 100 000 and, based upon this extrapolation, would become 18.024 per 100 000.

▶ **Dose estimations of usual X-ray examinations**

The usual conventional X-ray examinations, including examination of the lower abdomen, all give a dose of less than 5 rem. In most cases, in a single X-ray of the abdominal, pelvic, and lumbar spine region (without shielding of the uterus), the dose will be well under 200 mrem, provided that examinations are conducted with current and correctly adjusted equipment. Longer screening times, as used in intestinal explorations or urographies, can lead to a dose to the uterus of 2 rem. Endoscopic retrograde cholangio-pancreatography (ERCP) was evaluated in 17 pregnant women (Kahaleh 2004), and the mean fetal radiation exposure was 40–46 mrad (range 1–180 mrad). Computerized tomography (CT scan) delivers higher doses; however, these mostly stay below 5 rem. The secondary irradiation owing to examinations of other body regions, such as the upper abdomen, thorax, extremities or teeth, is negligible, because the doses delivered to the uterus lie well below 10 mrem – even as low as 1 mrem.

Recommendation. As a woman may not be aware of her pregnancy at the beginning, radiologists should not rely on a negative answer from a woman asked about a possible pregnancy before a radiological exploration. Any necessary X-ray examination of the lower abdomen should be performed only during the first half of the menstrual cycle. If X-ray examinations are indispensable during pregnancy, only the most modern devices should be used, with optimal protection of the uterus. In any case of X-ray examination during pregnancy that (inadvertently) includes the uterus, the uterine dose should be assessed and documented; this is especially important in cases of X-ray screening for more than 15 seconds, or a CT scan.

Neither radiographs outside the genital region and the uterus, nor the usual X-ray examinations (including standard CT scan) inadvertently including the pregnant uterus, require termination of pregnancy or any additional diagnostic procedures.

2.20.2   Ultrasound

For about 30 years, ultrasound has been used during all phases of pregnancy. Numerous animal experiments were reviewed by Jensh and Brent (1999), but little has been published regarding adverse fetal effects in humans (epidemiologic studies are reviewed in Ziskin 1999).

Ultrasound waves passing through living tissue have at least two effects: increased temperature (thermal effect) and tissue/molecular movements (mechanical effect). Negative effects may be suspected because of local induced hyperthermia. Although several hypotheses regarding the association of ultrasound with increased fetal activity, decreased birthweight or delayed speech development have been discussed in a few studies (Newnham 2004, Visser 1993), none of them have been verified. This applies particularly to the usual range of diagnostics and the application of modern devices, which are much improved, compared with those of the 1970s, with respect to performance. Follow-up studies of about 1500 infants could not demonstrate developmental differences at the ages of 1–8 years among infants exposed to five examinations between gestational weeks 18 and 38, compared to a control group exposed only once during pregnancy (Newnham 2004).

Kieler (2001) undertook a cohort study that included men born in Sweden from 1973 to 1978 who enrolled for military service. They found that when ultrasonography was offered more widely (1976–1978), the risk of left-handedness was higher among those exposed to ultrasound compared with those unexposed (OR 1.32, 95% CI 1.16–1.51), while during the introduction phase (1973–1975) there was no difference in lateralization between ultrasound-exposed and the unexposed. They conclude that ultrasound exposure in fetal life increases the risk of left-handedness in men, suggesting that prenatal ultrasound affects the fetal brain. To assess a possible association between prenatal ultrasound and intellectual performance, the same authors studied the intellectual scores of the same men born in Sweden from 1973 to 1978 (Kieler 2005). They were measured by a test battery at enrollment for military service, and the study failed to demonstrate a clear association between ultrasound scanning and intellectual performance.

However, the acoustic output of machines has increased almost eight-fold since then: in 1992, the maximal permissible output for fetal use was increased (at least in the USA) from 94 to 720 mW/cm^2 (Miller 1998). Higher energy is of particular concern for pulsed-Doppler color-flow first-trimester ultrasound with a long transvesical path (> 5 cm), and for second- or third-trimester examinations when bone is in the focal zone, as well as when scanning tissue with minimal perfusion (embryonic) or in patients who are febrile (Bly 2005, Barnett 2000).

> **Recommendation.** Ultrasonographic studies in pregnancy should be limited to medically necessary investigations. On this condition, and according to the available data, the risk of negative effects on fetal development is remote.

2.20.3   Magnetic resonance imaging

Magnetic resonance imaging (MRI) provides multiplanar large field-of-view images of the body with excellent soft-tissue contrast, and without ionizing radiation. As a result, MRI is increasingly being used to image the maternal abdomen and pelvis during pregnancy. During MRI, electromagnetic fields (EMF) are produced which do not differ from those produced by other electric appliances, including radiowaves. The magnetic field strength given to the patient is 2 Tesla (T); for the examination staff it is 5–100 mT. MRI has been applied for about 20 years in the second and third trimesters of pregnancy, for an increasing number of indications: localization of the placenta; measurements of the pelvis (when vaginal delivery seems questionable); examination of the fetal brain, lungs, and kidneys; and examination of unidentified masses (de Wilde 2005). No negative effects on the mother or newborn seem to be attributable to MRI, and visual and hearing tests at the ages of 3 and about 8 years also showed no negative effects (Kok 2004, Baker 1994). Nonetheless, experience during the first trimester is lacking (for review of the effects of EMF, see Robert 1999, Brent 1993). Epidemiological studies on occupational exposures to MRI have raised no indication of a reproductive risk (Evans 1993).

> **Recommendation.** Until more conclusive safety data become available, MRI should be reserved for cases in which results of ultrasonography are inconclusive and patient care depends on further imaging. Weighing the potential risks of X-rays against those of MRI, preference is to be given to MRI at any stage of pregnancy.

2.20.4   Barium sulfate

Barium sulfate is a contrast medium used for radiologic opacification of the stomach and intestinal tract. Barium sulfate is insoluble, and is not absorbed by the digestive tract. Therefore, no damage to the fetus can be expected in cases of exposure to this contrast medium during pregnancy.

2.20.5   Iodine-containing contrast media

Pharmacology and toxicology

Iodine-containing contrast agents include *iobitridol, iodamide, iodixanol, iohexol, iomeprol, iopamidol, iopanoic acid, iopentol, iopodate, iopromide, iotalamine acid, iotrolan, iotroxine, ioversol, ioxagline acid, ioxitalamine acid, lysine amido-trizoate, meglumine amido-trizoate* and *sodium amido-trizoate, metrizamide, metrizoate,* and *sodium iodine.*

Those iodinated, low molecular weight radiographic non-ionic contrast agents cross the human placenta and enter the fetus in significant concentrations (Moon 2000). Among these contrast media, renal and biliary preparations are to be distinguished. Biliary contrast media are lipophilic. This facilitates their elimination by the liver, but also aids the transplacental passage. More than 80% of biliary contrast media is rapidly eliminated through the bile in the digestive tract. Urinary contrast media, as well as those used for angiography, are hydrophilic, intravenously applicable, and poorly bound to plasma proteins. They are eliminated quickly by the kidney. In one case, the presence of iopromide was reported in the bowel and urine of a preterm infant born 10 days after intravenous administration of the non-ionic monomer to his mother (Vanhaesebrouck 2005). Excessive urinary iodine excretion and borderline hyperthyrotropinemia were observed in the infant. Moreover, crossing of the fetal blood–brain barrier was demonstrated by detection of the angiographic material in CSF, and thus direct fetal neurotoxic effects cannot be excluded. Therefore, the perinatal safety of these diagnostic agents might be questioned, especially in preterm infants.

The amount of free iodine in the contrast medium is less than 0.1% of the total. The amount of the free iodide depends on the compound, and can increase during storage. The Contrast Media Safety Committee of the European Society of Urogenital Radiology reviewed the literature and developed guidelines (Webb 2005). Free iodide can reach the fetal thyroid and be stored there. The danger with iodine in excess is transient fetal hypothyroidism, particularly from the twelfth week of pregnancy onward, when the fetal thyroid starts its endocrine function (Webb 2005).

> **Recommendation.** In particular during the second and third trimesters, iodine-containing contrast agents should only be used for compelling diagnostic indications. Neonatal thyroid function should be checked carefully during the first week.

2.20.6   Ultrasonographic and magnetic resonance contrast media

Pharmacology and toxicology

D-galactose has been used in Europe, mainly in the UK and Finland, as a contrast medium in ultrasound diagnostic procedures (Schroeder 1999). No studies could be found regarding the use of this contrast enhancer in pregnancy ultrasound examinations.

Gadolinium derivatives such as *gadopentetate dimeglumine, gadobene acid, gadodiamide, gadoteridol, gadoter acid*, and *gadoxetic acid* are ionic paramagnetic contrast media, which are used for MRI. Animal studies have shown no indication of fetal or maternal toxic effects of these contrast media when applied antenatally. Also, none of the currently available case reports regarding the application of gadolinium in humans (Webb 2005, Marcos 1997), although representing predominantly post-first trimester exposures, found any indication of fetotoxicity.

Ferristen is considered to be safe. No accurate risk estimation is possible for the manganiferous *mangafodipir*, because of insufficient experience.

> **Recommendation.** No effect on the fetus has been seen after the use of gadolinium contrast media, and therefore it may be used if necessary. Mangafodipir should not be used, because of insufficient experience.

2.20.7   Radioactive isotopes

Pharmacology and toxicology

The radiation dose reaching the embryo within the framework of scintigraphy or positron emission tomography (PET) is dependent on the isotope used, its half-life, and the amount applied. In scintigraphy, *technetium* has largely replaced the iodine, and *18FDG*

(2-fluoro-2-deoxy-D-glucose) is applied intravenously in PET. The dose to the uterus will, after administration for diagnostic purposes, generally be within the μCi (microcurie) range (being less than 10 mGy), and will cause no embryo- or fetotoxicity (Adelstein 1999).

In contrast, when radioactive isotopes (mainly the radioiodine I^{131}) are used as therapeutics, as in hyperthyroidism or thyroid carcinoma, doses may be above 100 mCi (millicurie), and this can induce fetal hypothyroidism or even athyroidism (Bentur 1991).

According to larger studies covering in total several hundred women exposed to I^{131} for thyroid carcinoma or hyperthyroidism before becoming pregnant, the results have revealed no evidence that exposure to radioiodine affects the outcome of subsequent pregnancies and offspring (Bal 2005, Chow 2004, Read 2004, Schlumberger 1996). Several children were observed until adulthood without indications for an increased risk of carcinogenesis or mutagenic insults. The observed increase of miscarriages in those women who were treated within 1 year before the index pregnancy could be related to gonadal irradiation or to insufficient control of the hormonal thyroid status (Schlumberger 1996). Read (2004) found no birth defects among 36 infants fathered by men with an I^{131} treatment history.

> **Recommendation.** Diagnostic and/or therapeutic administration of radioisotopes during pregnancy is contraindicated. An exposure for diagnostic purposes is, nevertheless, not an indication for termination of pregnancy or for any additional diagnostic procedures. In cases of therapeutic dosage administration of I^{131} for treatment of hyperthyroidism or thyroid carcinoma, the fetal risk and resulting consequences must be discussed individually, based upon gestational age at exposure as well as dose exposure.

2.20.8   Stable isotopes

Pharmacology and toxicology

For different trace elements, stable isotopes have been developed, which are not radioactive and differ from the original element in their atomic weight. So far, no embryotoxic effects have been observed, either in animal experiments (Spielmann 1986) or in humans.

> **Recommendation.** There is no indication of a reproductive risk linked with the application of diagnostic procedures with stable isotopes.

2.20.9   Dyes

Pharmacology and toxicology

Specially developed dyes are used for the determination of heart, liver, and kidney function. Among them are *bromosulfthalein, Evans blue, indigo carmine, Congo red, methylene blue, phenol red, toluidine blue, tricarbocyanin,* and *trypaflavin.*

Methylene blue is used for the therapy of methemoglobinemia, and has also been used in twin pregnancies to mark one twin during amniocentesis, and for prepartum localization of amniotic fluid leakage. Small gut atresias have been described as fetotoxic effects from methylene blue. These are likely a consequence of disturbed perfusion in the small intestine, which is either due to hemolysis or can be explained by the vasoactivity of methylene blue. In cases of administration late in pregnancy, hemolysis and neonatal hyperbilirubinemia have been described together, with skin discoloration and respiratory distress syndromes (reviewed in Gauthier 2000, Cragan 1999). A case of jejunal atresia in twins was observed after injection of toluidine blue (Dinger 2003).

Indigo carmine and, to a lesser extent, *Evans blue* and *Congo red* have been administered in numerous cases with good marking results for amniocentesis as well as maternal blood volume. However, indigo carmine is an analog of serotonin, and therefore an indirect vasoactive effect cannot be excluded. Nevertheless, no effects comparable to those of methylene blue have been reported in over 150 documented pregnancies (Cragan 1993). There is insufficient experience on any of the other compounds.

> **Recommendation.** Diagnostic dyes should only be used in pregnant women for vital indications. Methylene blue and toluidine blue should not be used during amniocentesis. Inadvertent administration, nevertheless, does not justify a termination of pregnancy.

2.20.10   Other diagnostic agents

Fluorescein may be administered as a diagnostic agent in the eye, orally and intravenously (angiography). A case series with over 100 pregnant women who had angiography with fluorescein failed to demonstrate any unwanted fetal effects (Halperin 1990). Animal experiments also showed no teratogenic effects. The substance was retrieved in the amniotic fluid of a pregnant woman after application in the eye.

A mailing survey was conducted by Fineman (2001) to assess the general knowledge among ophthalmologists regarding the use of *indocyanine green* (ICG) angiography during pregnancy, and the literature was reviewed. Of respondents, 89% withheld fluorescein angiography and 24% withheld ICG angiography, largely because of fear of teratogenicity or lawsuit. Diabetic retinopathy and choroidal neovascular membrane were the most common indications for fluorescein angiography, and choroidal neovascular membrane and choroidal tumor were the most common indications for ICG angiography. Only 24% thought that it was safe to use ICG angiography in a pregnant patient, and only 5% thought it was safer than fluorescein angiography. The authors conclude that despite the documented safety of ICG when used for retinal angiography and the extensive experience with the use of intravenous ICG to measure hepatic blood flow in pregnant women, this survey shows widespread hesitation regarding the use of ICG for retinal angiography in pregnant women. Current practice patterns regarding the use of ICG angiography in pregnant patients may be unnecessarily restrictive.

Skin tests such as *tuberculin or allergy tests* are considered to be safe. This applies also to enzyme tests, for example with secretin.

Metyrapone is a competitive inhibitor of cortisol biosynthesis, used for evaluation of ACTH secretion in the rare cases when Cushing disease is suspected (Morris 2003). There is no indication for its use during pregnancy, as other diagnostic methods exist, but no congenital abnormalities were reported after exposure to metyrapone during pregnancy.

> **Recommendation.** Fluorescein and skin tests may be used in pregnancy when required. Inadvertent administration of metyrapone never justifies termination of pregnancy.

References

Adelstein SJ. Administered radionuclides in pregnancy. Teratology 1999; 59: 236–9.

Baker PN, Johnson IR, Harvey PR et al. A three-year follow-up of children imaged in utero with echo-planar magnetic resonance. Am J Obstet Gynecol 1994; 170: 32–3.

Bal C, Kumar A, Tripathi M et al. High-dose radioiodine treatment for differentiated thyroid carcinoma is not associated with change in female fertility or any genetic risk to the offspring. Intl J Radiat Oncol Biol Phys 2005; 63: 449–55.

Barnett SB, ter Haar GR, Ziskin MC et al. International recommendations and guidelines for the safe use of diagnostic ultrasound in medicine. Ultrasound Med Biol 2000; 26: 355–66.

Bentur Y, Horlatsch N, Koren G. Exposure to ionizing radiation during pregnancy: perception of teratogenic risk and outcome. Teratology 1991; 43: 109–12.

Bly S, van den Hof MC. Diagnostic Imaging Committee, Society of Obstetricians and Gynaecologists of Canada. Obstetric ultrasound biological effects and safety. J Obstet Gynaecol Can 2005; 27: 572–80.

Boice JD, Miller RW. Childhood and adult of cancer after intrauterine exposure to ionizing radiation. Teratology 1999; 59: 227–33.

Boice JD Jr, Stovall M, Mulvihill JJ et al. Dental X-rays and low birth weight. J Radiol Prot 2004; 24: 321–3.

Brent RL, Gordon WE, Bennett WR et al. Reproductive and teratogenic effects of electromagnetic fields. Reprod Toxicol 1993; 7: 535–80.

Brent RL. Utilization of developmental basic science principles in the evaluation of reproductive risks from pre- and postconception environmental radiation exposures. Teratology 1999; 59: 182–204.

Brent RL. Commentary on JAMA article by Hujoel et al: Antepartum dental radiography and infant low birth weight. Health Phys 2005; 88: 379–81.

Chow SM, Yau S, Lee SH et al. Pregnancy outcome after diagnosis of differentiated thyroid carcinoma: no deleterious effect after radioactive iodine treatment. Intl J Radiat Oncol Biol Phys 2004; 59: 992–1000.

Cragan JD, Martin ML, Khoury MJ et al. Dye use during amniocentesis and birth defects. Lancet 1993; 341: 1352.

Cragan JD. Teratogen update: methylene blue. Teratology 1999; 60: 42–8.

de Santis M (A), di Gianantonio E, Straface G et al. Ionizing radiations in pregnancy and teratogenesis: a review of literature. Reprod Toxicol 2005; 20: 323–9.

de Santis M (B), Straface G, Cavaliere AF et al. First trimester maternal thyroid X-ray exposure and neonatal birth weight. Reprod Toxicol 2005; 20: 3–4.

de Wilde JP, Rivers AW, Price DL. A review of the current use of magnetic resonance imaging in pregnancy and safety implications for the fetus. Prog Biophys Mol Biol 2005; 87: 335–53.

Dinger J, Autenrieth A, Kamin G et al. Jejunal atresia related to the use of toluidine blue in genetic amniocentesis in twins. J Perinatal Med 2003; 31: 266–8.

Evans JA, Savitz DA, Channel E et al. Infertility and pregnancy outcome among magnetic resonance imaging workers. J Occup Med 1993; 35: 1191–5.

Fineman MS, Maguire JI, Fineman SW et al. Safety of indocyanine green angiography during pregnancy: a survey of the retina, macula, and vitreous societies. Arch Ophthalmol 2001; 119: 353–5.

Gauthier TW. Methylene blue-induced hyperbilirubinemia in neonatal glucose-6-phosphate dehydrogenase (G6PD) deficiency. J Matern Fetal Med 2000; 9: 252–4.

Halperin LS, Olk RJ, Soubrane G et al. Safety of fluorescein angiography during pregnancy. Intl J Ophthalmol 1990; 109: 563–6.

Hamilton PM, Roney PL, Keppel KG et al. Radiation procedures performed on US women during pregnancy: findings from two 1980 surveys. Public Health Rep 1984; 99: 146–51.

Harvey EB, Bolce JD, Honeyman M et al. Prenatal X-ray exposure and childhood cancer in twins. N Engl J Med 1985; 312: 541–5.

Hujoel PP, Bollen AM, Noonan CJ et al. Antepartum dental radiography and infant low birth weight. J Am Med Assoc 2004; 28(291): 1987–93.

Jensh RP, Brent RL. Intrauterine effects of ultrasound: animal studies. Teratology 1999; 59: 240–51.

Kahaleh M, Hartwell GD, Arseneau KO et al. Safety and efficacy of ERCP in pregnancy. Gastrointest Endosc 2004; 60: 287–92.

Kieler H, Cnattingius S, Haglund B et al. Sinistrality – a side-effect of prenatal sonography: a comparative study of young men. Epidemiology 2001, 6: 618–23.

Kieler H, Haglund B, Cnattingius S et al. Does prenatal sonography affect intellectual performance? Epidemiology 2005; 16: 304–10.

Kok RD, de Vries MM, Heerschap A et al. Absence of harmful effects of magnetic resonance exposure at 1.5 T in utero during the third trimester of pregnancy: a follow-up study. Magn Reson Imaging 2004; 22: 851–4.

Marcos HB, Semelka RC, Worawattanakul S. Normal placenta: gadolinium-enhanced, dynamic MR imaging. Radiology 1997; 205: 493–6.

Miller MW, Brayman AA, Abramowicz JS. Obstetric ultrasonography: a biophysical consideration of patient safety – the "rules" have changed. Am J Obstet Gynecol 1998; 179: 241–54.

Moon AJ, Katzberg RW, Sherman MP. Transplacental passage of iohexol. J Pediatr 2000; 136: 548–9.

Morris DG, Grossman AB. Dynamic tests in the diagnosis and differential diagnosis of Cushing's syndrome. J Endocrinol Investb 2003; 26(Suppl 7): S64–73.

Neel JV. Changing perspectives on the genetic doubling box of ionizing radiation for humans, mice, and drosophila. Teratology 1999; 59: 216–21.

Newnham JP, Doherty DA, Kendall GE et al. Effects of repeated prenatal ultrasound examinations on childhood outcome up to 8 years of age: follow-up of a randomised controlled trial. Lancet 2004; 364: 2038–44.

Patton T, Olshan AF, Neglia JP et al. Parental exposure to medical radiation and neuroblastoma in offspring. Paediatr Perinatal Epidemiol 2004; 18: 178–85.

Read CH Jr, Tansey MJ, Menda Y. A 36-year retrospective analysis of the efficacy and safety of radioactive iodine in treating young Graves' patients. J Clin Endocrinol Metab 2004; 89: 4229–33, 4227–8.

Robert E. Intrauterine effects of electromagnetic fields (low frequency, mid frequency RF, and microwave): review of epidemiologic studies. Teratology 1999; 59: 292–8.

Schlumberger M, de Vathaire F, Ceccarelli C et al. Exposure to radioactive iodine-131 for scintigraphy or therapy does not preclude pregnancy in thyroid cancer patients. J Nucl Med 1996; 37: 606–12.

Schroeder RJ, Maeurer J, Vogl TJ et al. D-galactose-based signal-enhanced color Doppler sonography of breast tumors and tumorlike lesions. Invest Radiol 1999; 34: 109–15.

Spielmann H, Nau H. Embryotoxicity of stable isotope and use of stable isotope in studies of teratogenic mechanisms. J Clin Pharmacol 1986; 26: 474–80.

Sternberg J. Radiation risk in pregnancy. Clin Obstet Gynecol 1973; 16: 235–78.

Vanhaesebrouck P, Verstraete AG, de Praeter C et al. Transplacental passage of a nonionic contrast agent. Eur J Pediatr 2005; 164: 408–10.

Visser GH, de Vries JI, Mulder EJ et al. Effects of frequent ultrasound during pregnancy. Lancet 1993; 342: 1359–60.

Wakeford R, Little MP. Risk coefficients for childhood cancer after intrauterine irradiation: a review. Intl J Radiat Biol 2003; 79: 293–309.

Webb JA, Thomsen HS, Morcos SK and the Members of Contrast Media Safety Committee of European Society of Urogenital Radiology (ESUR). The use of iodinated and gadolinium contrast media during pregnancy and lactation. Eur Radiol 2005; 15: 1234–40.

Ziskin MC. Intrauterine effects of ultrasound: human epidemiology. Teratology 1999; 59: 252–60.

Recreational drugs

Paul Peters and Christof Schaefer

2.21

2.21.1   Alcohol (ethanol)

About 30 years ago, a clinical picture that has been well-known for centuries (and was noted during the "gin epidemic" in England between 1720 and 1750) was "rediscovered". Alcoholism during pregnancy causes a specific complex of congenital organic and functional developmental defects known as *fetal alcohol syndrome* (FAS) (Jones 1973, Lemoine 1968, Rouquette 1957). The milder version, in which there is primarily functional damage, is referred to as *fetal alcohol effects* (FAE). There is still debate regarding the terminology (Aase 1995). At the center of all functional alcohol damage to the fetus are the effects on the central nervous system, referred to as alcohol-related neurodevelopment disorder (ARND). Alcohol is the most widely used teratogen, and causes birth defects more often than any medication. Refraining from alcohol during pregnancy is the most effective way to prevent birth defects.

2 Pregnancy

2.21 Recreational drugs

Pharmacology

Alcohol (ethanol, ethyl alcohol) is quickly absorbed from the gastro-intestinal tract. Owing to the lipid solubility and the rapid and even distribution of ethanol, the concentration in the blood is, for the most part, the same as in the brain. It is this latter concentration that is decisive for an acute alcohol effect. The maximum concentrations are reached 30–60 minutes after intake (Brien 1983).

Up to 90% of ethanol is metabolized in the liver by the enzyme, alcohol dehydrogenase, to acetaldehyde, and then via aldehyde dehydrogenase, to acetic acid, produced via the citric acid cycle CO_2 and H_2O (Wilkinson 1980). The maximal amount of ethanol that can be metabolized human body is estimated to be in the range of 100–300 mg/kg per hour. This is usually translated as 6–9 g ethanol per hour for a healthy subject. Considerable interindividual variations in ethanol metabolism rate have been reported (Jones 1984). Both environmental and genetic factors influence the rate of ethanol degradation – for example, gender and race (Kopun 1977).

Prenatal damage as a result of chronic alcoholism comes about primarily because of the direct action of ethanol or acetaldehyde on the fetus. The exact damaging mechanism is not understood. There is no doubt that the FAS risk for the baby is correlated with the severity of the mother's alcoholism. Although the damaging effect of alcohol is different in the various phases of pregnancy, it is by no means limited to the first trimester. Acetaldehyde has been discussed as being possibly more relevant than alcohol because its kinetic varies more, depending on individual metabolism, than does the kinetic of alcohol itself. This could explain why only some heavy drinkers give birth to children with FAS. Since some FAS features are also characteristic of pyruvate dehydrogenase deficiency, it has been speculated (and supported by some experimental results) that the inhibition of the pyruvate dehydrogenase caused by acetaldehyde also contributes to the alcohol damage (Hard 2000). Maternal malnutrition and disturbances of the liver function can also affect fetal development.

In most studies, alcohol consumption is expressed as the average amount consumed per day or week, leaving the pattern of alcohol consumption out of consideration. To make the average amount of alcohol consumed comparable between the different studies, the intake is recalculated here with the help of a recent report of the Netherlands Health Council (HCNL 2006) to grams of ethanol per day, where necessary. Internationally, different standard sizes are used for the amount of ethanol in one drink (e.g. 12 g in the USA; 10 g in Germany and The Netherlands) and the amount of ethanol in one unit (8 g/drink in the UK). It should, however, be kept in mind that oral alcohol intake is a discrete parameter (a multiple of units) rather than a continuous parameter. Apart from the total dose per week or day, the drinking pattern might also be of great importance (Bailey 2004). Some effects are thought to be associated with the total dose (AUC), while others are thought to be associated with the blood-alcohol concentration, which is dependent on the consumption pattern. Unfortunately, information on the drinking pattern – e.g. binge drinking versus regular daily drinking – was often not collected in the studies. If available, information on the influence of the drinking pattern on each effect will be discussed here. Finally, for the same level of alcohol consumption, the internal dose is approximately 50% higher for women than for men, due to differences in body weight and amount of body water per kilogram of body weight (HCNL 2006). This should be taken into account when comparing the results from the epidemiological studies among women and men.

Both ethanol and acetaldehyde cross the placenta and the blood-brain barrier of the unborn. Ethanol inhibits the secretion of oxytocin and vasopressin from the posterior pituitary gland. This physiologic effect was used in the 1970s in tocolysis; with high blood levels, after both intravenous and oral administration, ethanol leads to an inhibition of contractions in two-thirds of all pregnant women (Fuchs 1967). This therapy is now judged as being obsolete (see also Chapter 2.14).

Toxicology

Alcohol has effects on fertility; the rates of spontaneous abortion, fetal death, and preterm delivery; the length of gestation; fetal behavior; and the newborn's birth weight, size, and growth. It can also cause FAS, anomalies, and neurobehavioral effects.

Fertility
Based on three studies on female fertility (Eggert 2004, Tolstrup 2003, Jensen 1998), it is concluded that there is a dose–effect relationship between alcohol consumption effects and female fertility. There are indications that consumption of less than 10 g/d ethanol might decrease female fertility (e.g. time to pregnancy). For effects on male fertility, only one published study (Hassan 2004) is available in which effects on fertility are described. Earlier, Rouquette (1957), in Paris, wrote an unpublished thesis on this topic. Based on this study, it can be concluded that there are indications that consumption of less than 10 g/d of ethanol might also decrease male fertility.

Spontaneous abortion and fetal death
When evaluating the effects of moderate alcohol consumption (by both men and women), before and during pregnancy, on spontaneous abortion and fetal death, it can be concluded that drinking alcoholic

beverages might increase the incidence. Several human studies by Rasch (2003), Kesmodel (2002A, 2002B), Windham (1995, 1992), Armstrong (1992), Kline (1980), and Harlap (1980) have demonstrated this effect in pregnant women drinking an average of at least 10 g/d of ethanol. Drinking less than 10 g/d of ethanol also revealed these effects in some of the studies; however, these data are less consistent.

Preterm delivery and length of gestation

Consumption of alcoholic beverages during pregnancy might increase the incidence of preterm delivery (birth before 37 weeks of pregnancy) and decrease the length of gestation. Several cohort studies by Parazzini (2003), Kesmodel (2000), Lundsberg (1997), and Sulaiman (1988) demonstrate an increased incidence of preterm delivery and shorter gestational length after drinking more than 17 g/d of ethanol. It has been suggested that this effect is predominantly related to consumption of alcohol in the second and third trimesters of pregnancy (Sulaiman 1988, Lundsberg 1997, Kesmodel 2000). The cohort study by Lundsberg (1997) also found effects on preterm delivery and length of gestation after drinking 1–8 g/d of ethanol. This, however, was not confirmed by the other studies.

Fetal behavior

Acute oral exposure to 12–30 g/d of ethanol in the third trimester of pregnancy influences fetal behavior and suppresses human fetal breathing movements (Akay 1996, McLeod 1983, Lewis 1979, Fox 1978). This effect is observed during the first 2 hours after consumption. In addition, there are indications (Little 2002) that the consumption of 1–10 g/d of ethanol might affect the fetal startle behavior (Hanson 1991).

Birth weight, size, and growth

The effects on birth weight, size, and growth are among the most studied developmental endpoints caused by ethanol. These effects also belong to the spectrum of adverse effects characteristic to FAS. It might be concluded that the human data concerning the effects of drinking alcohol on fetal growth are not consistent. The studies of Whitehead (2003), Passaro (1996), Ogston (1992), and Marbury (1983) suggest a relationship between alcohol consumption and decreased fetal growth and birth weight. There are no clear indications that drinking 10–20 g/d of ethanol might affect fetal growth and birth weight; however, there are sufficient indications that drinking more than 20 g/d of ethanol might increase the risk for this effect.

Fetal alcohol syndrome and anomalies
The definition of fetal alcohol syndrome (FAS), which was first
described more than 30 years ago (see earlier), has been repeatedly
discussed. One of the points of discussion is whether or not the diagnosis should include the criterion of chronic alcoholism of the
mother. However, as supported by several evaluations, the full spectrum of physical and mental handicaps of FAS is only seen in offspring of female heavy drinkers (Aase 1992). Whether an individual
anomaly which is a characteristic of FAS may be the result of a lower
intake of alcohol is not clear. The diagnosis of FAS is made if there are
signs of the following three categories:

1. Growth restriction – reduction of birth weight, body length, and
   head circumference (lowest tertile)
2. Central nervous system involvement – neurological abnormalities,
   developmental delay, intellectual impairment
3. Craniofacial dysmorphological stigmata – microcephaly, narrow
   palpebral fissures, shorter and broader bridge of the nose, flat
   mid-face with maxillary hypoplasia, narrow upper lip margin,
   smooth philtrum.

Further, non-specific malformations in the heart, kidney, and limbs
(among them camptodactyly, clinodactyly, and hypoplasia of distal
phalanges) may occur. In addition, inhibition of intellectual and
motor development with permanent retardation has been observed.
Other less-specific birth defects are also involved, such as those of
the thorax and genitalia, and oral clefts (Jones 1973). When only
some of the above signs are present, the term "fetal alcohol effect"
(FAE) is used (Sokol 1989). The risk for FAS is increased after long-
term consumption of more than 90 g/d of ethanol (Moore 1997).
There are no convincing indications that consumption levels lower
than 60 g/d increase the incidence of individual anomalies.

Neurobehavioral development
From many studies, it is suggested that exposure to alcohol *in utero*
has an adverse effect on the neurobehavioral development of the offspring (summarized in HCNL 2006). A meta-analysis performed by
Testa (2003) confirmed that prenatal exposure to more than 12 g/dof
ethanol will result in a lower mental development index in 1-year-old
children. This effect was not observed in younger or older children.
Two large cohort studies (from Seattle and from Detroit) showed
that maternal alcohol consumption (5 g/d or more) during pregnancy
has an adverse effect on the neurological behavior of 6–7-year-old
children (Day 2002, Jacobson 2002, 1994, Sood 2001, Sampson
2000, 1994, Kaplan-Estrin 1999, Streissguth 1994A, 1994B, 1994C,
1990, 1989A, 1989B, 1989C, 1984, 1981, Hanson 1978). Hence, the
conclusion is that just one unit of alcohol per day (1–10 g/d) might

influence the neurobehavioral development of children. Effects at higher consumption levels have already been confirmed.

Consumption behavior

Regular consumption of small amounts
With regular consumption of approximately 15 g/d of ethanol during pregnancy, the first concrete statistical effects on mental development are seen. A case-control study (Yang 2000) of about 700 children with intrauterine growth restriction (IUGR) showed a slight, but statistically insignificant, increase in the IUGR risk among moderate drinkers (fewer than 14 drinks a week).

An increase in the risk of spontaneous abortion, especially in the first 10 weeks of pregnancy, as a result of limited alcohol consumption (three or more drinks a week), has been discussed (Windham 1995). A meta-analysis of the risk of birth defects, which included 24 000 pregnant women who had 2–14 drinks a week, did not give any indication of this sort of effect (Polygenis 1998). A European action study (EUROMAC 1992) determined the alcohol consumption habits of 6000 pregnant women and the pediatric outcome of the children. A significant difference was found in the length of the newborn children (who were shorter) from mothers who had consumed 120 g/week ethanol, in comparison with non-drinking mothers. No other differences were seen in this study.

Binge drinking
Binge drinking in early pregnancy – that is, the occasional drinking of large quantities of alcohol (more than five drinks at a sitting) without regular consumption – can lead to some inhibition of central nervous system development. This would seem to manifest itself not as a reduction in intelligence, but more likely as behavioral deviations such as distractibility, and a lowered inhibition threshold in preschool and school-aged children. The level of remarkable behavior correlates with the frequency and the quantity of binging (Nulman 2004, 2000).

"Severe" alcoholism
In the presence of pronounced alcoholism, symptoms of FAS can be expected. A 30–45% likelihood of FAS in the case of severe alcoholism has been mentioned in older publications, although newer ones estimate it as being less than 10% when other teratogenic cofactors are ruled out (Abel 1999, 1995).

Long-term development
Long-term studies over more than 10 years show that the alcohol-related morphological features disappear or are minimized in most of

the children with FAS (Spohr 1995). This is particularly so for the craniofacial stigmata. There also tends to be moderate "catch-up" growth in body length and weight. By contrast, microcephaly and limitations of intellectual and psychosocial development – including psychiatric symptoms – tend, for the most part, to be permanent (Autti-Ramo 2006). The majority of the children observed in a long-term study attended special educational needs schools (Steinhausen 1995). Additional follow-up studies of 30 children of alcoholics through adulthood have confirmed that permanent mental and psychiatric developmental disorders must be expected. These are not related to the existence of physical stigmata. It is likely that more than a few children of alcoholics will be overlooked at birth, and that their development will not be appropriately encouraged, because they are morphologically unremarkable (Spohr 2000, personal communication).

The developmentally toxic effect of paternal alcohol exposure observed in some animal experiments and postulated in individual case reports cannot (yet) be proven in humans (Passaro 1998). However, the negative effects on male fertility as a result of alcohol abuse have been proven (see above).

It is often difficult to determine the exposure to alcohol in the mother and/or newborn based upon blood alcohol levels, due to the very brief half-life of ethanol. However, recent techniques that measure the ethyl esters of fatty acids in the newborn meconium and hair can provide a history of maternal alcohol exposure (Chan 2003).

> **Recommendation.** Primary prevention of developmental and reproductive (fertility) disorders is the main issue. This can be achieved by education, planning a pregnancy, and alcohol abstinence. Because alcohol is a proven teratogen, there must be a warning against regular or excessive use. Alcoholism is one of the few situations in which pregnancy interruption may be discussed with the patient. Lying about an alcohol problem during pregnancy has (life-long) consequences for the mother and child. The use of alcohol-containing tonics and medications with an alcohol base cannot be compared with alcohol abuse, but should nevertheless be avoided (see also Chapter 2.19). This applies to medications with an alcohol base, at least when the concentration exceeds 10%.

2.21.2   Caffeine and other xanthine derivatives

Pharmacology and toxicology

The methyl xanthine derivatives *caffeine* and *theobromine* act as stimulants on the central nervous system as well as on the heart, circulation, and respiration. They are the pharmacologically effective components in a number of drinks, such as coffee, tea, cocoa, and cola beverages. Caffeine is also an ingredient in many over-the-counter pain and cold medications (see also Chapter 1.19).

Theophylline is one of the methyl xanthines. The action of this asthma medication is described in Chapter 2.3. These xanthines are well absorbed from the gastrointestinal tract; they cross the placenta, and cause increased fetal activity and a significant increase in its heart frequency. In animal studies, extremely high doses of caffeine (200 mg/kg per day) caused minor development anomalies of the phalanges. For this reason, in 1980 studies were conducted in the USA, with the support of the health authorities, consumer organizations, and coffee and cola manufacturers, on whether caffeine-containing drinks could also cause birth defects in humans. Unlike the animal studies mentioned, adults usually do not consume more than 3–6 mg/kg of caffeine daily. Extensive epidemiological studies in several countries gave no indication for any reproductive toxicity or teratogenicity under these conditions (Browne 2006, Castellanos 2002, Christian 2001). A meta-analysis involving about 50 000 pregnant women indicated a slightly increased rate of spontaneous abortion and intrauterine growth restriction (IUGR) in babies when the mother consumed more than 150 mg of caffeine a day (Signorello 2004, Vik 2003, Leviton 2002). However, the authors were not able to rule out the effect of other factors, such as the mother's age, smoking, and alcohol intake (Fernandes 1998). A population-based case-control study in Uruguay found that the category with a mean caffeine intake (Brazilian mate) of 300 mg/d or more showed a significantly increased risk of fetal death (OR 2.33, CI 1.23–4.41) compared with the category of no caffeine consumption during pregnancy (Matijasevich 2006), and hence, caffeine intake in the Brazilian drink "mate" was identified as a preventable risk factor. The effect on fertility as a result of regular use of larger quantities of caffeine has also been discussed.

> **Recommendation.** There is no objection to the consumption of normal amounts of caffeine and theobromine in pregnancy – that is, three cups of normal-strength coffee with 50–100 mg of caffeine, or the equivalent amounts of other caffeine-containing drinks. If significantly higher amounts have been consumed, this does not require any additional diagnostic procedures. However, consumption should be reduced for the rest of the pregnancy.

2.21.3   Tobacco and smoking

Toxicology

Tobacco smoke is a mixture of different gases (primarily carbon monoxide) and a drop- and particle-containing phase in which the primary ingredients are water, nicotine, and the so-called tobacco tar (consisting of all the other ingredients together). *Nicotine* is the primary toxin in tobacco. A cigarette weighing 1 g contains about 10 mg of nicotine, of which about 10–15% (1–1.5 mg) is contained in the smoke. Nicotine is absorbed through the mucosa in the mouth cavity, the respiratory system, and the gastrointestinal tract. Only about 25–50% is absorbed through the mouth. When smoke is inhaled deeply into the lungs, absorption is about 90%. Nicotine has a half-life of 2 hours; 90% of the nicotine absorbed is metabolized in the liver to hydroxynicotine and cotinine (which has a half-life of 20 hours).

Nicotine crosses the placenta unimpeded, and causes the fetal heart frequency to increase. Elevated placental levels are noted for the heavy metal cadmium (see Chapter 2.23), and also for the organochlorine pesticide hexachlorbenzene (HCB) and polychlorinated biphenyls (PCBs). Potential carcinogens – such as *benzo(α) pyrene* and 4-(methylnitrosamino)-1-(3-pyridyl)-1-butanon – were detected in the serum of newborns before the first oral feed (Lackmann 2000, 1999). The respective differences in concentrations among children of active and passive smokers, as well as women from non-smoking households, were statistically significant.

Smoking is embryo- and fetotoxic, but apparently does not represent a significant risk of birth defects. However, associations between smoking during the first trimester and risks of non-syndromal orofacial clefts (Deacon 2005, Little 2004A, 2004B, Zeiger 2004, Chung 2000) are still under debate. These studies indicate that the risk for genetically predisposed fetuses to develop clefts is increased from 1 in 500 (the general population prevalence) to about 1 in 183.

The following effects of smoking during pregnancy have been discussed (see also Werler 1997):

- Smoking only marginally increases the risk for spontaneous abortion when other risk factors such as alcohol consumption, pregnancy history, social status, and karyotype are considered and decrease uterine receptivity (Soares 2006).
- Smoking contributes to placenta previa and placenta abruption. The risk increases with the number of cigarettes and the history of smoking. Perinatal mortality as a result of abruptio is two to three times higher among the children of smokers than among those of non-smokers. Smoking causes 10% of these two placental function disturbances. The mechanism is not yet entirely clear.
- Smoking lowers the birth weight by, on average, about 200 g. This effect is dependent on the number of cigarettes smoked daily. The rate of low birth weight (<2500 g) children among smokers is double that among non-smokers. This risk is increased among primiparas and older smokers. Twenty percent of low birth weight children are so because of smoking. If the birth weight is related to

the week of pregnancy, and the number of children with intrauterine growth restriction is examined, this percentage is 2.5 times higher among smokers. Here, too, primiparas and older women are most at risk. Thirty percent of all IUGR children are children of smokers. Women who stop smoking in the early weeks of pregnancy can expect to have children with a normal birth weight.

- Prematurity (birth at <37 weeks) is still 30% higher among smokers even when the above-mentioned placental disturbances are not considered. Here, too, the number of cigarettes is decisive. Women who smoke 20 cigarettes a day double their risk of a premature rupture of the membranes before the thirty-third week of pregnancy. About 5% of all premature births are a consequence of smoking. A study on the effect of passive smoking in pregnancy found, even among non-smokers, a significantly increased risk of premature birth if they were exposed to smoke for at least 7 hours a day (Hanke 1999). Experimental study results support the hypothesis that passive smoking can lead to histological and general structural fetotoxic damage (Nelson 1999A, 1999B).

- Perinatal mortality (fetal death after the twentieth week and infant death up to 28 days after birth) is increased by about 30% as a result of low birth weight, prematurity, and placental disturbances. When the birth weight is standardized according to the week of pregnancy and the respective average weight, children of smokers have a higher risk at the same weight as children of non-smokers. Ten percent of perinatal mortality is the result of smoking. By contrast, there is no increased mortality among the children of mothers who live at high altitudes – i.e. also under conditions of limited oxygen availability.

- Morbidity and mortality in childhood in connection with smoking is hard to judge, because in almost every case there has been both pre- and postnatal exposure. As far as we know, smoking in pregnancy does not seem to have any long-term effect on postnatal growth. However, sudden infant death syndrome (SIDS) appears to occur more frequently, and a significantly increased risk of SIDS (Shah 2006) was found when the babies were exposed to smoke not only after birth but also prenatally (Anderson 2005, Alm 1998). In addition, one study of newborns who were not directly exposed to smoke after birth showed that children of mothers who smoke more often have respiratory function limitations. A combined effect of pre- and postnatal exposure on the occurrence of food allergies in the first 3 years of life was observed in one study group (Kulig 1999). Another publication stressed the predictive value of the cotinine concentration in meconium for the risk of early childhood respiratory infections (Nuesslein 1999). In a prospective follow-up study, an increased risk of being overweight in children born to mothers who had smoked during pregnancy at the age of 8 years

(Chen 2005). Moreover, otitis and gastrointestinal dysfunction, such as colic (Shenassa 2004), have been accepted as occurring more frequently in children born to mothers who smoked.

- Comments on the effect of smoking before birth on cognitive and behavioral development are not conclusive, although the effects are mentioned repeatedly – for example, when the mother smokes 10 or more cigarettes a day, the risk doubles that the children will be unable to babble at 8 months (Obel 1998). A higher risk for language and other moderate cognitive impairments in older children was observed by other authors (Cornelius 2001, Fried 1998, Lassen 1998). A connection between lower IQ and maternal smoking could not be confirmed; such associations were more linked with other effects, such as lower birth weights (Breslau 2005). From Linnet's (2005) observations, an association between maternal smoking during pregnancy and a hyperkinetic offspring was seen. Association between smoking during pregnancy and the risk of congenital urinary tract anomalies was discussed by Li (1996).

- Chromosomal anomalies do not appear to occur more frequently. Teratogenic damage to the central nervous system, the heart and the extremities, and gastroschisis could not be clearly proven. Gastroschisis has been discussed as a consequence of vascular disruption, a mechanism which is also attributed to nicotine.

- Cleft lip and palate have been discussed extensively in connection with smoking in early pregnancy (Chung 2000), especially in the presence of transforming growth factor-α (TGF-α)-deficiency. Depending on the type of cleft, the risk can be up to four times the average. This is one of the few examples where epidemiological data support the hypothesis of a multifactorial etiology of genetic predisposition and teratogenic factors. Two other studies discuss a weak connection between some forms of craniosynostosis and smoking (Honein 2000, Källén 1999), and maternal smoking and talipes (Skelly 2002) and heart defects (Wasserman 1996).

- The possible carcinogenic action on the children of mothers who smoke during pregnancy has been studied in different ways. The results do not indicate a high risk (Brooks 2004). There are, however, indications of an association with childhood brain tumors, leukemia, and lymphoma. Some studies assign a relative risk of this of 1.5–2 or beyond (surveyed in Sasco 1999). Other studies (such as Brondum 1999) find no indication of transplacental carcinogenesis. In any case, metabolites of the tobacco-specific carcinogen 4-(methylnitrosamino)-1-(3-pyridyl)-1-butanon (NNK) can be detected in the newborns of mothers who smoke. The average concentration in the first urine was about 10% of that found in active adult smokers. There was a correlation between the number of cigarettes smoked and the nicotine and cotinine concentrations in the urine. In addition, somatic mutations in the HPRT gene of the babies' T-lymphocytes were observed, which are similar to the changes in childhood leukemia and lymphoma (Lackmann 1999).

■ In areas with marginal iodine deficiency, smoking can cause neonatal thyroid enlargement (Chanoine 1991).

> **Recommendation.** Since smoking during the entire period of prenatal development endangers the fetus, women should be advised to abstain from smoking throughout pregnancy. The often repeated recommendation to limit smoking to five cigarettes a day has no scientific basis, and should be viewed, at most, as a very unhappy compromise for heavy smokers who are unable to abstain. Passive smoking should also be avoided as much as possible. No invasive diagnostics are indicated in the case of heavy smoking during pregnancy; immediate cessation of smoking is the best recommendation.

2.21.4   Drugs of abuse in general (excluding alcohol)

Drugs can be divided into the following groups:

■ Opiates, such as *heroin, opium, morphine*, and *codeine*
■ Stimulants, such as *cocaine* and *amphetamines*
■ Hallucinogens, such as *marijuana* or *hashish, lysergic acid diethylamide (LSD), phencyclidine, mescaline*, and *psilocybin*
■ "Sniffed" substances – e.g. solvents (toluene, gasoline), glue.

In the case of the "hard drugs" heroin and cocaine, it must be considered that the effects on the unborn baby's health are frequently intensified due to polytoxicomania, including alcohol and nicotine. Under socially deprived conditions, malnutrition, infections, and trauma may also have an additional developmental toxic effect. For this reason, miscarriages, prematurity, intrauterine growth restriction, and intrauterine death cannot easily be attributed to a single substance. Drugs in the newborn can be detected not only in the urine, but also just as reliably in the meconium, using radioimmunological procedures (Dahlem 1992) and hair samples (Bar-Oz 2003).

2.21.5   Opiates

Toxicology

Opiate dependency is not a rarity among pregnant women. There is extensive experience with pregnant *heroin* addicts (see survey by Schardein 2000). The intrauterine growth of children of heroin-dependent mothers can be inhibited. Low birth weight in the newborn, together with premature rupture of the membranes, prematurity, and the respiratory depression characteristic with opiates, can increase perinatal mortality.

However, the circumstances during the pregnancy – that is, the use of other drugs (including alcohol), the mother's nutritional status and lifestyle, infections (HIV, hepatitis B and C), and trauma ("drug-related crime") – are at least as decisive for the outcome of the pregnancy as is the level of opiate consumption.

In contrast to alcohol and cocaine, heroin and other opiates do not appear to have any teratogenic potential. In contrast to those children who are damaged by alcohol, problems with neurological development (including cognitive abilities) in the children whose mothers who have abused drugs seems to be more a consequence of the deprived social environment in the first years of life. In such instances, intact family relationships as a result of prompt adoption after birth appear to permit broadly normal development (Ornoy 2001, Coles 1993). Only attention deficits and hyperactivity (ADHD) were noted more often in adopted children than in the unexposed control group. However, there were significant differences between adopted children (37%) and those children who remained in a drug-taking environment (67%). This was the result of a follow-up study of 6- to 11-year-old children exposed prenatally (Ornoy 2001).

Severe withdrawal symptoms beginning, for the most part, within 24–72 hours postpartum, such as respiratory distress, hyperirritability, tremor, diarrhea, vomiting, disturbances in the sleep–wake rhythm, and, to some extent, therapy-resistant seizures, can quickly lead to death if they are not treated (Boobis 1986). In 10% of the children, the occurrence of seizures and other withdrawal symptoms are delayed up to 10–36 days after birth. The risk of life-threatening withdrawal symptoms is particularly high when the mother's dependency is unknown and careful monitoring and phenobarbital prophylaxis are not started in time. Whether or not exclusive breastfeeding from birth onwards can minimize the withdrawal symptoms by passing opiates to the infant via the milk and should therefore be recommended is controversial – particularly if it does not involve controlled methadone withdrawal in the mother without further additional drug abuse, see also Chapter 4.16.

Permanent damage following successful therapy for the withdrawal symptoms should apparently not be expected. However, sudden infant death syndrome (SIDS) does seem to occur more often among babies exposed to opiates prenatally than among those in an unexposed control group.

Acute withdrawal of opiates during pregnancy can cause fetal death and, in the last trimester, premature labor. There have been successes in substituting *naltrexone* (Hulse 2004), *levomethadone*, or *methadone* (Berghella 2003), which, with long half-lives of

15–60 hours, are more appropriate for this purpose than *buprenorphine* or *codeine* (half-lives 2–4 hours). Nevertheless, many physicians prescribe up to 2000 mg/d of codeine as a heroin substitute. The goal of methadone therapy is reduction of the maintenance dosage to 40 mg a day at most. Neonatal respiratory depression and withdrawal symptoms also occur with methadone. Most effective is neonatal therapeutic treatment with an oral opiate (see recommendation) in order to prevent acute and severe withdrawal effects (Arlettaz 2005, Jackson 2004, Siddappa 2003).

Recommendation. Acute opiate withdrawal should be avoided during pregnancy. In heroin dependency, substitution with methadone is recommended. Other opioids (e.g. codeine) do not have any proven advantage as a substitution therapy, and should not be used for this purpose. Substitution requires exact dosage titration, and should not be undertaken by inexperienced physicians. The daily methadone dosage must be oriented both to prior drug consumption and to the severity of the withdrawal symptoms. Additional drug consumption can be detected with urine screening.

Comprehensive social support should be provided in an attempt to put an end to drug-related (criminal) behavior. In hopeless cases, timely efforts should be made to facilitate adoption or permanent foster care (see above).

In some cases, newborns must be observed for many weeks to ensure that delayed severe withdrawal symptoms can be treated. Phenobarbital is the drug of choice for this treatment. In resistant cases, a special newborn preparation of *tincture opii per os* is recommended (American Academy of Pediatrics 1983). For full-term newborns, the dosage of tincture opii, based on a 0.04% morphine equivalent, is 0.2–0.5 ml every 3–4 hours. This represents 0.08–0.2 mg morphine equivalent.

2.21.6   Stimulants

Cocaine

Toxicology

Cocaine (coke, snow) is an alkaloid (benzoecgonine methyl ester) of the coca bush (*Erythroxylon coca*), which grows primarily in the Andes. The leaves contain about 1% cocaine. Cocaine was first used as an anesthetic in 1884. It is chemically related to local anesthetics, but has only been proven to be of value for external use in treating eyes, ears, nose, and throat conditions. *Crack* is the free base of cocaine; this is smoked.

Cocaine blocks the reuptake of noradrenaline and dopamine at the synapse, and in this way increases the catecholamine concentration. This leads to a sympathicomimetic and central stimulating effect.

When cocaine is taken orally, it is absorbed very slowly because of its vasoconstrictive action and the hydrolytic breakdown in the stomach. It is metabolized in the liver within 2 hours to the ineffective primary metabolite, benzoecgonine. About 20% is excreted unchanged via the kidneys. Intranasal absorption occurs within 20 minutes (there is a delay as a result of vasoconstriction). Intravenous administration or crack smoking cause an effect within a few minutes.

In the USA, 4–20% of all pregnant women were said to have experience with cocaine (Fantel 1990). Until the beginning of the 1980s, cocaine was considered to be non-toxic prenatally. Since then, countless developmental disturbances have been attributed to repeated use of cocaine or crack during pregnancy. In the light of the available experience to date, sporadic use in early pregnancy when social relationships are intact and there is no additional damaging factor (such as alcohol, other drugs, infections, malnutrition, or trauma) does not seem to involve any noteworthy increased risk for birth defects.

Documented consequences of cocaine use itself – independent from other drugs – are placenta abruptio and premature rupture of the membranes (Addis 2001). An increased rate of miscarriage, prematurity, stillbirths, intrauterine growth restriction, and microcephaly could not be specifically attributed to cocaine. In addition, there have been reports of cerebral seizures, necrotizing enterocolitis in newborns, birth defects of the urogenital and skeletal systems, as well as intestinal atresia and infarction (Eyler 1998A, Hoyme 1990, Schaefer 1990, Mercado 1989, Chasnoff 1988). A typical "cocaine syndrome" cannot be defined (Little 1996). Furthermore, a meta-analysis covering 33 studies did not find higher risks of major malformations compared with children exposed to poly-drug use but no cocaine (Addis 2001). The wide spectrum of morphological changes that have been attributed to cocaine have been explained as a result of vasoconstriction with reduced circulation both in the area of the placenta and in the fetal organs. As a result, (focal) differentiation and growth disturbances could be induced during all phases of pregnancy.

Cocaine and crack cause more severe heart, circulatory, and neurological effects in pregnant women than in those who are not pregnant. It has been discussed whether the damage to the embryo following decreased perfusion may not in fact be the direct consequence of oxygen deprivation, but rather may be caused by a highly reactive toxic oxygen radical following reperfusion of the ischemic tissue. In the first trimester, the fetoplacental unit does not have sufficient protective antioxidants.

Cocaine is found in relatively high concentrations in the amniotic fluid and, due to limited clearance, the level decreases very slowly.

For this reason, the fetus can take in significant amounts of cocaine by swallowing and through its skin, which is quite permeable until the twenty-fourth week of pregnancy (Woods 1998).

The acute symptoms observed in the newborn are less marked than those associated with heroin, and are more apt to be of a toxic nature than related to withdrawal – for example, sleep disturbances, tremor, weak suck, hypertonia, vomiting, high-pitched crying, sneezing, tachypnea, soft stools, and fever. Beyond this, in some studies noticeable deviations from the norm were observed in neurological tests in newborns, EEG changes, and sudden infant death, as well as later behavioral deviations and (motor) developmental disturbances (Eyler 1998B). However, a review covering 36 publications concluded that among children aged 6 years or younger there is no convincing evidence that prenatal cocaine exposure is associated with morphological and functional (e.g. language) developmental toxic effects that are independent from prenatal exposure to tobacco, marijuana or alcohol (Beeghly 2006, Schiller 2005, Bandstra 2004, 2002, Messinger 2004, Frank 2001).

> **Recommendation.** Because cocaine has potentially toxic effects on development, it should not be used during pregnancy. However, cocaine use does not necessarily justify interruption of the pregnancy. In the case of repeated use, especially when living conditions are problematic, the normal development of the fetus should be confirmed with detailed ultrasound.

Amphetamines

Toxicology

Due to their vasoconstrictive effects in high doses, *amphetamine* derivatives such as in "speed" and "ecstasy" can, similar to cocaine, lead to lowered perfusion of the fetoplacental unit or of individual fetal organs. There has as yet been no consistent indication that sporadic use, when the living conditions are otherwise intact, increases the risk of congenital anomalies. However, some older publications from the 1970s describe birth defects in connection with the use of amphetamines during pregnancy (surveyed in Schardein 2000). In addition, in a prospectively collected series of cases of 136 pregnant women exposed to ecstasy (without a control group), 12 developmental anomalies were described among the 78 live-born babies. However, some of these were minor anomalies, (i.e. foot deformities). No typical pattern could be discerned. Just about half of the mothers had also consumed alcohol or other drugs in quantities that were not defined (McElhatton 1999). In a further study of 228 pregnant users, the rate of minor developmental anomalies was double that observed in an unexposed control group. There was an increase, in the newborn period, of neurological symptoms, including disturbances of muscle tone and hyperexcitability. The rate of spontaneous abortion was not increased, but there were three stillborn babies in the exposed group (Felix 2000). In this study, too, tobacco and alcohol and, to some extent, other drugs were also consumed. For an overview of developmental casuistics and maternal exposure to amphetamines, see Golub (2005).

Among 65 children followed-up until 14 years of age, a significant number had learning difficulties at school. However, a large percentage of the mothers not only abused amphetamines during their pregnancies, but also consumed opiates and alcohol, smoked more than 10 cigarettes a day, and were in problematic psychosocial situations. At the age 14 years, only 22% of the children still lived with their mothers (Cernerud 1996).

A Thai study of 47 newborns born to mothers who were methamphetamine abusers during pregnancy concluded that such *in utero* exposure caused a wide variety of withdrawal symptoms and significantly smaller-for-date infants. No gross malformations were found (Chomchai 2004). Similar fetal growth restriction was noted in a US population (Smith 2006).

> **Recommendation.** Pregnant women should avoid amphetamines under all circumstances. However, exposure does not justify interruption of the pregnancy. If there has been significant consumption during the first trimester, the normal development of the fetus should be monitored with detailed ultrasound.

2.21.7 Hallucinogens

▶ Marijuana

Toxicology

Marijuana (cannabis, Indian hemp, hashish), along with alcohol, nicotine, and ecstasy, is among the drugs most commonly used during pregnancy. The carbon monoxide concentration in the blood caused by marijuana is thought to be five times higher than that caused by tobacco, and the coal tar content in the blood is three times higher. *Tetrahydrocannabinol*, the active ingredient in marijuana, crosses the placenta and can lead to a decline in the baby's heart frequency. The rate of birth defects is not increased after using marijuana during pregnancy, but perinatal morbidity probably is. One long-term study found that speech and thought capabilities at the age of 4 years were significantly affected in children whose mothers had consumed marijuana regularly – i.e. ranging from several times a week to daily – during the pregnancy (Fried 1990). This study also found a significantly smaller head circumference in the older children, although the difference at birth had not been noticeable (Fried 1999). A meta-analysis on the effect on the birth weight did not give any conclusive indication that it was lower, at least when the cannabis use was moderate or only occasional (English 1997). There is, as yet, no indication that the chromosome breaks attributed to marijuana in earlier animal studies have any clinical relevance.

2

Pregnancy

Recommendation. Pregnant women should avoid using marijuana in all circumstances. However, if it has been consumed, this does not justify inter-ruption of the pregnancy, and neither does sporadic use justify any addi-tional diagnostic procedures.

▶ Lysergic acid diethylamide (LSD)

Toxicology

No specific embryotoxic effects have been proven in humans after using the hallucinogen LSD. Epidemiologic studies have not been performed. Thus, published data on LSD use during pregnancy are insufficient for a detailed risk assessment. The accumulated reports, according to the Reprotox database of abnormal human births that included the ingestion of LSD early in gestation, involve defects of the limbs (Lilienfeld 1970, Zellweger 1967, Carakushansky 1969), eyes (Margolis 1980, Chan 1978, Apple 1974, Boddanof 1972), and central nervous system (Jacobsen 1972). Some small prospective stud-ies have reported normal births following first-trimester use of LSD (Chan 1978, Aase 1970), but a possible increase in spontaneous abor-tions has been suggested (Jacobsen 1972, McGlothlin 1970). A small number of patients who received LSD therapeutically did not have an increased incidence of abnormal or low birth weight babies (Cohen 1968). People who use LSD as a recreational drug during pregnancy are likely to use other drugs as well (e.g. cannabis, alcohol, tobacco) (McGlothlin 1970, Cohen 1968), and to engage in a variety of activi-ties that may compromise their reproductive health. Therefore, iden-tifying specific reproductive effects of this or any recreational drug is difficult. Available reports do not suggest there are persistent repro-ductive effects from LSD used in the past. There have been reports of chromosome breaks (Cohen 1968).

2.21 Recreational drugs

> **Recommendation.** Pregnant women should avoid LSD under all circumstances. However, if it has been used, this does not justify interruption of the pregnancy. When there has been repeated exposure during the first trimester, detailed ultrasound should be carried out to confirm the normal development of the fetus.

▶ Phencyclidine

Toxicology

Phencyclidine piperidine (PCP, Angel dust) is an arylcyclohexylamine, and is one of the hallucinogens. It was introduced in 1957 as an intravenously administered anesthetic, but was then removed from the market because of undesirable side effects. Until 1979 it was available as a veterinary drug, which was also used in the drug scene. Phencyclidine is easily produced and is a cheap extender for other drugs (LSD, mescaline, cocaine). Phencyclidine is taken by mouth or smoked, mixed with marijuana, tobacco, and oregano.

Phencyclidine inhibits the reuptake of dopamine, noradrenaline, and serotonin in the central nervous system, and blocks postsynaptic acetylcholine. Depending on the dose and the site of action, phencyclidine can act either as a stimulant or as a depressant. With severe intoxication, sympathomimetic action and depression of the central nervous system are the most prominent symptoms.

After oral intake, phencyclidine is quickly absorbed in the small intestine and, following excretion, reabsorbed in the stomach. The effects are noticed 15 minutes after oral intake, or within 2–5 minutes after smoking. Lipophylic characteristics encourage accumulation in the fatty tissue and in the central nervous system. For this reason, the effects last for 4–6 hours despite a plasma half-life of only 1 hour.

In case reports, a connection has been noted between phencyclidine abuse and microcephaly, as well as facial asymmetry and a complex intra- and extracranial birth defect syndrome. A causal relationship has not yet been proven. Intrauterine growth restriction and postnatal interaction deficits, as well as other neurological deviations and opiate-like withdrawal symptoms, have been reported (Wachsmann 1989). Follow-up studies at 1 year on 62 children exposed *in utero* did not reveal anything remarkable compared with a control group (Wachsmann 1989). Animal experiments indicate that it may cause degeneration of fetal cortex neurons (surveyed in Schardein 2000).

2

Recommendation. Pregnant women should avoid the use of phencyclidine under all circumstances. However, its use does not justify interruption of pregnancy interruption. A detailed ultrasound should be performed to confirm normal fetal development.

Mescaline

Toxicology

Mescaline is a hallucinogen made from Mexican cacti. Animal studies on the teratogenic potential of mescaline are contradictory (Hirsch 1981, Geber 1967). There is insufficient experience on prenatal toxicity in humans. Chromosome anomalies were not observed in one study (Dorrance 1975).

Recommendation. Pregnant women should avoid mescaline under all circumstances. However, its use does not justify an interruption of pregnancy. If there has been repeated exposure during the first trimester, detailed ultrasound should be performed to confirm normal fetal development.

Psilocybin

Toxicology

Psilocybin is a hallucinogen made from mushrooms ("magic mushrooms"). There is insufficient experience in humans to allow a risk assessment on its use in pregnancy.

Recommendation. Pregnant women should avoid psilocybin under all circumstances. However, its use does not justify interruption of the pregnancy. If there has been repeated use in the first trimester, detailed ultrasound should be carried out to confirm normal fetal development.

2.21.8   "Sniffed" substances

Toxicology

The toxic effect of higher doses of organic solvents such as *toluene, gasoline, "nitro thinner"*, and *chlorinated hydrocarbons* on the central nervous system, liver, and kidneys is known. Because of the similarity of the effects on the fetus of toluene, gasoline, and ethanol, a fetal solvent syndrome may include all three solvents at abusive/intoxicating chronic dosing.

In a case-control study of 104 ten-year-old children with severe mental retardation, an association was observed with a maternal history of occupational exposure to gasoline, natural gas, or fuel products (OR 4.6, 95% CI 1.1–19.3) (Decoufle 1993). No assessment of the magnitude or precise nature of the exposure was provided, however, and this association is based on just four exposed cases.

Two children with profound mental retardation, neurological dysfunction, and minor dysmorphic features, whose mothers had abused gasoline to "get high" during pregnancy, have been reported (Hunter 1979). No causal inference can be made on the basis of this anecdotal observation, but the resemblance of the abnormalities in these children to those reported in children born to women who abused toluene during pregnancy suggests a causal relationship (Arnold 1994, Pearson 1994).

All of these effects on the embryo/fetus have been at abusive intoxicating chronic exposure levels of toluene and gasoline, which are well above the occupational PEL/TLV exposures (for more information on toluene, see Chapter 2.23). Furthermore, there are notable effects on the mother, demonstrating ataxia and shrinkage of the brain as measured by MRI.

> **Recommendation.** Sniffing solvents in pregnancy should be avoided under all circumstances. Sporadic abuse does not necessarily require interruption of pregnancy. However, in severe maternal debilitating cases, a complete discussion of all options should be discussed. Fetal development should be monitored with detailed ultrasound.

References

Aase JM, Laestadius N, Smith DW. Children of mothers who took LSD in pregnancy. Lancet 1970; 1: 100–101.

Aase JM. Dysmorphologic diagnosis for the pediatric practitioner. Pediatr Clin North Am, 1992; 39: 135–56.

Aase JM, Jones KL, Clarren SK. Do we need the term "FAE"? Pediatrics 1995; 95: 428–30.

Abel EL. An update on the incidence of FAS: FAS is not an equal opportunity birth defect. Neurotoxicol Teratol 1995; 17: 437–3.

Abel EL. What really causes FAS? Teratology 1999; 59: 4–6.

Addis A, Moretti ME, Syed FA et al. Fetal effects of cocaine: an updated meta-analysis. Reprod Toxicol 2001; 15: 341–69.

Akay M, Mulder EJ. Investigating the effect of maternal alcohol intake on human fetal breathing rate using adaptive time-frequency analysis methods. Early Hum Dev 1996; 46: 153–64.

Alm B, Milerad J, Wennergren G et al. A case-control study of smoking and sudden infant death syndrome in the Scandinavian countries, 1992–1995. The Nordic Epidemiological SIDS Study. Arch Dis Childhood 1998; 78: 329–34.

American Academy of Pediatrics, Committee on Drugs. Neonatal drug withdrawal. Pediatrics 1983; 72: 895–902.

Anderson ME, Johnson DC, Batal HA. Sudden Infant Death Syndrome and prenatal maternal smoking: rising attributed risk in the Back to Sleep era. BMC Med 2005; 3: 4.

Apple DJ, Bennett TT. Multiple systemic and ocular malformations associated with maternal LSD usage. Arch Ophthalmol 1974; 92: 301–3.

Arlettaz R, Kashiwagi M, das Kundu S et al. Methadone maintenance in a Swiss perinatal center: II. Neonatal outcome and social resources. Acta Obstet Gynecol Scand 2005; 84: 145–50.

Armstrong BG, McDonald AD, Sloan M. Cigarette, alcohol, and coffee consumption and spontaneous abortion. Am J Public Health 1992; 82: 85–7.

Arnold GL, Kirby RS, Langendoerfer S et al. Toluene embryopathy: clinical delineation and developmental follow-up. Pediatrics, 1994; 93: 216–20.

Autti-Ramo I, Fagerlund A, Ervalahti N et al. Fetal alcohol spectrum disease in Finland: Clinical delineation of 77 older children and adolescents. Am J Med Genet A 2006; 140: 137–43.

Bailey BN, Delaney-Black V, Covington JH et al. Prenatal exposure to binge drinking and cognitive and behavioral outcomes at age 7 years. Am J Obstet Gynecol, 2004; 191: 1037–43.

Bandstra ES, Morrow CE, Vogel AL et al. Longitudinal influence of prenatal cocaine exposure on child language functioning. Teratology 2002; 24: 297–308.

Bandstra ES, Vogel AL, Morrow CE et al. Severity of prenatal cocaine exposure and child language functioning through age seven years: a longitudinal latent growth curve analysis. Subst Use Misuse 2004; 39: 25–59.

Bar-Oz B, Klein J, Karaskov T et al. Comparison of meconium and neonatal hair analysis for detection of gestational exposure to drugs of abuse. Arch Dis Child Fetal Neonatal Ed 2003; 88: F98–100.

Beeghly M, Martin B, Rose-Jacobs R et al. Prenatal cocaine exposure and children's language functioning at 6 and 9.5 years: moderating effects of child age, birthweight, and gender. J Pediatr Psychol 2006; 31: 98–115.

Berghella V, Lim PJ, Hill MK et al. Maternal methadone dose and neonatal withdrawal. Am J Obstet Gynecol 2003; 189: 312–17.

Boddanoff B, Rorke LB, Yanoff M et al. Brain and eye abnormalities: possible sequelae to prenatal use of multiple drugs including LSD. Am J Dis Child 1972; 123: 145–8.

Boobis S, Sullivan FM. Effects of lifestyle on reproduction. In: S Fabro, A Scialli (eds), Drug and Chemical Action in Pregnancy. New York: Marcel Dekker, 1986, pp. 373–5.

Breslau N, Paneth N, Lucia VC et al. Maternal smoking during pregnancy and offspring IQ. Intl J Epidemiol 2005; 34: 1047–53.

Brien JF, Loomis CW, Tranmer J et al. Disposition of ethanol 9 in human maternal venous blood and amniotic fluid. Am J Obstet Gynecol 1983; 146: 181–6.

Brondum J, Shu XO, Steinbuch M et al. Parental cigarette smoking and the risk of acute leukemia in children. Cancer 1999; 85: 1380–88.

Brooks DR, Mucci LA, Hatch EE et al. Maternal smoking during pregnancy and risk of brain tumors in offspring. Cancer Causes Control 2004; 15: 997–1005.

2

Pregnancy

2.21 Recreational drugs

Browne ML. Maternal exposure to caffeine and risk of congenital anomalies: a systematic review. Epidemiology 2006; 17: 324–31.

Carakushansky G, Neu RL, Gardner LI. Lysergide and cannabis as possible teratogens in man. Lancet 1969; 1: 150–51.

Castellanos FX, Rapoport JL. Effects of caffeine on development and behavior in infancy and childhood: a review of the published literature. Food Chem Toxicol 2002; 40: 1235–42.

Cernerud L, Eriksson M, Jonsson B et al. Amphetamine addiction during pregnancy: 14 year follow-up of growth and school performance. Acta Paediatr 1996; 85: 204–8.

Chan CC, Fishman M, Egbert PR. Multiple ocular anomalies associated with maternal LSD ingestion. Arch Ophthalmol 1978; 96: 282–4.

Chan D, Bar-Oz B, Pellerin B et al. Population baseline of meconium fatty acid ethyly esters among infants of nondrinking women in Jerusalem and Toronto. Ther Drug Monit 2003; 25: 271–8.

Chanoine JP, Toppet V, Bordoux P et al. Smoking during pregnancy: a significant cause of neonatal thyroid enlargement. Br J Obstet Gynaecol 1991; 98: 65–8.

Chasnoff IJ, Chisum GM, Kaplan WE. Maternal cocaine use and genitourinary tract malformations. Teratology 1988; 37: 201–4.

Chen A, Penell ML, Klebanoff MA et al. Maternal smoking during pregnancy in relation to child overweight: follow-up to age 8 years. Intl J Epidemiol. 2005; 35: 121–30.

Chomchai C, Na Manorom N, Watanarungsan P. Methamphetamine abuse during pregnancy and its health impact on neonates born at Siriraj Hospital, Bangkok, Thailand. SE Asian J Trop Med Public Health 2004; 35: 228–31.

Christian MS, Brent RL. Teratogen update: evaluation of the reproductive and developmental risks of caffeine. Teratology 2001; 64: 51–78.

Chung KC, Kowalski CP, Kiim HY et al. Maternal cigarette smoking during pregnancy and the risk of having a child with cleft lip/palate. Plast Reconstr Surg 2000; 105: 485–91.

Cohen MM, Hirschhorn K, Verbo S et al. The effect of LSD-25 on the chromosomes of children exposed in utero. Pediat Res 1968; 2: 486–92.

Coles CD, Platzman KA. Behavioral development in children prenatally exposed to drugs and alcohol. Intl J Addictions 1993; 28: 1393–433.

Cornelius MD, Ryan CM, Day NL et al. Prenatal tobacco effects on neuropsychological outcomes among preadolescents. J Dev Behav Pediatr 2001; 22: 217–25.

Dahlem P, Bucher HU, Ursprung Th et al. Nachweis von Drogen im Mekonium. Monatsschr Kinderheilkd 1992; 140: 354–6.

Day NL, Leech SL, Richardson GA et al. Prenatal alcohol exposure predicts continued deficits in offspring size at 14 years of age. Alcohol Clin Exp Res 2002; 26: 1584–91.

Deacon S. Maternal smoking during pregnancy is associated with a higher risk of non-syndromic orofacial clefts in infants. Evid Based Dent 2005; 6: 43–4.

Decoufle P, Murphy CC, Drews CD et al. Mental retardation in ten-year-old children in relation to their mothers' employment during pregnancy. Am J Indust Med, 1993; 24: 567–86.

Dorrance DL, Janiger O, Teplitz RL. Effect of peyote on human chromosomes. Cytogenetic study of the Huichol Indians of Northern Mexico. J Am Med Assoc. 1975; 20(234): 299–302.

Eggert J, Theobald H, Engfeldt P. Effects of alcohol consumption on female fertility during an 18-year period. Fertil Steril 2004; 81: 379–83.

English DR, Hulse GK, Milne E et al. Maternal cannabis use and birth weight: a meta-analysis. Addiction 1997; 92: 1553–60.

EUROMAC. A European Concerned Action: Maternal alcohol consumption and its relation to the outcome of pregnancy and child development at 18 months. Intl J Epidemiol 1992; 21: 1–87.

Eyler FD (A), Behnke M, Conlon M et al. Birth outcome from a prospective, matched study of prenatal crack/cocaine use: I. Interactive and dose effects on health and growth. Pediatrics 1998; 101: 229–37.

Eyler FD (B), Behnke M, Conlon M et al. Birth outcome from a prospective, matched study of prenatal crack/cocaine use: II. Interactive and dose effects on neurobehavioral assesment. Pediatrics 1998; 101: 237–41.

Fantel AG, Shepard TH. Prenatal cocaine exposure. Reprod Toxicol 1990; 4: 83–5.

Felix RJ, Chambers CD, Dick LM et al. Prospective pregnancy outcome in women exposed to amphetamines. Teratology 2000; 61: 441.

Fernandes O, Sabharwal M, Smiley T et al. Moderate to heavy caffeine consumption during pregnancy and relationship to spontaneous abortion and abnormal fetal growth: a meta-analysis. Reprod Toxicol 1998; 12: 435–44.

Fox HE, Steinbrecher M, Pessel D et al. Maternal ethanol ingestion and the occurrence of human fetal breathing movements. Am J Obstet Gynecol 1978; 132: 354–8.

Frank DA, Augustyn M, Knight WG et al. Growth, development, and behavior in early childhood following prenatal cocaine exposure. A systematic review. J Am Med Assoc 2001; 285: 1613–25.

Fried PA, Watkinson B. 36- and 48-month neurobehavioral follow-up of children prenatally exposed to marijuana, cigarettes and alcohol. Dev Behav Pediatrics 1990; 11: 49–58.

Fried PA, Watkinson B, Gray R. Differential effects on cognitive functioning in 9- to 12-year olds prenatally exposed to cigarettes and marijuana. Neurotoxicol Teratol 1998; 20: 293–306.

Fried PA, Watkinson B, Gray R. Growth from birth to early adolescence in offspring prenatally exposed to cigarettes and marijuana. Neurotox Teratol 1999; 21: 513–25.

Fuchs F, Fuchs AR, Poblette VF Jr et al. Effect of alcohol on threatened premature labor. Am J Obstet Gynecol 1967; 99: 627–37.

Geber WF: Congenital malformations induced by mescaline, lysergic acid diethylamide and bromolysergic acid in the hamster. Science 1967; 158: 265–6.

Golub M, Costa L, Crofton K et al. NTP-CERHR Expert Panel Report on the reproductive and developmental toxicity of amphetamine and methamphetamine. Birth Def Res B 2005; 74: 471–84.

Hanke W, Kalinka J, Florek E, Sobala W. Passive smoking and pregnancy outcome in central Poland. Human Exper Toxicol 1999; 18: 265–71.

Hanson JW, Streissguth AP, Smith DW. The effects of moderate alcohol consumption during pregnancy on fetal growth and morphogenesis. J Pediatr 1978; 92: 457–60.

Hanson MA. The Fetal and Neonatal Brain Stem: Developmental and Clinical Issues. Cambridge: Cambridge University Press, 1991.

Hard M, Raha S, Robinson BH et al. The role of acetaldehyde. The Motherisk Newsletter, Hospital for Sick Children Toronto 2000; 12: 5.

Harlap S, Shiono PH. Alcohol, smoking, and incidence of spontaneous abortions in the first and second trimester. Lancet 1980; 2: 173–6.

Hassan MA, Killick SR. Negative lifestyle is associated with a significant reduction in fecundity. Fertil Steril 2004; 81: 384–92.

2

Pregnancy

2.21 Recreational drugs

HCNL. Ethanol (ethyl alcohol); Evaluation of the health effects from occupational exposure. The Hague: Health Council of the Netherlands, 2006; publication 2006/06OSH. www.healthcouncil.nl.

Hirsch KS, Fritz HI. Teratogenic effects of mescaline, epinephrine, and norepinephrine in the hamster. Teratology, 1981; 23: 287–91.

Honein MA, Rasmussen SA. Further evidence for an association between maternal smoking and craniosyostosis. Teratology 2000; 62: 145–6.

Hoyme HE, Jones KL, Dixon SD et al. Prenatal cocaine exposure and fetal vascular disruption. Pediatrics 1990; 85: 743–51.

Hulse GK, O'Neil G, Arnold-Reed DE. Methadone maintenance vs. implantable naltrexone treatment in the pregnant heroin user. Intl J Gynaecol Obstet 2004; 85: 170–71.

Hunter AGW, Thompson D, Evans JA. Is there a fetal gasoline syndrome? Teratology, 1979; 20: 75–9.

Jackson L, Ting A, McKay S et al. A randomised controlled trial of morphine versus phenobarbitone for neonatal abstinence syndrome. Arch Dis Child Fetal Neonatal Ed 2004; 89: F300–4.

Jacobsen CB, Berlin CM. Possible reproductive detriment in LSD users. J Am Med Assoc 1972; 222: 1367–73.

Jacobson SW, Jacobson JL, Sokol RJ. Effects of fetal alcohol exposure on infant reaction time. Alcohol Clin Exp Res 1994; 18: 1125–32.

Jacobson SW, Chiodo LM, Sokol RJ et al. Validity of maternal report of prenatal alcohol, cocaine, and smoking in relation to neurobehavioral outcome. Pediatrics 2002; 109: 815–25.

Jensen TK, Hjollund NH, Henriksen TB et al. Does moderate alcohol consumption affect fertility? Follow-up study among couples planning first pregnancy. Br Med J 1998; 317: 505–10.

Jones AW. Interindividual variations in the disposition and metabolism of ethanol in healthy men. Alcohol 1984; 1: 385–91.

Jones HE, Balster RL. Inhalant abuse in pregnancy. Obstet Gynecol Clin North Am 1998; 25: 153–67.

Jones KL, Smith DW. Recognition of the fetal alcohol syndrome in early infancy. Lancet 1973; 2: 999–1001.

Källén K. Maternal smoking during pregnancy and limb reduction malformations in Sweden. Am J Public Health 1997; 87: 29–32.

Källén K. Maternal smoking and craniosynostosis. Teratology 1999; 60: 146–50.

Kaplan-Estrin M, Jacobson SW, Jacobson JL. Neurobehavioral effects of prenatal alcohol exposure at 26 months. Neurotoxicol Teratol 1999; 21: 503–11.

Kesmodel U, Olsen SF, Secher NJ. Does alcohol increase the risk of preterm delivery? Epidemiology 2000; 11: 512–18.

Kesmodel U (A), Wisborg K, Olsen SF et al. Moderate alcohol intake in pregnancy and the risk of spontaneous abortion. Alcohol 2002; 37: 87–92.

Kesmodel U (B), Wisborg K, Olsen SF et al. Moderate alcohol intake during pregnancy and the risk of stillbirth and death in the first year of life. Am J Epidemiol 2002; 155: 305–12.

Kline J, Shrout P, Stein Z et al. Drinking during pregnancy and spontaneous abortion. Lancet 1980; 2: 176–80.

Kopun M, Propping P. The kinetics of ethanol absorption and elimination in twins and supplementary repetitive experiments in singleton subjects. Eur J Clin Pharmacol 1977; 11: 337–44.

Kulig M, Luck W, Wahn U. Multicenter Allergy Study Group, Germany. The association between pre- and postnatal tobacco smoke exposure and allergic sensitization during early childhood. Human Exper Toxicol 1999; 18: 241–4.

Lackmann GM, Salzberger U, Chen M et al. Tabakspezifische trans-plazentare Kanzerogene, Nikotin und Cotinin im Urin von Neugeborenen rauchender Mütter. Monatsschr Kinderheilkd 1999; 147: 333–8.

Lackmann GM, Angerer J, Töllner U. Parental smoking and neonatal serum levels of polychlorinated biphenyls and hexachlorobenzene. Pediatr Res 2000; 47: 598–601.

Lassen K, Oei TP. Effects of maternal cigarette smoking during pregnancy on long-term physical and cognitive parameters of child development. Addict Behav 1998; 23: 635–53.

Lemoine P, Harousseau H, Borteyru J-P et al. Les enfants de parents alcooliques. Anomalies observées. A propos de 127 cas. Paris Ouest Medical 1968; 21: 476–82.

Leviton A, Cowan L. A review of the literature relating caffeine consumption by women to their risks of reproductive hazards. Food Chem Toxicol 2002; 40: 1271–310.

Lewis PJ, Boylan P. Alcohol and fetal breathing. Lancet 1979; 1: 388.

Li DK, Mueller BA, Hickok DE et al. Maternal smoking during pregnancy and the risk of congenital urinary tract anomalies. Am J Public Health 1996; 86: 249–53.

Lilienfeld AM. Population difference in frequency of malformations at birth. In: FC Fraser, VA McKinsick VA (eds), Congenital Malformations. Amsterdam: Excerpta Medicus, 1970, pp. 251–63.

Linnet KM, Wisborg K, Obel C et al. Smoking during pregnancy and the risk for hyperkinetic disorder in offspring. Pediatrics 2005; 116: 462–7.

Little BB, Wilson GN, Jackson G. Is there a cocaine syndrome? Dysmorphic and anthropometric assessment of infants exposed to cocaine. Teratology 1996; 54: 145–9.

Little J, Hepper PG, Dornan JC. Maternal alcohol consumption during pregnancy and fetal startle behavior. Physiol Behav 2002; 76: 691–4.

Little J (A), Cardy A, Arslan MT et al. United Kingdom-based case-control study. Smoking and orofacial clefts: a United Kingdom-based case-control study. Cleft Palate Craniofac J 2004; 41: 381–6.

Little J (B), Cardy A, Munger RG. Tobacco smoking and oral clefts: a meta-analysis. Bull WHO 2004; 82: 213–18.

Lundsberg LS, Bracken MB, Saftlas AF. Low-to-moderate gestational alcohol use and intrauterine growth retardation, low birthweight, and preterm delivery. Ann Epidemiol 1997; 7: 498–508.

Marbury MC, Linn S, Monson R et al. The association of alcohol consumption with outcome of pregnancy. Am J Public Health 1983; 73: 1165–8.

Margolis S, Martin L. Anophthalmia in an infant of parents using LSD. Ann Ophthalmol 1980; 12: 1378–81.

Matijasevich A, Barros FC, Santos IS et al. Maternal caffeine consumption and fetal death: a case-control study in Uruguay. Paediatr Perinat Epidemiol 2006; 20(2): 100–109.

McElhatton PR, Bateman DN, Evans C et al. Congenital anomalies after prenatal ecstasy exposure. Lancet 1999; 354: 1441–2.

McGlothlin WH, Sparkes RS, Arnold DO. Effect of LSD on human pregnancy. J Am Med Assoc 1970; 212: 1483–7.

McLeod W, Brien J, Loomis C et al. Effect of maternal ethanol ingestion on fetal breathing movements, gross body movements, and heart rate at 37 to 40 weeks' gestational age. Am J Obstet Gynecol 1983; 145: 251–7.

Mercado A, Johnson G, Calver D et al. Cocaine, pregnancy and postpartum intracerebral hemorrhage. Obstet Gynecol 1989; 73: 467–72.

2

Pregnancy

2.21 Recreational drugs

Messinger DS, Bauer CR, Das A et al. The maternal lifestyle study: cognitive, motor, and behavioral outcomes of cocaine-exposed and opiate-exposed infants through three years of age. Pediatrics 2004; 113: 1677–85.

Moore CA, Khoury MJ, Liu Y Does light-to-moderate alcohol consumption during pregnancy increase the risk for renal anomalies among offspring? Pediatrics 1997; 99: E11.

Nelson E (A), Jodscheit K, Guo Y. Maternal passive smoking during pregnancy and fetal developmental toxicology. Part 1: Gross morphological effects. Hum Exper Toxicol 1999; 18: 252–6.

Nelson E (B), Goubet-Wiemers C, Guo Y et al. Maternal passive smoking during pregnancy and fetal developmental toxicology. Part 2: Histological changes. Hum Exper Toxicol 1999; 18: 257–64.

Nuesslein TG, Beckers D, Rieger CHL. Cotinine in meconium indicates risk for early respiratory tract infections. Hum Exper Toxicol 1999; 18: 283–90.

Nulman I, Kennedy D, Rovet J et al. Neurodevelopment of children exposed in utero to maternal binge alcohol consumption: a prospective, controlled study. The Motherisk Newsletter, Hospital for Sick Children Toronto 2000; 12: 2–3.

Nulman I, Rovet J, Kennedy D et al. Binge alcohol consumption by non-alcohol dependent women during pregnancy affects child behavior, but not general intellectual functioning; a prospective controlled study. Arch Women's Mental Health 2004; 7: 173–81.

Obel C, Henriksen TB, Heedegard M et al. Smoking during pregnancy and babbling abilities of the 8-month-old infant. Paed Perinatal Epidemiol 1998; 12: 37–48.

Ogston SA, Parry GJ. EUROMAC. A European concerted action: maternal alcohol consumption and its relation to the outcome of pregnancy and child development at 18 months. Results–strategy of analysis and analysis of pregnancy outcome. Intl J Epidemiol 1992; 21(Suppl 1): S45–71.

Ornoy A, Segal J, Bar-Hamburger R et al. Developmental outcome of school-age children born to mothers with heroin dependency: importance of environmental factors. Dev Med Child Neurol 2001; 43: 668–75.

Parazzini F, Chatenoud L, Surace M et al. Moderate alcohol drinking and risk of preterm birth. Eur J Clin Nutr 2003; 57: 1345–9.

Passaro KT, Little RE, Savitz DA et al. The effect of maternal drinking before conception and in early pregnancy on infant birthweight. The ALSPAC Study Team. Avon Longitudinal Study of Pregnancy and Childhood. Epidemiology 1996; 7: 377–83.

Passaro KT, Little RE, Savitz DA et al. Effect of paternal alcohol consumption before conception on infant birth weight. Teratology 1998; 576: 294–301.

Pearson MA, Hoyme HE, Seaver LH et al. Toluene embryopathy: delineation of the phenotype and comparison with fetal alcohol syndrome. Pediatrics 1994; 93: 211–15.

Polygenis D, Wharton S, Malmberg C et al. Moderate alcohol consumption during pregnancy and the incidence of fetal malformations: a meta-analysis. Neurotox Teratol 1998; 20: 61–7.

Rasch V. Cigarette, alcohol, and caffeine consumption: risk factors for spontaneous abortion. Acta Obstet Gynecol Scand 2003; 82: 182–8.

Rouquette J. Influence of paternal alcoholic toxicomania on the psychic development of young children {in French}. Unpublished Medical Thesis, 1957, University of Paris, Paris, France.

Sampson PD, Bookstein FL, Barr HM et al. Prenatal alcohol exposure, birthweight, and measures of child size from birth to age 14 years. Am J Public Health 1994; 84: 1421–8.

Sampson PD, Streissguth AP, Bookstein FL et al. On categorizations in analyses of alcohol teratogenesis. Environ Health Perspect 2000; 108(Suppl 3): S421–8.

Sasco AJ, Vainio H. From in utero and childhood exposure to parental smoking to childhood cancer: a possible link and the need for action. Hum Exper Toxicol 1999; 18: 192–201.

Schaefer C, Spielmann H. Kokain in der Schwangerschaft: ein zweites Contergan? Geburtsh Frauenheilk 1990; 50: 899–900.

Schardein JL. Chemically Induced Birth Defects, 3rd edn. New York: Marcel Dekker, 2000.

Schiller C, Allen PJ. Follow-up of infants prenatally exposeed to cocaine. Pediatr Nurs 2005; 5: 427–36.

Shah T, Sullivan K, Carter J. Sudden infant syndrome and reported maternal smoking during pregnancy. Am J Publ Health 2006; 96: 1757–9.

Shenassa ED, Brown MJ. Maternal smoking and infantile gastrointestinal dysregulation: the case of colic. Pediatrics 2004; 114: 497–505.

Siddappa R, Fletcher J, Heard A et al. Methadone dosage for prevention of opioid withdrawal in children. Paediatr Anaesth 2003; 13: 805–10.

Signorello LB, McLaughlin JK. Maternal coffeine consumption and spontaneous abortion: a review of the epidemiologic evidence. Epidemiology 2004; 15: 229–39.

Skelly AC, Holt VL, Mosca VS et al. Talipes equinovarus and maternal smoking: a population-based case-control study in Washington State. Teratology 2002; 66: 91–100.

Smith LM, LaGasse LL, Drauf C et al. The Infant Development, Environment, and Life Study: Effects of Prenatal Methamphetamine exposure, Polydrug Exposure and Poverty on Intrauterine Growth, Pediatrics 2006; 118: 1149–56.

Soares SR, Simon C, Remhi A et al. Cigarette smoking affects uterine receptiveness. Human Reprod 2006; 21 (in press).

Sokol RJ, Clarren SK. Guidelines for use of terminology describing the impact of prenatal alcohol on the offspring. Alcohol Clin Exp Res 1989; 13: 597–8.

Sood B, Delaney-Black V, Covington C et al. Prenatal alcohol exposure and childhood behavior at age 6 to 7 years: I. dose-response effect. Pediatrics 2001; 108: E34.

Spohr HL, Willms J, Steinhausen H-C. Die Berliner Verlaufsstudie von Kindern mit einem Fetalem Alkoholsyndrom (FAS). 1. Pädiatrische Befunde. Monatsschr Kinderheilkd 1995; 143: 149–56.

Steinhausen H-C, Willms J, Spohr HL. Die Berliner Verlaufsstudie von Kindern mit einem Fetalem Alkoholsyndrom (FAS). 2. Psychiatrische und psychologische Befunde. Monatsschr Kinderheilkd 1995; 143: 157–64.

Streissguth AP, Martin DC, Martin JC et al. The Seattle longitudinal prospective study on alcohol and pregnancy. Neurobehav Toxicol Teratol 1981; 3: 223–33.

Streissguth AP, Barr HM, Martin DC. Alcohol exposure in utero and functional deficits in children during the first four years of life. Ciba Found Symp 1984; 105: 176–96.

Streissguth AP (A), Barr HM, Sampson PD et al. Neurobehavioral effects of prenatal alcohol: Part I. Research strategy. Neurotoxicol Teratol 1989; 11: 461–76.

Streissguth AP (B), Bookstein FL, Sampson PD et al. Neurobehavioral effects of prenatal alcohol: Part III. PLS analyses of neuropsychologic tests. Neurotoxicol Teratol 1989; 11: 493–507.

Streissguth AP (C), Sampson PD, Barr HM. Neurobehavioral dose–response effects of prenatal alcohol exposure in humans from infancy to adulthood. Ann NY Acad Sci 1989; 562: 145–58.

Streissguth AP, Barr HM, Sampson PD. Moderate prenatal alcohol exposure: effects on child IQ and learning problems at age 7 1/2 years. Alcohol Clin Exp Res 1990; 14: 662–9.

Streissguth AP (A), Barr HM, Olson HC et al. Drinking during pregnancy decreases word attack and arithmetic scores on standardized tests: adolescent data from a population-based prospective study. Alcohol Clin Exp Res 1994; 18: 248–54.

Streissguth AP (B), Sampson PD, Olson HC et al. Maternal drinking during pregnancy: attention and short-term memory in 14-year-old offspring – a longitudinal prospective study. Alcohol Clin Exp Res 1994; 18: 202–8.

Streissguth AP (C), Barr HM, Sampson PD et al. Prenatal alcohol and offspring development: the first fourteen years. Drug Alcohol Depend 1994; 36: 89–99.

Sulaiman ND, Florey CD, Taylor DJ et al. Alcohol consumption in Dundee primigravidas and its effects on outcome of pregnancy. Br Med J (Clin Res Ed) 1988; 296: 1500–1503.

Testa M, Quigley BM, Eiden RD. The effects of prenatal alcohol exposure on infant mental development: a meta-analytical review. Alcohol 2003; 38: 295–304.

Tolstrup JS, Kjaer SK, Holst C et al. Alcohol use as predictor for infertility in a representative population of Danish women. Acta Obstet Gynecol Scand 2003; 82: 744–9.

Vik T, Bakketeig LS, Trygg KU et al. High caffeine consumption in the third trimester of pregnancy: gender-specific effects on fetal growth. Paediatr Perinat Epidemiol 2003; 17: 324–31.

Wachsman L, Schuetz S, Chan LS et al. What happens to babies exposed to phencyclidine (PCP) in utero? Am J Drug Alcohol Abuse 1989; 15: 31–9.

Wasserman CR, Shaw GM, O'Malley CD et al. Parental cigarette smoking and risk for congenital anomalies of the heart, neural tube, or limb. Teratology 1996; 53: 261–7.

Werler MM. Teratogen update: smoking and reproductive outcomes. Teratology 1997; 55: 382–8.

Whitehead N, Lipscomb L. Patterns of alcohol use before and during pregnancy and the risk of small for-gestational-age birth. Am J Epidemiol 2003; 158: 654–62.

Wilkinson PK. Pharmacokinetics of ethanol: a review. Alcohol Clin Exp Res 1980; 4: 6–21.

Windham GC, Fenster L, Swan SH. Moderate maternal and paternal alcohol consumption and the risk of spontaneous abortion. Epidemiology 1992; 3: 364–70.

Windham GC, Fenster L, Hopkins B et al. The association of moderate maternal and paternal alcohol consumption with birthweight and gestational age. Epidemiology 1995; 6: 591–7.

Windham GC, von Behren J, Fenster L et al. Moderate maternal alcohol consumption and risk of spontaneous abortion. Epidemiology 1997; 8: 509–14.

Woods JR. Maternal and transplacental effects of cocaine. Ann NY Acad Sci 1998; 846: 1–11.

Yang QH, Witkiewicz BB, Olney RS et al. Maternal alcohol consumption and intrauterine growth retardation: a population-based case-control study. Teratology 2000; 61: 441.

Zeiger JS, Beaty TH, Liang KY. Oral clefts, maternal smoking, and TGFA: a meta-analysis of gene-environment interaction. Cleft Palate Craniofac J 2005; 42: 58–63.

Zellweger H, McDonald JS, Abbo G. Is lysergic-acid diethylamide a teratogen? Lancet 1967; 2: 1066–8.

Poisonings and toxins

Christof Schaefer

2.22

2.22.1   The general risk of poisoning in pregnancy

Experience involving the effects of toxins and poisoning during pregnancy is principally based on case reports and smaller case series (see, for example, Bailey 2003, McElhatton 2001, Little 1998, Czeizel 1997, 1988, Tenenbein 1994). Therefore, a differentiated evaluation of the risk for the unborn is difficult.

A study from Hungary investigated 109 women who were treated in hospitals because of acute poisoning during different phases of pregnancy. In 70% of these cases, suicide was attempted, mostly with drugs (Czeizel 1988). Of 96 children born alive, seven had malformations, but only in two of them a causal association could not be eliminated. The only significant deviation in development was a slightly higher proportion (6.5%) of mentally retarded children. This finding, though, should not be generalized, as the number of cases is too small. However, an investigation based on larger figures, which the same author published later, showed no significantly increased rate of birth defects. This was also valid for the 27 women who had taken high doses of drugs during early pregnancy between weeks 5 and 10 (Czeizel 1997). In a more recent Danish study of 122 pregnant women, a doubled rate of spontaneous abortions was found, but no higher risk of birth defects and no increase in premature deliveries (Flint 2002). These data should not be used to say that poisoning in pregnancy does not affect the fetus. However, there is some indication that the majority of poisonings do not result in a high malformation risk, at least if the mother was adequately treated. Therefore, termination of pregnancy should not be decided without careful individual evaluation.

2.22.2   Treatment of poisoning in pregnancy

Frequently, questions arise about the developmental toxicity of both a particular toxicant and the treatment with antidotes. In general, it can be assumed that the fetus is more endangered by the toxicant than by the treatment. For instance, this was observed with poisoning by *methanol* (Hantson 1997) as well as with overdoses of *paracetamol* and *iron* compounds.

On the other hand, there are practically no epidemiological studies focusing on fetal outcome after antidote use during the first trimester. There are only case reports and case series which until now have not indicated any teratogenicity, the only exception being the chelating agent *penicillamin, ethanol*, and *methylene blue* (after intra-amnotic injection).

With regard to the chelating agent *dimercaprol* (*2,3-dimercapto-propanol*, also known as *British Anti-Lewisite*, or *BAL*), there are several case reports regarding the treatment of poisoning with *arsenic* and *lead*, and these do not reveal any embryotoxic risk (Bailey 2003). The chemically related chelating agent *2,3-dimercapto-1-propansulfon acid* (DMPS) can be evaluated similarly. However, any chelate therapy has to take into account that essential components of nutrition, such as zinc and copper, are also eliminated, so deficiencies can result for the fetus.

Most experience exists with antidotes which are mainly used for other than toxicological indications (e.g. *atropine, pyridoxine*).

Concerning paracetamol overdose, which is frequently described in pregnancy, there is a risk of liver toxicity in both mother and fetus. Therapy with the antidote *acetylcysteine* is either determined by the amount of paracetamol which the woman (pregnant or not) has probably taken, or by the concentration of paracetamol in her blood (McElhatton 1996). Acetylcysteine crosses the placenta and functions as antidote for the fetus, too (Horowitz 1997).

To refrain from therapy with *deferoxamine* antidote in the case of iron poisoning would endanger mother and child (McElhatton 1991, Olenmark 1987).

Recommendation. Generally, every pregnant woman suffering from an intoxication should be treated in the same way as a non-pregnant woman, which means that all the therapeutic measures that are clinically and toxicologically indicated should be applied. Treatment, however, should follow updated guidelines. As a result of recent findings, the recommendations for therapy have in parts been changed substantially in the last few years. As it would go beyond the scope of this book to integrate these, in the case of necessity, competent Poison Control Centers or relevant textbooks (e.g. Brent 2005) should be consulted. The following case reports do not necessarily follow actual guidelines, because they are in parts "historical".

2.22.3   Chemicals

Arsenic

Several reports have described *arsenic* poisoning of pregnant women after the first trimester. In most cases the newborn babies were healthy, even if the mother developed toxic encephalopathy. However, premature delivery of newborns who died shortly after being born has also been reported (Bollinger 1992, Daya 1989, Lugo 1969, Kantor 1948). Recently, elevated arsenic in drinking water has been associated with a higher risk for anemia in pregnancy and reduced birth weight (Hopenhayn 2006, 2003, Yang 2003). Exposed populations in Chile (40 µg/l) and Taiwan (up to 3 mg/l) were compared to non-exposed (<1 µg/l). Such elevated levels of arsenic in drinking water are often associated with pollution from rock formations in the region, e.g. granite. Other sources of arsenic can be from manufacturing processes – for example, the production of copper.

Carbon monoxide

Carbon monoxide (CO) crosses the placenta and can reach concentrations in the fetal blood comparable to those in the mother's. Empirical observations, animal experiments, and theoretical models show that a delay of several hours can be expected in fetuses accumulating and also reducing CO levels. Only after about 14–24 hours is a balance reached. The elimination half-life in a fetus is four to five times longer than in the mother (survey in Barlow 1982).

The risk for CNS damage in a fetus is increased if the mother was somnolent or lost consciousness, symptoms corresponding to intoxication stages 4 or 5, even if she recovered soon afterwards. Mental and motor retardation or even severe cerebral damage is possible in such infants. The mature fetus reacts more sensitively to CO intoxication than does the embryo during organogenesis.

A slight acute exposure of the mother with transitory light symptoms like headache and nausea (corresponding to stages 1–2), or chronic exposure to CO (such as is measured in smokers who use one packet of cigarettes per day, or occurs with a concentration of 30 ppm in a room or in city air resulting from a working place or environmental sources), is associated with a COHb-concentration of 2–10% in the mother and does not distinctly correlate with fetal damage (Koren 1991, survey in Barlow 1982). The fetus of a smoker, however, does not tolerate additional CO exposure; its capacity to compensate might already be exhausted.

For almost 80 years (see Maresch 1929) there have been reports about CO poisoning in pregnancy that describe inconspicuous courses as well as fetal deaths and CNS defects (Aubard 2000, Kopelman 1998, own observations). A recent study covered 582 women, of whom 54% had not experienced any loss of consciousness. All were treated with hyperbaric oxygen. The maternal outcome was death in two patients and long-term manifestations in four – no different from the outcome in non-pregnant CO-poisoned women. An evaluation of fetal outcome was possible in 515 cases. Fetal death occurred in 15 cases, and 486 pregnancies ended with the delivery of a normal baby. Malformations were observed in 13 babies, which is not a significantly increased rate (Mathieu-Nolf 2006).

In summary, apart from CNS damage, teratogenic effects resulting from CO intoxication are unlikely.

Concerns about oxygen toxicity (retinopathy, premature closure of ductus arteriosus, etc.) resulting from (hyperbaric) oxygen treatment after CO poisoning were discussed, but not confirmed (Mathieu-Nolf 2006, Silverman 1997). In any case, not treating severe CO intoxication would be a far greater risk for the fetus.

Recommendation. Because of the much delayed kinetics of CO in the fetal organism and the higher risk of hypoxic CNS damage to the child resulting from this delay, hyperbaric oxygen treatment of pregnant women with severe CO intoxication must be considered at an early stage. The therapy should be performed for longer than suggested by the symptoms and the CO concentration. Every pregnant woman with reduced consciousness resulting from CO and with a COHb-concentration >20%, or with a deviant fetal heart rate (decelerations, tachycardy, loss of modulation), must be treated with hyperbaric oxygen as quickly as possible and be given 100% oxygen until the start of therapy. As CO reaches the fetus with a considerable delay and phases out only slowly, treatment should be started even after a delay of many hours and after spontaneous improvement of maternal symptoms.

Methanol

Poisoning with *methanol* during pregnancy can secondarily damage the fetus, if the acidosis is of long duration. Although methanol crosses the placenta, the fetus seems to be relatively well-protected at first owing to its slower metabolism of methanol into its toxic metabolites like formaldehyde. The classical therapy with intravenous ethanol exposes the fetus to alcohol, and is therefore not totally harmless because of the possible neurological consequences seen with binge drinking and tocolysis with alcohol (Nulman 2004). This is why *fomepizol* has been suggested more recently as an alternative antidote (Velez 2003). At any rate, neither with methanol nor with *ethylene glycol* intoxication should (alcohol) therapy be withheld because of a pregnancy (Tenenbein 1997). A report on a case of methanol intoxication during late pregnancy describes a healthy newborn after the treatment of the mother with ethanol, hemodialysis, and alkalinization (Hantson 1997). In another case report, the mother and the child (who was delivered by cesarean section in week 30) died some days after the birth. Alcohol therapy was started in the acidotic mother (pH 7.17) after 36 hours, and only on the third day was she treated with fomepizol. The blood of the acidotic newborn (pH 6.9) had 61.6 mg/dl of methanol – a concentration similar to that in the mother (Belson 2004).

Organophosphorus pesticides

Some reports describe accidental and suicidal overdoses with different outcomes. One mother in her nineteenth week of pregnancy reported that she had no longer felt any movements of the baby 2 hours after having taken *chlorpyrifos* with suicidal intent. Not earlier than 10 hours after the initial gastric lavage, intensive therapy was started. In the meantime, the fetus had died. Besides a low level of pseudocholinesterase in the mother, the fetal blood contained a high concentration of chlorpyrifos. Some further cases of *organophosphorus* intoxication of pregnant women ended with the delivery of healthy children. In these cases, therapy with (among others) *atropine* and *pralidoxime* was quickly initiated (Kamha

2005, Sebe 2005A). One of these children developed without any problems until at least the age of 4 years.

▶ Paraquat

In reports on nine pregnant women who had taken larger amounts of the herbicide *paraquat*, no fetus and only two mothers survived the intoxication. The concentration of paraquat was higher in the fetus' than in the mother's serum (Talbot 1988). Another report describes the intake of 80–100 ml paraquat with suicidal intent in the sixth week of pregnancy. The mother was treated with hemodialysis. The pregnancy seemed to progress without problems; however, it was terminated in the ninth week. Paraquat was found in the fetal tissues (0.25 µg/g) and in the amniotic fluid (0.05 µg/ml). The concentration in the mother's serum was said to be clearly lower at this time (initially 4.8 µg/ml was measured). The authors discuss the higher protection of the embryo against paraquat in comparison to the mature fetus. They point out that, especially with intoxication during later pregnancy, the fetus (who is at that stage more endangered anyway) represents an at-risk "reservoir" of paraquat which could return to the mother, and that under these circumstances a therapeutic abortion should be considered (Tsatsakis 1996). One exception is the report about a term birth of a healthy girl, who developed normally until at least the age of 5 years, and whose mother had taken an overdose of paraquat in the twenty-seventh week of pregnancy. She was treated with carbon hemoperfusion, high-dose cyclophosphamide, and methylprednisolone (Jenq 2005).

▶ Thallium

About 20 cases of *thallium* ingestion, with suicidal intent or to provoke an abortion, have been reported. A case of chronic intoxication by a rodenticide containing thallium at the workplace has also recently been described. Most of the children survived the poisoning of their mother, if she was treated adequately. Apart from alopecia, premature delivery and intrauterine growth retardation (but no birth defects) seem to be possible effects of prenatal exposure, including the first trimester (Hoffmann 2000).

▶ Water intoxication

There are some sporadic reports about water intoxication during delivery – for example, the case of a baby aged 6 hours presenting with seizures and hyponatremia (121 mmol/l; mother, 126 mmol/l). The mother had consumed 3 l of water shortly before delivery. The further development of the child was uneventful (West 2004).

2.22.4   Medicines

Acetylsalicylic acid

There are few data available on the effects of *acetylsalicylic acid* (ASA) overdose in pregnancy. A report about a mother having taken 16 g ASA in week 38 describes a concentration of salicylic acid of 31.7 mg/dl after having been admitted to hospital. Because of fetal distress with bradycardia down to 60/min, and late decelerations, cesarean delivery was performed. The ASA concentration in the mother directly before this was 14 mg/dl. In the newborn, however, it amounted to 35.2 mg/dl. The umbilical artery pH was 7.49, pCO_2 27 mmHg, and bicarbonate 18 mmol/l. The further development of the child until its discharge was uneventful (Anonymous 2001).

The National Teratology Information Service (NTIS) in Newcastle, UK, has follow-up data on 101 pregnancies. Of these, 26 involved aspirin only, and 75 involved aspirin compound preparations (or other drugs in addition). Only one child showed a birth defect (a foot deformity); 82 newborn babies were normal (McElhatton 2001). The concentration of ASA measured in some mothers ranged above that which had induced teratogenic effects in animal experiments. In the absence of severe maternal toxicity, there was no increase in the incidence of fetal hemorrhage, spontaneous abortion, or intrauterine death. These results are in contrast to some other studies that describe an increase of spontaneous abortions after therapeutic dosage of nonsteroidal antipholgistics (NSAIDs) like ASA and ibuprofen (Li 2003, Nielsen 2001). Palatnick (1998) postulated that, due to increased sensitivity to ASA, the fetus is at greater risk than the mother.

> **Recommendation.** Generally, a pregnant woman with high concentration of ASA should be treated in the same way as a woman who is not pregnant. In general, termination of pregnancy owing to fear that the fetus could be damaged is not justified.

Antidepressants

Tricyclic antidepressants like *amitriptyline* and *dothiepin* can cause severe maternal toxicity, including cardiac arrhythmia and seizures, thus endangering the fetus too. In a series of reports of the NTIS in Newcastle, UK, on 18 women who had taken between 150 and 1000 mg of amitriptyline, in 16 cases a normal baby was born, 1 intrauterine death occurred, and 1 pregnancy was terminated (McElhatton 2001). Among the mothers of the 16 normal newborns, 6 had taken the overdose during the first trimester, 8 during the second (3 of whom had medium to severe toxic symptoms), and 2 in the third. The intrauterine death occurred shortly after mixed intoxication with severe symptoms at 24 weeks' gestation.

Again in an NTIS report, of 21 pregnant women who had taken overdoses of *dothiepin*, 10 had taken it during the first trimester, eight during the second, and three during the third. Two mothers developed severe toxic symptoms; one of them had convulsions. The outcomes were 18 normal newborns and 1 showing a systolic murmur (overdose at 23 weeks, additional maternal alcohol problem); 1 pregnancy aborted spontaneously and 1 was terminated. There are no further data regarding the aborted fetuses.

In another study, an overdose of the selective serotonin reuptake inhibitor (SSRI) *fluoxetine* was ingested in 21 pregnancies; 16 of these were exposed in the first trimester. Among these, 13 infants were normal and 3 demonstrated anomalies – 1 cavernous hemangioma, 1 birthmark on the left cheek and an ear tag, and 1 severe CNS defect. However, a causal relationship cannot be established because all three pregnant women took multiple drug overdoses (McElhatton 2001). In the meantime, the NTIS in Newcastle has collected data on 160 pregnancies with overdoses of antidepressants that do not reveal any evidence of specific effects (McElhatton, personal communication 2003).

> **Recommendation.** As serious maternal ASA poisoning (especially where the mother has had seizures or lost consciousness) is likely to be associated with pregnancy complications, the mother should be treated in the same way as a non-pregnant woman. Termination of pregnancy owing to fear that the fetus might be damaged is generally not justified.

▶ **Bromides**

A neonatal *bromide* intoxication with hypotonia after the mother had taken a high dose at the end of pregnancy indicates the substantial transfer of this drug to the fetus. The further development of the infant was described as normal (Pleasure 1975).

Carbamazepine

Following intoxication with *carbamazepine* in week 33, with suicidal intent, the mother was comatose and was treated with activated carbon and plasmapheresis. The baby did not show any damage after birth; the Apgar score and umbilical artery pH were normal (Saygan-Karamursel 2005).

Colchicine

In week 34 of pregnancy, a woman took 8 mg/kg *colchicine*. A healthy child was born 10 hours later by cesarean section; it showed only very little colchicine in its serum (<5 ng/ml). Although given intensive care, the mother died (Blache 1982).

Diazepam

To date, case reports concerning intoxication with *diazepam* have not shown a specific toxic risk for the fetus (Cerqueira 1988). One report describes a pregnant woman in week 33 who had taken about 100 mg of a *benzodiazepine*, probably diazepam. Her serum contained 175 μg/l benzodiazepine, her urine 303 μg/l. Kinetocardiotocography about 8 hours after ingestion showed, as expected, decreased modulation of the fetal heart rate. Furthermore, immediately after the patient had been admitted to the hospital, decelerations were observed that did not correspond to uterine contractions but to increased fetal movement. The basic heart rate was not noticeable. After about 6 hours, fetal heart rate modulation had normalized – i.e. accelerations followed fetal movements. This phenomenon, being independent from the pregnant woman's position, was interpreted as transitory hypoxemia resulting from intoxication (Heinrich 1996).

Digitalis

One report deals with intoxication with *digitalis* (8.9 mg *digitoxin*) in month 7. After spontaneous delivery in week 30, the child died on its third day of life. Hemorrhagic infarctions in both kidneys and degenerative changes in the CNS were found, which were interpreted as hypoxic due to continuous intrauterine bradycardia (Sherman 1960).

▶ **Ibuprofen**

In a case series of 60 pregnancies exposed to *ibuprofen* overdose, 1 child had a malformation of the soft palate (which could not be attributed to the drug as exposure was in week 27), and there were 4 spontaneous abortions and 16 terminations of pregnancy (McElhatton 2001). The same author has collected information on 100 pregnant women exposed to overdoses of ibuprofen. Of the 73 children who were born alive, 3 had cardiac anomalies. Although this is more than expected, it is not enough to conclude a causal relationship (McElhatton, personal communication 2003). The higher rate of spontaneous abortion after the therapeutic use of NSAIDs discussed by other authors (Li 2003) was not confirmed by McElhatton.

> **Recommendation.** Pregnant women with ibuprofen overdose must be treated in the same way as non-pregnant women. There is no indication for termination of pregnancy owing to fear of malformations.

▶ **Iron compounds**

There are several publications on *iron* overdose during pregnancy (Tran 2000, 1998, McElhatton 1998, 1993, Lacoste 1992, Dugdale 1964). In a case series, 85 pregnancies were evaluated; 6 were exposed in the first trimester, 37 in the second, and 41 in the third. There were 73 live-born infants without congenital malformations. Five of these infants were delivered prematurely, one had genital herpes, and one had severe jaundice following exposure at week 36/37. Five infants, all exposed in the second and third trimesters, had malformations. Two fetal deaths, in weeks 22 and 29, were observed, one of them immediately after intoxication and another following abdominal trauma. Five pregnancies were terminated.

Serum iron levels were available in 51 patients; 21 were in the moderately toxic range (60–89 μmol/l) and 8 were in the severely toxic range (>90 μmol/l) (McElhatton 1998).

Chelation therapy with intravenous *desferoxamine* is indicated if the serum iron level is >55 μmol/l or if an overdose was clearly taken and the pregnant woman develops seizures, is unconscious, or presents with circulatory shock. In these cases, there is not time to wait for serum iron levels.

In the NTIS series, 41 women received deferoxamine and another 20 underwent other elimination procedures (ipecacuanha 10, gastric lavage 6, activated charcoal 3, bicarbonate 1). All the mothers survived. No maternal or fetal toxicity was observed following treatment of the mother with desferoxamine. Similar results have been reported in other studies (Khoury 1995, Turk 1993).

> **Recommendation.** There is no substantial risk for the fetus if a mother with iron intoxication is treated in the same way as a non-pregnant woman. However, as experience with first-trimester overdose is limited, specific statements regarding teratogenicity are not possible. Termination of pregnancy owing to fear that the fetus might be damaged is not indicated.

Haloperidol

After an overdose of 300 mg *haloperidol* in week 34, a decrease of fetal movement was observed for some days. The child was born in week 39 and developed normally until at least month 18 (Hansen 1997).

Paracetamol

In adults, *paracetamol* is metabolized to an active metabolite which, in high concentration, is hepatotoxic. There is only a limited capacity of detoxifying by conjugation with glutathione. The fetal capacity to conjugate increases with age. The metabolism of paracetamol by the fetal liver is estimated to be 10 times slower than in the adult; therefore it produces the toxic metabolite much more slowly, which affords some protection to the fetus.

The NTIS in Newcastle, UK, has prospective follow-up data on 450 pregnancies in which paracetamol overdoses occurred (McElhatton 2001), including 40 who took combination compounds which also contained *dextropropoxyphene*. There were 140 first-trimester exposures. Eleven infants had various malformations, but a causal relationship could not be established, particularly as exposure was beyond the first trimester.

The spontaneous abortion rate was not increased (8–10%). Furthermore, neither the aborted fetuses, which underwent post-mortem examinations, nor the live infants showed signs of liver or kidney damage. This included one infant born to a mother considered for liver transplant following two large paracetamol overdoses at 32–33 weeks (Rosevear 1989).

The available data on *acetylcysteine* used as an antidote do not indicate that it is associated with fetal toxicity.

> **Recommendation.** Treatment is similar to that for overdoses in non preg-
> nant women. According to the level of serum concentration of paracetamol,
> therapy with the antidote has to be started at once due to the needs of the
> mother and fetus. Postponing this therapy has in some cases led to the
> death of fetus and mother. On the other hand, there is no evidence of fetal
> toxicity, if toxic symptoms of the mother do not appear and the concentra-
> tion in the serum is not toxic. Therefore, in general, paracetamol overdose is
> no indication for termination of pregnancy owing to the fear of malformations.

▶ Podophyllotoxin

Podophyllotoxin, externally applied in high doses, led to psychiatric
symptoms in a few pregnant women. Furthermore, there was one
maternal death, one fetal death (Stoudemire 1981, Slater 1978,
Montaldi 1974, Chamberlain 1972, Ward 1954), and one malformation of extremities, heart and ear after exposure between weeks 5
and 9 of pregnancy (Karol 1980).

2.22.5   Animal toxins

More than 90 cases of *snake bites* in pregnant women have been
reported in the literature, although only in a few have clinical data
been described in detail (Sebe 2005B, Langley 2004, Nasu 2004,
Dao 1997, Pantanowitz 1996). In addition, there are a very few case
reports on *spider bites* (see below; Pantanowitz 1996). Not much is
known about the effects on the fetus of the various neurotoxins,
cytotoxins, and hematotoxins. There is a report concerning four
women in Sri Lanka, of whom two were bitten by cobras and two
by vipers (James 1985). Three of the women had no symptoms, but
noticed a significant decrease in fetal activity. The fetal heart rate also
diminished. Following administration of antitoxins, the fetal movements and heart rate were normal within 24 hours. These three
mothers delivered healthy full-term infants. The fourth woman also
noticed a decrease in fetal activity in the first 24 hours, but was
only treated with the antitoxin after a severe toxic state with hemolysis and renal failure had developed. Shortly afterwards, the baby
was stillborn. The observation by all four women of diminished fetal
activity indicates that small doses of snake toxin apparently reach
the fetus even when no toxic symptoms are observed in the mother.
In another case series of four pregnant women in Burkina Faso,
there were two cases of fetal death. One of the two mothers also died,
as a result of a severe coagulopathy and anemia (Dao 1997). Another

fetus died in a mother whose leg was extremely swollen and who suffered from oculomotorius paresis and rhabdomyolysis after being bitten by a viper in week 10, although she was treated intensively (Nasu 2004).

Only in one case a birth defect was reported, after the mother had been bitten by a viper in her third month of pregnancy. The baby, who was hydrocephalic and had many other anomalies, died shortly after birh (Pantanowitz 1996). A teratogenic potential in humans cannot be deduced from this case report. In about half of the published case descriptions, spontaneous abortion or fetal death occurred. The percentage is actually higher among those treated with antitoxins; however, this may be due to the underlying severe illness. Premature birth and placental abruption – with or without coagulopathy – may also result from snake bites.

Two case reports on *spider bites* (black widow) during pregnancy described healthy newborns. The mothers were treated symptomatically and received antitoxin (survey in Pantanowitz 1996).

Antitoxins against bites of poisonous animals have not been suspected of having any toxic effect on prenatal development. However, maternal anaphylaxis can indirectly endanger the fetus.

A case report on a baby with multiple birth defects whose mother was stung by a *bee* in the third month (Schneegans 1961) has only anecdotal character and does not, of course, verify any causality.

> **Recommendation.** Treatment with antitoxins following snake or poisonous spider bites should not be withheld because of pregnancy. It may also be indicated when the mother has no toxic symptoms herself, but fetal activity or heart rate is irregular.

2.22.6   Mushrooms

Following poisoning with *Amanita phalloides* (death cap), spontaneous abortion occurred in the first trimester (Kaufmann 1978). The cyclic octapeptide toxin, *alpha-amanitin*, blocks the synthesis of protein and can damage the fetal liver through the placenta. A woman treated with plasmapheresis for *Amanita phalloides* poisoning in the eighth month delivered a healthy baby (Belliadro 1983). Alpha-amanitin was found in her blood, but not in the amniotic fluid. In further reports on more than 20 poisonings with *Amanita phalloides* in pregnancy, there was no indication of fetotoxic effects if the mother was treated adequately (Schleufe 2003, Timar 1997). Compared to a control group, a relatively low birth weight was observed (Timar 1997). However, the number of cases is not high enough to interpret this as intrauterine growth retardation caused by poisoning.

> **Recommendation.** Ingestion of poisonous mushrooms, especially *Amanita phalloides* (death cap), must be treated as in non-pregnant women, which means that all the therapeutic measures indicated should be applied.

2.22.7 Other plant toxins

Although a large number of plant toxins have shown teratogenic effects on certain species in animal experiments (for example, *aflatoxins* and *cytochalasin* B and D), to date there is no evidence that these toxins are causing malformations in humans too (see survey in Schardein 2000). However, in one report there was found to be a correlation between lower birth weight and aflatoxin in the maternal blood (De Vries 1989).

Potato blight is caused by a fungus, *Phytophthora infestans*. In 1972, Renwick published a hypothesis that neural tube defects (NTD; i.e. anencephaly and spina bifida) were associated with maternal exposure to some component from potatoes, possibly *cytochalasins*. A higher incidence of these defects among lower socioeconomic groups was suggested. Although the hypothesized potato–NTD association stimulated many research projects, it remained unproven (Allen 1977, Lemire 1977, Poswillo 1973, Roberts 1973).

2.22.8 Bacterial endotoxins

There are no reports regarding embryotoxic effects in humans of either bacterial toxins in *food poisoning* (e.g. staphylococcal, *E. coli*, and salmonella), or about other toxins (such as in diphtheria) (see survey in Schardein 2000). There are, however, reports about four mothers with *botulism* in the second or third trimester (Polo 1996, Robin 1996, St Clair 1975). None of the children were damaged by this illness, which is life-threatening to the mother. In one case (Polo 1996), it is explicitly mentioned that the only movements in the mother (who was totally paralyzed) were those of the fetus. Obviously, the botulinum toxin does not cross the placenta.

References

Allen JR, Marlar RJ, Chesney CF et al. Teratogenicity studies on late blighted potatoes in non-human primates (*Macaca mulatta* and *Saguinus labiatus*). Teratology 1977; 15: 17–24.

Anonymous. Aspirin overdose in mother and fetus. North American Conference of Clinical Toxicology (NACCT) Abstract Review 2001.

Aubard Y, Magne I. Carbon monoxide poisoning in pregnancy. Br J Obstet Gynaecol 2000; 107: 833–8.

Bailey B. Are there teratogenic risks associated with antidotes used in the acute management of poisoned pregnant women? Birth Def Res A 2003; 67: 133–40.

Barlow SM, Sullivan FM. Reproductive Hazards of Industrial Chemicals. London: Academic Press, 1982.

Belliadro E, Massano G, Accomo S. Amatoxins do not cross the placental barrier. Lancet 1983; 1: 1381.

Belson M, Morgan BW. Methanol toxicity in a newborn. J Toxicol 2004; 42: 673–7.

Blache JL, Jean Ph, Vigouroux C et al. Fatal colchicine poisoning. Two particular cases {Abstract}. Intensive Care Med 1982; 8: 249.

Bollinger CT, van Zijl P, Louw JA. Multiple organ failure with the adult respiratory distress syndrome in homicidal arsenic poisoning. Respiration 1992; 59: 57–61.

Brent J, Wallace K, Burkhart K. Critical Care Toxicology: Diagnosis and Management of the Critically Poisoned Patient. St Louis, MO: Mosby, 2005.

Cerqueira MJ, Olle C, Bellart J et al. Intoxication by benzodiazepines during pregnancy. Lancet 1988; 1: 1341.

Chamberlain MJ, Reynolds AL, Yeoman WB. Toxic effect of podophylline application in pregnancy. Br Med J 1972; 3: 391–2.

Czeizel A, Szentesi I, Szekeres I et al. A study of adverse effects on the progeny after intoxication during pregnancy. Arch Toxicol 1988; 62: 1–7.

Czeizel AE, Tomcsik M, Timar L. Teratologic evaluation of 178 infants born to mothers who attempted suicide by drugs during pregnancy. Obstet Gynecol 1997; 90: 195–201.

Dao B, Da E, Koalaga AP et al. Morsures de serpents au cours de la grossesse. Méd Trop 1997; 57: 100–1.

Daya MR, Irwin R, Parshley MC et al. Arsenic ingestion in pregnancy. Vet Hum Toxicol 1989; 31: 347.

De Vries HR, Maxwell SM, Hendrickse RG. Foetal and neonatal exposure to aflatoxins. Acta Paediatr Scand 1989; 78: 373–8.

Dugdale AE, Powell LW. Acute iron poisoning: its effects and treatment. Med J Aust 1964; 11: 990–92.

Flint C, Larsen H, Nielsen GL et al. Pregnancy outcome after suicide attempt by drug use: a Danish population-based study. Acta Obstet Gynecol Scand 2002; 81: 516–22.

Hansen LM, Megerian G, Donnenfeld AE. Haloperidol overdose during pregnancy. Obstet Gynecol 1997; 90: 659–61.

Hantson P, Lambermont J-Y, Mahieu P. Methanol poisoning during late pregnancy. J Toxicol Clin Toxicol 1997; 35: 187–91.

Heinrich J. Kinetocardiotocography – follow-up of diazepam poisoning {in German}. Zentralblatt Gynäkol 1996; 118: 689–92.

Hoffmann RS. Thallium poisoning during pregnancy: a case report and comprehensive literature review. J Toxicol Clin Toxicol 2000; 38: 767–75.

Hopenhayn C, Ferreccio C, Browning SR et al. Arsenic exposure from drinking water and birth weight. Epidemiology 2003; 14: 593–602.

Hopenhayn C, Bush HM, Bingcang A et al. Association between arsenic exposure from drinking water and anemia during pregnancy. J Occup Environ Med 2006; 48: 635–43.

Horowitz RS, Dart RC, Jarvie DR et al. Placental transfer of N-acetylcysteine following human maternal acetaminophen toxicity. J Toxicol Clin Toxicol 1997; 35: 447–51.

2

Pregnancy

2.22 Poisonings and toxins

James RF. Snake bite in pregnancy. Lancet 1985; 2: 731.

Jenq CC, Wu CD, Lin JL. Mother and fetus both survive from severe paraquat intoxication. Clin Toxicol 2005; 43: 291–5.

Kamha AA, al Omary IY, Zalabany HA et al. Organophosphate poisoning in pregnancy: a case report. Basic Clin Pharmacol Toxicol 2005; 96: 397–8.

Kantor HI, Levin PM. Arsenic encephalopathy in pregnancy with recovery. Am J Obstet Gynecol 1948; 56: 370–74.

Karol MC, Connor CS, Murphey KJ. Podophyllum: suspected teratogenicity from topical application. Clin Toxicol 1980; 16: 283–6.

Kaufmann MM, Müller A, Paweletz N et al. Fetal damage due to mushroom poisoning with Amanita phalloides during the first trimester of pregnancy. Geburtsh Frauenheilk 1978; 38: 122–4.

Khoury S, Odeh M, Oettinger M. Deferoxamine treatment for acute iron intoxication in pregnancy. Acta Obstet Gynecol Scand 1995; 74: 756–7.

Kopelman AE, Plaut TA. Fetal compromise caused by maternal carbon monoxide poisoning. J Perinat 1998; 18: 74–7.

Koren G, Sharav T, Pastuszak A. A multicenter, prospective study of fetal outcome following accidental carbon monoxide poisoning in pregnancy. Reprod Toxicol 1991; 5: 397–405.

Lacoste H, Goyert GL, Goldman LS et al. Acute iron intoxication in pregnancy: case report and review of the literature. Obstet Gynecol 1992; 80: 500–501.

Langley RL. A review of venomous animal bites and stings in pregnant patients. Wilderness Environ Med 2004; 15: 207–15.

Lemire RJ, Beckwith JB, Warkany J. Anencephaly, Incidences, Etiology and Epidemiology. New York: Raven Press, 1977, pp. 12–47.

Li D-K, Liu L, Odouli R. Exposure to non-steroidal anti-inflammatory drugs during pregnancy and risk of miscarriage: population-based cohort study. Br Med J 2003; 327: 368–72.

Little BB, Gilstrap LC, van Beveren TT. Drug overdoses during pregnancy. In: LC Gilstrap and BB Little (eds), Drugs and Pregnancy, 2nd edn. New York: Chapman & Hall, 1998, pp. 377–404.

Lugo G, Cassady G, Palmisano P. Acute maternal arsenic intoxication with neonatal death. Am J Dis Child 1969; 117: 328–30.

Maresch R. Über einen Fall von Kohlenoxydgasschädigung des Kindes in der Gebärmutter. Wien Med Wochenschr 1929; 79: 454–6.

Mathieu-Nolf M, Mathieu D, Durak C et al. Acute carbon monoxide poisoning during pregnancy. Materna land fetal outcome {Abstract}. Reprod Toxicol 2006; 22: 279.

McElhatton PR, Roberts JC, Sullivan FM. The consequences of iron overdose and its treatment with desferrioxamine in pregnancy. Hum Exper Toxicol 1991; 10: 251–9.

McElhatton PR, Sullivan FM, Volans GN. Outcome of pregnancy following deliberate iron overdose by the mother. Hum Exper Toxicol 1993; 12: 579.

McElhatton PR, Sullivan FM, Volans GN. Paracetamol overdose in pregnancy: analysis of the outcomes of 300 cases referred to the Teratology Information Service. Reprod Toxicol 1996; 11: 85–94.

McElhatton PR, Bateman DN, Evans C et al. The outcome of pregnancy following iron overdose by the mother. Br J Clin Pharmacol 1998; 45: 212–13.

McElhatton PR, Garbis H, Schaefer C. Poisons and overdoses. In: C Schaefer (ed.), Drugs During Pregnancy and Lactation. Amsterdam: Elsevier, 2001, pp. 206–13.

Montaldi D, Giambrone JP, Courney NG. Podophyllin poisoning associated with the treatment of condyloma accuminatum. A case report. Am J Obstet Gynecol 1974; 119: 1130–31.

Nasu K, Ueda T, Miyakawa I. Intrauterine fetal death caused by pit viper venom poisoning in early pregnancy. Gynecol Obstet Invest 2004; 57: 114–16.

Nielsen GL, Sorensen T, Larsen H et al. Risk of adverse birth outcome and miscarriage in pregnant users of non-steroidal anti-inflammatory drugs: population based observational study and case-control study. Br Med J 2001; 322: 266–70.

Nulman I, Rovet J, Kennedy D et al. Binge alcohol consumption by non-alcohol dependent women during pregnancy affects child behavior, but not general intellectual functioning; a prospective controlled study. Arch Women's Mental Health 2004; 7: 173–81.

Olenmark M, Biber B, Dottori O et al. Fatal iron intoxication in late pregnancy. J Toxicol Clin Toxicol 1987; 25: 347–59.

Palatnick W, Tenenbein M. Aspirin poising during pregnancy: increased fetal sensitivity. Am J Perinatol 1998; 15: 39–41.

Pantanowitz L, Guidozzi F. Management of snake and spider bite in pregnancy. Obstet Gynecol Rev 1996; 51: 615–20.

Pleasure JR, Blackburn MG. Neonatal bromide intoxication: prenatal ingestion of a large quantity of bromides with transplacental accumulation in the fetus. Pediatrics 1975; 55: 503–6.

Polo JM, Martin J, Berciano J. Botulism and pregnancy. Lancet 1996; 348: 195.

Poswillo DE, Sopher D, Mitchell SJ et al. Further investigations into the teratogenic potential of imperfect potatoes. Nature 1973; 244: 367–8.

Renwick JH. Spina bifida, anencephaly, and potato blight. Lancet 1972; 2: 976–86.

Roberts CJ, Revington CJ, Lloyd S. Potato cultivation and storage in South Wales and its relation to neural tube malformation prevalence. Br J Prevent Soc Med 1973; 27: 214–16.

Robin L, Herman D, Redett R. Botulism in a pregnant woman. N Engl J Med 1996; 335: 823–4.

Rosevear SK, Hope PL. Favourable neonatal outcome following maternal paracetamol overdose and severe fetal distress. Case report. Br J Obstet Gynaecol 1989; 96: 491–3.

Saygan-Karamursel B, Guven S, Onderoglu L et al. Mega-dose carbamazepine complicating third trimester of pregnancy. J Perinat Med 2005; 33: 72–5.

Schardein JL. Chemically Induced Birth Defects, 3rd edn. New York: Marcel-Dekker, 2000.

Schleufe P, Seidel C. Amanita poisoning during pregnancy {in German}. Anasthesiol Intensivmed Notfallmed Schmerzther 2003; 38: 716–18.

Schneegans E, Keller R, Kohmer A et al. Mort néonatale par malformations multiples a la suite de l'action du poison d'abeilles. Ann Pédiatr 1961; 37: 376–9.

Sebe A (A), Satar S, Alpay R. Organophosphate poisoning associated with fetal death: a case study. Mount Sinai J Med 2005; 72: 354–6.

Sebe A (B), Satar S, Acikalin A. Snakebite during pregnancy. Hum Exper Toxicol 2005; 24: 341–5.

Sherman JL Jr, Locke RV. Transplacental neonatal digitalis intoxication. Am J Cardiol 1960; 6: 834–7.

Silverman RK, Montano J. Hyperbaric oxygen teatment during pregnancy in acute carbon monoxide poisoning. J Reprod Med 1997; 42: 309–11.

Slater GE, Rumack BH, Peterson RG. Podophllin poisoning: systemic toxicity following cutaneous application. Obset Gynecol 1978; 52: 94–6.

2

Pregnancy

2.22 Poisonings and toxins

St Clair EH, di Liberti JH, O'Brien ML. Observations of an infant born to a mother with botulism. J Pediatr 1975; 87: 658.

Stoudemire A, Baker N, Thompson TL. Delirium induced by topical application of podophyllin: a case report. Am J Psychiatry 1981; 138: 1505–6.

Talbot AR, Fu CC, Hsieh MF. Paraquat intoxication during pregnancy: a report of 9 cases. Vet Hum Toxicol 1988; 30: 12–17.

Tenenbein M. Poisoning in pregnancy. In: G Koren (ed.), Maternal & Fetal Toxicology, 2nd edn. New York: Marcel Dekker, 1994, pp. 223–52.

Tenenbein M. Methanol poisoning during pregnancy – prediction of risk and suggestions for management. J Toxicol Clin Toxicol 1997; 35: 193–4.

Timar L, Czeizel AE. Birth weight and congenital anomalies following poisonous mushroom intoxication during pregnancy. Reprod Toxicol 1997; 11: 861–6.

Tran T, Wax JR, Steinfeld JD et al. Acute intentional iron overdose in pregnancy. Obstet Gynecol 1998; 92: 678–80.

Tran T, Wax JR, Philput C et al. Intentional iron overdose in pregnancy – management and outcome. J Emerg Med 2000; 18: 225–8.

Tsatsakis AM, Perakis K, Koumantakis E. Experience with acute paraquat poisoning in Crete. Vet Human Toxicol 1996; 38: 113–17.

Turk J, Aks S, Ampuero F et al. Successful therapy of iron intoxication in pregnancy with intravenous deferoxamine and whole bowel irrigation. Vet Hum Toxicol 1993; 35: 441–4.

Velez LI, Kulstad E, Shepherd G et al. Inhalational methanol toxicity in pregnancy treated twice with fomepizole. Vet Hum Toxicol 2003; 45: 28–30.

Ward JW, Clifford WS, Monaco AR. Fatal systemic poisoning following podophylline treatment of condyloma accuminatum. South Med J 1954; 47: 1204–6.

West CR, Harding JE. Maternal water intoxication as a cause of neonatal seizures. J Paediatr Child Health 2004; 40: 709–10.

Yang CY, Chang CC, Tsai SS et al. Arsenic in drinking water and adverse pregnancy outcome in an arseniasis-endemic area in northeastern Taiwan. Environ Res 2003; 91: 29–34.

Occupational, industrial, and environmental agents

2.23

Richard K. Miller, Paul Peters, and Patricia R. McElhatton

It is ambitious to describe the risk assessment of environmental agents being the sum total of all the substances capable of producing an effect, whether physical, chemical or biological, which make up the surroundings and influence the development of an individual. Synthetic but also naturally occurring substances sometimes have significant pharmacological and toxicological properties; but how many are there? For example, toxins such as chemicals from microorganisms, fungi, plants, and animals have not been analyzed systematically. Millions of synthetic chemicals are registered, but fewer than 100 000 are currently in commercial or industrial use, and most of these chemicals have not been tested for developmental toxicity. The number of synthetic chemicals is likely to continue to increase. Hence, agents selected here might be of importance if there is occupational exposure for women who are pregnant or are in their reproductive years, and include:

- substances in the home or garden environment
- those agents we know that do have actions on reproduction (mostly pollutants)

■ those chemicals about which there are frequent inquiries at teratology information services.

In principle, it is difficult to distinguish between industrial and
environmental chemicals. Environmental pollutants are usually
industrial chemicals released as pollutants into the environment during production, use, recycling, and combustion processes, or into air,
water or soil from naturally high sources – for example, arsenic in
regions with substantial granite deposits. However, the concentration of industrial chemicals may normally be higher in a particular
workplace than in the general environment. Moreover, when an
accident occurs, the environmental pollution may exceed the usual
workplace exposure. Thus, biomonitoring is important in all settings.
A number of reviews have been published on the reproductive
toxicity of industrial chemicals (see overviews in Miller 2004,
Schardein 2000, Gilstrap 1998, Paul 1993, Sullivan 1993, Barlow
1982), but these cover only a small fraction of the total number of
chemicals to which women may be exposed in the workplace.
There is an EU requirement in the Pregnant Workers Directive
(92/85/EC) for the production of materials safety datasheets. These
sheets should include what information exists on the reproductive
toxicity of the chemical, but in practice these MSDS datasheets
rarely provide a useful reference source other than identification of
the constituents of the product; the same situation holds true for
physical and biological agents.
As there is legislation in most developed countries preventing
gender discrimination in employment and protecting the rights of
women to work during pregnancy, there is a need for adequate information on the possible risks of exposure to chemicals in the workplace. Among the most widely known is the Johnson Controls case in
the US, where the US Supreme Court ruled that since there was
reproductive toxicity of lead in both males and females, battery production had to accommodate both genders, and also to reduce the
exposure to lead levels appropriate for both genders. Thus, women
gained equal access to better pay, since working in the battery production area was the route to those higher-paid positions. (UAW *v*
Johnson Controls US Supreme Court 89-1215).
However, individual risk characterization is much more difficult
with chemical and physical exposure than with a particular drug
treatment, because:

■ a pregnant woman is rarely exposed to a single compound
■ measuring workplace or environmental/household contamination levels is often expensive and time-consuming
■ workplace measures are often feared because of conflicts with
the employer

- quantifying exposure via inhalation, oral intake or dermal absorption is difficult
- there is a lack of data regarding kinetic properties (absorption, distribution, metabolism, excretion)
- fetal exposure and kinetic are even less well known
- reference data in the literature (e.g. no observed adverse effect levels – NOAELs) are mostly derived from animal experiments, which have limited relevance for human exposure. There are few substances where NOAELs can be supported with epidemiological data.

Since it is difficult to specify the upper limits of workplace exposure for pregnant women because of the lack of data, the general Occupational Exposure (Standards and Maximum Exposure) Limits (OELs) of the chemical in question are often used. For an overview of global occupational exposure limits (OELs) for over 5000 specific chemicals, see Brandys (2006). OELs are regularly updated in Canada, France, Germany, Japan, Russia, and the United Kingdom; the OEL is the amount of a workplace health hazard that most workers can be exposed to without harming their health. OELs are not, in the main, based upon reproductive health demands. In the USA, the Occupational & Safety Health Administration (OSHA) sets enforceable permissible exposure limits (PELs) to protect workers against the health effects of exposure to hazardous substances. PELs are regulatory limits on the amount or concentration of a substance in the air. They may also contain a skin designation (see www.osha.gov/SLTC/pel). PELs are based on an 8-hour time-weighted average (TWA) exposure.

In accordance with the maternal protection laws in many countries, pregnant women should not be exposed to toxic, infectious, ionizing or carcinogenic substances. However, in practice many workplaces require pregnant women to handle potentially toxic compounds and do not take into account the possibility that workers might already be pregnant. In addition, non-specific symptoms have to be considered when discussing the tolerability of a certain workplace or household contaminant. If pregnant women complain of repeated symptoms in the workplace – such as headaches, emesis, vertigo – this should be taken seriously. Such recurrent disorders can endanger the normal course of pregnancy. As will be noted later in this chapter, pregnant women may have exaggerated responses to exposure simply because they are pregnant. This is often reported in relationship to the nausea and vomiting of pregnancy. For evaluating approaches to exposure during pregnancy, see Miller (2004).

With respect to awareness of an increased risk for birth defects from environmental pollution, birth defect monitoring systems would be of help. However, birth defect monitoring and surveillance systems

2

Pregnancy

2.23 Occupational, industrial, and environmental agents

seldom methodically measure environmental exposure. Only in the case of a cluster with suggestions for pollution-related causation might such studies be performed. Absence of a change in the prevalence of birth defects in a population is not an observation useful to exclude a (new) environmental developmental toxicant *per se*, since these monitoring systems are considered too insensitive. On the other hand, in case of a linkage of occupational exposure with reproductive hazards, the epidemiologist has to demonstrate that, without reasonable doubt, reproductive outcome is worse than expected when the mother has a specific occupational exposure, and that this is not due to a confounder such as disease, maternal age, cigarette smoking, etc. (Källén 1988).

2.23.1   Solvent exposure in general

Toxicology

Organic solvents are chemicals that dissolve other chemicals. Common organic solvents include *alcohols* (see Chapter 2.21), *ethylether, hexane, tetrachloroethane, toluene, and xylene*. Other degreasers, such as paint thinners, varnish removers, lacquers, silk-screening inks, and paints also contain these chemicals. Exposure is frequently to mixed solvents by the inhalatory or dermal route. Exposure to one single solvent is rare. Hence, much of the epidemiology has been conducted on mixed or unspecified solvent exposure both at work and at home. In a series of early studies (Holmberg 1982, 1979), excessive solvent exposure among mothers who gave birth to children with CNS defects was reported, but this was not supported by later studies on the same population (Kurppa 1983). A 1999 Canadian study found that 125 women who were exposed to solvents while working and who were seen by their physician during the first trimester of pregnancy were about 13 times more likely than unexposed women to have a baby with a major malformation (e.g. open spina bifida, clubfoot, heart defects, deafness). The women in the study included factory workers, laboratory technicians, artists, graphic designers, and printing industry workers. The number of these exposed women who had suffered previous miscarriages while working with organic solvents was greater than in workers who were not exposed to solvents. The conclusion was that occupational exposure to organic solvents during pregnancy is associated with an increased risk of fetal malformations. Symptomatic exposure appears to predict a higher fetal risk for malformations (Khattak 1999); however, this data set was very small, and the types of solvents were not identified (Brent 1999A). From a meta-analysis report on pregnancy outcome following maternal organic solvent exposure for major malformations (including five studies with 7036 patients) and for spontaneous abortions (including five studies with 2899 patients), the conclusions were that maternal occupational exposure to organic solvents is associated with a tendency toward increased risk for spontaneous abortion, and that there is a significant association with major malformations (McMartin 1998).

Spontaneous abortions were studied among women working in the Finnish pharmaceutical industry. The study population was taken from the company records of eight pharmaceutical factories from 1973 to 1980. The odds ratio of spontaneous abortion was significantly increased when the women were exposed to four or more solvents, but not in those exposed to one to three solvents. No data were given on the actual levels of solvent exposure (Taskinen 1994, 1989).

Spontaneous abortions and congenital malformations of offspring among wives of men exposed to organic solvents have been studied in Finland (Taskinen 1989). Data on exposure of the males covered a time period of 80 days prior to the onset of pregnancy, and for the females covered the first trimester of pregnancy. An odds ratio of 2.7 ($p < 0.05$) was found for spontaneous abortions related to organic solvent exposure of the males, but no significant effect was found when the women were exposed. A meta-analysis to assess the risks of spontaneous abortions and major malformations after paternal exposure to organic solvents concluded that paternal exposure was associated with an increased risk for neural tube defects, but not for spontaneous abortions (Logman 2005).

In summary, chronic exposure to hydrocarbon solvents, especially if associated with maternal toxicity, has been reported to cause an increased risk of spontaneous abortion and IUGR. There is an association with an increased malformation risk. Additional reports are available for specific solvents below.

> **Recommendation.** In general, exposure to hydrocarbon solvents should be avoided during pregnancy. At a minimum, exposure should be well below the PELs or OELs. Acute exposure is not an indication for termination of pregnancy; neither are additional prenatal diagnostic tests required as long as the mother demonstrates no symptoms. If continuous and significant exposure has occurred, a detailed fetal ultrasound may be offered and fetal growth should be monitored.

Acetone (solvent)

Toxicology

Acetone is an organic solvent used in the home and in industry. Acetone is produced in an uncontrolled diabetic patient. A number of small studies on workers exposed to acetone have not indicated an increased risk of spontaneous abortions at exposure levels of up to 350 ppm, but the numbers of subjects studied were too small to draw any definite conclusions (Axelsson 1984).

In a case report on sacral agenesis, acetone was one of five solvents involved in exposure of five pregnant women (Kufera 1968). Such studies do not permit causal relationships to be established for any individual chemical. There are inadequate data for human risk assessment.

> **Recommendation.** Exposure to acetone should be avoided in pregnancy wherever possible. Nevertheless, when there has been significant exposure, this is not an indication for the termination of pregnancy. However, if the mother has had symptoms of toxicity and/or continuous exposure, she may be offered additional prenatal diagnostic measures – e.g. a detailed fetal ultrasound may be offered and fetal growth should be monitored. The patient should be removed from exposure, as well as having the workplace monitored for acetone levels. For the diabetic, optimizing control of her glucose level is important (see Chapter 2.15).

▶ **Carbon disulfide (solvent)**

Toxicology

Carbon disulfide is widely encountered in the textile industry. There are equivocal data on its potential reproductive toxicity. Carbon disulfide-exposed women have been reported to have alterations in their menstrual cycles suggestive of hormonal abnormalities (Zhou 1988). Placental transfer in human pregnancy has been demonstrated (Cai 1981). The results of one study suggested that female rayon workers exposed to carbon disulfide have an increased incidence of spontaneous abortion (Hemminki 1980). However, a subsequent study by the same group found that although female rayon workers and the wives of male rayon workers appeared to have a higher incidence of spontaneous abortion, no causal relationship with carbon disulfide exposure levels could be established (Hemminki 1982A). These data are of doubtful biological significance. A higher incidence of congenital anomalies (e.g. heart defects, inguinal hernia, and CNS abnormalities) has been briefly reported in a Chinese study of female workers exposed to carbon disulfide (Bao 1991). The malformation rate among exposed women was 2.4%, compared with 1.4% in the controls – a rather low rate when compared with the 3–4% background incidence of malformations in the general population in Europe and the US.

No pattern of malformations was reported. The data are inadequate to assess its reproductive toxicity in humans. There is no clear evidence to indicate that maternal exposure is associated with an increased risk of fetal toxicity.

Recommendation. Exposure to carbon disulfide should be avoided in pregnancy. Nevertheless, when there has been significant exposure, this is not an indication for the termination of pregnancy. However, if the mother has had symptoms of toxicity and/or continuous exposure, she may be offered additional prenatal diagnostic measures – e.g. a detailed fetal ultrasound – and should also be removed from exposure, as well as having the workplace monitored for carbon disulfide.

Carbon tetrachloride (tetrachloromethane)

Toxicology

Carbon tetrachloride is a chlorinated organic solvent. In a prospective cohort study (Seidler 1999), the association between maternal occupational exposure to specific chemical substances (among these carbon tetrachloride) and the birth of small-for-gestational-age (SGA) infants was evaluated. From a total of 3946 pregnant women in Germany working in the leather industry, no association with carbon tetrachloride and SGA was found. However, the power of the study is limited. There are inadequate data for human risk assessment. Data from animal studies indicate that embryotoxicity and gonadal toxicity occur only at exposure levels that produce significant general toxicity (Sullivan 1993).

Recommendation. Exposure to carbon tetrachloride should be avoided in pregnancy wherever possible, and the workplace should be monitored for carbon tetrachloride. Nevertheless, when there has been significant exposure, this is not an indication for termination of pregnancy. However, if the mother has had symptoms of toxicity and/or continuous exposure, she may be offered additional prenatal diagnostic measures, such as a detailed fetal ultrasound.

Chloroform (trichloromethane)

Toxicology

Chloroform is a widely used industrial and laboratory solvent. Interference with implantation and fetal growth retardation has been reported after exposure to chloroform in human pregnancy.

2 Pregnancy

2.23 Occupational, industrial, and environmental agents

There are a small number of epidemiological studies of pregnancy outcomes following chloroform exposure, but they are difficult to interpret (Williams 1998, Reif 1996). Exposure in these studies is usually to chloroform and a varying number of other chemicals. In a study of 492 children of laboratory workers exposed to organic solvents during the first trimester of pregnancy, 148 were exposed to chloroform. The frequency of congenital anomalies was no greater than expected compared with the general population (Axelsson 1984). However, with multi-chemical exposure, establishing a cause–effect relationship is difficult. Similarly, no increase in risk for spontaneous abortion was found in 206 women exposed to chloroform in the pharmaceutical industry (Taskinen 1994). In both of the above studies, because of the inherent methodological limitations, the data are inadequate to draw any definite conclusions.

In recent years, reports have raised concerns about possible pregnancy risks from by-products of chlorinated drinking water. Chlorides are added to drinking water to kill disease-causing microorganisms. However, when chlorine combines with other substances in water, it may form chloroform and related chemicals (*trihalomethanes*). The level of these chemicals in water supplies varies. There are conflicting data concerning the possible adverse effects of chloroform and trihalomethanes in drinking water; a few studies suggest that the risk of miscarriage and poor fetal growth may be increased when levels of these chemicals are high, while other studies have not found an increased risk. In a case-control study of 1039 infants with congenital anomalies, no association with maternal consumption of chlorinated drinking water during pregnancy was found (Aschengrau 1993). In contrast, data from an ecological study found an association with maternal residence in an area in which the water supply contained more than $80\,\mu g/l$ of trihalomethanes. However, the data set was small (Bove 1995). A weak association with maternal residence in communities with drinking water chloroform concentrations above $10\,\mu g/l$ was reported in a case-control study of 187 growth-retarded infants (Kramer 1992).

In a prospective study of 5144 pregnant women, there was an association between spontaneous abortion and maternal consumption of five or more glasses per day of water that contained $= 75\,\mu g/l$ of trihalomethanes (Waller 1998). There was no such association with the chloroform content of the water, or in the group with low trihalomethane consumption. The miscarriage rate was 9.5% (10–20% was expected).

Low birth weight was reported in term infants whose mothers drank water with a trihalomethane concentration greater than $0.3\,\mu g/l$ during the third trimester (Gallagher 1998). In contrast, no association with low birth weight was seen in another study (Savitz 1995).

Significantly higher frequencies of acquired chromosomal aberrations were noted in the lymphocytes of women occupationally exposed to chloroform and other organic solvents (Funes-Craioto 1977). Similar findings were observed in the children of these women. This study has not been independently confirmed, and the relevance of acquired somatic chromosomal aberrations to the risk of malformations or any other disease in the offspring is unknown.

Recommendation. Exposure to chloroform should be avoided in pregnancy wherever possible. Certainly, atmospheric levels should be kept to a minimum well below the recommended Occupational Exposure Limits (OELs). In cases where there is chronic exposure and/or severe maternal toxicity, a detailed fetal ultrasound should be offered and fetal growth monitored. Exposure *per se* is not an indication for termination of pregnancy. In areas with known higher levels of trihalomethanes, pregnant women who are concerned about chlorine in drinking water may choose to drink bottled water.

Dichloroethane (1,2-dichloroethylene; ethylene chloride; glycol dichloride)

Toxicology

Dichloroethane is used mainly as a solvent. The general reproductive toxicity effects in man have been reviewed by Sullivan (1993). No relevant published data were found on the effects of dichloroethane in human pregnancy.

Recommendation. Exposure to dichloroethane should be avoided in pregnancy. Nevertheless, when there has been significant exposure this is not an indication for termination of pregnancy. However, if the mother has had symptoms of toxicity and/or continuous exposure, she may be offered additional prenatal diagnostic measures – e.g. a detailed fetal ultrasound. Patients, especially those who have symptoms, should be removed from exposure, and the workplace should be monitored.

Dichloromethane (methylene chloride)

Toxicology

The main uses of *dichloromethane*, a halogenated organic solvent, are as a solvent in paint removers and degreasing fluids, and in

2

Pregnancy

2.23 Occupational, industrial, and environmental agents

aerosol propellants and hair lacquers. As a consequence of its wide-spread use, many workers may be exposed for prolonged periods (Sullivan 1993). Dichloromethane is metabolized readily to carbon monoxide, which may have toxic effects on the developing fetal brain (see section 2.20.1).

There are three published studies on the effects of occupational exposure to dichloromethane in human pregnancy (Taskinen 1986, Axelsson 1984, Kurppa 1983). Data from these studies indicate that there was no overall increase in the incidence of congenital malformations rate or any syndrome of defects. However, there was a slight but not significant increased incidence of miscarriages.

> **Recommendation.** Exposure to dichloromethane should be avoided in pregnancy wherever possible. Nevertheless, when there has been significant exposure this is not an indication for termination of pregnancy. However, if the mother has had symptoms of toxicity and/or continuous exposure, she may be offered additional prenatal diagnostic measures, such as a detailed fetal ultrasound. The patient should be removed from exposure, and the workplace monitored for dichloromethane.

▶ Methylethylketone (MEK, 2-butanone)

Toxicology

Methylethylketone is a solvent that is commonly used in industry and in pharmaceutical and cosmetic manufacturing. No relevant published data on any aspect of human reproductive toxicity were found. There is limited evidence from studies in rats that MEK is not embryolethal, but it is teratogenic (major malformations and retarded ossification) at exposure levels of around 3000 ppm. There was no maternal toxicity seen at these levels. An increase in fetal anomalies was reported at exposure levels of 1000 ppm with a no-effect level of 400 ppm.

The National Teratology Information Service in Newcastle, UK, has prospective follow-up data (unpublished) on seven pregnancies in which occupational exposure to MEK occurred. Four were exposed during the first 6–9 weeks, two during the first 14 weeks, and one during the first 19 weeks of gestation. Six of these women delivered normal babies, one of whom was premature (36 weeks). One mother who was exposed to multiple chemicals prior to pregnancy and during the first 6 weeks of pregnancy had a termination of pregnancy because multiple malformations were seen on ultrasound scan. However, exposure measurements were absent.

Recommendation. Exposure to MEK should be avoided in pregnancy wherever possible. Atmospheric levels should be kept to a minimum, well below the recommended OELs. Monitoring of the workplace should be available. If there has been chronic exposure and/or severe maternal toxicity, a detailed fetal ultrasound should be offered and fetal growth monitored. Exposure *per se* is not an indication for termination of pregnancy.

Tetrachloroethylene (perchloroethylene, PERC)

Toxicology

Tetrachloroethylene is widely used in the dry-cleaning industry, and so exposure of women is common, especially in small businesses where industrial hygienic practices may be inadequate.

There are experimental data suggesting a carcinogenic potential of PERC. A number of studies have shown an increased risk for spontaneous abortion of about two-fold in women exposed to tetrachloroethylene in the laundry and dry-cleaning industry, and the risk is increased in more heavily exposed women (Doyle 1997, Windham 1991, Olsen 1990, Kyyrönen 1989, Bosco 1987, Hemminki 1980). No increase in the incidence of low birth weight children or congenital malformations was found in the Canadian study (McDonald 1987). None of the other studies were adequate to draw any conclusions about these outcomes.

Maternal exposure to volatile organic compounds, such as PERC, was found to influence the immune status of the newborn according to a specific Lifestyle–Immune System–Allergy cohort study (Lehman 2002).

In summary, however, there are consistent data indicating that high levels of exposure, especially if associated with maternal toxicity, are associated with an increased risk of intrauterine growth restriction.

Recommendation. Exposure to tetrachloroethylene should be avoided during pregnancy wherever possible. Nevertheless, when there has been significant exposure this is not an indication for termination of pregnancy. However, if the mother has had symptoms of toxicity and/or continuous exposure, she may be offered additional prenatal diagnostic measures, such as a detailed fetal ultrasound including control of fetal growth.

2.23 Occupational, industrial, and environmental agents

▶ **Toluene**

Toxicology

Toluene (*toluol, methylbenzene*) is a widely used solvent in the paint, metal-cleaning products and adhesive applications (shoes) industries. Besides the industrial applications, toluene has been used as a recreational drug as an alternative to ethanol (see Chapter 2.21). Toluene is a difficult product to regulate in the workplace and elsewhere because an individual can detect the sweet odor at approximately 3 ppm and the TLV is 25 ppm. Thus, only solvent monitoring of the workplace can establish exposure levels.

Symptoms in the pregnant woman can be the first evidence of substantive exposure – dizziness and hallucinations can be one sign associated with the workplace or with use of the product. It is often difficult to separate the symptoms of pregnancy nausea and vomiting from toxic effects of the solvent. In either case, it will be necessary, if the symptoms persist, to remove the woman from the specific work area. As with ethanol, dose is a principal concern. In more than 30 cases of exposure to toluene via chronic recreational use to the point of "getting high", both maternal effects (e.g. acute intoxication, chronic ataxia, and atrophy of the cerebellum upon MRI examination) and effects similar to the fetal alcohol syndrome have been regularly noted (Bowen 2006). In 56 patients with reported solvent abuse, 12 patients (21.4%) delivered preterm infants. Nine infants (16.1%) had major anomalies, seven (12.5%) had fetal solvent syndrome facial features, and six (10.7%) had hearing loss (Scheeres 2002).

Questions have been raised about solvent exposure during pregnancy and the risk for childhood leukemia. In a recent study of 790 exposed pregnancies, no relationship was found between solvent exposure in the workplace during pregnancy and childhood leukemia (Infante-Rivard 2005). Unfortunately, even with this number of subjects, the power was limited.

Recommendation. The difficulty with occupational and environmental exposure to toluene compared with its abuse is similar to the use of alcohol (ethanol). Chronic abusive high levels resulting in persistent and acute symptoms, for both ethanol and toluene, result in impaired children. Chronic exposure in the workplace to levels resulting in substantive maternal symptoms is thought to place the offspring and mother at risk. Thus, it is recommended that if the pregnant woman is having symptoms (whether exaggerated responses to noxious odors during pregnancy or intoxication because of the excessive levels of solvent), she should not return to the workplace in her usual capacity until environmental monitoring data demonstrate that levels of toluene and any other solvents are well below the regulated levels (PEL, TLV). Even if the levels of toluene are below the acceptable 8-hour threshold, the patient still may have to be moved to a non-solvent area because of her enhanced sensitivity to odors and her persistent and regular vomiting and nausea. It is recommended that the status of both mother and conceptus be more closely monitored throughout the pregnancy. Return to the workplace will be dependent upon the monitoring reports and, if the levels are low enough, on how the pregnant women responds to the odors – remembering that odor detection is very low at 3 ppm, while regulatory levels are 25 ppm.

Nevertheless, when there has been significant exposure this is not an indication for termination of pregnancy. However, if the mother has had symptoms of toxicity and/or continuous exposure, she may be offered additional prenatal diagnostic measures, such as a detailed fetal ultrasound including control of fetal growth.

2.23.2   Formaldehyde and formalin

Toxicology

Formaldehyde is a hydrocarbon that is widely used as a disinfectant and tissue preservative. *Formalin* is a solution of formaldehyde in water, often with 10–15% methanol to prevent polymerization. Data on the potential reproductive toxicity of formaldehyde exposure in human pregnancy are limited. One study that reported on the effects of occupational exposure to formaldehyde in hospital workers did not demonstrate an increased incidence of spontaneous abortions or birth defects when compared with employees who were not exposed (Hemminki 1982B). Furthermore, no significant association was observed with maternal occupational exposure to formaldehyde during the first 3 months of pregnancy in a case-control study of 34 nurses whose infants had congenital anomalies (Hemminki 1985).

However, in a cohort study of 316 operating-room nurses who were exposed to formalin during early pregnancy, a significant increase in spontaneous abortions was reported. Furthermore, it was reported that among the 271 infants born to these nurses there was a significant increase in the overall malformation rate, although not of major defects (Saurel-Cubizolles 1994). This study population was exposed to volatile anesthetics and ionizing radiation as well as formalin. Therefore, the adverse effects cannot be directly attributed to formalin *per se*.

Two case-control studies also reported weak associations with occupational exposure to formaldehyde during the first trimester of pregnancy in 61 cosmetologists and 206 female laboratory workers who had miscarriages (John 1994, Taskinen 1994). However, no significant association was observed with maternal occupational exposure to formaldehyde during the first 3 months of pregnancy in another case-control study that involved 164 nurses who had miscarriages (Hemminki 1985). Another Finnish study (Taskinen 1999) investigated whether exposure to formaldehyde affected the fertility of female woodworkers. Exposure to formaldehyde was significantly associated with delayed conception. Additionally, an association was observed between exposure to formaldehyde and an increased risk of spontaneous abortion. A possible relationship between environmental risk factors and cardiac malformations was studied in a case-control study. Residential exposure to ambient formaldehyde ($>2.42\,\mu g/m^3$) tended to increase the risk of unspecified congenital heart defects (Dulskiene 2005).

> **Recommendation.** Exposure to chronic or high concentrations of formaldehyde and formalin should be avoided in pregnancy wherever possible. Atmospheric levels should be kept to a minimum, well below the recommended OELs. Exposure *per se* is not an indication for termination of pregnancy; as a rule, additional prenatal diagnostic tests are also not required.

2.23.3   Chloroprene (chlorobutadiene)

Toxicology

Chloroprene is used primarily in the manufacture of rubber. It readily oxidizes in air to form polyperoxides, which are considerably more toxic than pure chloroprene.

The majority of the published information on the reproductive effects of chloroprene comes from the Russian literature (reviewed by Sullivan 1993, Barlow 1982). The data are inadequate to assess its reproductive toxicity in humans.

> **Recommendation.** Exposure to chloroprene should be avoided in pregnancy wherever possible. Even though a large risk for chloroprene is unlikely for low exposure levels, a small risk cannot be excluded. When there has been significant exposure, this is not an indication for termination of pregnancy. However, if the mother has had symptoms of toxicity and/or continuous exposure, she may be offered additional prenatal diagnostic measures, such as a detailed fetal ultrasound.

2.23.4   Cyanide

Toxicology

In industry, *cyanide* is used as a fumigant (hydrogen cyanide gas) and a sterilizing agent. Cyanide toxicity is due to the affinity of cyanide for the ferric iron in mitochondrial cytochrome oxidase. It inhibits cellular respiration, and oxygen utilization is impaired. If tissue cyanide levels accumulate rapidly, death can occur within minutes. Exposure to lower concentrations of cyanide results in toxic effects similar to those caused by carbon monoxide poisoning, i.e. due to brain hypoxia.

Cyanide and some cyanogenic compounds can cross the placenta. Embryotoxicity, including teratogenicity, has been induced by administration of cyanide in several species (see overview in Schardein 2000), but the clinical relevance of the data is unclear. There have been no syndromes of human malformations attributed to cyanide-containing compounds.

Recommendation. Exposure to cyanide should be avoided during pregnancy because of its inherent toxicity. Workplace exposure should be monitored. Nevertheless, when there has been significant exposure, this is no indication for the termination of pregnancy. Even though a large risk for low-level exposure to cyanide is unlikely, a small risk cannot be excluded. If the mother has had symptoms of toxicity and/or continuous exposure she may be offered additional prenatal diagnostic measures, such as a detailed fetal ultrasound.

2.23.5   Photographic/printing chemicals

Toxicology

Many of these substances are highly irritant and corrosive (see overview in Schardein 2000, Gilstrap 1998, Paul 1993). The most commonly used chemicals are: *acetic acid, ammonium sulfate, ammonium thiocyanate, ammonium thiosulfate, bromine/potassium bromide, citric acid, diethylenetriaminepenta acetic acid (DTPA), ethylenediamine tetra acetic acid (EDTA; ferric ammonium salt of EDTA), glycol ethers, hydrocarbon solvents, hydroxylamine, 3-phenylenediamine, 4-phenylenediamine, potassium carbonate, sodium benzoate, sodium sulfite,* and *sulfur dioxide.*

High doses of *bromine salts* are toxic. There is one case report concerning an infant who was found to have high serum bromide levels at birth. The mother had handled photographic chemicals during her pregnancy. At birth the child was hypotonic, but once the bromism had resolved the early childhood development was normal (Mangurten 1982). There are no data available on the potential toxic effects in human pregnancy for the majority of chemicals used in the photographic/printing industry.

Ammonia gas exposure is another common exposure, due to accidental spills in photographic processing. Because ammonia is an irritant odor, it is difficult for workers to remain in the workplace. Therefore, most exposure to ammonia is acute. Ammonia is rapidly metabolized in humans with normal liver function. If there is liver failure, ammonia levels can increase in the body. Ammonia concentrations have been found in the umbilical cord to be approximately twice the normal levels in 96 deliveries studied (de Santo 1993).

> **Recommendation.** Based on the very limited data available, exposure to high concentrations of photographic and printing chemicals should be avoided in pregnancy. If spills do occur, it is recommended that pregnant women avoid the area and allow others with appropriate protective gear to clean up the spillage. It is important that the atmospheric levels are well below the recommended OELs. Exposure *per se* is not an indication for termination of pregnancy.

2.23.6   Pesticides

▶ Carbamate pesticides

Toxicology

Bendiocarb (ficam) is a derivative of *carbamic acid*. The carbamates are rapidly metabolized by mammals and inactive acetylcholinesterase by carbamylating the enzyme. *Benomyl (carbendazim)* is a benzimidazole carbamate that is widely used as a fungicide in agriculture and home gardening, and as an antihelminthic in veterinary medicine (IPCS 1993). Benomyl acts as a mitotic poison by altering tubulin binding and microtubule formation. This has been proposed as a possible mechanism of action for the developmental abnormalities seen in animal studies with high concentrations.

In 1993, small clusters of births of children with eye defects (anophthalmia or microphthalmia) allegedly related to garden and agricultural use of benomyl was reported in the UK. Following this report, a working party was set up by the Department of Health (DH) to investigate the prevalence and the clinical characteristics of anophthalmia and severe microphthalmia in England and Wales

(Dolk 1993, Gilbert 1993). No evidence for geographic clustering was found in England among 444 cases of anophthalmia or microphthalmia using National Registry of Birth Defects data (Dolk 1998A). However, this study did find a higher prevalence of anophthalmia or microphthalmia in rural rather than urban areas. Evaluation of data from several National Birth Defects Registries showed no secular changes in the frequency of anophthalmia or microphthalmia that would support such an association with benomyl exposure (Bianchi 1994, Castilla 1994, Kristensen 1994, Spagnolo 1994, Gilbert 1993). Furthermore, the epidemiological evidence suggests that the background incidence of anophthalmia or microphthalmia originally used for comparison in the English clusters had limitations because of substantial under-ascertainment (Busby 1998, Källén 1996). A relatively small Italian study of 63 children with anophthalmia or microphthalmia showed no association between parental (either maternal, paternal or both) occupation in agriculture (Spagnolo 1994).

As a result of the working party investigation in 1993, and data from other European Birth Defects Monitoring Programs, the UK DH concluded that there was insufficient evidence to warrant setting up a prospective study (EUROCAT 1994).

> **Recommendation.** Exposure to carbamate pesticides should be avoided in pregnancy wherever possible. Nevertheless, when there has been significant exposure this is not an indication for termination of pregnancy. Even though a large risk for the carbamate pesticides is unlikely, a small risk cannot be excluded. If the mother has had symptoms of toxicity and/or continuous exposure, she may be offered additional prenatal diagnostic measures such as a detailed fetal ultrasound.

Organochlorine pesticides

Toxicology

Lindane (γ-benzene hexachloride, γ-BHC), a γ-isomer of hexachlorohexane, is an organochlorine pesticide used to control houseflies and agricultural insects. In medicine, dilute concentrations are used topically to treat lice and scabies. Among the theoretical concerns about fetal exposure to lindane is the possibility that it may possess mild estrogenic properties, or induce hepatic microsomal enzymes and alter fetal steroid metabolism (Uphouse 1989, Saxena 1980). Despite the widespread use of this drug in the treatment of lice and scabies for more than 40 years, clinical reports supportive of these concerns were not located. Intoxications following the use of topical 1% lindane are associated with excessive use and overexposure to the product. Symptoms induced by overexposure include restlessness, muscle spasms, convulsions, and coma.

No epidemiological studies of congenital anomalies in infants whose mothers were exposed to lindane during pregnancy were found (see overview in Schardein 2000, Gilstrap 1998). Dermal absorption is increased by conditions that damage the skin. Once absorbed, lindane crosses the placenta (Saxena 1981). One study reported that maternal and placental concentrations of lindane and other organochloride insecticides were higher among 10 women with spontaneous abortions than among women with term pregnancies (Saxena 1981). This observation has not been verified or refuted by other studies. Another study reported a higher than expected serum lindane concentration in women who had a history of four or more previous spontaneous abortions (Gerhard 1998). There is one report of the death of twin fetuses in a woman who ingested a toxic dose of lindane in a suicide attempt (Konje 1992). When used in the recommended manner, there is no conclusive evidence to suggest that there is a significant increase in spontaneous abortions or in the incidence of congenital anomalies.

Other organochlorine pesticides, such as *dichlordiphenyl-trichlorethan* (DDT), *hexachlorbenzene* (HCB), *dieldrin*, and α- *and* β-*hexachlorcyclohexan* (α- and β-*HCH*) were removed from the market several years ago because of their long persistence in nature with resulting accumulation in the human food chain, including high levels in body fat and mother's milk (see Chapter 4.18). Data from an Australian cross-sectional study (Khanjani 2006) of organochlorines in breast milk indicated that there was no association between low birth weight/small-for-gestational-age babies, and organochlorine (DDT and *dichlorodiphenyldichloroethylene (DDE)* contamination. Bhatia (2005) re-evaluated the Child Health and Development Study, a longitudinal cohort of pregnancies occurring between 1959 and 1967 in the US. Sera were available from the mothers of 75 children born with cryptorchidism, 66 with hypospadias, and four with both. The results of this study did not support an association of DDT or DDE with hypospadias or cryptorchidism. In a study of a birth cohort in California of 385 low-income Latinas living in an agricultural community (Fenster 2006), no adverse associations between maternal serum organochlorine levels and birth weight or crown–heel length was observed. A reduction of gestational length was only associated with HCB. It was concluded that this association did not have a clinical implication, given its relatively low rate of preterm delivery (6.5%).

For details of another group of persistent organochlorine compounds, the *polychlorinated biphenyls* (PCB), see Chapter 4.18.

Recommendation. Exposure to organochlorine pesticides should be avoided in pregnancy wherever possible. Nevertheless, when there has been exposure, this is not an indication for termination of pregnancy. Even though a large risk of these organochlorine pesticides is unlikely, a small risk cannot be excluded. If the mother has had symptoms of toxicity and/or continuous exposure, she may be offered additional prenatal diagnostic measures such as a detailed fetal ultrasound. For therapeutic lindane administration, see Chapter 2.17.15.

Organophosphorous (OP) pesticides

Toxicology

Organophosphorous pesticides such as *carbophenothion, endothion, malathion*, and *triamiphos* exert their toxic effects by long-lasting inhibition of cholinesterases (ChE) at many sites in the body. There are limited data available on the effects of OPs during human pregnancy. Some reports have linked exposure to organophosphates with birth defects in humans; however, none of these studies have implicated carbophenothion, endothion or triamiphos specifically (overview in Schardein 2000, Gordon 1981). These studies are of limited value because of inherent design faults. They often report on exposure to multiple or unidentified pesticides, and fail to account for other possible causes. There is a single case report describing an amyoplasia congenita-like condition following maternal exposure to malathion during the eleventh to twelfth week of pregnancy (Lindhout 1987); a possible causal relationship was considered because of the action of malathion on the neuromuscular system, but this opinion is not universally accepted (Hall 1988).

Normal infants were born to two women who had attempted suicide by ingesting organophosphates during the second and third trimesters (Karalliedde 1988). The National Teratology Information Service in Newcastle, UK, has unpublished prospective follow-up data on 20 pregnancies in which exposure to OP compounds occurred. There was no clinical toxicity in any of the mothers, and all the infants were normal.

No controlled human studies on the possible reproductive toxicity of malathion were found, but there are two large cohort studies involving agricultural use. There was no significant increase in the incidence of congenital anomalies in a cohort of 22 465 infants born to women who lived in areas where aerial malathion spraying had occurred during the first trimester of pregnancy (Grether 1987). In the other case-cohort study of 7450 women potentially exposed to malathion during the 1981–1982 aerial spraying of large areas of San Francisco Bay, similar results were reported (Thomas 1992).

When OPs are used in the recommended way, there is no conclusive evidence to suggest that there is a significant increase in spontaneous abortions or in the incidence of congenital anomalies. In general, OPs used in concentrations that do not cause maternal toxicity are unlikely to increase the risks of fetal toxicity.

> **Recommendation.** Exposure to organophosphorous pesticides should be avoided in pregnancy wherever possible. Occupational or environmental exposure to malathion at or below accepted safety limits is unlikely to produce a substantial teratogenic risk, but the data are insufficient to state that there is no risk. Nevertheless, when there has been significant exposure, this is not an indication for the termination of pregnancy. However, if the mother has had symptoms of toxicity and/or continuous exposure, she may be offered additional prenatal diagnostic measures, e.g. a detailed fetal ultrasound. Severe poisoning, especially if associated with features of cholinesterase inhibition, requires urgent medical attention.

▶ **Pyrethrin (pyrethrum, pyrethroid) pesticides**

Toxicology

Pyrethrins (*cypermethrin, delta-methrin, permethrin, tetramethrin*) are a group of synthetic analogs of the natural substance *pyrethrum*, which comes from dried chrysanthemum flowers. The pyrethrins are widely used as both domestic and agricultural insecticidal sprays and dusting powders. They have also been used in topical preparations for the treatment of pediculosis (see overview in Schardein 2000).

There are few data on the effects of the pyrethroids in human pregnancy. Low toxicity for human subjects has been reported following pyrethroid exposure. No epidemiological studies of congenital abnormalities amongst the children of women exposed to pyrethroids have been reported.

The National Teratology Information Service in the UK has obtained follow-up data (unpublished) on the outcomes of pregnancy in 48 women exposed to this group of pesticides during pregnancy (35 permethrin, 5 deltamethrin, 4 cypermethrin and 4 tetramethrin). There were 41 normal babies, 2 spontaneous abortions (no postmortem data available), and 5 children with anomalies (mild talipes, unilateral inguinal hernia, an abnormal right little toe, bilateral talipes, a heart murmur). No cause–effect relationship with the pyrethroid exposure could be established in any of these infants. A teratogen information program in Australia (Kennedy 2005) published about the safety of permethrin exposure. The data on 113 pregnancies where the mothers had used 1% creme permethrin in the treatment of lice some time during pregnancy indicated that the use of such products was relatively safe. Obviously, the study is insufficient to draw final conclusions.

When pyrethrins are used in the recommended way, there is no conclusive evidence to suggest that there is a significant increase in spontaneous abortions or congenital anomalies. In general, pyrethrins used in concentrations that do not cause maternal toxicity have demonstrated low fetotoxicity.

> **Recommendation.** Exposure to pyrethrins should be minimized in pregnancy. However, exposure is not an indication for termination of pregnancy, and additional prenatal diagnostic tests are not required. Occupational or environmental exposure to pyrethrins at or below accepted safety limits is unlikely to produce a substantial teratogenic risk, but the data are insufficient to state that there is no risk for therapeutic pyrethrum/pyrethroid administration, see Chapter 2.17.

2.23.7   Phenoxyacetic acid derivatives and chlorinated dibenzo-dioxins

Toxicology

Agent Orange, the active constituents of which *are 2,4-dichlorophenoxyacetic acid* (2,4-D) and *2,4,5-trichlorophenoxyacetic acid* (2,4, 5-T), was widely used as a defoliant in the USA, and in Southeast Asia during the Vietnam War. There is particular concern about one of its trace contaminants, *2,3,7,8-tetrachlorodibenzo-p-dioxin* (*TCDD*, often referred to as *dioxin*, see below).

There is conflicting evidence of an association between Agent Orange and birth defects (see overview in Schardein 2000). There are three reports that suggest that there is an association with congenital malformations. The US Environmental Protection Agency (EPA) reported an increase in the incidence of spontaneous abortion in an area sprayed with herbicides including Agent Orange, compared with that found in two control areas (EPA Federal Register 1979). However, there are serious methodological limitations in this study which make interpretation of the data very difficult (Tognoni 1982). The other two studies describe the incidence of neural tube defects (Field 1979) and congenital anomalies (Hanify 1981) in agricultural areas using 2,4,5-T herbicides.

There are several reports of investigations where no association between 2,4,5-T exposure and an increased incidence of either spontaneous abortions or any specific type of congenital anomalies was observed (Smith 1982, Townsend 1982, Thomas 1980, Nelson 1979).

Concerns have been raised regarding the possibility that paternal exposure to Agent Orange/TCDD may have increased the incidence of congenital anomalies among the offspring of Vietnam veterans. Although there have been several reports of children with malformations allegedly due to paternal exposure to Agent Orange during the Vietnam War, the results of three comprehensive case-control studies indicate that no causal relationship could be established. No pattern of congenital anomalies was observed (Wolfe 1995, Donovan 1984, Erickson 1984). Compared with the plentiful studies on paternal exposure of US Vietnam veterans, there is little published material about the health of the exposed (pregnant) population of Vietnam. Moreover, a biologic plausibility regarding paternal teratogenicity, for example by indicating a mutagenic effect of Agent Orange/TCDD on spermatogonia and further developing sperm, has not been demonstrated.

Chlorinated dibenzodioxins are contaminants formed during the manufacture and combustion of organochlorine compounds. In July 1976, at Seveso in Italy, there was an accident at a pesticide manufacturing plant resulting in the release of TCDD into the environment. Numerous investigations followed this incident, involving the exposure of approximately 37 000 people, some of whom developed chloracne. The majority of studies found no association between exposure to TCDD/Agent Orange and an increased incidence of congenital anomalies (see overview in Schardein 2000, Smith 1982, Townsend 1982, Thomas 1980, Nelson 1979). Only one investigation indicated that the TCDD release was associated with an increase in adverse pregnancy outcome (Commoner 1977). Detailed analysis of this report indicates serious flaws in data collection, with no assessment of the relationship between exposure and stage of fetal development (Friedman 1984). Furthermore, none of the reports provide clear proof of exposure to TCDD/Agent Orange in the populations studied.

Recommendation. Exposure to TCDD/Agent Orange must be strictly avoided in pregnancy. However, if exposure has accidentally occurred this is not an indication for termination of pregnancy. It has to be decided upon individually as to whether additional diagnostic measures should be undertaken.

2.23.8   Metals

▶ Arsenic (see also Chapter 2.22)

Toxicology

Arsenic (As) is an element. Some commonly encountered inorganic arsenic salts include the trivalent *sodium arsenite* and the pentavalent *sodium arsenate*. Arsenic is a by-product of smelting, and a contaminant in hazardous waste sites. Furthermore, arsenic can naturally leach from certain types of rock – e.g. granite – resulting in substantially elevated levels of arsenic in the aquifers used for drinking water. This is a particular problem for unfiltered well water. Organic arsenicals have been used in the past for the treatment of syphilis. *Arsine* (AsH3) is an arsenical that is used as a gas in manufacturing semiconductors. Monomethylarsonic acid is used in some herbicides.

Both the inorganic arsenic salts and the organic arsenicals cross the human placenta and have been shown to accumulate in the placenta and the fetus. Trivalent arsenite demonstrates enhanced cytotoxicity compared with the pentavalent arsenate.

Occupational and environmental exposure to arsenic has been associated with adverse events in the conceptus. Nordstrom (1978) studied spontaneous abortions, birth weight of offspring, and congenital defects in Swedish workers in and around a smelter. Significant increases in malformation rates in the fetuses and newborns of the female workers, as compared to other women living in the region, were found. There were 13 malformations among 253 women who worked in the plant, compared to 694 among 24 018 in the region ($p < 0.05$). Birth weights were reduced, and spontaneous abortions increased.

Environmental exposure, as noted by elevated levels in soil and water, to arsenic resulted in the birth of low birth-weight babies. In 2003, associations between elevated water levels of arsenic (40 μg/l) in communities and an increased incidence of fetal growth restriction (FGR) were reported in Taiwan (Yang 2003) and in South America (Hopenhayn 2003).

> **Recommendation.** Evidence is developing that arsenic can increase the incidence of pregnancy loss and fetal growth restriction. If arsenic is a known or potential contaminant of soil or water (especially private wells), both the water/soil and blood/urine levels should be monitored. Eliminating exposure is the recommended intervention (e.g. using filtered water or bottled water in cases of water contamination), and following the pregnancy closely to monitor fetal growth and development.

▶ Cadmium

Toxicology

Cadmium is widely distributed in industrialized countries. Besides occupational exposure, some of the most common incidents are exposure to tobacco smoke and to old and poorly coated cookware, and from ingesting shellfish and kidney. For example, using an old silver-plated pitcher for an acidic drink like lemonade can lead to acute gastritis (Miller 2004), while 2–4 µg of cadmium can accumulate in a one-pack-a-day smoker. Cadmium levels are significantly increased in placentas from women who smoke during pregnancy (Eisenmann 1996). In the past, most toxicologists have considered cadmium to be initially a renal toxicant; however, evidence in both animal and human *in vitro* and *in utero* studies have demonstrated that the placenta is more sensitive to the toxic effects of cadmium than is the kidney (Miller 2004, Wier 1990). Occupational exposure is usually found in welders, and workers in foundries and cadmium battery factories. Two case reports identified cadmium intoxication in women who taught welding. They lost multiple pregnancies, and could not carry a child beyond the second trimester (Eisenmann 1996).

Animal studies demonstrate that cadmium is concentrated in the placenta and appears to damage it, resulting in the demise of the fetuses (White 1990, Levin 1980, Parizek 1964). Such was the observation for the two human case reports. Malformations (hydrocephalus) were only noted when the rat fetuses were directly injected, bypassing the rodent placenta (White 1990).

> **Recommendation.** Exposure to cadmium has certainly been noted in humans. During pregnancy, the apparent concern is the bioaccumulation in the placenta, leading to compromise and possible necrosis that is dose-dependent. Current limited human studies would suggest that if a pregnant woman is demonstrating signs of renal toxicity – increased beta-microglobulins and cadmium in their urine – then very close monitoring of the pregnancy, with determination of the source of cadmium to eliminate any further exposure, is required to reduce risk of pregnancy loss. Cadmium has a half-life of 30 years.

▶ Lead

Toxicology

Lead toxicity has been recognized for over 1000 years. Poisoning by organic lead (*tetraethyl lead*) is associated primarily with CNS toxicity which is distinguishable from that produced by inorganic lead. The overall toxicity of the organic form would seem to be due to the molecular species as a whole, rather than the metallic constituent alone.

Organic lead is much more rapidly absorbed than inorganic salts, by all routes, and is highly lipid-soluble, rapidly passing the blood–placenta barrier from 12 weeks onwards, and the fetal blood–brain barrier (Rabinowitz 1988). The effects on human reproduction are not unique. There have many unsubstantiated reports that women who worked in occupations with high lead exposure (white lead industries, potteries) had high miscarriage and stillbirth rates and gave birth to stunted, abnormal babies, but there are no epidemiological studies or case reports specifically on organic lead. It was a commonly held belief that lead was an abortifacient; however, as lead is a cumulative poison and is ubiquitously distributed in the environment, it is potentially a reproductive hazard for men and women (Schardein 2000, Miller 1993, Manton 1992, Bornschein 1984, Barlow 1982, Scanlon 1975). There is no conclusive evidence to suggest that maternal exposure to lead is associated with an increased risk of major structural malformations. There have, however, been some unconfirmed indications that there may be an increased risk of minor anomalies in women with high blood lead levels, which in some instances seemed to be a dose-related effect (Schardein 2000, Miller 1993, Rabinowitz 1988, Bornschein 1984, Needleman 1984, Barlow 1982, Scanlon 1975).

Other forms of fetal lead toxicity have been reported. Some studies have shown a significant association between chronic exposure to high concentrations of lead and premature delivery, decreased gestational maturity, low birth weight (Kaul 2002), and reduced postnatal growth. Exposure to high concentrations of lead in the third trimester has been associated with an increased risk of macrocephaly.

There are a number of case reports indicating neurological deficits and poor IQ scores in the offspring of lead-exposed mothers, even with a moderate increase of maternal lead level ($<300\,\mu g/l$) (see overview in Schardein 2000, Miller 1993, Bellinger 1992, 1991, Davis 1990, Barlow 1982). However, other workers have reported no adverse effects on language development in children studied from birth to 3 years old (Dietrich 1993, Ernhart 1989). Two other studies have found no association between prenatal lead exposure and intelligence at 4 years of age (Dietrich 1993, Davis 1990). Iron deficiency anemia often occurs in populations with high lead exposure, and has also been associated with lower scores on mental and psychomotor indices.

The results of two large prospective studies in the smelter town Port Pirie (Australia) and in Boston showed no significant association between prenatal lead exposure and child intelligence during the preschool period (Bellinger 1991, McMichael 1988).

A third prospective study of lead exposure and early postnatal development was performed in two groups of pregnant women, one group from a smelter town and the other group from a non-lead-exposed town in Yugoslavia (Wasserman 1994). The children were followed to 4 years of age. The authors concluded that continuing lead exposure is associated with cumulative losses in cognitive function, particularly those involving perceptual-motor integration, during the preschool years. Collectively, the findings of these three prospective studies indicate that the most sensitive period for exposure to lead occurs from the age of 18 months onwards.

One of the difficulties in trying to assess the risk of fetal toxicity for an individual pregnant woman is that the amount of lead to which she (and the fetus) are exposed is not always known. Thus, the majority of the published data refer to low, medium, and high exposure.

In general, maternal blood lead concentrations within the normal range (i.e. $<10\,\mu g/dl$) have not been associated generally with an increased risk of fetal toxicity. However, questions continue to be raised for values $>5\,\mu g/dl$. In adults, the blood lead concentrations regarded as toxic and requiring chelation therapy are in the range of $>60\,\mu g/dl$. In pregnant women, blood lead concentrations $>30\,\mu g/dl$ would be cause for concern. At concentrations which cause severe maternal toxicity ($>100\,\mu g/dl$), an increased risk of fetal loss may occur. In such circumstances, the uterine muscles relax and the fetus is expelled from the uterus. It is not known whether this is due entirely to the high concentrations of lead *per se*, or whether it is secondary to the maternal toxicity (see overview in Schardein 2000, Rabinowitz 1988, Barlow 1982, Scanlon 1975). In children with brain dysfunction following *in utero* exposure to lead, the blood concentrations of lead are usually $>35\,\mu g/dl$. Lead concentrations of $>40\,\mu g/dl$ in children are regarded as toxic, and require chelation therapy.

Women who live in older homes may be exposed to higher levels of lead due to deteriorating lead-based paint. If paint needs to be removed (preferably by experts) from a home, pregnant women and children should remain out of the way. Lead crystal glassware and some ceramic dishes may contain lead, and pregnant women and children should avoid frequent use of these items. Other unexpected sources of lead in the home may include such items as the wicks of scented candles and the plastic (polyvinylchloride) grips on some hand tools. Jobs that are related to lead, and thus contamination with lead, include painters, smelters, and workers in auto repair shops, battery manufacturing plants, and certain types of construction (Sallmen 1992).

Of particular concern regarding lead exposure are specialty food products produced in the homes – for example, ethnic foods cooked in lead pots brought into the US by family members. These foods have a sweet taste provided by the lead (NYCDH 2004). Further, women are obtaining elevated levels of lead from aryvedic medicines produced in non-health-inspected sites. Careful monitoring of all cookware and knowing the origins of prepared foods and medicines can assist in reducing lead exposure. In New York (USA), there are mandatory requirements for all pregnant women to be screened for lead at their first prenatal visit (Miller 2004).

At a minimum, pregnant women should be screened for lead (by questionnaire or blood lead level). A factor that influences judgment regarding lead exposure is whether the lead exposure is acute or chronic. Measuring bone lead with K-X ray fluorescence (K-XRF) can provide a history of chronic exposure (Miller 2006). Tibia and patellar bone lead provides the index for chronic versus acute exposure to lead. This assessment can be helpful in predicting whether large amounts of lead will be mobilized from the bone as the pregnancy continues.

> **Recommendation.** All (occupational, environmental, home, medicines, foods) exposure to lead should be avoided. If there is any known exposure to lead, women who are planning a pregnancy or currently pregnant should have, at a minimum, their blood lead level checked. Also, low exposure levels have been shown to influence mental development. A water supply running through lead pipes with the usual water pH value is not a major concern; however, standing water in lead-sealed containers can lead to significant exposure. Accidental exposure is not an indication for termination of pregnancy. If significant (continuous) exposure has occurred before or during pregnancy, maternal blood lead concentrations should be determined, along with the possibility of the use of KXF screening, which is now just considered for pregnant women.

Mercury

Toxicology

Mercury enters the environment from natural and man-made sources (such as coal-burning, and other industrial pollution). There are two main types of mercury; inorganic (metallic mercury, used in thermometers and sphygmomanometers), and converted by bacteria (organic mercury, e.g. *methyl mercury*, as accumulated in the fatty tissues of fish or used in seed dressings as an antifungal agent). While trace amounts of mercury are present in many types of fish, mercury is most concentrated in large fish that eat other fish, such as swordfish and shark; these fish contain more than 1 mg/kg of mercury (EFSA 2004). There is an extensive literature on the reproductive toxicology of mercury both in man and animals (Clarkson 2006). One of the main problems with the published data is that often there is no distinction made between inorganic and organic mercury, and the results are based on total mercury measured (Barlow 1982). However, more recently, species differentiation has been reported (Clarkson 2006).

The effects of accidental exposure to high-dose methyl mercury on pre- and postnatal development have been well documented as Minamata disease, including CNS damage. Ingestion of contaminated fish in Japan, ingestion of flour made from treated grain in Iraq, and ingestion of pork contaminated with phenyl mercuric acetate have all resulted in poisoning. An interesting publication concerned two heavily contaminated Minamata areas – Modo (M) and Akasaki (A) – comparing stillbirth and spontaneous abortion before and between 1956 and 1968, when the mercury contamination became serious (Itai 2004). Before contamination, the "abnormal pregnancy" rate was 7.0% in M and 5.4% in A; this rose to 18.1% (M) and 14.2% (A) after contamination.

The evidence linking metallic mercury and its inorganic ions to birth defects in humans is less clear (Cox 1999). Furthermore, it is often difficult to interpret the results of studies where exposure to mercury salts has occurred, because the uptake and distribution of the salts may differ from that of metallic mercury.

While there are many studies showing that mercury is available to the fetus, there are conflicting data regarding whether or not the placenta concentrates mercury (Yoshida 2002, Barlow 1982). Acute inhalation of mercury vapor by pregnant women has resulted in comparable levels of mercury in maternal and neonatal blood samples (Lien 1983). The blood level of mercury in populations differs according to the food intake: in Germany it is $<1\,\mu g/l$; the level is higher in Sweden and Japan; and in the Inuit the level may be $16\,\mu g/l$ (maternal blood level) and $35\,\mu g/l$ (cord blood), according to Bjerregard (2000).

There is also conflicting evidence whether or not metallic mercury causes birth defects, such as CNS anomalies, cleft palate, and skeletal defects (Stewart 2003, Ratcliffe 1996, Ericson 1989, Brodsky 1985, de Rosis 1985). The same conflict exists regarding cognitive shortcomings after maternal normal-to-moderate fish intake (Trasande 2006, Oken 2005, Myers 2003, Grandjean 1997). In a 2006 report, the Seychelles research team (Davidson 2006) determined that with low doses of meHg in fish, there was a bell-shaped curve in performance as the meHg level increased in the children. Such a result supports the importance of other constituents of fresh fish which contribute to the overall well-being of the child – e.g. 3-omega fatty acids.

Regarding *thiomersal* (see also Chapter 2.7), a convincing publication by Heron (2004) found no evidence that early exposure to mercury in thiomersal had any deleterious effect on neurologic or psychological outcome.

No association with possible occupational exposure to mercury during early pregnancy was seen in a case-control study of 4915 children with congenital anomalies (Matte 1993). No increase in the incidence of either spontaneous abortion or birth defects was found in the postal survey of 3212 pregnancies in dental workers who prepared more than 40 mercury amalgams per week (Brodsky 1985). No significant increase in the frequency of congenital anomalies was observed among 120 pregnancies in women who were occupationally exposed to mercury vapor in a lamp factory (de Rosis 1985).

Furthermore, there were no consistent patterns of adverse effects among 8157 infants born to women who worked during pregnancy as dentists, dental assistants, or dental technicians (Ericson 1989).

The results of another study in dentists and dental assistants has indicated that women with high occupational exposure (i.e. who prepare >30 amalgams per week and have poor occupational hygiene practices) were less fertile and took longer to conceive (Rowland 1994). This again is in contrast with the negative outcome of an epidemiological study regarding dental filling placement during pregnancy and low birth weight (Hujoel 2005). There is evidence that there is an increased risk of spontaneous abortion amongst the wives of males occupationally exposed to metallic mercury (Cordier 1992). There is no evidence of a teratogenic risk related to maternal dental amalgams. Absorption of mercury from dental amalgams has been found to be low (see Eley 1997, Larsson 1992).

The clinical data and experimental results of studies concerning the potential teratogenic risks associated with the inhalation of mercury vapor from dental amalgam do not warrant restriction of amalgams in pregnant women. The results also indicate that dental personnel are at no greater risk, provided that they have good occupational hygiene (Larsson 1990).

Recommendation. All (occupational) exposure to mercury should be avoided. Low exposure levels have been shown to influence mental development. Acute, inadvertent exposure to inorganic/metallic mercury is not necessarily grounds for termination of pregnancy, and, as a rule; no additional prenatal diagnostic tests are required.

Dental mercury

If indicated, dental amalgam fillings may be restored during pregnancy. However, if it is available and applicable, substitute material may be preferred. Dental amalgam fillings are by no means grounds for "detoxification" with chelating agents!

Consumption of seafood known for having higher levels of mercury contamination (shark, swordfish, tile fish, whaleblubber, and, to a lesser degree, tuna) should be avoided. If chronic significant mercury exposure has occurred before or during pregnancy, maternal blood levels should be monitored.

In 2004, the US FDA (Food and Drug Administration) and EPA (Environmental Protection Agency) made three recommendations for women who might become pregnant, women who are pregnant, and nursing mothers (see also Chapter 4.18) so they can gain the benefit from eating fish while reducing exposure to the harmful effects of mercury:

1. Do not consume fish that contain high levels of mercury, e.g. shark, swordfish, king mackerel or tilefish.
2. Consume up to 12 ounces (2 average meals) a week of a variety of fish and shellfish that are lower in mercury, e.g. shrimp, canned light tuna, salmon, pollock and catfish. Albacore ("white") tuna has more mercury than canned light tuna. Consume no more than 6 ounces (one average meal) of albacore tuna per week.

Otherwise, women are advised not to eat more than one average meal per week of locally caught fish.

2.23.9 Hazardous waste landfill sites

Toxicology

Waste disposal sites are a potential hazard to health. There has been a series of publications to assess reproductive disorders and birth defects in communities near hazardous chemical sites (Boyle 1997, Goldman 1997, Holmes 1997, Kimmel 1997, Savitz 1997, Scialli 1997, Wyrobek 1997). These studies investigated structural anomalies, genetic changes, mutagenesis, stillbirth and infant death, functional deficits, and growth retardation. Menstrual dysfunction, infertility, pregnancy loss, pregnancy complications, and effects on lactation were also investigated (Scialli 1997). Problems involved in epidemiological studies of congenital anomalies incorporating measurements of both environmental and genetic factors have also been reviewed by Shaw (1997) and Kipen (1996). Such studies are difficult to perform and interpret because of the numerous confounding factors.

The results of a multicenter case-control study (EUROHAZCON) of the risks of congenital anomalies associated with residents near hazardous landfill sites in Europe was reported by Dolk (1998B). The results of this study indicated that residents living within 3 km of a landfill site were at a significantly increased risk of having a child with congenital anomalies.

The study group consisted of 1089 live births, stillbirths, and terminations of pregnancy with non-chromosomal congenital anomalies, and 2366 control births without malformations whose mothers resided within 7 km of a landfill site. Twenty-one sites were included in the study. A zone within a 3-km radius of each site was defined as the "proximate" zone of most likely exposure to teratogens. Of the study group, 295 cases and 511 controls lived within 0–3 km of the site, and 794 cases and 1855 controls lived within 3–7 km of the sites, giving a combined odds ratio of 1.33, adjusted for maternal age and socioeconomic status. The risk decreased considerably with distance away from the sites.

The malformations found were neural tube defects, cardiac septal defects, and anomalies of the great arteries and veins. There was borderline significance for tracheoesophageal anomalies, hypospadias, and gastroschisis. There was little evidence of a difference in risks between any of the landfill sites, but the authors point out that the powers to detect such differences were low.

A study surrounded with comments and erratum was published in 2001, dealing with the results of adverse birth outcomes in populations living near landfills (Elliott 2001). Over 8.2 million live births, nearly 125 000 congenital anomalies (including terminations of pregnancy) and more than 40 000 stillbirths were involved. The conclusion was a small excess of congenital anomalies and low and very low birth weight in populations living near landfill sites without causal mechanisms available to explain the findings. Alternative explanations conferred data artefacts and residual confounding, to name but a few. Hence, for primary prevention interventions there are no indications. The dispute was enriched by Vrijheid (2002), who suggested an increase in risk of chromosomal anomalies similar to that found for non-chromosomal anomalies from 245 cases of chromosomal anomalies who lived within 0–3 km of 23 hazardous landfill sites in Europe. It should be noted, regarding this issue, that their findings suggested that previously reported results for congenital anomalies should not be extrapolated to a wider range of pregnancy outcomes, but should be evaluated separately for each (Staff 1998).

Recommendation. The studies have not conclusively indicated causative factors. Therefore, no advice can be given other than the obvious: no dwellings should be built on or near a (hazardous) landfill site.

2.23.10   Radiation associated with the nuclear industry

Adverse effects

Although background ionizing radiation is a known mutagen, few studies have examined transgenerational effects in human beings.

Chernobyl

Chernobyl, in the former USSR, was the site in 1986 of probably the worst accident ever to have occurred at a nuclear plant. Considerable quantities of radioactivity were released into the atmosphere, much of which was dispersed over the former Soviet Union and Western and Northern Europe. The radioactivity from the accident was washed from the skies and entered the food chain, notably in areas of high rainfall. Subsequent to the accident, people in the area around Chernobyl were evacuated. They have not been allowed to return.

Although not apparent for the first 3 years after the accident, by the end of 1994 a clear increase in childhood thyroid cancers was being seen in children from the surrounding areas. As the data available so far cover only approximately 10 years since the incident, it is too early for there to be significant information concerning other cancers. No relevant data were found regarding whether there was any change in the incidence of reproductive toxicity or in the incidence of congenital anomalies in the surrounding areas.

Sellafield

A study was performed using the workforce at the Sellafield nuclear reprocessing plant in Cumbria in the UK, which is considered to be the most highly exposed workforce in Western Europe and North America (Parker 1999). The aims of this study, which is part of a larger program investigating the health of the children of the Sellafield workforce, were to determine whether there was evidence of an association between stillbirth risk and paternal exposure to ionizing radiation.

Data from birth registration documents for all singleton live births (248 097) and stillbirths (3715) in Cumbria between 1950 and 1989 were analyzed. Within this cohort, the 9078 live births and 130 stillbirths to partners of male radiation workers employed at Sellafield were identified. A significant positive association was found between the risk of a baby being stillborn and the father's total exposure to external ionizing radiation before conception. There was a higher risk for stillbirths with congenital anomalies; (nine stillbirths with neural tube defects). Although the possibility of an unmeasured risk factor for stillbirth being confounded with paternal preconception irradiation cannot be excluded, extensive checks confirmed that the statistical models were a good fit to the data and there was not statistical evidence of unmeasured factors (Parker 1999).

UK Atomic Energy Authority, Atomic Weapons Establishment and British Nuclear Fuels Study

In contrast, another study of a similarly exposed workforce to that at Sellafield showed no increase in fetal death and congenital malformations in babies born to nuclear industry employees (Doyle 2000). This study analyzed pregnancies reported by an occupational cohort of nuclear industry workers in the UK. Employment and radiation monitoring data supplied by the employers was linked to each pregnancy conceived after the first employment within the nuclear industry. The men reported a total of 23 676 singleton pregnancies and the women reported 3585 pregnancies.

Among the pregnancies in female workers, the risk of early miscarriage before 13 weeks' gestation was higher if the mother had been monitored before conception, but this was not dose-related. The risk of stillbirth was also higher if the mother had been monitored before conception, but this finding was based on a small number of cases, of which 13 of 29 were exposed. The risk of any major malformation or of specific groups of malformations was not associated with maternal monitoring, the dose received during pregnancy, or the dose received before conception.

Overall, no evidence of a link between exposure to low-level ionizing radiation before conception and an increased risk of adverse reproductive outcome in men working in the nuclear industry was found. Similarly, there was no evidence of an association for women between monitoring before conception and malformations in the babies. The findings relating maternal preconceptual monitoring to increased risk of fetal death remain equivocal, and require ongoing investigation (Doyle 2000). In a second study, the hypothesis linking exposure to low-level ionizing radiation among men with primary infertility was not supported (Doyle 2001).

In a critique of the first study, it was pointed out that 12% of the pregnancies reported by male radiation workers and 15% reported by female workers ended in fetal death. However, the female workers were on average 10 years younger than the male workers at the time of the survey. Moreover, pregnancies reported by female workers were more recent than those reported by the men. Both of these factors contribute to a much lower expected fetal death rate in female workers than in male workers, especially for late events such as stillbirths (Parker 2001). However, Doyle and co-workers did not accept the statement that men are less likely than women to report stillbirths (fetal deaths after 24 weeks' gestation).

> **Recommendation.** Environmental ionizing radiation will have an effect; however, no realistic primary prevention method is realistic. This is also evident with the higher levels of ionizing radiation linked with travel flights, radon, and other background radiation. If a new nuclear power accident happens, exposing a population to low-level radiation in a way similar to that after Chernobyl, data from UNSCEAR, the United Nations study group evaluating the measures and decisions taken after Chernobyl, may help to make the right decisions – including, for example, restricting food intake from an exposed area.

2.23.11 Video display terminals (VDTs)

Adverse effects

The potential reproductive hazards of being exposed to electromagnetic radiation emitted from VDTs has been the subject of debate for many years (Paul 1993, Scialli 1990). The major concern started in Canada in 1980, where a cluster of four infants with severe malformations was described. The mothers worked at the same place – a newspaper department in Toronto. The cluster was linked to the fact that the women had worked with VDTs during pregnancy. The publication of this cluster in the lay press (TGM 1980) soon brought forward reports on other clusters of reproductive failure from different parts of Canada and the US (Bergquist 1984). Many of these reports concluded that significant levels of ionizing radiation were not emitted by VDTs. Furthermore, the non-ionizing radiation and magnetic fields associated with these units are not produced in biologically significant amounts (see, for example, Blackwell 1988). There have been reports of a number of adverse pregnancy outcomes allegedly associated with exposure to VDTs. Four case-control studies report no association between congenital anomalies and maternal exposure to VDTs (Tikkanen 1990, McDonald 1986, Ericson 1986A, 1986B, Kurppa 1985).

At the General Telephone Company of Michigan, a cluster of miscarriages was investigated when 6 of 29 pregnancies in VDT-exposed women spontaneously miscarried, compared with 8 of 97 pregnancies in those not exposed to VDTs (Lichty 1985). Although this difference was statistically significant, the author commented that it may not be biologically significant. There was a possibility that other work-related factors might be involved, because the jobs of women working with VDTs and non-exposed women were considerably different. Mathematical models of clusters have been published showing that a number of random groups of pregnant women should have higher than "normal" rates of adverse outcome, regardless of exposure status (Abenhaim 1991, Bergqvist 1984).

The results of a large case-control study have suggested a small but significantly increased incidence of miscarriage for women who work on VDTs for more than 20 hours per week during the first trimester of pregnancy (Goldhaber 1988). A degree of recall bias cannot be excluded in this retrospective investigation, because the women were questioned about their VDT use more than 2 years after the pregnancies in question (Robinson 1989). A causal relationship with other unmeasured parameters, such as job-related stress, long working hours, and poor ergonomic conditions, may have been a contributory factor (see, for example, McDiarmid 1994).

The U.S. National Institute for Occupational Safety and Health (NIOSH) monitored the incidence of spontaneous abortion in 882 pregnancies that included occupational use of VDTs during gestation (Schnorr 1991). The data from this very comprehensive investigation do not indicate any association between the use of VDTs, exposure to the accompanying electromagnetic fields, and an increased risk of spontaneous abortion. These findings were consistent with the results of two other studies in Finland (Lindbohm 1992) and in Italy (Grasso 1997). The Finnish study did find an increased risk of spontaneous abortion for women who worked with VDTs that emitted a high level of extremely low-frequency magnetic field, but the numbers involved were low (<20 per group), so the clinical significance of this observation is questionable.

Similar negative results were reported in a case-control study that was designed to minimize a possible role of non-occupational factors relating to the incidence of spontaneous abortions (Roman 1992). Another study also reported no significant increased risk of reduced birth weight or premature deliveries among women working with VDTs (Grajewski 1997). Overall, from the investigations to date, the risks (if any) associated with VDT exposure are low (Parazzini 1993). The VDT events have at least been useful as a warning of how society can come to conclusions despite scientific facts. Källén (1988) quotes the pertinent remark from Foster (1986) about the VDT debate: "Controversy about possible hazards from video display terminals is unavoidable when the data are ambiguous and the stakes are high."

> **Recommendation.** There is, to date, no evidence to indicate that pregnant women working with VDTs have an increased risk of spontaneous abortion, congenital anomalies, reduced birth weight, or premature deliveries. Pregnant women may continue working with VDTs. However, ergonomic conditions, working hours, and job-related stress should be carefully considered.

2   Pregnancy

2.23 Occupational, industrial, and environmental agents

2.23.12   Mobile phones

Adverse effects

Mobile phones are low-power radio devices that transmit and receive radio-frequency (RF) radiation in the microwave range of 900–1800 MHz through an antenna used close to the user's head (Maier 2000). Analog systems have been replaced by digital models. Concerns have been expressed that microwaves might induce or promote cancer, along with symptoms such as sleep disturbance, memory problems, headaches, nausea, and dizziness. Changes in the permeability of the blood–brain barrier, blood pressure, and electroencephalographic activity have also been reported. There is uncertainty about the validity of many of these findings and the underlying mechanism of action. One report states that radio-frequency radiation below guideline thresholds has a demonstrable effect on cells and tissues, which suggests that a precautionary approach is warranted (Rothman 2000). In children, the brain is smaller and still developing, the skull is thinner, and there is a longer potential exposure time to RF radiation from phones. No relevant data were found on the use of mobile phones in pregnancy or their impact on fetal development.

> **Recommendation.** As there is no clear evidence from the data available to indicate that pregnant women who use mobile phones are likely to have an increased risk of adverse pregnancy outcomes, such use requires no specific measures during pregnancy.

2.23.13   Other sources of electromagnetic radiation

Adverse effects

Proximity to *electric current* involves exposure to weak *electromagnetic fields*. Very low-frequency magnetic fields are generated by a large number of electrical appliances in the home and office (Breysse 1994).

One of the highest exposure sources, both in homes and factories, is the sewing machine (Sobel 1994). There is a report of a weak association between childhood diagnosis of acute lymphoblastic leukemia and maternal work at home during pregnancy (Infante-Rivard 1995). Most of the pregnant women were thought to have used electric sewing machines, and thus exposed the fetus to electromagnetic fields. Childhood exposure to sewing machines or other factors in the home was also mentioned.

In a survey of 372 married couples in which the man worked at one of two Swedish power companies between 1953 and 1979, an increase in the incidence of congenital anomalies was found, but no pattern of anomalies (Nordstrom 1983). The mechanism by which these anomalies might have been transmitted via paternal exposure is not clear. However, in this study the finding could not be explained by confounding or reporting biases (Coleman 1988).

A seasonally related increase in spontaneous pregnancy loss was reported in users of electric blankets and heated waterbeds (Wertheimer 1986). The authors concluded that either thermal or electromagnetic field effects might be involved. Similar results were reported by the same authors following exposure to ceiling heating coils (Wertheimer 1989). A small increase in risk of pregnancy loss associated with electric blanket use at the time of conception and in early pregnancy has also been reported (Belanger 1998). A brief report on pregnant women with a history of subfertility implied that there was an association between electric blanket use and congenital urinary tract anomalies (Li 1995). However, an increased risk of congenital anomalies or fetal loss associated with electric bed heating was not confirmed by the results of an epidemiological study in New York State (Jansson 1993, Dlugosz 1992). Similarly, a comprehensive prospective study of 2967 pregnant women that included some use of personal monitors to measure exposure to electromagnetic fields did not find a biologically significant increase in risk in relation to birth weight and fetal growth retardation associated with the use of electrically heated beds (Bracken 1995). Overall, the majority of evidence indicates that reproductive and teratogenic effects of electromagnetic fields are unlikely to occur in women under normal exposure conditions (Brent 1999B).

Concern has been expressed about the possible adverse effects on fetal development of living in an area close to high-voltage power lines. However, the results of studies in France and Norway did not identify an excess of congenital anomalies among children whose parents lived within 500 m of a high-voltage power line (Blaasaas 2004, Robert 1999, 1996, 1993). It was emphasized that the field strength drops rapidly with distance from the line, and that few people live directly below a power line. Therefore, most of the index children were exposed to electromagnetic field levels *in utero* that were not much different from those to which the non-exposed children were subjected. No significant association with residence within 100 or 50 m of a high-voltage power line was found in a subsequent study (Robert 1996).

2

Pregnancy

2.23 Occupational, industrial, and environmental agents

> **Recommendation.** As the majority of evidence indicates that reproductive
> and teratogenic effects of electromagnetic fields are unlikely to occur in
> women under normal exposure conditions, such exposures do not require any
> additional prenatal diagnostic intervention.

2.23.14   Electric shocks and lightning strikes

Adverse effects

There are published data on 15 pregnant women who received electric shocks when their fetuses were between 12 and 40 weeks' gestation (Mehl 1992, Leiberman 1986, Peppier 1974). Only one mother, who had been shot with a Taser (electro-weapon), lost consciousness and sustained injuries and burns (Mehl 1992). Fetal death occurred in 11 (73%) of the pregnancies, possibly due to changes in fetal heart conduction leading to cardiac arrest. The adverse outcomes may also be due to lesions to the uteroplacental bed. Two of the surviving fetuses had oligohydramnios, a clinical sign that is also consistent with impaired cardiac function (Leiberman 1986). In cases of accidental electric shock, the most common sign of adverse fetal effects was immediate cessation of fetal movements. It is possible that there is a reporting bias with these cases, in that only those with the most serious adverse outcomes are more likely to be reported. Nevertheless, these reports do indicate that even an apparently harmless maternal electric shock may cause fetal death.

In 1997, the results were published of a small case-control study of 31 women who received electrical shocks during pregnancy, matched with control subjects (Einarson 1997). Of these women, 26 had been exposed to 110 V, 2 to 220 V, 2 to high voltage (from electrified fences), and 1 to 12 V (from a telephone wire). In the exposed group there were 28 normal infants, 1 infant with ventricular septal defect, and 2 miscarriages. In the unexposed control, there were 30 normal infants and 1 miscarriage. The authors reported that in this study the pathway of electric current was only likely to have passed through the uterus in 3 of the 31 women, in contrast with previously published case reports. Adverse effects on the fetus seem more likely to occur when the current is reported to have passed from hand to foot, or electrical burn marks suggest such a route.

Eleven case reports of lightning strikes of pregnant women were found (Flannery 1982, Chan 1979, Guha-Ray 1979, Weinstein 1979, Rees 1965). There was a wide range of maternal symptoms reported, such as no loss of consciousness, brief loss of consciousness in those in whom the electrical injury caused maternal cardiovascular collapse, and uterine rupture at 6 months' gestation. Five (45%) of the exposed fetuses died.

> **Recommendation.** Any work that could expose a pregnant woman to the risk of electrical shock must be avoided during pregnancy. If an electrical shock has occurred, the fetal status should be evaluated immediately.

References

Abenhaim L, Lert F. Methodological issues for the assessment of clusters of adverse pregnancy outcomes in the workplace: the case of video display terminal users. J Occup Med 1991; 33: 1091–6.

Aschengrau A, Zierler S, Cohen A. Quality of community drinking water and the occurrence of late adverse pregnancy outcomes. Arch Environ Health 1993; 48: 105–13.

Axelsson G, Lutz C, Rylander R. Exposure to solvents and outcome of pregnancy in university laboratory employees. Br J Ind Med 1984; 41: 305–12.

Bao YS, Cai S, Zhao SF et al. Birth defects in the offspring of female workers occupationally exposed to carbon disulfide in China. Teratology 1991; 43: 451–2.

Barlow SM, Sullivan FM. Reproductive Hazards of Industrial Chemicals. London: Academic Press, 1982.

Belanger K, Leaderer B, Hellenbrand K et al. Spontaneous abortion and exposure to electric blankets and heated water beds. Epidemiology 1998; 9: 36–42.

Bellinger D, Sloman J, Leviton A et al. Low level lead exposure and children's cognitive function in the pre school years. Pediatrics 1991; 87: 219–27.

Bellinger D, Needleman HL. Neurodevelopmental effects of low level lead exposure in children. In: HL Needleman (ed.), Human Lead Exposure. Ann Arbor, MI: CRC Press, 1992, pp. 191–208.

Bergqvist UO. A model study on the occurrence of adverse pregnancy outcomes in clusters of workers using video display terminals. Scand J Work Environ Health 1984; 10: 80–82.

Bhatia R, Shiau R, Petreas M et al. Organochlorine pesticides and male genital anomalies in the child health and development studies. Environ Health Persp 2005; 113: 220–24.

Bianchi F, Calabro A, Calzolari E et al. Clusters of anophthalmia. No link with benomyl in Italy or in Norway. Br Med J 1994; 308: 205.

Bjerregard P, Hansen JC. Organochlorines and heavy metals in pregnant women from the Disko-Bay area in Greenland. Science Total Environm 2000; 245: 195–202.

Blaasaas KG, Tynes T, Lie RT. Risk of selected birth defects by maternal residence close to power lines during pregnancy. Occup Envon Med 2004; 61: 174–6.

Blackwell R, Chang A. Video display terminals and pregnancy. A review. Br J Obstet Gynaecol 1988; 95: 446–53.

Bornschein RL, Rabinowitz MB (eds). The Second International Conference on Prospective Studies of Lead. Cincinnati, Ohio, April 1984. Environmental Res 1985; 38.

Bosco MG, Figa-Talamanca I, Salerno S. Health and reproductive status of female workers in dry cleaning shops. Intl Arch Occup Environ Health 1987; 59: 295–301.

Bove FJ, Fulcomer MC, Klotz JB et al. Public drinking water contamination and birth outcomes. Am J Epidemiol 1995; 141: 850–62.

Bowen SE, Hannigan JH. Developmental toxicity of prenatal exposure to toluene. AAPS J 2006; 8: E419–24.

Boyle CA. Surveillance of developmental disabilities with an emphasis on special studies. Reprod Toxicol 1997; 11: 271–4.

Bracken MB, Belanger K, Hellenbrand K et al. Exposure to electromagnetic fields during pregnancy with emphasis on electrically heated beds: association with birthweight and intrauterine growth retardation. Epidemiology 1995; 6: 263–70.

Brandys RC, Brandys GM. Global occupational exposure limits for over 5,000 specific chemicals. Hinsdal: OEHCS Inc., 2006.

Brent RL (A), Chambers CD, Chernoff GF et al. Pregnancy outcome following gestational exposure to organic solvents: a response [Letter to Editor] Teratology. 1999; 60: 328–9.

Brent RL (B). Reproductive and teratologic effects of low-frequency electromagnetic fields: a review of in vivo and in vitro studies using animal models. Teratology 1999; 59: 261–86.

Breysse P, Lees PS, McDiarmid MA et al. ELF magnetic field exposures in an office environment. Am J Indust Med 1994; 25: 177–85.

Brodsky JB, Cohen EN, Whitcheret C et al. Occupational exposure to mercury in dentistry and pregnancy outcome. J Am Dent Assoc 1985; 111: 779–80.

Busby A, Dolg H, Collin R et al. Compiling a national register of babies born with anophthalmia/microphthalmia in England 1988–94. Arch Dis Child Fetal Neonatal Ed 1998; 79: F168–73.

Cai SX, Bao YS. Placental transfer secretion into mothers' milk of carbon disulfide and the effects on maternal function of female viscose rayon workers. Indust Health 1981; 19: 15–30.

Castilla EE. Clusters of anophthalmia. No further clues from global investigation. Br Med J 1994; 308: 206.

Chan Y-F, Sivasamboo R. Lightning accidents in pregnancy. J Obstet Gynecol Br Commonw 1979; 79: 761–2.

Chapin R, Gulati D, Hope E et al. Chloroform. Environ Health Perspect 1997; 105(Suppl 1): 285–6.

Clarkson TW, Magos L. The toxicology of mercury and its chemical compounds. Crit Rev Toxicol 2006; 36: 609–62.

Coleman M, Beral V. A review of epidemiological studies of the health effects of living near or working with electricity generation and transmission equipment. Intl J Epidemiol 1988; 17: 1–13.

Commoner B. Seveso. The tragedy lingers on. Clin Toxicol 1977; 11: 479–82.

Cordier S, Deplan F, Mandereau L et al. Paternal exposure to mercury and spontaneous abortions. Obstet Gynecol Survey 1992; 47: 152–4.

Cox C, Breaza A, Davidson PW et al. Prenatal and postnatal methylmercury exposure and neurodevelopmental outcomes. J Am Med Assoc 1999; 282: 1333–44.

Davidson PW, Myers GJ, Cox C et al. Methylmercury and neurodevelopment: longitudinal analysis of the Seychelles child development cohort. Neurotoxicol Teratol 2006; 28: 529–35.

Davis JM, Otto DA, Weil DE et al. The comparative developmental neurotoxicity of lead in humans and animals. Neurotoxicol Teratol 1990; 12: 215–29.

De Rosis F, Anastasio SP, Selvaggi L et al. Female reproductive health in two lamp factories: effects of exposure to inorganic mercury vapour and stress factors. Br J Indust Med 1985; 42: 488–94.

De Santo JT, Nagomi W, Liechty EA et al. Blood ammonia concentration in cord blood during pregnancy. Early Hum Dev 1993; 33: 1–8.

Dietrich KN, Succop PA, Berger OG et al. Lead exposure and the cognitive development of urban pre school children: The Cincinnati lead study cohort at 4 years. Neurotoxicol Teratol 1991; 13: 203–11.

Dietrich KN, Berger OG, Succop PA et al. The developmental consequences of low to moderate prenatal and postnatal lead exposure: intellectual attainment in the Cincinnati lead study cohort following school entry. Neurotoxicol Teratol 1993; 15: 37–44.

Dlugosz L, Vena J, Byers T et al. Congenital defects and electric bed heating in New York State: a register-based case-control study. Am J Epidemiol 1992; 135: 1000–1011.

Dolk H, Elliott P. Evidence for "clusters of anophthalmia" is thin. Br Med J 1993; 307: 203.

Dolk H (A), Busby A, Armstrong BG et al. Geographical variation in anophthalmia and microphthalmia in England, 1988–94. Commentary: clustering of anophthalmia and microphthalmia is not supported by the data. Br Med J 1998; 317: 905–10.

Dolk H (B), Vrijheid M, Armstrong B et al. Risk of congenital anomalies near hazardous-waste landfill sites in Europe: the EUROHAZCON study. Lancet 1998; 352: 423–7.

Donovan JW, MacLennan R, Adena M. Vietnam service and the risk of congenital anomalies a case-control study. Med J Aust 1984; 140: 394–7.

Dowty BJ, Laseter JL, Storer J. The transplacental migration and accumulation in blood of volatile organic constituents. Ped Res 1976; 10: 696–701.

Doyle P, Roman DP, Beral V et al. Spontaneous abortion in dry cleaning workers potentially exposed to perchloroethylene. Occup Environ Med 1997; 54: 848–53.

Doyle P, Maconochie N, Roman E et al. Fetal death and congenital malformation in babies born to nuclear industry employees: report from the nuclear industry family study. Lancet 2000; 356: 1293–9.

Doyle P, Roman E, Maconochie N et al. Primary infertility in nuclear industry employees: report from the nuclear industry family study. Occup Environ Med 2001; 58: 535–9.

Duggal H, Ray S. Notification of congenital anomalies. Lancet 1998; 352: 1477.

Dulskiene V, Grazuleviciene R. Environmental risk factors and outdoor formaldehyde and risk of congenital heart malformations. Medicina {Lith.} 2005; 41: 787–95.

EFSA. European Food Safety Agency, Rome 2004 Mercury risk assessment in fish (www.efsa.eu.int/science/contam-panel/catindex-en.html).

Einarson A, Bailey B, Inocencion G et al. Accidental electric shock in pregnancy: a prospective cohort study. Am J Obstet Gynecol 1997; 176: 678–81.

Eisenmann CJ, Miller RK. Placental transport, metabolism and toxicity of metals. In: LW Chang (ed.), Toxicology of Metals. Boca Raton, Fla, CRC Press, 1996, pp. 1003–26.

Eley BM. The future of dental amalgam: a review of the literature. Part 5: Mercury in the urine, blood and body organs from amalgam fillings; and Part 6: Possible harmful effects of mercury from dental amalgam. Br Dent J 1997; 182: 413–17, 455–9.

Elliott P, Briggs D, Morris S et al. Risk of adverse birth outcomes in populations living near landfill sites. Br Med J 2001; 323: 363–8.

Epidemiology Studies Division, US EPA. Six years' spontaneous abortion rates in Oregon areas in relation to forest 2,4,5-T spray practices. Fed Register 1979; 44: 874.

2 Pregnancy

2.23 Occupational, industrial, and environmental agents

Erickson JD. Vietnam veterans' risk for fathering babies with birth defects. J Am Med Assoc 1984; 252: 903–12.

Ericson A (A), Källén B. An epidemiological study of work with video screen and pregnancy outcomes: a registry study. Am J Indust Med 1986; 9: 447–57.

Ericson A (B), Källén B. An epidemiological study of work with video screens and pregnancy outcomes: II. A case-control study. Am J Indust Med 1986; 9: 459–75.

Ericson A, Källén B. Pregnancy outcome in women working as dentists, dental assistants or dental technicians. Intl Arch Occup Environm Health 1989; 61: 329–33.

Ernhart C. Low lead level exposure and early pre school periods: intelligence prior to school entry. Neurotoxicol Teratol 1989; 11: 161–70.

EUROCAT Newsletter 8, 1994.

Feldmann RJ, Maibach HI. Percutaneous penetration of some pesticides and herbicides in man. Toxicol Appl Pharmacol 1974; 28: 126–32.

Fenster L, Eskenazi B, Anderson B et al. Association of in utero organochlorine pesticide exposure and fetal growth and fetal length of gestation in agricultural population. Environ Health Perspect 2006; 114: 597–602.

Field B, Kerr C. Herbicide use and incidence of neural tube defects. Lancet 1979; 1: 1341–2.

Flannery DB, Wiles H. Follow-up of a survivor of intrauterine lightning exposure. Am J Obstet Gynecol 1982; 142: 238–9.

Foster KR. The VDT debate. Am Sci 1986; 74: 163.

Friedman JM. Does Agent Orange cause birth defects? Teratology 1984; 29: 193–221.

Funes-Cravioto F, Kolmodin-Hedman B, Lindsten J et al. Chromosome aberrations and sister-chromatid exchange in workers in chemical laboratories and a rotoprinting factory and in children of women laboratory workers. Lancet 1977; 2: 322–5.

Gallagher MD, Nuckols JR, Stallones L et al. Exposure to trihalomethanes and adverse pregnancy outcomes. Epidemiology 1998; 9: 484–9.

Gerhard I, Daniel V, Link S et al. Chlorinated hydrocarbons in women with repeated miscarriages. Environ Health Perspect 1998; 106: 675–81.

Gilbert R. "Clusters" of anophthalmia in Britain. Difficult to implicate benomyl on current evidence. Br Med J 1993; 307: 340–41.

Gilstrap LC, Little BB. Drugs and Pregnancy, 2nd edn. London: Chapman & Hall, 1998.

Goldhaber K, Polen MR, Hiatt RA et al. The risk of miscarriage and birth defects among women who use visual display terminals during pregnancy. Am J Indust Med 1988; 13: 695–706.

Goldman LR. New approaches for assessing the etiology and risks of developmental abnormalities from chemical exposure. Reprod Toxicol 1997; 11: 443–51.

Gordon JE , Shy CM. Agricultural chemical use and congenital cleft lip and/or palate. Arch Environ Health 1981; 36: 213–20.

Grajewski B, Schnorr TM, Reefhuis J. Work with video display terminal and the risk of reduced birth-weight and preterm birth. Am J Indust Med 1997; 32: 681–8.

Grandjean P, Weihe P, White RF et al. Cognitive deficit in 7-year-old children with prenatal exposure to methylmercury. Neurotoxicol Teratol 1997; 19: 417–28.

Grasso P, Parazzini F, Chatenoud L et al. Exposure to video display terminals and risk of spontaneous abortion. Am J Indust Med 1997; 32: 403–7.

Grether JK, Harris JA, Neutra R et al. Exposure to aerial malathion application and the occurrence of congenital anomalies and low birthweight. Am J Public Health 1987; 77: 1009–10.

Guha-Ray DK. Fetal death at term due to lightning. Am J Obstet Gynecol 1979; 134: 103–5.

Hall JG. Comments on "Amyoplasia congenita-like condition and maternal malathion exposure": is all amyoplasia amyoplasia? Teratology (letter) 1988; 38: 493–5.

Hanify JA, Metcalf P, Nobbs CL et al. Aerial spraying of 2,4,5-T and human birth malformations: an epidemiological investigation. Science 1981; 212: 349–51.

Hemminki K, Franssila E, Vainio H et al. Spontaneous abortions among female chemical workers in Finland. Intl Arch Occup Environ Health 1980; 46: 93–8.

Hemminki K (A), Niemi ML. Community study of spontaneous abortions: relation to occupation and air pollution by sulfur dioxide, hydrogen sulfide, and carbon disulfide. Intl Arch Occup Environ Health 1982; 51: 55–63.

Hemminki K (B) et al. Spontaneous abortions in hospital staff engaged in sterilizing instruments with chemical agents. Br Med J 1982; 285: 1461–3.

Hemminki K, Kyyronen P, Lindbohm M-L. Spontaneous abortions and malformations in the offspring of nurses exposed to anaesthetic gases, cytostatic drugs, and other potential hazards in hospitals, based on registered information of outcome. J Epidemiol Commun Health 1985; 39: 141–7.

Heron J, Golding J; ALSPAC Study Team. Thimerosal exposure in infants and developmental disorders: a prospective cohort study in the United Kingdom does not support a causal association. Pediatrics 2004; 114: 577–83.

Holmberg PC. Central-nervous-system defects in children born to mothers exposed to organic solvents during pregnancy. Lancet 1979; 2: 177–9.

Holmberg PC, Hernberg S, Kurppa K et al. Oral clefts and organic solvent exposure during pregnancy. Intl Arch Occup Environ Health 1982; 50: 371–6.

Holmes LB. Impact of the detention and prevention of developmental abnormalities in human studies. Reprod Toxicol 1997; 11: 267–9.

Hopenhayn C, Ferreccio C, Browning SR et al. Arsenic exposure form drinking water and birth weight. Epidemiology 2003; 14: 592–602.

Hujoel PP, Lydon-Rochelle M, Bollen AM et al. Mercury exposure from dental filling placement during pregnancy and low birth weight risk. Am J Epidemiol 2005; 161: 734–40.

Infante-Rivard C. Electromagnetic field exposure during pregnancy and childhood leukaemia. Lancet 1995; 346: 177.

Infante-Rivard C, Siemiatycki J, Lakhani R et al. Maternal exposure to occupational solvents and childhood leukemia. Environ Health Perspect 2005; 113: 787–92.

IPCS (International Programme on Chemical Safety): Benomyl Environ Health Criteria 1993; 148: 13–18.

Itai Y, Fujino T, Ueno K et al. An epidemiological study of the incidence of abnormal pregnancy in areas heavily contaminated with methylmercury. Environ Sci 2004; 1: 83–97.

Jansson E Re. Congenital defects and electric bed heating in New York State: a register-based case-control study {Letter; comment}. Am J Epidemiol 1993; 137: 585–7.

John EM, Savitz DA, Shy CM. Spontaneous abortions among cosmetologists. Epidemiology 1994; 5: 147–55.

Källén, B. Epidemiology of Human Reproduction. Boca Raton, FL: CRC Press, 1988.

Källén B, Robert E, Harris J. The descriptive epidemiology of anophthalmia and microphthalmia. Intl J Epidemiol 1996; 25: 1009–16.

Karalliedde L, Senanayake N, Ariaratnam A. Acute organophosphorus insecticide poisoning during pregnancy. Hum Toxicol 1988; 7: 363–4.

Kaul PP, Srivastava R, Srivastava SP. Relationships of maternal blood lead and disorders of pregnancy to neonatal birthweight. Vet Hum Toxicol 2002; 44: 321–3.

2

Pregnancy

2.23 Occupational, industrial, and environmental agents

Kennedy D, Hurst V, Konradsdottir E et al. Pregnancy outcome following exposure to permethrin d use of teratogen information. Am J Perinatol 2005; 22: 87–90.

Khanjani N, Sim MR. Maternal contamination with dichlorophenyltrichloroethane and reproductive outcomes in an Australian population. Environ Res 2006; 101: 37–9.

Khattak S, K-Moghtader G, McMartin K et al. Pregnancy outcome following gestational exposure to organic solvents: a prospective controlled study. J Am Med Assoc 1999; 281: 1106–9.

Kimmel CA. Introduction to the symposium. Reprod Toxicol 1997; 11: 261–3.

Kipen HM. Assessment of reproductive health effects of hazardous waste. Toxicol Indust Health 1996; 12: 211–24.

Konje JC, Otolorin E, Sotunmbi PT et al. Insecticide poisoning in pregnancy: a case report. J Reprod Med 1992; 37: 992–4.

Kramer MD, Lynch CF, Isacson P et al. The association of waterborne chloroform with intrauterine growth retardation. Epidemiology 1992; 3: 407–13.

Kristensen P, Irgens LM. Clusters of anophthalmia. No link with benomyl in Italy… or in Norway. Br Med J 1994; 308: 205–6.

Kufera J. Exposure to fat solvents: a possible cause of sacral agenesis in man. J Pediatr 1968; 72: 857–9.

Kurppa K, Holmberg PC, Hernberg S et al. Screening for occupational exposures and congenital malformations. Scand J Work Environ Health 1983; 9: 89–93.

Kurppa K, Holmberg PC, Rantala K et al. Birth defects and exposure to video display terminals during pregnancy. Scand J Work Environ Health 1985; 11: 353–6.

Kyyrönen P, Taskinen H, Lindbohm ML et al. Spontaneous abortions and congenital malformations among women exposed to tetrachloroethylene in dry cleaning. J Epidemiol Commun Health 1989; 43: 346–51.

Larsson KS, Sagulin G-B. Placental transfer of mercury from amalgam. Lancet 1990; 336: 25.

Larsson KS. Teratological aspects of dental amalgam. Adv Dent Res 1992; 6: 114–19.

Lehman I, Thoelke A, Rehwagen M. et al. Environ Toxicol. 2002; 17: 203–10.

Leiberman JR, Mazor M, Macho J et al. Electrical accidents during pregnancy. Obstet Gynecol 1986; 67: 861–3.

Levin AA, Miller RK. Fetal toxicity of cadmium in the rat. Teratology 1980; 22: 1–5.

Li D-K, Checkoway H, Mueller BA. Electric blanket use in relation to the risk of congenital urinary tract anomalies among women with a history of subfertility. Teratology 1995; 51: 190.

Lichty PD. Health Hazard Evaluation Report No. HETA-84-297-1609. NIOSH, Department of Health and Human Services, 1985.

Lien DC, Todoruk DN, Rajani HR et al. Accidental inhalation of mercury vapor: respiratory and toxicologic consequences. Can Med Assoc J 1983; 129: 591–5.

Lindbohm ML, Hietanen M, Kyyronen P et al. Magnetic fields of video display terminals and spontaneous abortion. Am J Epidemiol 1992; 136: 1041–51.

Lindhout D, Hageman G. Amyoplasia congenita-like condition and maternal malathion exposure. Teratology 1987; 36: 7–10.

Logman JF, de Vries LE, Hemels ME et al. Paternal organic solvent exposure and adverse pregnancy ourtcomes: a meta-analysis. Am J Indust Med 2005; 47: 37–44.

Maier K Sr. Mobile phones: are they safe? Lancet 2000; 355: 1793.

Mangurten HM, Kaye CI. Neonatal bromism secondary to maternal exposure in photographic laboratory. J Pediatr 1982; 100: 596–8.

Manton WI. Postpartum changes to maternal blood lead concentrations {Letter}. Br J Indust Med 1992; 49: 671–2.

Matte TD, Mulinare J, Erickson JD. Case-control study of congenital defects and parental employment in health care. Am J Indust Med 1993; 24: 11–23.

McDiarmid MA, Breysse P, Lees PS et al. Investigation of a spontaneous abortion cluster: lessons learned. Am J Indust Med 1994; 25: 463–75.

McDonald AD, Cherry NM, Delorme C et al. Visual display units and pregnancy: evidence from the Montreal survey. J Occup Med 1986; 28: 1226–31.

McDonald AD, McDonald JC, Armstrong B et al. Occupation and pregnancy outcome. Br J Indust Med 1987; 44: 521–6.

McMartin KI, Chu M, Kopecky E et al. Pregnancy outcome following maternal organic solvent exposure: a meta-analysis of epidemiologic studies. Am J Indust Med 1998; 34: 288–92.

McMichael AJ, Baghurst PA, Wigg NR et al. Port Pirie cohort study: environmental exposure to lead and children's abilities at the age of four years. N Engl J Med 1988; 319: 468–75.

Mehl LE. Electrical injury from tasering and miscarriage. Acta Obstet Gynecol Scand 1992; 71: 118–23.

Miller RK, Bellinger D. Metals: occupational and environmental. In: M Paul (ed.), Reproductive Hazards: A Guide for Clinicians. Baltimore, MD: Williams & Wilkins, 1993.

Miller RK. Environmental and occupational exposures involving reproduction. In: P. Leppert (ed.), Primary Care for Women, 2nd edn. New York: Lippincott, 2004.

Miller RK, Hu H, Peterson J et al. Lead Exposures During Pregnancy: Importance of Blood Leads and K-XRF Assessments. OTIS Annual Meeting, 2006, p. 2.

Myers GJ, Davidson PW, Cox C et al. Prenatal methylmercury exposure from ocean fish consumption in the Seychelles child development study. Lancet 2003; 361: 1686–92.

Needleman H, Rabinowitz M, Leviton A et al. The relationship between prenatal exposure to lead and congenital anomalies. J Am Med Assoc 1984; 251: 2956–9.

Nelson CJ, Holson JF, Green HG et al. Retrospective study of the relationship between agricultural use of 2,4,5-T and cleft palate occurrence in Arkansas. Teratology 1979; 19: 337–84.

Nordstrom S, Beckman L, Nordenson I. Occupational and environmental risks in and around a smelter in northern Sweden. VI. Congenital malformations. Hereditas 1978; 90: 297–307.

Nordstrom S, Birke E, Gustavsson L et al. Reproductive hazards among workers at high voltage substations. Bioelectromagnetics 1983; 4: 91–101.

NYCDH (New York City Department of Health) Report: Guidelines for the Identification and Management of Pregnant Women with Elevated Lead Levels in New York City, October 4, 2004.

Oken E, Wright RO, Kleinman KP et al. Maternal fish consumption, hair mercury, and infant cognition in a US Cohort. Environ Health Perspect 2005; 113: 1376–80.

Olsen J, Hemminki K, Ahlborg G et al. Low birthweight, congenital malformations, and spontaneous abortions among dry-cleaning workers in Scandinavia. Scand J Work Environ Health 1990; 16: 163–8.

Parazzini F, Luchini L, la Vecchia C et al. Video display terminal use during pregnancy and reproductive outcome – a meta-analysis. J Epidemiol Commun Health 1993; 47: 265–8.

Parizek J. Vascular changes at the sites of oestrogen biosynthesis produced by parenteral injection of cadmium salts: the destruction of placenta by cadmium salts. J Reprod Fertil 1964; 17: 559–562.

2

Pregnancy

2.23 Occupational, industrial, and environmental agents

Parker L, Pearce MS, Dickinson HO et al. Stillbirths among offspring of male radiation workers at Sellafield nuclear reprocessing plant. Lancet 1999; 354: 1407–14.

Parker L. Fetal death and radiation exposure. Lancet 2001; 357: 556–7.

Paul M. Occupational and Environmental Reproductive Hazards. Baltimore, MD: Williams & Wilkins, 1993.

Peppler RD, Labranche FJ, Comeaux JJ. Intrauterine death of a fetus in a mother shocked by an electric current: a case report. J LA State Med Soc 1974; 124: 37–8.

Rabinowitz M. Lead and pregnancy. Birth 1988; 15: 236–41.

Ratcliffe HE, Swanson GM, Fischer LJ. Human exposure to mercury – a critical assessment of the evidence of adverse health effects. J Toxicol Environ Health 1996; 49: 221–70.

Rees WD. Pregnant woman struck by lightning. Br Med J 1965; 1: 103–4.

Reif JS, Hatch MC, Bracken M et al. Reproductive and developmental effects of disinfection byproducts in drinking water. Environ Health Perspect 1996; 104: 1056–61.

Robert E. Birth defects and high voltage power lines: an exploratory study based on registry data. Reprod Toxicol 1993; 7: 283–7.

Robert E. Intrauterine effects of electromagnetic field-(low frequency, mid frequency RF, and microwave): review of epidemiologic studies. Teratology 1999; 59: 292–8.

Robert E, Harris JA, Robert O et al. Case-control study on maternal residential proximity to high voltage power lines and congenital anomalies in France. Paediatr Perinat Epidemiol 1996; 10: 32–8.

Robinson H. The risk of miscarriage and birth defects among women who use visual display terminals during pregnancy {Letter}. Am J Indust Med 1989; 15: 357–8.

Roman E, Beral V, Pelerin M et al. Spontaneous abortion and work with visual display units. Br J Indust Med 1992; 49: 507–12.

Rothman KJ. Epidemiological evidence on health risks of cellular telephones. Lancet 2000; 356: 1837–40.

Rowland AS, Baird DD, Weinberg CR et al. The effect of occupational exposure to mercury vapour on the fertility of female dental assistants. Occup Environ Med 1994; 51: 28–34.

Sallmen M, Lindbohm ML, Anttila A et al. Paternal occupational lead exposure and congenital malformations. J Epidemiol Commun Health 1992; 46: 519–22.

Saurel-Cubizolles MJ, Hays M, Estryn-Behar M. Work in operating rooms and pregnancy outcome among nurses. Intl Arch Occup Environ Health 1994; 66: 235–41.

Savitz DA, Andrews KW, Pastore LM. Drinking water and pregnancy outcome in central North Carolina: source, amount and trihalomethane levels. Environ Health Perspect 1995; 103: 592–6.

Savitz DA, Bornschein RL, Amler RW et al. Assessment of reproductive disorders and birth defects in communities near hazardous chemical waste sites. I. Birth defects and developmental disorders. Reprod Toxicol 1997; 11: 223–30.

Saxena MC, Siddiqui MK, Bhargava AK et al. Role of chlorinated hydrocarbon pesticides in abortions and premature labor. Toxicology 1980; 17: 323–31.

Saxena MC, Siddiqui MKJ, Seth TD et al. Organochlorine pesticides in specimens from women undergoing spontaneous abortion, premature or full-term delivery. J Anal Toxicol 1981; 5: 6–9.

Scanlon JW. Dangers to the human fetus from certain heavy metals in the environment. Rev Environ Health 1975; 2: 39–64.

Schardein J. Chemically Induced Birth Defects, 3rd edn. New York: Marcel Dekker, 2000.

Scheeres JJ, Chudley AE. Solvent abuse in pregnancy: a perinatal perspective. J Obstet Gynaecol Can 2002; 24: 22–6.

Schnorr TM, Grajewski B, Hornung R et al. Video display terminals and the risk of spontaneous abortion. N Engl J Med 1991; 324: 727–33.

Scialli AR. The history of concerns about VDTS. Reprod Toxicol 1990; 4: 43–4.

Scialli AR, Swan SH, Amler RW et al. Assessment of reproductive disorders and birth defects in communities near hazardous chemical waste sites. II. Female reproductive disorders. Reprod Toxicol 1997; 11: 231–42.

Seidler A, Raum E, Arabin B et al. Maternal occupational exposure to chemical substances and the risk of infants small-for-gestational-age. Am J Indust Med 1999; 36: 213–22.

Shaw GM, Lammer EJ. Incorporating molecular genetic variation and environmental exposures into epidemiological studies of congenital anomalies. Reprod Toxicol 1997; 11: 275–80.

Smith AH, Fisher DO, Pearce N et al. Congenital defects and miscarriages among New Zealand 2,4,5-T sprayers. Arch Environ Health 1982; 37: 197–200.

Sobel E, Davanipour Z, Sulkava R et al. Occupational exposure to electromagnetic fields as a risk factor for Alzheimer's disease. Proceeding of the Annual Review of Research on Biological Effects of Electric and Magnetic Fields from the Generation, Delivery and Use of Electricity. US Dept of Energy, 6–10 November 1994, Albuquerque, NM.

Spagnolo A, Bianchi F, Calabro A et al. Anophthalmia and benomyl in Italy: a multicenter study based on 940,615 newborns. Reprod Toxicol 1994; 8: 397–403.

Staff MG. Landfill sites and congenital abnormalities. Lancet 1998; 352: 1705.

Stewart PW, Reihman J, Lonky EI et al. Cognitive development in preschool children prenatally exposed to PCBs and MeHg. Neurotoxicol Teratol 2003; 25: 11–22.

Sullivan FM, Watkins WJ, van der Venne M-Th. The Toxicology of Chemicals – Series Two. Reproductive Toxicology, Vol 1. Commission of European Communities. EUR. 14991 EN 1993, pp. 81–91.

Taskinen H, Anttila Lindbohm ML et al. Spontaneous abortions and congenital malformations among the wives of men occupationally exposed to organic solvents. Scand J Work Environ Health 1989; 15: 345–52.

Taskinen H, Kyyrönen P, Hemminki K et al. Laboratory work and pregnancy outcome. J Occup Med 1994; 36: 311–19.

Taskinen H, Kyyrönen P, Sallmen M et al. Reduced fertility among female wood workers exposed to formaldehyde. Am J Indust Med 1999; 36: 206–12.

TGM, *Toronto Globe and Mail* (Canada). Work conditions probed at Star as defects found in 4 employees. 23 July 1980.

Thomas DC, Petitti DB, Goldhaber M et al. Reproductive outcomes in relation to malathion spraying in the San Francisco Bay Area, 1981–1982. Epidemiology 1992; 3: 32–9.

Thomas HE 2,4,5-T use and congenital malformation rates in Hungary. Lancet 1980; 2: 214–15.

Tikkanen J, Heinonen OP, Kurppa K et al. Cardiovascular malformations and maternal exposure to video display terminals during pregnancy. Eur J Epidemiol 1990; 6: 61–6.

Tognoni G, Bonaccorsi A. Epidemiological problems with TCDD (a critical view). Drug Metab Rev 1982; 13: 447–69.

Townsend JC, Bodneri K, van Peenen PFD et al. Survey of reproductive events of wives of employees exposed to chlorinated dioxins. Am J Epidemiol 1982; 115: 695–713.

2

Pregnancy

2.23 Occupational, industrial, and environmental agents

Trasande L, Schechter CB, Haynes KA et al. Mental retardation and prenatal methylmercury toxicity. Am J Indust Med 2006; 49: 153–8.

Uphouse L, Williams J. Diestrous treatment with lindane disrupts the female rat reproductive cycle. Toxicol Letts 1989; 48: 21–28.

Vrijheid M, Dolk H, Armstrong B et al. Chromosomal anomalies and residence near hazardous waste landfill sites. Lancet 2002; 359: 320–22.

Waller K, Swan SH, de Lorenze G et al. Trihalomethanes in drinking water and spontaneous abortion. Epidemiology 1998; 9: 134–40.

Wasserman GA, Graziano JH, Factor-Litvak P et al. Consequences of lead exposure and iron supplementation on childhood development at age 4 years. Neurotoxicol Teratol 1994; 16: 233–40.

Weinstein L. Lightning: a rare cause of intrauterine death with maternal survival. South Med J 1979; 72: 632–3.

Wertheimer N, Leeper E. Possible effects of electric blankets and heated waterbeds on fetal development. Bioelectromagnetics 1986; 7: 13–22.

Wertheimer N, Leeper E. Fetal loss associated with two seasonal sources of electromagnetic field exposure. Am J Epidemiol 1989; 129: 220–24.

White TEK, Baggs RB, Miller RK. Central nervous system lesions in the Wistar rat fetus following direct fetal injections of cadmium. Teratology 1990; 42: 7–13.

Wier PJ, Miller RK, Maulik D et al. Cadmium toxicity in the perfused human placenta. Toxicol Appl Pharm 1990; 105: 156–71.

Williams MA, Weiss NS. Drinking water and adverse reproductive outcomes. Epidemiology 1998; 9: 113–14.

Windham GC, Shusterman D, Swan SH et al. Exposure to organic solvents and adverse pregnancy outcome. Am J Indust Med 1991; 20: 241–59.

Wolfe WH, Michalek JE, Miner JC et al. Paternal serum dioxin and reproductive outcomes among veterans of Operation Ranch Hand. Epidemiology 1995; 6: 17–22.

Wyrobek AJ, Schrader SM, Perreault SD et al. Assessment of reproductive disorders and birth defects in communities near hazardous chemical waste sites. III. Guidelines for field studies of male reproductive disorders. Reprod Toxicol 1997; 11: 243–59.

Yang CC, Chang CC, Tsai SS et al. Arsenic in drinking water and adverse pregnancy outcome in an arseniasis-endemic area in northeastern Taiwan. Environ Res 2003; 91: 29–34.

Yoshida M. Placental to fetal transfer of mercury and fetotoxicity. Tohoku J Exp Med 2002; 196: 79–88.

Zhou SY, Liang YX, Chen ZQ et al. Effects of occupational exposure to low-level carbon disulfide on menstruation and pregnancy. Indust Health 1988; 26: 203–14.

General commentary on drug therapy and drug risk during lactation

Ruth Lawrence and Christof Schaefer

3.1   The advantages of breastfeeding versus the risks of maternal medication

No discussion of the risks of maternal medications can be undertaken without an understanding of the benefits of being breastfed for the child. Advantages to breastfeeding have been recognized in general terms for decades. However, new information and evidence-based studies following breastfed infants for months and even years have identified many additional advantages and protections provided by human milk and the process of breastfeeding.

The nutrient advantages can be simply stated by "species specificity" (see Table 3.1). The nutrient needs of the human infant are specifically met by the nutrient content of human milk. The most dramatic evidence of this is demonstrated by the comparative advantages to brain growth, visual acuity, auditory acuity, and scores on

Table 3.1 Composition of human breast milk and of cow's milk

	Cow's milk	Colostrum	Mature milk
Total protein (g/l)	33	23	11
Casein (g/l)	25	12	3.7
Lactalbumin (g/l)	2.4	–	3.6
Lactoglobulin (g/l)	1.7	35	–
Secretory IgA (g/l)	0.03	6	1
Lactose (g/l)	47	57	71
Fat (g/l)	38	30	45
Polyunsaturated fatty acids (%)	20	70	80
Calories (kcal/l)	701	671	747

Mean values; adopted from Behrman (2000).

developmental tests related to infants who are exclusively breastfed, compared to infants who receive traditional formulas. These data are substantiated by multiple studies in both prematures and full-term infants. Along with the ideal nutrients, such as omega-3 fatty acids, whey protein, and high levels of lactose, the energy for the brain, are the presence of enzymes and ligands that facilitate the digestion and absorption of nutrients, including the micronutrients.

The other well-documented advantages of human milk are the infection-protection qualities that protect the breastfed infant from respiratory infections, otitis media, gastrointestinal infections, and even urinary tract and meningeal infections (Hanson 2004). The study of the immunologic properties of human milk has shown that infants who are exclusively breastfed for at least 4 months have a reduced risk of childhood onset diabetes, Crohn's disease, celiac disease, and childhood-onset cancers – especially leukemia. Hundreds of articles testing the allergy protection of human milk have shown a clear advantage in being breastfed for potentially allergic children.

There are many advantages to breastfeeding for the mother herself. The process facilitates the rapid recovery postpartum, with a reduced loss of blood and the prompt involution of the uterus to its pre-pregnant state (Labbok 2001). Further breastfeeding prevents post-partal depression (Groer 2005), and reduces the long-term risk of obesity and osteoporosis for the nursing mother. Studies of specific diseases show that there is a reduced risk of breast cancer and ovarian cancer for women who breastfeed (Lawrence 2005, Collaborative Group 2002). Finally, the special relationship between mother and infant that develops while the infant suckles at the breast has always been a prime reason to breastfeed.

Determining the risk–benefit ratio, for a given infant, of maternal medication requires taking all of the tremendous advantages under consideration and understanding the specific risk of the medication to a given child. For example, if the child is in a developing country where the risk of dying of an infectious disease in the first year of life is 50% for those infants who receive formula, then the risk of a maternal medication is relatively insignificant by comparison.

The World Health Organization (WHO) and the Innocenti Declaration state clearly the importance of infants being breastfed. The Innocenti Declaration was reaffirmed in 2006 at its fifteenth-year anniversary, once again urging exclusive breastfeeding for the first 6 months of life followed by continued breastfeeding with the addition of solid foods through to 12 months of age, and for as long thereafter as mother and child wish.

The incidence of breastfeeding decreased significantly throughout the 1970s and 1980s and is now slowly increasing worldwide because of a vigorous effort on the part of many supportive organizations to reverse the trend of bottle feeding. The most extensive program is the Baby Friendly Hospital Initiative (BFHI), which was begun by the United Nations International Children's Emergency Fund (UNICEF). The Baby Friendly Hospital Initiative has spread throughout most of the developing world, but is only slowly being accepted in Western cultures. BFHI requires that all hospitals have a breastfeeding policy and that all staff be thoroughly trained in the introduction and management of breastfeeding. In addition to adequate training of the staff, all infants should be put to breast within the first hour of life. It is also required that dummies or pacifiers not be provided to breastfeeding infants, and that BFHI hospitals pay for any formula utilized, accept no free samples, and distribute no free samples to their patients.

While encouraging mothers and babies to breastfeed in the hospital, support needs to be provided at home as well by the mother's physician, the pediatrician, the nurse midwife, and office staff, as well as licensed, board-certified lactation consultants. With respect to medications, however, proper information is essential. Many mothers are told to wean because of the medication that they must take. This is actually very rarely necessary. The information available to the practitioner, however, is often incorrect. Package inserts and the physician's desk reference, for instance, almost always suggests that the drug is not recommended during lactation, not because there is negative information but because the manufacturer has not provided any studies or information that would permit them to say it is safe. This may also lead to poor compliance – that is, the mothers do not follow medical advice. In a prospective study carried out at a counseling center among 203 breastfeeding mothers who were prescribed an antibiotic compatible with breastfeeding, 15% of the women did not take the medication prescribed and 7% stopped breastfeeding (Ito 1993A). It therefore becomes the responsibility of the practitioner to adequately inform the breastfeeding mother using relevant medical literature, and to determine the probability that the drug will enter the milk in a relevant quantity and present any problem for the child.

3.2   The passage of medications into the mother's milk

It is important to be aware of the characteristics of the drug itself, the ability of a given mother to absorb, metabolize, and excrete the medication, and the infant's ability to absorb, detoxify, and excrete the agent. The infant's age influences the latter ability, and no decision can be made about a given drug without knowing the age of the infant.

The characteristics of the drug that are significant include the route of administration, the absorption rate, the half-life or peak serum time, the dissociation constant, and the volume of distribution. The passage of a drug is influenced by the size of the molecule, its ionization, and the pH of the substrate (plasma 7.4, milk 6.8), the solubility in water and in lipids, and the protein binding. The distribution of a compound may follow one of several pathways (Figure 3.1).

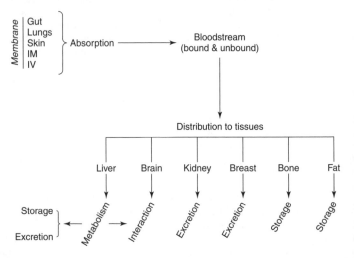

Figure 3.1 Distribution pathways for drugs absorbed during lactation (Lawrence 2005)

Table 3.2 Predicted distribution ratios of drug concentrations in milk and plasma

General drug type	Milk/plasma (M/P) ratio
Highly lipid-soluble drugs	~1
Highly protein-bound drugs in maternal serum	<1
Small (mol wt <200) water-soluble drugs	~1
Weak acids	=1
Weak bases	=1
Actively transported drugs	>1

Modified from Lawrence (2005).

The solubility of a drug is important because the alveolar and epithelial layer of the breast is a lipid barrier that is most permeable in the first few days of lactation, when colostrum is being produced. The solubility of a compound in water and in lipid is a determining factor for its transfer throughout lactation (see Table 3.2).

Drugs pass into milk by five identified pathways. Simple diffusion, carrier mediated diffusion and active transport, pinocytosis and reverse pinocytosis. If it is assumed that the body is a single compartment and the blood is distributed in the compartment uniformly, then an important characteristic of the drug is the volume of distribution which can be calculated as the volume of distribution = the total amount of drug in the body/concentration of drug in the plasma. Thus, drugs with a large volume of distribution do not get into the milk in any amount as compared to drugs with a low volume of distribution which pass into the milk from the plasma in greater amounts.

3.3   Infant characteristics

In addition to the parameters of the drug and the dose in mother's serum, and the amount in the milk, the characteristics of the infant are essential. The most important is the age and maturity of the infant, because the infant's ability to absorb, metabolize, and excrete the drug are dependent on this. Therefore, medications in the milk are of greater concern in the first few days of life than they will be at a week, a month or a year of age. For example, when a mother is taking a medication that is poorly excreted by a neonate, such as

3

Lactation

3 General commentary on drug therapy and drug risk during lactation

aminophylline, it may be well excreted by a 1-year-old and is not accumulated.

Absorption from the infant's gastrointestinal tract is dependent on the bioavailability of the drug, the effect of gastric pH and gastric enzymes, and the presence of food, which may impair absorption. Obviously, drugs in breast milk are present with food. If a medication can be given directly to an infant (for example, acetaminophen), it can be given to the nursing mother. Infants tolerate acetaminophen very well, detoxifying it in the sulfhydryl pathway rather than the glucuronidase pathway.

Infants' liver and kidneys are immature at birth. Thus, a drug that depends on liver metabolism, such as sulfadiazine, will compete with the bilirubin metabolism. A drug such as aspirin competes for albumin-binding sites in the infant, displacing bilirubin in the first month of life. However, clinical relevance may be questionable, due to the small amounts of a drug transferred via breast milk. In the case of aspirin, it is salicylic acid that passes into the milk and not acetylsalicylic acid; thus, it does not interfere with platelets in the infant.

Renal excretion is also immature early in life and a drug that depends on renal excretion, such as caffeine, theophylline, and some antibiotics, will accumulate in the infant in the first weeks and months of life but will gradually be better tolerated as the infant excretes it more effectively. These same drugs when given to an infant directly are given less frequently (daily instead of twice daily) in the first week of life.

3.4   Milk plasma ratio

The milk/plasma (M/P) ratio for drugs has been measured and reported for a number of medications. The milk plasma ratio is the concentration of the drug in the milk at the same moment that the concentration in maternal plasma is measured. It assumes that the relationship that between the two remains constant, but in most cases it does not. Therefore, the M/P ratio is often calculated from the average concentrations in the blood and milk over a longer period of several hours. These average concentrations are the area under the respective concentration curves (area under curve, or AUC), which are constructed from individual concentrations reported over the course of the time interval. The latter method is preferred in the newer studies because the M/P values they establish are more representative. Nevertheless, to some extent there are considerable variations in the M/P ratios calculated, not only between different studies and subjects, but also with the same mother: the colostrum has different concentrations than the milk some weeks later, and the first milk of a breastfeed is different from a sample taken later in the same feed. Thus, the M/P ratios cited in the following chapters should be viewed only as approximate values. They represent the mean values of present experience, and are useful only for a rough comparison with other medications.

The M/P ratio is not suitable for comparison of drug risks. A milk/plasma ratio of 1 assumes that the levels are the same in both plasma and milk. If, however, the level is very low in the plasma, it will also be low in the milk, even though the milk plasma ratio is 1. Low M/P ratios (<1) indicate that there is no accumulation in the mother's milk. However, significant concentrations in the milk can be reached even with low M/P ratios when there is a high maternal plasma value. On the other hand, relevant or even toxic amounts of medication cannot necessarily be assumed from a high M/P ratio with those drugs where the concentration in the maternal serum is very limited because of a high distribution volume typical for the particular medication. In such a case, even an M/P ratio of 8, which indicates a relative accumulation in the milk compared to the maternal plasma, means only a limited concentration of the medication in the milk, and consequently only a limited relative dosage (see above).

3.5   Amount of medication in the milk and relative dose

The simple calculation to determine the amount of the drug which the infant would consume via the milk in a day's time can be calculated by multiplying the concentration in the mother's milk (C_M) by the volume of milk consumed (V_M).

The amount of milk produced daily is between 500 and 900 ml. This amount is achieved about 4 days after birth. In order to better compare the different medications, the average daily amount per kg bodyweight that the infant takes in, rather than the individual total amount of milk consumed, is used as a basis for calculation. It is presumed that an infant receives about 150 ml/kg per day ($=0.15$ l/kg per day).

If, for example, the concentration of a medication in the milk is 50 µg/l, the exclusively breastfed baby receives:

50 µg/l $\times$ 0.15 l/kg daily = 7.5 µg/kg daily.

Sometimes there is also information about how much medication a child takes in with each meal. This method of calculating can make sense in the case of a single dosage of a drug with a short half-life. Based on the assumption of five breastfeeds a day, a child would drink 150/5 = 30 ml/kg per breastfeed (= 0.03 l/kg per breastfeed).

The amount of ingested drug is calculated analogous to the formula above (see also Bennett 1996):

$(50 \, \mu g/l \times 0.15 \, l/kg \text{ daily})/5 = 1.5 \, \mu g/kg$ per breastfeed.

The relative dose is the proportion of the maternal dosage per kg bodyweight that the breastfed baby takes in from the milk per kg of his bodyweight – i.e. the percentage of the maternal weight-related dosage:

$$\text{Relative dosage (\%)} = \frac{\text{dosage via mother's milk/kg}}{\text{maternal dosage/kg}} \times 100$$

Assuming in the above example that the maternal daily dosage of medication is 150 mg (= 150 000 μg), the mother weighs 60 kg, and the baby takes in 7.5 $\mu g/kg$ daily as calculated above, then the relative dosage is:

$$\text{Relative dosage} = \frac{7.5 \, \mu g/kg \text{ daily}}{150\,000 \, \mu g \text{ daily}/60} \times 100 = 0.3\%$$

Compared to the M/P ratio, the "Relative dose" is more appropriate for estimating the exposure risk for the child via breast milk because it considers the distribution volume of the drug (see Table 3.3).

Table 3.3 Comparison of the M/P ratio and relative drug dose

Drug	M/P ratio	Relative dose (%)
Atenolol	3	8–19
Chlortalidone	0.06	15.5
Captopril	0.03	0.014
Sotalol	4	42
Iodine	15–65	49
Pentoxyverin	10	1.4
Propylthiouracil	0.1	1.5
Carbimazole	1	27
Valproic acid	0.05	7
Lithium	1	80

3.6   Toxicity of medications in the mother's milk

Via breast, most medications reach the child milk in limited amounts of under 3% of a therapeutic dosage per kg bodyweight. Thus a toxic effect is unlikely. However, some aspects have to be considered: first, metabolites of the medication may also have pharmacological effects; and secondly, medications with longer half-lives can accumulate, especially in younger or premature newborns (Hale 2003). In such cases, a relative dosage of 3% may cause serum concentrations in the child that by far exceed 3% of the therapeutic serum concentration in the mother.

When the baby's feeding behavior changes while the mother is taking medication, this does not necessarily mean that there has been a toxic effect. Just like maternal diet, a medication can alter the sensory qualities of the milk and lead to "feeding problems".

Most medications reach concentrations in the mother's milk far below a therapeutic level for an infant. Only very rarely are toxic amounts measured. However, when medication is taken over a long period, even drugs with a low relative dosage may accumulate as a result of the prolonged half-life in infancy, and lead to symptoms. For this reason, the repeated administration of a medication must be more critically viewed than a single dosage.

Of a group of 838 mothers who had drug therapy while breastfeeding, about 11% reported symptoms in their infants that were possibly caused by the medication. In no case did this involve serious symptoms needing therapeutic intervention. The following associations were observed by the mothers (Ito 1993 B):

- Antibiotics decreased stool consistency
- Analgesics, narcotics, sedatives, antidepressants, antiepileptics: sedation
- Antihistamines: irritability.

Toxic effects need to be considered more with very young infants than with those above 2 months of age, or even with an older baby who is only breastfed once or twice a day. Newborns and especially premature infants are more at risk because neither the clearance nor the functional competency of barriers such as the blood–brain barrier is completely developed (Hale 2003). Particularly in the case of long-term therapy, attention must be paid to symptoms in the infant.

In a review of all published reports on toxic symptoms in breastfed infants, Anderson (2003) evaluated 100 eligible case descriptions. Causality between maternal exposure and symptoms in the infant was categorized as "possible" in 53 cases, and "probable" in 47. In 3 of 100 cases the infants died; their mothers were all exposed to psychotropic substances and to additional risk factors like drugs of abuse. Of the 100 children, 63 were younger than 1 month, 78 were a maximum of 2 months old, and only 4 were older than 6 months.

In some cases, an interruption of breastfeeding following the administration of medication may make sense. This may be easier to adhere to if the mother chooses, for instance, to take the medication in the evening after the last breastfeed. By avoiding the peak plasma times, the maternal drug levels that reach the milk can be minimized. In the case of paracetamol, it was even demonstrated that there was a higher concentration of medication if the breast had been frequently pumped (Notarianni 1987).

The risk of an increased icterus in the newborn as a result of medication in the milk is often overestimated. For example, bilirubin measurement does not reflect the amount of free bilirubin; the minimal amounts of medication and today's established control and phototherapy make the possibility of any damage less likely. In an otherwise healthy newborn, the risk for bilirubin encephalopathy as a result of medication in the mother's milk is low, even in the presence of the rare metabolic disorder glucose-6-phosphate-dehydrogenase deficiency, in which patients are disposed to hemolysis.

There is very little experience regarding the question of the long-term effects of medications that the baby receives through the milk. It is theoretically possible, for example, for specific sensitization through antibiotics and an increase of allergies as a result of various sorts of chemicals. Psychotropic medications and drugs could have a negative effect on later behavior and intellectual development, and potentially carcinogenic substances could promote the development of a tumor at a later stage. At present, however, there is no serious suspicion of such damage resulting exclusively from the mother's milk, and independently from intrauterine exposure or direct postnatal exposure. However, studies of long-term effects are rare.

The following exposures are known to be problematic in breastfeeding:

- Antineoplastic drugs
- Radionuclides
- Combination therapy with several psychotropic drugs or antiepileptics
- Iodine-containing contrast media, iodine-containing expectorants, and broad-based iodine-containing disinfectants.

When administration cannot be avoided in an individual case, it must be decided whether to abandon breastfeeding temporarily or permanently. For details, see the appropriate chapters.

3.7   Medications that affect lactation

Medications with an antidopamine effect, such as *phenothiazine, haloperidol,* and other neuroleptics, such as *sulpiride* and *risperidone,* as well as the antihypertensive α-*methyldopa,* and medications used to stimulate intestinal peristalsis, *domperidone* and *metoclopramide,* can, as a result of increasing the secretion of prolactin, stimulate milk production. The sympatholytic action of *reserpine* can have the same effect. Growth hormone and thyrotrophin-releasing hormone can also enhance milk production. Domperidone and metoclopramide are occasionally used for this purpose – for example, 10 mg metoclopramid three times a day (for a maximum of 7–10 days) and then tapering off the dosage for 2–5 days is sometimes recommended. Domperidone (not available in the USA) is less capable of crossing the blood–brain barrier, and therefore the risk of extrapyramidal symptoms is remote. Due to a molecular mass of 426, protein binding >90%, and poor oral bioavailability, the relative dose for a fully breastfed child is only 0.4% (see section 4.3.3). A dose of 50 mg of *sulpiride* two to three times a day, or 10 mg of *chlorpromazine* three times a day, have also been tried (Hallbauer 1997). Extrapyramidal symptoms and tiredness in the mother make the use of the latter two medications questionable. In addition, it has been repeatedly reported that individual psychological and technical support of the mother is as successful as prolactin-activating medication in resolving breastfeeding problems, or even with relactation (see, for example, Seema 1997).

Oxytocin stimulates the milk ejection reflex (also called the let-down reflex). For this reason, and because it also encourages uterine involution, it is the drug of choice for the often painful engorgement. *Amphetamines, diuretics, estrogen* and *dopamine agonists* from the group of *ergotamine derivatives* – such as, for instance, *bromocriptine, cabergolin, lisuride, methylergometrine (methylergonovine), pergolide,* and the drug *quinagolide,* all of which have an antiprolactin action – can reduce the production of milk. The various *prostaglandins* have been observed both to enhance and impede milk production. *Alcohol* and *opiates* cause a decline in the milk ejection due to reduction in the release of oxytocin.

Bromocriptine is used especially for weaning. However, the possible risks for the mother should lead to its cautious use. Because of the possible cardiovascular side effects, the American Food and Drug Administration (FDA) has rescinded the (earlier) permission to prescribe bromocriptine for weaning. Physical measures such as well-fitted supportive clothing, cooling, and emptying the breast until the mother feels relieved are preferable to ergotamine derivatives. In the case of mastitis, recommendations are bed rest, frequent emptying of the breast (after first using heat), and cooling it afterwards, as well as antibiotic therapy in some cases. Binding the breasts is no longer

3

Lactation

3 General commentary on drug therapy and drug risk during lactation

recommended because of the danger of engorgement. However, mothers are instructed to wear firm-fitting brassieres.

High-dosage *estrogen* is no longer used for weaning because of the risk of thromboembolism. The low estrogen content in the oral contraceptives which are available today limit milk production, if at all, only then when lactation is already poorly established. Pure gestagen contraceptives have no influence on the amount of milk produced.

3.8   Breastfeeding support

Inquiries from breastfeeding mothers about regional lactation consultants and self-help groups for questions and problems connected with breastfeeding can be addressed to the organizations listed in Appendix B.

References

Anderson PO, Pochop SL, Manoguerra AS. Adverse drug reaction in breastfed infants: less than imagined. Clin Pediatrics 2003; 42: 325–40.

Behrman RE, Kliegman RM, Jenson HB (eds). Nelson Textbook of Pediatrics, 16th edn. Philadelphia, PA: Saunders, 2000.

Bennett PN (ed.). Drugs and Human Lactation, 2nd ed. Amsterdam: Elsevier, 1996.

Collaborative Group on Hormonal Factors in Breast Cancer. Breast cancer and breastfeeding: collaborative reanalysis of individual data from 47 epidemiological studies in 30 countries, including 50 302 women with breast cancer and 96 973 women without the disease. Lancet 2002; 360: 187–95.

Groer M, Davis M, Casey K et al. Neuroendocrine and immune relationships in postpartum fatigue. MCN Am J Matern Child Nurs 2005; 30: 133–8.

Hale TW. Medications in breastfeeding mothers of preterm infants. Pediatric Annals 2003; 32: 337–47.

Hallbauer U. Sulpiride (Eglonyl) – use to stimulate lactation. SA Med J 1997; 87: 774–5.

Hanson L. Immunobiology of human milk. Amarillo, TX: Pharmasoft Publishing, 2004.

Ito S (A), Koren G, Einarson TR. Maternal noncompliance with antibiotics during breastfeeding. Ann Pharmacother 1993; 27: 40.

Ito S (B), Blajchman A, Stephenson M et al. Prospective follow-up of adverse reactions in breast-fed infants exposed to maternal medication. Am J Obstet Gynecol 1993; 168: 1393–9.

Labbok MH. Effects of breastfeeding on the mother. Pediatr Clin North Am 2001; 48: 143–58.

Lawrence R, Lawrence M. Breastfeeding: A Guide for the Medical Profession. St Louis, MI: Mosby, 2005.

Notarianni LJ, Oldham HG, Bennett PN. Passage of paracetamol into breast milk and its subsequent metabolism by the neonate. Br J Clin Pharmacol 1987; 24: 63–7.

Seema, MD, Patwari AK, Satyanarayana L. Relactation: an effective intervention to promote exclusive breastfeeding. J Trop Pediatrics 1997; 43: 213–16.

Specific drug therapies during lactation

4

Christof Schaefer and Ruth Lawrence

Please note that in the following chapters drugs are discussed under their generic names. For trade names, refer to the Physician's Desk Reference or comparable pharmacopoeias of your country.

Only a limited number of drugs have been studied with respect to their quantitative passage into mother's milk. Over the years, analytic methods have been considerably refined. Results of older studies (such as for propylthiouracil) needed to be revised. In the following sections, medications, arranged according to indications, are evaluated with the proviso that the currently available results are by no means definitive. Wherever possible, the amount of medication that the infant receives with the milk is given as a percentage of the maternal therapeutic daily dosage (per kilogram bodyweight; see Chapter 3). The terms "percentage of weight-related maternal dosage" and "relative dosage" used in the text are synonymous. Sometimes the percentage of the drug that the baby takes in per feeding is given. This way of calculating can make sense in the case of a single dose with active ingredients that have a short half-life. When there is a recommended dosage for therapeutic use in infancy or childhood, the relative dosage will, in some cases, be compared to this instead of to the maternal dosage.

Presuming an average daily breastmilk intake of 150 ml/kg of the child's bodyweight, the infant's weight-related exposure to the medication is identical to the amount of medication in 150 ml of milk (again, see Chapter 3). When protein binding and the half-life of a particular drug are mentioned, these values refer to the relationships in adults (i.e. in the mother) unless otherwise indicated. For some medications, the reference "Bennett 1996" is given for the sake of an overview. This is a standard publication of the European WHO Working Group. We refer less often to the classification of the American Academy of Pediatrics, Committee on Drugs (2001), cited more frequently in other places, because there is, for the most part, no additional information in this source.

References

American Academy of Pediatrics, Committee on Drugs. The transfer of drugs and other chemicals into human milk. Pediatrics 2001; 108: 776–89.
Bennett PN (ed.). Drugs and Human Lactation, 2nd edn. Amsterdam: Elsevier, 1996.

4.1.1   Paracetamol

Experience

The half-life of *paracetamol* in both mother's plasma and milk is 2.6 hours. After a dose of 650 mg, maximum concentrations of 15 mg/l were measured in the milk. Thus, an infant can get as much as 0.45 mg/kg at a feed. This is about 4% of the weight-related individual therapeutic dose in infancy. The M/P ratio is 1. Beyond one report of a reproducible maculopapular exanthema after 1 g of paracetamol, no undesirable effects have been reported following breastfeeding (survey in Bar-Oz 2003, Bennett 1996). No side effects were observed among 43 breastfed infants of mothers treated with paracetamol (Ito 1993). Since metabolism and renal excretion are not fully developed in the newborn, accumulation cannot be ruled out in the case of long-term treatment (Notarianni 1987).

> **Recommendation.** Apart from ibuprofen, paracetamol belongs to the group of analgesics of choice during breastfeeding.

4.1.2   Acetylsalicylic acid

Experience

The half-life of salicylates in mother's milk is more than 7 hours, which is decidedly longer than in plasma. The highest values are reached in just about 3 hours. Following a single dose of 500 mg *acetylsalicylic acid*, a maximum of 7.8 mg/l was measured in the milk; after 1000 mg this rose to 21 mg/l, and after 1500 mg it was 48 mg/l (Jamali 1981). If these high concentrations apply, an infant can consume between 0.2 and 1.4 mg acetylsalicylic acid per kg bodyweight at each breastfeed. This represents 2–14% of an antipyretic infant dosage of 10 mg/kg. There is very little experience for long-term antiphlogistic therapy with a daily dosage of up to 5 g. In one case, a near-therapeutic concentration of 65 mg/l was found in the infant's plasma despite supplementary feeding (Unsworth 1987). The 16-day-old infant of another mother who took 4 g of acetylsalicylic acid daily, as antiphlogistic therapy, showed toxic symptoms with a salicylate concentration of 240 mg/l in the plasma (Clark 1981). However, other reports do not describe any toxic effects – for example, a report on 15 breastfed infants under maternal aspirin therapy (Ito 1993).

Disturbances of coagulation or Reye's syndrome would not be expected as a result of analgesic dosing via the mother's milk (Hurwitz 1985).

> **Recommendation.** The occasional use of acetylsalicylic acid as a measure against pain seems justifiable, up to 1.5 g/daily. Paracetamol is, however, the analgesic of first choice. Taking acetylsalicylic acid regularly – especially in antiphlogistic (antirheumatic) dosages – is not acceptable. Here, ibuprofen is preferable. Low-dose acetylsalicylic acid treatment with 100–300 mg daily to inhibit thrombocyte aggregation is not problematic. External, short-term use of salicylates is no cause for concern.

4.1.3   Opioid analgesics and other centrally acting analgesics

Experience

Alfentanil, buprenorphin, butorphanol, codeine, dextropropoxyphene, fentanyl, morphine, nalbuphine, pethidine, and *sufentanil* have been analyzed with respect to their passage into the mother's milk.

In one study of a total of five mothers, a maximum of 500 μg of *morphine* per liter was found in the milk of the mothers after they had received first 10 mg i.v. and then 5 mg i.m. following the birth (Feilberg 1989). Another report describes concentrations of up to 100 μg/l of milk following a daily intake of four times 5 mg in a mother who had already received morphine in the third trimester of pregnancy. Her infant was calculated to have received up to 12% of the maternal weight-related dosage; with 4 μg/l, there were near analgesic values in the serum (Robieux 1990). Neither toxic symptoms nor withdrawal was observed. The authors explain this as the habituation of the infant, who was already exposed prenatally, or as the slow reduction of his serum values because of the extended half-life in newborns. Jacobson and colleagues (1990) point to possible "imprinting," as a result of prenatal morphine exposure, that could lead to dependency later in adult life. Other authors also mentioned the potential effects on behavioral and cognitive development, but these are unlikely with the temporary use of opiates. The limited oral availability of about 26% speaks against substantial drug transfer to the breastfed infant (Bar-Oz 2003). There are no reports to date on severe side effects via breast milk (American Academy of Pediatrics 2001). The concentration of morphine and its metabolite morphin-6-glucuronide in colostrum were very low in seven women receiving patient-controlled analgesia (PCA) after cesarean section (Baka 2002).

Buprenorphine enhances the pain-relieving action of *bupivacaine* when they are both administered epidurally. Furthermore, it is increasingly used in opioid replacement therapy (see also Chapter 4.16).

Buprenorphine and *norbuprenorphine* levels were determined from 10 random breast-milk samples collected over 4 successive days from a lactating woman during buprenorphine maintenance therapy with 8 mg/d. Concentrations ranged from 1.0–14.7 and 0.6–6.3 ng/ml, respectively. Considering the peak concentrations, a fully breastfed child would ingest 3.2 μg/kg daily – i.e. approximately 2% of the weight-adjusted maternal dose (Grimm 2005). Another case report of a mother taking 4 mg/d calculated a relative dose of 1% (Marquet 1997). A study of 20 mother–child pairs observed lower milk production and weight gain of the breastfed newborn of mothers receiving a 3-day course of epidural buprenorphine analgesia (Hirose 1997). Although clearance may be slower

4

Lactation

4.1 Analgesics, antiphlogistics and anesthetics

in the neonatal period because the drug is metabolized by glucuronidation, the low relative dose and oral availability do not contraindicate continuous breastfeeding.

Butorphanol has a half-life of up to 4 hours and an M/P ratio of 1–2. The results of studies of 12 women who received 2 mg i.m. or 8 mg orally after birth lead us to expect a relative dosage of under 1% for a breastfed baby (cited in Bennett 1996).

For *codeine*, see Chapter 4.2.

After administering 665 mg *dextropropoxyphene* to six study subjects, using the highest concentration in the milk as a basis, a dosage of 1.9% of the maternal weight-related daily dosage was calculated for the infant (Kunka 1984).

Four hours after delivery, a maximum of 0.15 µg/l of milk was measured in 10 study subjects who had received up to 400 µg *fentanyl* subpartu. Thus, an infant would receive a maximum of 22.5 ng/kg per day (Leuschen 1990). In another study of 13 mothers, a maximum of 19 ng/kg via the colostrum was calculated (Steer 1992). Five lactating women underwent induction of anesthesia with propofol and fentanyl (Nitsun 2006). Fentanyl pharmacokinetics were consistent with reports of others. In 24 hours of milk collection, averages of 0.033% (0.006–0.073%) of the fentanyl dose were collected in milk. All studies indicate less than 1% of the mother's weight-related dosage as a realistic exposure for the breastfed child. However, immediately after the injection, distinctly higher concentrations could be measured in the milk, although they decline rapidly. In no cases were any toxic effects described.

Alfentanil and *sufentanil* can, apparently, be similarly evaluated (Madej 1987, Giesecke 1985). Alfentanil, with a half-life of about 1 hour, has a shorter half-life than fentanyl and sufentanil. The transfer of sufentanil (20 µg together with 0.5% bupivacaine), administered epidurally during a cesarean section, was studied in 29 mothers who were treated after birth with patient-controlled analgesia. Up to the third day postpartum, measurement of sufentanil in the milk indicated values of 0.1–0.2 µg/l. All of the children were unremarkable neurologically (Cuypers 1995).

With *nalbuphine*, there is an M/P ratio of about 1. It would seem that only minimal amounts – about 1% of the maternal weight-related dosage – are transferred into the milk. This was determined in seven mothers who received a single 20-mg dosage i.m. (Wischnik 1988).

Following a single injection of 50 mg of *pethidine*, a maximum of 0.21 mg/l of milk was measured in nine mothers. For the infant, about 0.03 mg/kg per day, or 4% of the maternal weight-related dosage, is reached (Peiker 1980). Similar results were found by Borgatta (1997). There were no side effects reported in breastfed infants (American Academy of Pediatrics 2001). However, the long half-life of pethidine (up to 13 hours) and its metabolite norpethidine (63 hours) may result in cumulation in the infant's plasma, especially in pre-terms (Bar-Oz 2003). During postpartum patient-controlled analgesia (PCA), infants exposed to pethidine had significantly more noteworthy reactions in neurological testing than did those exposed to morphine (Wittels 1990). See Chapter 2.1 for the negative effects of pethidine, administered during labor, on early breastfeeding behavior.

For *tramadol*, only 0.1% of the weight-adjusted maternal dosage was calculated to be transferred via breast milk (Kmetec 2003).

Flupirtin, hydromorphone, meptazinol, nefopam, pentazocine, piritramide, remifentanil, and *tilidine* are not sufficiently studied. This applies also to the opiate antagonists *naloxone* and *naltrexone*. For *methadone* and *levomethadone*, see Chapter 4.16.

Recommendation. Opiate analgesics should only be used for short periods during breastfeeding. Because of their depressive effect on respiration, particular care should be taken with children with a tendency towards apnea.

Codeine (in combination with paracetamol or acetylsalicylic acid), fentanyl, and morphine are, depending on the indication, the opiate analgesics of choice during breastfeeding. However, these drugs also require close observation for somnolence in case of repeated dosages. If alfentanil, dextropropoxyphene, nalbuphine or pethidine are necessary, these are also acceptable. Other medications, such as buprenorphine, flupirtin, meptazinol, nefopam, pentazocine, piritramide, tilidine, and tramadol, as well as the opiate antagonists mentioned above, do not require any limitation on breastfeeding when they are given as single doses. The continuation of prenatally-initiated substitution for heroin addicts is viewed less critically than beginning a high-dosage opiate analgesia during breastfeeding (see Chapter 4.16).

4.1.4   Classic nonsteroid anti-inflammatory drugs

Experience

The group of acidic antiphlogistics shows only a very low M/P ratio – distinctly under 1 – because of its acidity and its high plasma binding (up to 99%). With a daily intravenous administration of 1200 mg *azapropazone*, the dosage that reaches the infant via the mother's milk is calculated to be 0.8 mg/kg, or 4% of the maternal weight-related dosage at maximum (Bald 1990).

Diclofenac and *flufenamic acid* also have short half-lives. The amount that passes into the mother's milk is, apparently, minimal. With flufenamic acid, it is a maximum of 0.2% (Buchanan 1969A). The importance of the active metabolites in diclofenac is unclear.

Ibuprofen has a half-life of only 2 hours. Following therapeutic administration of 800–1600 mg daily, it could not be detected in the mother's milk. The detection limit in both of the available studies was given as 1 or 0.5 mg/l. There have been no reports of any side effects on breastfed children (Townsend 1984, Weibert 1983), including in a prospective study covering 21 mother–child pairs (Ito 1993).

The half-life of *flurbiprofen* is 3 hours. After administration for 3 days postpartum, using 100–200 mg daily, it could only be detected at a maximum level of 0.08 mg/l in 3 milk samples during a study of 12 women. Thus, an infant receives 0.012 mg/kg per day or, at most, 0.5% of the maternal dosage per kg of bodyweight. No toxic effects have been described (Smith 1989, Cox 1987).

Indoprofen and *suprofen* can be similarly rated.

Following the ingestion of *indomethacin*, a seizure attack was observed in one breastfed infant (Eeg-Olofsson 1978). However, in a study of 16 mothers who received 75–300 mg daily for several days, only a maximum of 1% of the maternal weight-related dosage was calculated for the children. They showed no symptoms (Lebedevs 1991).

For *ketorolac*, a maximum of 0.3% of the maternal weight-related dosage is calculated for the infant (Wischnik 1989).

In the case of long-term therapy of a mother with *naproxen*, a maximum relative dosage of 3.6% was indicated for the infant (Jamali 1983). In another case of long-term therapy, a prolonged aggregation time for prothrombin and thrombocytes was found (Fidalgo 1989). Of 20 treated mothers, 10 reported slight sedation in their breastfed infants (Ito 1993).

With *piroxicam*, there is a transfer of about 8%. However, no substance could be detected in the serum of the clinically unremarkable infant (Østensen 1988). Half-lives of *naproxen* and *piroxicam* are 14 and up to 60 hours respectively – considerably longer than those in the antiphlogistics previously mentioned.

Mefenamic acid and *tenoxicam* pass into the milk at a maximum level of 0.8% of the relative dosage (Heintz 1993, Buchanan 1969B).

There is insufficient experience to evaluate the other nonsteroid antirheumatics, including *acemetacin, dexketoprofen, etofenamat, fenbufen, ketoprofen, lonazolac, lornoxicam, meloxicam, nabumetone, niflumic acid, nimesulide, proglumetacin, sulindac,* and *tiaprofen.*

Recommendation. Among the nonsteroid antirheumatics, the acidic antiphlogistics ibuprofen and flurbiprofen are the drugs of choice during breastfeeding. Occasional use of azapropazon, diclofenac, and flufenamic acid is also permissible. Accidental administration of one of the other nonsteroid antirheumatics does not require any limitation of breastfeeding, although the medication should be changed.

4.1.5   Selective cyclooxygenase-2 (COX-2) inhibitors

Experience

This group of drugs includes *celecoxib, etoricoxib, lumiracoxib, parecoxib, rofecoxib,* and *valdecoxib*. Their half-lives range from 8 to 17 hours.

Celecoxib is a lipophilic substance, of which 97% is bound to plasma protein, and it exhibits a high distribution volume. A peak concentration of 133 ng/ml was measured in the milk 5 hours after the administration of 100 mg, which corresponds to 20 µg/kg per day to a breastfed infant, or a weight-adjusted dose of approximately 1% (Knoppert 2003). A more recent publication studied oral administration of celecoxib 200 mg to six lactating volunteers. The median M/P ratio was 0.18 (0.15–0.26). The median infant dose was 0.23% (0.17–0.30%) of the maternal dose, adjusted for weight (Gardiner 2006).

After the application of 25 mg *rofecoxib*, an M/P ratio of 0.25 was determined. A relative dose of 1.8–3.2% was calculated (Gardiner 2005). Because cardiotoxic side effects were suspected, rofecoxib was withdrawn from the market. *Valdecoxib* was also withdrawn because of dermatological side effects. There is insufficient experience with the other COX-2-inhibitors during lactation.

> **Recommendation.** Because of the lack of experience with these substances during breastfeeding, selective COX-2 inhibitors should be avoided. Single doses do not require cessation of breastfeeding.

4.1.6   Pyrazolone- and phenylbutazone derivatives

Experience

There is very little experience of using these medications during breastfeeding. Taking its four main metabolites into consideration, an M/P ratio of about 1 was calculated for *metamizol*. In one case, very similar serum concentrations were found in both mother and child (Zylber-Katz 1986). Another report describes cyanotic attacks in an infant after his mother took metamizol (Rizzoni 1984).

Phenylbutazone has a half-life of 30–170 hours and an M/P ratio of 0.1–0.3. There have been no toxic effects reported, as yet, in breastfed infants. The American Academy of Pediatrics does not object to its occasional use during breastfeeding.

4   Lactation

4.1   Analgesics, antiphlogistics and anesthetics

A hemolytic anemia was described in an infant in connection with *propyphenazone* therapy in the mother (Frei 1985). Eight days after ending the therapy, phenazone could still be detected in the milk, but no longer in the plasma.

There are no data on *famprofazone, kebuzone, mofebutazone*, and *phenazone*.

> **Recommendation.** Famprofazone, kebuzone, metamizol, mofebutazone, phenazone, phenylbutazone, and propyphenazone should be avoided. Accidental intake does not require any limitations on breastfeeding, but the medication should be changed. Ibuprofen and paracetamol are the analgesics/antiphlogistics of choice.

4.1.7 Other antirheumatics

Experience

Gold derivatives such as *auranofin*, with a half-life of 70–80 days, and *sodium gold thiomalate*, with a half-life of 225–250 days, are detected in the mother's milk in large quantities, although a maximum M/P ratio of only 0.1 has been reported. With a monthly intramuscular injection of 10 mg, there were 15–30 μg/l in the milk. Assuming the highest levels, 4.5 μg of gold/kg daily or around 130 μg/kg per month is calculated for the exclusively breastfed baby. This is equivalent to the maternal, weight-related dosage! In the child's serum, 51 μg of gold per liter was found – which was about 10% of the maternal concentration (Bennett 1990).

Three other working groups have found comparable loads in the mother's milk, to some extent, but with higher maternal dosages and other gold derivatives. The calculated weight-related parts of the dosage for the infant were, however, markedly lower. There has, as yet, been no indication of toxic effects (survey in American Academy of Pediatrics 2001, Bennett 1996).

With a daily dosage of 400 mg *hydroxychloroquine* as a long-term therapy with steady-state conditions, a maximum of 1.5 mg/l of the drug was found in the milk of one mother. An exclusively breastfed baby could receive 4.3% of the weight-related dosage (Nation 1984). The half-life is 30–60 days.

There is no experience yet for the antirheumatic and immunosuppressant *leflunomide*, which has a half-life of 2 weeks.

Ademetionin, glucosamine, hyaluronic acid preparations, and *oxaceprol*, as well as *D-penicillamine*, are, to some extent, controversial because of their risk–benefit ratio. Passage into the mother's milk and tolerability during breastfeeding have not been studied sufficiently to assess risk. A case report describes two healthy babies who were breastfed for 3 months during maternal *penicillamine* therapy for Wilson's disease (Messner 1998).

For *glucocorticoids*, see Chapter 4.11.
For *methotrexate*, see Chapter 4.10.
For *sulfasalazine*, see Chapter 4.3.

4

Lactation

> **Recommendation.** Among the basic antirheumatics, sulfasalazine and glucocorticoids and, in some instances, hydroxychloroquine are acceptable during breastfeeding. The American Academy of Pediatrics considers taking gold preparations while breastfeeding to be acceptable. This should be looked at critically because of the above pharmacokinetic data. Single doses of the other medications do not require any limitation of breastfeeding.

4.1.8   Migraine medications

Experience

Ergotamine (tartrate) may be more likely than the less fat-soluble *dihydroergotamine* to cause symptoms of ergotism by passing into the milk. Milk production may decrease in the presence of ergotamine derivatives as a result of the antiprolactin action (see also section 3.7). This also applies to those ergotamines used for other indications – for example, *cabergoline, lisuride,* and *methysergide*. There are, as yet, no exact data on the passage of ergotamine alkaloids into the mother's milk.

Sumatriptan has an M/P ratio of about 5. Following subcutaneous injection of 6 mg (in five women studied), 3.5% of the weight-related dosage for an exclusively breastfed baby was calculated. Considering an oral bioavailability of only 14% and limited clearance in infancy, the weight-related dosage lies between 0.7 and 4.9% (Wojnar-Horton 1996). There is no information yet on any side effects of sumatriptan in the breastfed child, but due to its common short-term (single-dose) use, they would scarcely be expected.

There is insufficient experience with *almotriptan, cyclandelat, eletriptan, ethaverin, frovatriptan, iprazochrom, naratriptan, pizotifen, rizatriptan,* and *zolmitriptan*.

4.1 Analgesics, antiphlogistics and anesthetics

> **Recommendation.** If ibuprofen or paracetamol (in combination with codeine or caffeine) are not sufficiently effective even in the upper recommended dosage range, then combinations with acetylsalicylic acid or dihydroergotamine or sumatriptan or other "triptanes" can be tried. Antiemetics like dimenhydrinate, meclizine, and metoclopramide are also acceptable.

4.1.9   Local anesthetics

Experience

Lidocaine, even in intravenous treatment of cardiac arrhythmia, passes into the mother's milk only in limited amounts (see Chapter 4.6). In 27 patients who received epidural anesthesia for a cesarean section and had, on average 183 mg of lidocaine and 82 mg of *bupivacaine*, the drugs and their metabolites could be detected in the patient's serum and in the milk after 2, 6 and 12 hours. On average there were 860 µg/l of lidocaine in the milk and 90 µg/l of bupivacaine, as well as 140 µg/l of the metabolite PPX (Ortega 1999). The M/P quotients were 0.9, 0.4, and 1.3 respectively. The expected relative dosage for a breastfed baby is no more than 1% to, at maximum, 4% of the active ingredient, which has in any case a limited oral availability. The children observed were unremarkable. Comparable low weight-related dosages (73.4 µg/l lidocaine and 66.1 µg/l of its metabolite monoethylglycerinxylidide) were found after local lidocaine anesthesia (without adrenaline) during dental procedures (Giuliani 2001).

A continuous interpleural infusion of *bupivacaine* at a rate of 25 mg/h led to a maximum concentration in the mother's milk of 0.45 µg/ml. The substance was not detected in the infant's serum (detection limit <0.1 µg/ml). Toxic symptoms were not observed (survey by Spigset 1994).

There are no data on other local anesthetics. It may be assumed, however, that substances such as *articaine*, with a shorter half-life and higher plasma protein binding, will also reach only limited concentrations in the milk. The adrenaline addition that is common today acts as an inhibitor to the passage into the mother's milk in any case.

Prilocaine, to a greater extent than other local anesthesia, creates methemoglobin.

There are no data on anesthetics for topical use, like *benzocaine, chlorethane, oxybuprocaine*, and *tetracaine*. However, resorption and systemic availability is probably negligible.

> **Recommendation.** For normal use (dental treatment or minor surgery), local anesthesia may also be used during breastfeeding. This also applies to combinations with adrenaline. Prilocaine should be avoided, but if it is used accidentally there is no need to interrupt breastfeeding.

4.1.10   Other medications used in connection with anesthesia

Experience

With *methohexital*, 1–2 hours after administration of 120–150 mg, peak values of 470 ng/ml were measured in the milk of nine women. After 24 hours, there were no measurable concentrations (Borgatta 1997). A fully breastfed baby would receive about 1% of the maternal weight-adjusted dose.

Propofol, with a half-life of 30–60 minutes and an M/P ratio of about 1, appears only in limited amounts in colostrum when it is used preparatory to a cesarean section (Dailland 1989). Five lactating women underwent induction of anesthesia with propofol and fentanyl (Nitsun 2006). Plasma propofol pharmacokinetics were consistent with reports of others. In a 24-hour milk collection, averages of 0.027% (0.004–0.082%) of the propofol dose were collected in milk. Even assuming complete intestinal absorption by the infant, the percentage compared to placental transfer is apparently negligible. The available data indicate that an infant gets no more than 1% of the weight-related dosage with the milk.

Following a maternal intravenous injection of 5 mg/kg of *thiopental* (half-life about 10 hours and M/P ratio about 0.5), peak values of about 0.9 µg/ml milk were measured. According to this, an exclusively breastfed infant would get about 0.135 mg/kg, or about 2–3% of the intravenous, weight-related maternal dosage through the milk. Realistically, however, it is more likely to be less than 0.1% with the first feed following anesthesia. This has been indicated in studies on a total of 16 women. Because there is not continuous exposure, a toxic effect from thiopental is not to be expected, even considering the prolonged half-life in infancy (survey by Spigset 1994).

There are no systematic studies on tolerance during breastfeeding for other intravenous anesthetics, such as *etomidate, ketamine*, and *methohexital*, and the neuroleptic *droperidol*. However, no noteworthy symptoms have been reported to date when a mother breastfeeds after such anesthesia.

4

Lactation

4.1 Analgesics, antiphlogistics and anesthetics

Halothane in the milk of a breastfeeding anesthetist was found in the same concentration as in the air of the operating theatre where she worked (2 ppm). However, there were no toxic symptoms described via breast milk, either as a result of occupational exposure or as a result of receiving inhalation anesthesia (Coté 1976). Also, with respect to other inhalation anesthetics such as *desflurane*, *enflurane* and *isoflurane*, no undesirable effects on the infant have been reported (Lee 1993).

Muscle relaxants of the *curare* type are quaternary ammonia combinations which can scarcely pass into the milk because of their limited lipophilia, and they are, practically speaking, not absorbed intestinally. It has long been known that the consumption of game that has been killed with curare arrows does not cause any toxic symptoms.

For information on *midazolam* and the other benzodiazepines, see Chapter 4.9.

> **Recommendation.** As soon as the mother is able to put her child to breast again after anesthesia, she may breastfeed. Neither the pharmacokinetic qualities connected to drugs used today for anesthesia nor clinical experience is a reason for an additional interruption of breastfeeding. This also applies to anesthesia for a cesarean delivery – for which, in any case, the portion of the anesthetic which passes to the infant transplacentally is more significant than that which goes through the small amount of colostrum!

4.1.11   Myotonolytics

Experience

Among the myotonolytics, in the broadest sense, there are very different agents, such as *baclofen, carisoprodol, quinine ethyl carbonate, chlormezanone, clostridium botulinum toxin, dantrolene, fenyramidol, mephenesin, methocarbamol, orphenadrine, pridinol, tetrazepam, tizanidine*, and *tolperisone.* For antiepileptics used for the treatment of neuropathic pain, see Chapter 4.8.

There is one case report on *baclofen* in which a maximum of 0.13 mg/l was measured in the mother's milk following a single dose of 20 mg (Erikssons 1981). In one breastfeed, this would be 1.2% of the weight-related dosage for the child.

At steady-state conditions in one woman using *carisoprodol* 2100 mg/d, on average 0.9 mg/l was found in her milk plus 11.6 mg/l of the active metabolite *meprobamate*. The relative dose would be 4%. The child was unremarkable, but was only partly breastfed

(Nordeng 2001). No general conclusions for tolerance could be drawn from this.

There is also insufficient experience on the use of the other drugs while breastfeeding – some of them are therapeutically out of date, and a mild sedation of the breastfed child is conceivable.

> **Recommendation.** Apart from emergency treatment with dantrolene for malignant hyperthermia, the indications for using a myotonolytic should be considered very critically. Physiotherapeutic measures and antiphlogistics/ antirheumatics are preferable. In individual cases, the relaxant effect of low doses of the better-studied diazepam should be used in the short term.

4

Lactation

4.1.12   Gout therapy

Experience

Allopurinol reduces the uric acid concentration in the blood by inhibiting the enzyme *xanthin oxidase*. One report describes an unremarkable infant whose mother took 300 mg of allopurinol daily. The active metabolite, *oxypurinol*, could be detected in the milk at about 50 mg/l; in the child's serum it was 7 mg/l. The therapeutically effective serum concentration is 13–19 mg/l. The daily dosage that the infant received – just about 8 mg of oxypurinol/kg – just reaches the lower therapeutic dose level (Kamilli 1991). There is no experience with *benzbromaron*.

The uricosuric *probenecid* is an interval medication that promotes the excretion of uric acid by inhibiting renal reabsorption. In a case report where milk was collected over a dose interval at steady-state, the average concentration of probenecid in milk was 964 µg/l, corresponding to absolute and relative infant doses of 145 µg/kg per day and 0.7% (Illett 2006). The breastfed infant developed severe diarrhea, which was ascribed to the concomitant maternal cephalexin treatment for breast infection. Due to the low relative dose and the mechanism by which probenecid works, no disturbing effect on a breastfed child should be expected.

Medications for treating gout attacks include (in addition to non-steroid antiphlogistics such as ibuprofen) *phenylbutazone* and the mitosis inhibitor *colchicine*.

With long-term therapy of 1 mg colchicine daily in four women with *Familial Mediterranean Fever* (FMF), a maximum of 8.6 ng/ml was measured in the milk (M/P ratio of about 1). Six hours after intake, between 0.9 and 2.6 ng/ml of milk was detected. Assuming the maximum value mentioned, close to 10% of the maternal weight-related dosage would be calculated for the infant. These four infants and other exposed infants followed by the author for 2 years developed unremarkably (Ben-Chetrit 1996).

Phenylbutazone, which has a strong antiphlogistic effect and a weak analgesic and antipyretic effect, is distinguished by an immune toxic effect on hemopoiesis, fluid retention, and a long half-life of 30–170 hours.

> **Recommendation.** Probenecid is the drug of choice for interval treatment of gout during breastfeeding. Allopurinol should be avoided whenever possible. Ibuprofen is the drug of choice with gout attacks. Phenylbutazone and colchicine should not be taken. However, individual doses are not grounds for limiting breastfeeding. Whether women on a maintenance therapy with colchicine for FMF should breastfeed has to be decided upon individually.

References

American Academy of Pediatrics, Committee on Drugs. The transfer of drugs and other chemicals into human milk. Pediatrics 2001; 108: 776–89.

Baka NE, Bayoumeu F, Boutroy MJ et al. Colostrum morphin concentrations during postcesarean intravenous patient-controlled analgesia. Anesth Analg 2002; 94: 184–7.

Bald R, Bernbeck-Betthäuser E-M, Spahn H et al. Excretion of azapropazone in human breast milk. Eur J Clin Pharmacol 1990; 39: 271–3.

Bar-Oz B, Bulkowstein M, Benyamini L et al. Use of antibiotic and analgesic drugs during lactation. Drug Saf 2003; 26: 925–35.

Ben-Chetrit E, Scherrmann J-M, Levy M. Colchicine in breast milk of patients with familial mediterranean fever. Arthritis Rheum 1996; 39: 1213–17.

Bennett PN, Humphries SJ, Osborne JP et al. Use of aurothiomalate during lactation. Br J Clin Pharmacol 1990; 29: 777–9.

Bennett PN (ed.). Drugs and Human Lactation, 2nd edn. Amsterdam: Elsevier, 1996.

Borgatta L, Jenny RW, Gruss L et al. Clinical significance of methohexital, meperidine, and diazepam in breast milk. J Clin Pharmacol 1997; 37: 186–92.

Buchanan RA (A), Eaton CJ, Koeff ST et al. The breast milk excretion of flufenamic acid. Curr Ther Res 1969; 11: 533–8.

Buchanan RA (B), Eaton CJ, Koeff ST et al. The breast milk excretion of mefenamic acid. Curr Ther Res 1969; 10: 592–7.

Clark JH, Wilson WG. A 16-day old breast-fed infant with metabolic acidosis caused by salicylates. Clin Pediatr 1981; 20: 53–4.

Coté CJ, Kenepp NB, Reed SB et al. Trace concentrations of halothane in human breast milk. Br J Anaesth 1976; 48: 541–3.

Cox SR, Forbes BA. Excretion of flurbiprofen into breast milk. Pharmacotherapy 1987; 7: 211–15.

Cuypers L, Wiebalck A, Vertommen JD et al. Epidural sufentanil for post caesarean pain: breast milk level and effects on the baby. Acta Anaesth Belg 1995; 46: 104–5.

Dailland P, Cockshott ID, Lirzin JD et al. Intravenous propofol during caesarean section: placental transfer, concentrations in breast milk and neonatal effects. A preliminary study. Anesthesiology 1989; 71: 827–34.

Eeg-Olofsson O, Malmros I, Elwin CE et al. Convulsions in a breast-fed infant after maternal indomethacin. Lancet 1978; ii: 215.

Erikssons G, Swahn CF. Concentrations of baclofen in serum and breast milk from a lactating woman. Scand J Clin Lab Invest 1981; 41: 185–7.

Feilberg VL, Rosenborg D, Broen Christensen C et al. Excretion of morphine in human breast milk. Acta Anaesthesiol Scand 1989; 33: 426–8.

Fidalgo I, Correa R, Gomez Carrasco JA et al. Anemia aguda, rectorragia y hematuria asociadas a la ingestion de naproxén. An Esp Pediat 1989; 30: 317–19.

Frei H, Bühlmann U, Rudin O. Toxic hemolytic anemia in the newborn infant following ingestion of a phenazone derivative (Cibalgin) via breast milk {in German}. Z Geburtsh Perinatol 1985; 189: 11–12.

Gardiner SJ, Begg EJ, Zhang M et al. Transfer of rofecoxib into human milk. Eur J Clin Pharmacol 2005; 61: 405–8.

Gardiner SJ, Doogue MP, Zhang M et al. Quantification of infant exposure to celecoxib through breast milk. Br J Clin Pharmacol 2006; 61: 101–4.

Giesecke AH, Rice LJ, Lipton JM. Alfentanil in colostrum. Anesthesiology 1985; 63: A284.

Giuliani M, Grossi GB, Pileri M et al. Could local anesthesia while breast-feeding be harmful to infants? Paedr Gastroenterol Nutr 2001; 32: 142–4.

Grimm D, Pauly E, Poschl J et al. Buprenorphine and norbuprenorphine concentrations in human breast milk samples determined by liquid chromatography-tandem mass spectrometry. Ther Drug Monit 2005; 27: 526–30.

Heintz RC, Stebler T, Lunell NO et al. Excretion of tenoxicam and 5'-hydroxy-tenoxicam into human milk. J Pharmacol Med 1993; 3: 57–64.

Hirose M, Hosokawa T, Tanaka Y. Extradural buprenorphine suppresses breastfeeding after caesarean section. Br J Anaesth 1997; 79: 120–21.

Hurwitz ES, Barrett MJ, Bregmann D et al. Public Health Service study on Reye's syndrome and medications. N Engl J Med 1985; 313: 849–57.

Ilett KF, Hackett LP, Ingle B et al. Transfer of probenecid and cephalexin into breast milk. Ann Pharmacother 2006; 40: 986–9.

Ito S, Blajchman A, Stephenson M et al. Prospective follow-up of adverse reactions in breast-fed infants exposed to maternal medication. Am J Obstet Gynaecol 1993; 168: 1393–9.

Jacobson B, Nyberg K, Grönbladh L et al. Opiate addiction in adult offspring through possible imprinting after obstetric treatment. Br Med J 1990; 301: 1067–70.

Jamali F, Keshavarz E. Salicylate in breast milk. Intl J Pharmacol 1981; 8: 285–90.

Jamali F, Stevens RD. Naproxen in milk. Drug Intell Clin Pharmacol 1983; 17: 910–11.

Kamilli I, Gresser U, Schaefer C et al. Allopurinol in breast milk. Adv Experim Med Biol 1991; 309A: 143–5.

Kmetec V, Roskar R. HPLC determination of tramadol in human breast milk. J Pharm Biomed Anal 2003; 32: 1061–6.

Knoppert DC, Stempak D, Baruchel S et al. Celecoxib in human milk: a case report. Pharmacother 2003; 23: 97–100.

Kunka RL, Venkataramanan R, Stern RM et al. Excretion of propoxyphene and norpropoxyphene in breast milk. Clin Pharmacol Ther 1984; 35: 675–80.

Lebedevs TH, Wojnar-Horton RE, Yapp P et al. Excretion of indomethacin in breast milk. Br J Clin Pharmacol 1991; 32: 751–4.

4

Lactation

4.1 Analgesics, antiphlogistics and anesthetics

Lee JJ, Rubin AP. Breast-feeding and anaesthesia. Anaesthesia 1993; 48: 616–25.

Leuschen MP, Wolf LJ, Rayburn WF. Fentanyl excretion in breast milk. Clin Pharmacol 1990; 9: 336–7.

Madej TH, Strunin L. Comparison of epidural fentanyl with sufentanil. Analgesia and side effects after a single bolus dose during elective caesarean section. Anesthesia 1987; 42: 1556–61.

Messner U, Günter HH, Niesert S. Wilson disease and pregnancy. Review of the literature and case report {in German}. Z Geburtsh Neonatol 1998; 202: 77–9.

Nation RL, Hackett LP, Dusci LJ et al. Excretion of hydroxychloroquine in human milk. Br J Clin Pharmacol 1984; 17: 368–9.

Nitsun M, Szokol JW, Saleh HJ et al. Pharmacokinetics of midazolam, propofol, and fentanyl transfer to human breast milk. Clin Pharmacol Ther 2006; 79: 549–57.

Nordeng H, Zahlsen K, Spigset O. Transfer of carisoprodol to breast milk. Ther Drug Monitor 2001; 23: 298–300.

Notarianni LJ, Oldham HG, Bennett PN. Passage of paracetamol into breast milk and its subsequent metabolism by the neonate. Br J Clin Pharmacol 1987; 24: 63–7.

Ortega D, Viviand X, Lorec AM et al. Excretion of lidocaine and bupivacaine in breast milk following epidural anesthesia for cesarean delivery. Acta Anesthesiol Scand 1999; 43: 394–7.

Østensen M, Matheson I, Laufen H. Piroxicam in breast milk after long-term therapy Eur J Clin Pharmacol 1988; 35: 567–9.

Peiker G, Müller B, Ihn W et al. Excretion of pethidine in mother's milk {authors translation}. Zentralbl Gynäkol 1980; 102: 537–41.

Rizzoni G, Furlanut M. Cyanotic crises in a breastfed infant from mother taking dipyrone. Hum Toxicol 1984; 3: 505–7.

Robieux I, Koren G, Vandenbergh H et al. Morphine excretion in breast milk and resultant exposure of a nursing infant. J Toxicol Clin Toxicol 1990; 28: 365–70.

Smith IJ, Hinson JL, Johnson VA et al. Flurbiprofen in post-partum women: plasma and breast milk disposition. J Clin Pharmacol 1989; 29: 174–84.

Spigset O. Anaesthetic agents and excretion in breast milk. Acta Anaesthesiol Scand 1994; 38: 94–103.

Steer PL, Biddle CJ, Marley WS et al. Concentration of fentanyl in colostrum after an analgesic dose. Can J Anaesth 1992; 39: 231–5.

Townsend RJ, Benedetti TJ, Erickson SH et al. Excretion of ibuprofen into breast milk. Am J Obstet Gynecol 1984; 149: 184–6.

Unsworth J, d'Assis-Fonseca A, Beswick DT et al. Serum salicylate levels in a breast fed infant. Ann Rheumat Dis 1987; 46: 638–9.

Weibert RT, Townsend RJ, Kaiser DG et al. Lack of ibuprofen secretion into human milk. Clin Pharmacol 1983; 1: 457–8.

Wischnik A, Wetzelsberger N, Lücker PW. Elimination of nalbuphine in human milk {in German}. Arzneimittelforschung 1988; 38: 1496–8.

Wischnik A, Manth SM, Lloyd J et al. The excretion of ketorolac tromethamine into breast milk after multiple oral dosing. Eur J Clin Pharmacol 1989; 36: 521–4.

Wittels B, Scott DT, Sinatra RS. Exogenous opioids in human breast milk and acute neonatal neurobehaviour: a preliminary study. Anesthesiology 1990; 73: 864–9.

Wojnar-Horton RE, Hackett LP, Yapp P et al. Distribution and excretion of sumatriptan in human milk. Br J Clin Pharmacol 1996; 41: 217–21.

Zylber-Katz E, Linder N, Granit L et al. Excretion of dipyrone metabolites in human breast milk. Eur J Clin Pharmacol 1986; 30: 359–61.

Antiallergics, antiasthmatics, and antitussives

4.2

Christof Schaefer

4.2.1 Antihistamines (H$_1$-blockers)

Experience

Antihistamines are used to treat allergic illnesses, and as antiemetics (see Chapter 4.3). Rarely, mild restlessness, sedation or weak sucking – none of them needing treatment – are described in the breastfed baby (see, for example, Moretti 1995).

Loratadine and *cetirizine* are the most used new-generation H$_1$-blockers, which have practically no sedative effect, and do not cross the blood–brain barrier. The other (older) antihistamines discussed below are more or less sedative.

The plasma half-life of *astemizole* is 26 hours, and that of the metabolites up to 9 days. Passage into the milk has, as yet, only been studied in dogs. There was shown to be an accumulation of the substance when very high doses were administered (information from the manufacturer).

In connection with the use of *brompheniramine* plus *d-isoephedrine* during breastfeeding, a hyperexcitable infant was described (Mortimer 1977).

There are no published data on the passage of *cetirizine* into mother's milk, but the experience to date indicates no noteworthy symptoms during breastfeeding. The half-life of 9 hours is quite short and the medication has scarcely any sedative or atropine-like action

Stiff neck, hyperexcitability, and sleepiness were observed in the infant of a mother being treated with *clemastine*, and 5–10 μg of the substance per liter was detected in the milk. No clemastine was found in the infant's serum (Kok 1982).

There are, as yet, no data available on *dimetindene* during breast-feeding. This common H$_1$-blocker has a short half-life of 5–7 hours and there are recommended doses for children beginning at 1 year Dimetindene has relatively little sedative action, but has an atropine like effect that should not be overlooked.

Diphenhydramine was recommended by the American Academy of Pediatrics for the breastfeeding period. However, because of the strong sedative effect, its use as an antiallergic can no longer be justified. This also applies to *doxylamine*.

There is no information on *levocabastine* during breastfeeding However, local application of this drug is not expected to be of any risk.

Following a single dose of 40 mg of *loratadine*, a transfer to the infant of about 1% of the effective substance (including metabolites) was calculated, compared to the maternal weight-related dosage (Hilbert 1988). There were no symptoms observed among the breast-fed infants of 51 women treated with loratadine (Merlob 2002).

There are no data on *oxatomide* during breastfeeding. However treatment of 4-month-old infants with this drug was well tolerated (Boccazzi 2001).

With *pseudoephedrine*, a maximum relative dosage of 15% can be calculated (Findlay 1984).

Terfenadine, with an M/P ratio of 0.2, has a half-life of 20 hours A study of four breastfeeding women indicated less than 0.5% of the weight-related dosage goes to the infant. Only the active metabolites, but not the maternal substance, were detectable in the milk (Lucas 1995).

Following a single dosage of 2.5 mg *triprolidine*, with a plasma half-life of 4 hours and effectiveness for up to 12 hours, the dosage taken in by the infant was 0.36 μg/kg per day (Findlay 1984). That is less than 0.1% of the daily therapeutic dosage for infants (3 mg/d) given by Reynolds (1989). No toxic symptoms were observed. This substance is only available in combination with pseudoephedrine (see above).

There is no detailed knowledge about the effects on breastfeeding for the following substances: *alimemazine, azelastine, bamipin, carbinoxamine, chlorpheniramine, chlorphenoxamine, cyprohepta-dine, desloratadine, dexchlorpheniramine, ebastine, epinastin, fex-ofenadine, hydroxyzine, ketotifen, levocetirizine, mebhydroline, mequitazin, mizolastine, olopatadine, oxatomide, pheniramine,* and *tritoqualin*.

> **Recommendation.** The antiallergics of choice during breastfeeding are dimentindene, loratadine, cetirizine, and triprolidine. Symptoms such as rest-lessness or mild sedation cannot be ruled out with any of these medications when therapy is long term. However, this is no reason to neglect necessary therapy or to wean the child. If symptoms appear, there should be a change to another preparation. *Desensitization therapy* is acceptable during breast-feeding.

4.2.2   β₂-sympathomimetics for asthma treatment

Experience

The β₂-sympathomimetics *fenoterol, pirbuterol, reproterol, salbuta-mol,* and *terbutaline* are well-tolerated inhalable broncholytics with a plasma half-life of 3 hours.

Only for *terbutaline* are there data available regarding passage into the mother's milk: $3.5\,\mu g/l$ of milk were measured with oral medication of 2.5 or 5 mg, three times a day. The M/P ratio was between 1 and 2. The infant's intake was a maximum of $0.7\,\mu g/kg$ per day, which was about 0.7% of the maternal dosage per kg body-weight. No toxic effects were observed (Boreus 1982, Lönnerholm 1982). With inhalation, the passage is less than with oral treatment. Excessive overdosing, however, can lead to restlessness and tachy-cardia in the infant.

The new medications *formoterol* and *salmeterol*, which are effec-tive for longer than the other drugs, have not been systematically studied for their tolerability during breastfeeding. This also applies to *clenbuterol* and *tulobuterol*.

> **Recommendation.** Salbutamol and terbutaline are the drugs of choice among the fast-acting inhaled β₂-sympathomimetics. If a long-acting β₂-sympathomimetic is indicated, formoterol or salmeterol can be used. Oral

4

Lactation

4.2 Antiallergics, antiasthmatics, and antitussives

treatment with β_2-sympathomimetics is not part of standard asthma treatment (see Chapter 2.3), and should also not take place during breastfeeding. Nevertheless, neither individual oral doses of these medication nor the administration of the other active ingredients mentioned above justify any limitation on breastfeeding; however, therapy should be changed.

4.2.3   Other sympathomimetics

Experience

The non-selective β-sympathomimetics *isoprenaline, hexoprenaline*, and *orciprenaline* are reserved for exceptional circumstances and do not belong to asthma therapy. However, even if these were used, restlessness and tachycardia, at the worst, could be expected to be observed in the breastfed child.

Recommendation. Individual doses of isoprenaline, hexoprenaline, and orciprenaline do not require weaning; however, the therapy should be changed.

4.2.4   Anticholinergics for asthma treatment

Experience

The anticholinergic effect of *ipratropium bromide* and *oxitropium bromide* also causes bronchodilatation and can lead to a considerable reduction in the necessary β-sympathomimetic dosage. Documented experience on its use during breastfeeding is limited. However, good tolerance can be assumed with the well-tried ipratropium bromide.

Recommendation. Ipratropium bromide is acceptable for treating asthma while breastfeeding, and should be used in preference to oxitropium bromide.

4.2.5   Theophylline

Experience

Theophylline preparations are well tolerated during breastfeeding in moderate dosages and in the time-released form used so commonly oday. Increased restlessness in the infant can occur after the dministration of higher doses, especially when given by injection r rectally. Larger amounts of caffeine-containing drinks should be voided during therapy.

After administration of 300 mg of theophylline, maximum concentrations of 6 mg/l of milk were measured and an M/P ratio of .7 calculated. At most, 0.9 mg/kg daily passes to the infant. With ong-term therapy using 800 mg daily, 10% of the weight-related hild dosage could pass to the infant (survey in Bennett 1996). Due o the extended plasma half-life of 15–40 hours in the infant, an ccumulation in young babies is possible. Viewed realistically, lasma concentrations are not likely to exceed 4 mg/l. Even for the ewborn this does not indicate any risk, since theophylline used for pnea prophylaxis in premature infants is well-tolerated. Here, lasma concentrations of 6–13 mg/l are the goal.

After a one-time dosage of 5 mg/kg of *diprophylline*, a peak value f 14 mg/l was measured in the milk of 20 women and an M/P ratio f 2 was found. This is about 40% of the maternal weight-related osage. The authors calculate that the infant's serum level, at 4.6 mg/l, an reach almost 70% of the maternal values (survey in Bennett 996).

Recommendation. Theophylline can be used during breastfeeding. Diprophylline should be avoided.

.2.6 Cromoglycic acid and nedocromil

xperience

With *cromoglycic acid*, less than 10% of the inhaled substance is bsorbed; enterally, it is under 1%. The plasma half-life is about 0 minutes. Transfer into the mother's milk is practically out of the uestion. There is no published experience on *nedocromil*.

Recommendation. Cromoglycic acid can be used, and is preferable to nedocromil.

.2.7 Corticoids

ee Chapter 4.11.

4.2.8   Leukotrien-receptor antagonists

Experience

The leukotrien-receptor antagonists montelukast and *zafirlukast* as well as the lipoxygenase inhibitor *zileuton*, are intended to be used as supplementary treatment to prevent asthmatic complaints. There is insufficient experience with their use during breastfeeding.

> **Recommendation.** When conventional measures in asthma therapy do not work sufficiently, montelukast can be tried. There should be close observation of the breastfed infant.

4.2.9   Acetylcysteine and other mucolytics

Experience

Acetylcysteine, ambroxol, and *bromhexine* are widely used and well-tolerated during breastfeeding. There are no details available on their kinetics.

Carbocisteine, guaiacol, guaifenesin, mesna, and preparations with essential oils such as *cineol, myrtle, lime,* and *eucalyptus* are probably also well-tolerated during breastfeeding, but here too there are no systematic studies to date. Essential oils can change the taste of the milk and lead to feeding problems.

Iodine from *potassium iodate* accumulates to a great extent in the milk, and can in this way block the infant's thyroid (see Chapter 4.11).

> **Recommendation.** Acetylcysteine, ambroxol, and bromhexine are the mucolytics of choice during breastfeeding when non-drug procedures such as abundant fluid and inhalation are not really effective. Carbocisteine, guaiacol, guaifenesin, and mesna should be avoided.
>
> Potassium iodate as an expectorant is absolutely contraindicated during breastfeeding.

4.2.10   Antitussives

Experience

Codeine has a half-life of 3–4 hours; less than 25% is bound to the plasma protein, and the M/P ratio is 2. Bradycardia was observed in a 1-week-old infant after a single maternal dose of 30 mg codeine (Smith 1982). In another case, following a 60-mg single maternal dose, a maximum of 455 µg/l in milk was measured (Findlay 1981). Mathematically, for the infant this means a maximum of 7% of the weight-related maternal dosage. Here, and also in other studies, breastfed infants showed no symptoms when the daily maternal dosage remained under 240 mg, as recommended by some authors (Meny 1993). As an antitussive, and for sporadic analgesic use, this amount is not reached by any means. Recently, fatal consequences were reported in a newborn whose mother was prescribed 60 mg codeine twice daily, with 1000 mg paracetamol, for episiotomy pain following birth. She reduced the dosage by half from day 2 because she experienced somnolence and constipation. The full-term healthy male infant showed intermittent periods of difficulty with breastfeeding and lethargy starting on day 7. On day 12, he had gray skin and his milk intake had fallen. He was found dead on day 13. The postmortem blood concentration of morphine (the active metabolite of codeine) was 70 ng/ml, while a milk sample from day 10 showed 87 ng/ml. A familial polymorphism of the enzyme CYP2D6 was diagnosed, resulting in extensive or even ultra-rapid metabolization of codeine to morphine in the child and his mother, respectively (Koren 2006).

In the case of a codeine-dependent mother (300 mg daily), 1 mg/l of codeine was found in the urine of her neurologically remarkable infant. In the case of a heroin-dependent mother who took 625 mg of codeine daily as replacement, 1.5 mg dihydrocodeine/l was measured in the serum of her cyanotic and apneic child (author's observations).

There are no case reports on the use of *dextromethorphan* during breastfeeding. The substance is a d-isomer of the codeine analog *levorphanol*. It has no analgesic properties. Sedative action and the potential for dependency are said to be lower than with codeine.

The administration of 150 mg of *noscapin* led to a concentration of a maximum of 83 µg/l of milk (Olsson 1986). This represents 12.5 µg/kg daily for the infant, which is 0.5% of the maternal weight-related dosage. Following experimental results, mutagenic properties were attributed to noscapin.

In connection with *pentoxyverin*, a child with apnea episodes lasting up to 15 seconds was described (Stier 1998). The mother had taken 90 mg daily. The levels measured in the infant's serum were said to be higher than those in the maternal serum. The M/P ratio was given as 10; the half-life for the child was 5 days. Mathematically, 660 ml of mother's milk (the daily quantity) had only 93 µg pentoxyverin. Apnea, sometimes accompanied by cyanosis, had already been observed earlier in young infants when pentoxyverin had been administered therapeutically (Mühlendahl 1996).

There is no experience with *benproperine, clobutinol, dropropizine, eprazinone, isoaminil, menadiol,* and *pipacetate* in breast milk in lactating women.

> **Recommendation.** A cough suppressant should only be considered in the case of ongoing unproductive and severe coughing. Before considering this, inhalation therapy, abundant fluid, and the administration of expectorants should be tried.
> Single doses of dextromethorphan and codeine are allowed during breastfeeding. Repeated dosages require close observation for somnolence. Pentoxyverin is contraindicated. Benproperine, clobutinol, dropropizine, eprazinone, isoaminil, menadiol, noscapin, and pipacetate should not be used. However, the accidental administration of single doses of these medications requires only a change of therapy and no limitation on breastfeeding.

References

Bennett PN (ed.). Drugs and Human Lactation, 2nd edn. Amsterdam: Elsevier, 1996.

Boccazzi A, Pugni L, Cesuti R et al. Oxatomide in the treatment of atopic dermatitis in breast-fed and very young infants. Minerva Pediatr 2001; 53: 265–9.

Boréus LO, de Château P, Lindberg C et al. Terbutaline in breast milk. Br J Clin Pharmacol 1982; 13: 731–2.

Findlay JWA, de Angelis RL, Kearney MF et al. Analgesic drugs in breast milk and plasma. Clin Pharmacol 1981; 29: 625–33.

Findlay JWA, Butz RF, Sailstad JM et al. Pseudoephedrine and triprolidine in plasma and breast milk of nursing mothers. Br J Clin Pharmacol 1984; 18: 901–6.

Hilbert J, Radwanski E, Affrime MB et al. Excretion of loratadine in human breast milk. J Clin Pharmacol 1988; 28: 234–9.

Kok THHG, Taitz LS, Bennett MJ et al. Drowsiness due to clemastine transmitted in breast milk. Lancet 1982; 1: 914–15.

Koren G, Cairns J, Chitayat D et al. Pharmacogenetics of morphine poisoning in a breastfed neonate of a codeine-prescribed mother. Lancet 2006; 368: 704.

Lönnerholm G, Lindström B. Terbutaline excretion into breast milk. Br J Clin Pharmacol 1982; 13: 729–30.

Lucas BD, Purdy CY, Scarim SK et al. Terfenadine pharmacokinetics in breast milk in lactating women. Clin Pharmacol Ther 1995; 57: 398–402.

Meny RG, Naumburg EG, Alger LS et al. Codeine and the breastfed neonate. J Hum Lact 1993; 9: 237–40.

Merlob P. Prospective follow-up of adverse reactions in breast-fed infants exposed to maternal loratadine treatment (1999–2001). BELTIS-Newsletter 2002; 10: 43–51.

Moretti ME, Liau-Chu M, Taddio A et al. Adverse events in breastfed infants exposed to anti-histamines in maternal milk. Reprod Toxicol 1995; 9: 588.

Mortimer EA Jr. Drug toxicity from breast milk? Pediatrics 1977; 60: 780–81.

Mühlendahl KE, Oberdisse U, Bunjes R et al. Vergiftungen im Kindesalter, 2nd edn. Stuttgart: Enke, 1996.

Olsson B, Bolme P, Dahlström B et al. Excretion of noscapine in human breast milk. Eur J Clin Pharmacol 1986; 30: 213–15.

Reynolds EF. Martindale. The Extra Pharmacopoeia. London: The Pharmaceutical Press, 1989.

Smith JW. Codeine-induced bradycardia in a breastfed infant. Clinical Res 1982; 30: 2.

Stier BJ, Sieverding L, Moeller H. Pentoxyverine poisoning via maternal milk in a fully breast-fed newborn infant {in German}. Dtsch Med Wschr 1988; 113: 898–900.

4

Lactation

4.2 Antiallergics, antiasthmatics, and antitussives

Gastrointestinal drugs

4.3

Christof Schaefer

4.3.1   Antacids

Experience

Classic antacids, such as *aluminum hydroxide, aluminum phosphate, calcium carbonate*, and *magnesium carbonate*, are only absorbed to a limited extent. No toxic effects from aluminum, for instance, have as yet been described, nor would they be expected. However, since the chronic intake of small amounts of aluminum is considered problematic, *magaldrate, algeldrate, almasilate, hydrotalcite*, and *sucralfate*, from which only traces of aluminum (at most) are believed to be absorbed, or the aluminum-free preparations of calcium carbonate plus magnesium carbonate or hydroxide, are of more interest therapeutically.

Recommendation. Antacids and ulcer therapeutics of choice during breastfeeding are the newer aluminum combinations, such as magaldrate and sucralfate as well as aluminum-free antacids. Older aluminum and magnesium combinations are also acceptable. When higher doses are taken over a longer period of time, or in patients with impaired kidney function, it is generally recommended that the serum concentration of aluminum or magnesium be monitored.

4.3.2   H$_2$-receptor blockers and other ulcer therapeutics

4

Lactation

Experience

Among the ulcer medications of the H$_2$-receptor blocker type are *cimetidine, famotidine, nizatidine, ranitidine*, and *roxatidine*.

Cimetidine and *ranitidine* reach relatively high concentrations in mother's milk. According to a study on 12 women who received single doses of 100, 600 or 1200 mg, *cimetidine* was actively transported into the milk with an M/P ratio of about 5. The infant received, on average, 6.7% of the maternal weight-related dosage, although the maximum was 20% (Oo 1995).

With maternal therapy of 150–300 mg of *ranitidine* daily, a relative dosage of up to 20% can reach the infant. The M/P ratio varies between 1 and over 20 (survey in Bennett 1996, Kearns 1985).

According to a study of eight mothers receiving a single dose of 40 mg *famotidine*, the relative dosage in the milk was under 2% (Courtney 1988).

With *nizatidine* therapy, a maximum of 5% of the maternal weight-related dosage can be assumed (Obermeyer 1990). This was reported in five mothers who received 150 mg every 12 hours. Among 10 women studied following a single dose of 150 mg of *roxatidine*, this was on average 4%. However, a higher amount might reach the infant when therapy is ongoing (Bender 1989).

A case report on *omeprazole* calculated a weight-adjusted dosage for a fully breastfed infant of less than 7% (Marshall 1998). Another case report of *pantoprazole* (40 mg) found a weight-adjusted dosage of <1% (Plante 2004). There were no symptoms observed in the breastfed infants.

There is insufficient documented experience with the proton-pump inhibitors *esomeprazole, lansoprazole*, and *rabeprazole*. This also applies to the so-called M$_1$-receptor blocker *pirenzepine*, the gastrin receptor antagonist *proglumide*, as well as the bismuth combinations *bismuth nitrate, bismuth salicylate, dibismuth-tris*, and *bismuth (III)-citrate hydroxide complex*. For the prostaglandin derivative, see Chapter 4.11.13.

4.3 Gastrointestinal drugs

> **Recommendation.** H_2-blockers may be given during lactation. Those with low concentration in breast milk should be preferred – for example, famotidine or nizatidine. If proton-pump blockers are indicated, omeprazole or pantoprazole should be chosen. Single doses of other medications do not require any limitation of breastfeeding, but a change in therapy is desirable.
> For the eradication of *Helicobacter pylori*, see the appropriate substances and Chapter 2.5.

4.3.3   Peristaltic stimulators

Experience

The antiemetic *metoclopramide* eases the emptying of the stomach and increases the milk production via its central antidopaminergic action. It may be used for a few days at a dosage of 3×10 mg per day to promote milk production (see also section 3.7). The young infant whose mother takes 3×10 mg daily over many weeks receives a maximum of 4.7% of a weight-related child's dosage. Only in one case among more than 20 mother–child pairs could the substance be measured in the infant's plasma (Kauppila 1983). No symptoms or disturbances of pituitary regulation were observed in breastfed children (Kauppila 1985).

Hansen (2005), in a randomized double-blind study, investigated more than 60 mothers of preterm newborns, who received either metoclopramid or placebo. There were no significant differences with respect to the amount of milk and duration of lactation period. Other reports observed its successful use in, for example, the context of lactation stimulation in a woman with agenesis of the uterus. Although her pregnancy was carried by another woman, she wanted to breastfeed her child. Therefore, she started with 3×10 mg metoclopramide from week 28 until delivery (of the host-mother), and stimulated the nipples with an electric milk pump. The effect of this method was confirmed by serum prolactin and estradiol measures. She was ultimately able to breastfeed her child until 3 months of age; however formula was used as a supplement because of insufficient milk production (Biervliet 2001).

Cisapride and *domperidon* also have a stimulating effect on peristalsis. Both appear only in limited amounts in the milk. In a study of 10 women using cisapride, about 0.1% of a weight-related infant dosage was calculated via the mother's milk (Hofmeyr 1986); with domperidone it was, on average, 0.4% of the maternal weight-related dosage (Hofmeyr 1985). A double-blind study of mothers of preterm babies, 7 on domperidone and 9 on placebo, found an average increase of daily milk production of almost 50 ml (da Silva 2001). A high molecular mass of about 426 and protein binding of 90% are grounds for a low relative dose to the breastfed child. In comparison to metoclopramid, domperidone is less able to cross the blood–brain barrier. Therefore the risk for CNS symptoms is lower, and such symptoms have not as yet been observed in practice. A recent discussion on cardiac arrest associated with domperidone was based on events following high intravenous dosages, which is not comparable with the drug transfer to a breastfed child.

There are no data on *bromopride* and *dexpanthenol*.

4

> **Recommendation.** Domperidone, metoclopramide, and cisapride may be used for appropriate indications. The short-term use of other medications does not require limitation of breastfeeding.

4.3.4   Cholinergics

Experience

In a case of treatment with *neostigmine* for myasthenia, one child was observed with postprandial stomach cramps; others were unremarkable (Fraser 1963).

When using *pyridostigmine*, with a half-life of about 4 hours, the infant receives a maximum of 0.09% of the weight-related maternal dosage daily. In the case of two unremarkable infants described, there was no active ingredient found in their serum (detection level $2\,\mu g/l$). Maternal serum concentrations were 25 and $80\,\mu g/l$; a maximum of $25\,\mu g/l$ was found in the milk with intravenous application of 300 mg/day pyridostigmine (Hardell 1982).

There are no data on transfer via mother's milk regarding the other cholinergics, *anetholtrithion, bethanechol, carbachol, ceruletide, distigmine,* and *physostigmine*. There have been no reports of intolerance in breastfed infants.

When increased levels of circulating antibodies can be documented, many authors recommend that mothers with myasthenia gravis wean, because the antibodies received via the mother's milk may have a negative influence on neonatal myasthenia (survey by Burke 1993).

> **Recommendation.** The usual short-term therapy for (postoperative) atony of the intestine or bladder, or treatment of myasthenia with cholinergics, is permissible while breastfeeding.

4.3.5   Anticholinergic spasmolytics

Experience

Atropine-like preparations are considered to be contraindicated due to the extreme sensitivity of the infant to this group of substances. However, there have been no publications, as yet, in which negative effects on the baby have been described as a result of giving atropine-like drugs to a breastfeeding mother.

Butylscopolamine appears to be well-tolerated by the breastfed infant, either as a single parenteral dose or with repeated oral or rectal administration.

Experience with other anticholinergics such as *butinolin, denaverin, glycopyrrolate bromide, hymecromon, mebeverine, methanthelinium, oxybutynin, phenamazide, pipenzolate, pipoxolan, tiropramide, tolterodine, trospium chloride,* and *valethamate bromide* is insufficient with respect to breastfeeding.

> **Recommendation.** Butylscopolamine may be administered for appropriate indications. In the case of bladder incontinence, oxybutynin, which is equally widely used, also seems to be acceptable. Single administration of the other drugs mentioned does not require any limitation of breastfeeding. However, a critical look at the indications, and in some cases a change in therapy, should be undertaken.

4.3.6   Laxatives

Experience

Multiple studies of *senna* preparations that belong to the *anthraquinone* family, and which used to be considered contraindicated, have shown that the risk of causing diarrhea in breastfed infants is apparently quite low (survey by Bennett 1996).

Bulking agents such as *linseed* and *wheat bran* are not absorbed. *Bisacodyl* and osmotic agents such as *lactulose*, or saline agents such as *sodium sulfate*, are also scarcely absorbed. Although there is no documented experience available on *macrogol*, it seems acceptable because of low intestinal resorption.

The inhibition of the absorption of fat-soluble vitamins with *castor oil*, and the possible drastic action of *sodium picosulfate*, argue against their use.

> **Recommendation.** If a change in dietary habits is not successful, bulking agents, senna preparations, bisacodyl, and both saline and osmotic agents

> may be taken during breastfeeding. Changing the intestinal flora with bacterial cultures is also permissible.
>   A single administration of another laxative does not require any limitation of breastfeeding, but use of the laxative should be stopped.

4.3.7   Agents used for chronic inflammatory bowel diseases

4

Lactation

Experience

Sulfonamides, 5-aminosalicylic acid, glucocorticoids (e.g. oral prednisolone or locally applied budesonide), cytostatics (methotrexate, 6-mercaptopurine, thioguanine), immunosuppressive drugs (azathioprine), and, recently, monoclonal antibodies (e.g. infliximab) are used to treat chronic inflammatory bowel disease, ulcerative colitis, and Crohn's disease.

The sulfonamide *salazosulfapyridine* (= *sulfasalazine*) was, for a long time, the standard medication for treating ulcerative colitis. It has an M/P ratio of 0.4. With a maternal daily dosage of 3 g, up to 10% of the weight-related portion can reach the infant. One case report mentioned bloody diarrhea in a breastfed baby whose plasma concentration was 5.3 mg/l (the therapeutic range is 20–50 mg/l). With a maternal dosage of 2 g daily, a significantly lower level of the substance was reported to reach the infant via mother's milk (survey in Bennett 1996).

Mesalazine consists of *5-aminosalicylic acid*, the anti-inflammatory portion of sulfasalazine. With a daily intake of 1500 mg, 0.015 mg/kg daily was calculated for the infant. This is less than 0.1% of the maternal weight-related dosage (Klotz 1993, Jenss 1990). However, taking into consideration the metabolite, acetyl-5-aminosalicylic acid (about 12 mg/l of milk), it would be 7.5%. A further publication also reports 15 mg active ingredient per liter (Christensen 1994). Silverman (2005) found very low levels of 5-aminosalicylic acid in the milk of four lactating mothers; however, the content of the relatively inactive metabolite N-acetyl-5-aminosalicylic acid was 1000-fold higher. A case report described an infant who developed diarrhea following repeated rectal administration of mesalazine to his mother. The diarrhea ceased when therapy was ended (Nelis 1989). In a further group of eight breastfeeding women, there was also a report of a child with diarrhea (Ito 1993). However, the authors of this book have found no symptoms in the overwhelming majority of the infants observed, regardless of the dosage.

Olsalazine, which consists of two mesalazine molecules, has an intestinal absorption rate of about 2% and can only be detected

4.3 Gastrointestinal drugs

in mother's milk in the form of its acetylated metabolites (Miller 1993).

Considering its very widespread use, the absence of further publications regarding the toxic effects of these antidiarrheal medications on the infant argues for good tolerance of these drugs during breastfeeding.

> **Recommendation.** For chronic inflammatory bowel diseases, mesalazine is the drug of choice. Olsalazine may also be used for appropriate indications. If the sulfonamide effect of sulfasalazine is particularly desirable, this drug may also be used. Corticoids may be administered both rectally and systemically during breastfeeding. Methotrexate should not be prescribed.
>
> For immunosuppressive medications used for chronic inflammatory bowel disease, see Chapter 4.10.

4.3.8   Antidiarrheals for acute diarrhea

Experience

Diphenoxylate and *loperamide* decrease intestinal motility by interacting with opiate receptors. In a study on loperamide, less than 0.1% of the maternal weight-related dosage was reported for the infant following administration to the mother twice (Nikodem 1992). No toxic action has been described as yet.

There are no data on *diphenoxylate* or *tannin albumate*.

> **Recommendation.** When dietary measures are really insufficient, loperamide may be taken temporarily during breastfeeding.

4.3.9   Carminatives

Experience

Dimeticon and *simeticon* are not absorbed in significant amounts. Toxic effects are as unlikely, as with *caraway* or *anise* preparations. However, the essential oil could, in individual instances, affect the taste of the milk and lead to a (temporary) nursing strike.

> **Recommendation.** Dimeticon or simeticon and vegetable preparations can be given for flatulence without reservation.

4.3.10   Lipid reducers

Experience

Pravastatin appears only in negligible amounts in the milk (less than 0.4% of a weight-related dosage) (Pan 1988).

No toxic effects on the infant have been reported as yet in connection with maternal intake of lipid reducers. However, the documented experience with *acipimox, atorvastatin, bezafibrate, cerivastatin, clofibrate, colestipol, cholestyramine, etofibrate, etofyllinclofibrate, ezetimibe, fenofibrate, fluvastatin, gemfibrozil, inositol nicotinate, lovastatin, pitavastatin, pravastatin, probucol, rosuvastatin, simvastatin, β-sitosterin*, and *xantinol nicotinate* is insufficient for a risk assessment.

Due to the way they work, the lipid-binding resins *colestipol* and *cholestyramine*, which are not absorbed in significant amounts, are not considered to pose a risk to the breastfed infant.

> **Recommendation.** Lipid reducers should not be used during breastfeeding because their safety is not established, and there would seem to be no disadvantage for the mother when therapy is stopped during pregnancy and breastfeeding. Taking the medication, however, does not require any limitation of breastfeeding, although, with the exception of colestipol, cholestyramine, and pravastatin, the continuation of treatment should be critically reviewed.

4.3.11   Chenodeoxycholic acid and ursodeoxycholic acid

Experience

There is no documented experience on the tolerance of *chenodeoxycholic acid* and *ursodeoxycholic acid* during breastfeeding. Only limited amounts of ursodeoxycholic acid appear in the blood circulation, where they are overwhelmingly bound to albumin. Thus, a quantitative transfer into the milk is unlikely.

> **Recommendation.** Chenodeoxycholic acid and ursodeoxycholic acid should not be used while breastfeeding. The exception is therapy for primary biliary cirrhosis with ursodeoxycholic acid. In such a case, breastfeeding does not necessarily need to be limited.

4 Lactation

4.3 Gastrointestinal drugs

4.3.12   Appetite suppressants

Experience

Pharmacological effects on the infant of appetite suppressants such as *amfepramone* (= *diethylpropiorin*), *dexfenfluramine*, *fenproporex*, *mefenorex*, *norpseudoephedrine*, *sibutramine*, and *orlistat* have not been studied. Weight reduction in the mother releases contaminants from her fatty tissue, which results in an additional burden on the mother's milk (see Chapter 4.18).

> **Recommendation.** Appetite suppressants are contraindicated during breastfeeding. The accidental intake of a single dose does not require limitation of breastfeeding.

4.3.13   Antiemetics

Experience

Antihistaminics and other compounds are used as antiemetics. Very rarely, mild restlessness, sedation or weak sucking – none of which require treatment – have been described in the breastfed infant (see, for example, Moretti 1995).

There is no detailed knowledge regarding the effects during breastfeeding of the following substances: *betahistine, cinnarizine, dimenhydrinate, diphenhydramine, flunarizine, meclizine*, and *scopolamine* patches, nor of the newer serotonin-(5-HT3) antagonists *dolasetron, granisetron, ondansetron, palonosetron*, and *tropisetron*.

The brief half-life of 2–3 hours and the long effectiveness of up to 24 hours argue for good tolerance of meclizine during pregnancy. Metoclopramide is discussed in section 4.3.3.

For phenothiazine neuroleptics and sulpiride, see Chapter 4.9.

> **Recommendation.** The antiemetic of choice during breastfeeding is meclizine. Even with the other, older antiemetics, including the phenothiazine-neuroleptics which are used for this purpose, severe intolerance in the infant – especially after single dosages – would not be expected.
>
> If a serotonin antagonist such as ondansetron is indicated during lactation, the child should be observed for unexpected symptoms.

References

Bender W, Brockmeier D. Pharmacokinetic characteristics of roxatidine. J Clin Gastroenterol 1989; 11(Suppl 1): 6–9.

Bennett PN (ed.). Drugs and Human Lactation, 2nd edn. Amsterdam: Elsevier, 1996.

Biervliet FP, Maguiness SD, Hay DM et al. Induction of lactation in the intended mother of a surrogate pregnancy: case report. Hum Reprod 2001; 16: 581–3.

Burke ME. Myasthenia gravis and pregnancy. J Perinat Neonatal Nurs 1993; 7: 11–21.

Christensen LA, Rasmussen SN, Hansen SH. Disposition of 5-aminosalicylic acid and N-acetyl-5-aminosalicylic acid preparations. Acta Obstet Gynecol Scand 1994; 74: 399–402.

Courtney TP, Shaw RW, Cedar E et al. Excretion of famotidine in breast milk. Proc Br Paed Soc 1988; 9: 639.

da Silva OP, Knoppert DC, Angelini MM et al. Effect of domperidone on milk production in mothers of premature newborns: a randomized, double-blind, placebo-controlled trial. Can Med Assoc J 2001; 164: 17–21.

Fraser D, Turner JWA. Myasthenia gravis and pregnancy. Proc R Soc Med 1963; 56: 379–81.

Hansen WF, McAndrew S, Harris K et al. Metoclopramide effect on breastfeeding the preterm infant: a randomized trial. Obstet Gynecol 2005; 105: 383–9.

Hardell LI, Lindstrom B, Lonnerholm G et al. Pyridostigmine in human breast milk. Br J Clin Pharmacol 1982; 14: 565–7.

Hofmeyr GJ, van Iddekinge B, Blott JA. Domperidone: secretion in breast milk and effect on puerperal prolactin levels. Br J Obstet Gynecol 1985; 92: 141–4.

Hofmeyr GJ, Sonnendecker EWW. Secretion of the gastrokinetic agent cisapride in human milk. Eur J Clin Pharmacol 1986; 30: 735–6.

Ito S, Blajchman A, Stephenson M et al. Prospective follow-up of adverse reactions in breast-fed infants exposed to maternal infection. Am J Obstet Gynecol 1993; 168: 1393–9.

Jenss H, Weber P, Hartman F. 5-Aminosalicylic acid and its metabolite in breast milk during lactation. Am J Gastroenterol 1990; 85: 331.

Kauppila A, Arvela P, Koivisto M et al. Metoclopramide and breast-feeding: transfer into milk and the newborn. Eur J Clin Pharmacol 1983; 25: 819–23.

Kauppila A, Anunti P, Kivinen S et al. Metoclopramide and breast-feeding: efficacy and anterior pituitary responses of the mother and the child. Eur J Obstet Gynecol Reprod Biol 1985; 19: 19–22.

Kearns GL, McConnel Jr RF, Trang JM et al. Appearance of ranitidine in breast milk following multiple dosing. Clin Pharmacol 1985; 4: 322–4.

Klotz U, Harings-Kaim A. Negligible excretion of 5-aminosalicylic acid in breast milk. Lancet 1993; 342: 618–19.

Marshall JK, Thomson ABR, Amstrong D. Omeprazole for refractory gastro-sophageal reflux disease during pregnancy and lactation. Can J Gastroenterol 1998; 12: 225–7.

Miller LG, Hopkinson JM, Motil KJ et al. Disposition of olsalazine and metabolites in breast milk. J Clin Pharmacol 1993; 33: 703–6.

Moretti ME, Liau-Chu M, Taddio A et al. Adverse events in breastfed infants exposed to anti-histamines in maternal milk. Reprod Toxicol 1995; 9: 588.

Nelis GF. Diarrhea due to 5-aminosalicylic acid in breast milk. Lancet 1989; 1: 383.

Nikodem VC, Hofmeyr GJ. Secretion of the anti-diarrheal agent loperamide oxide in breast milk. Eur J Clin Pharmacol 1992; 42: 695–6.

4

Lactation

4.3 Gastrointestinal drugs

Obermeyer BD, Bergstrom RF, Callaghan JT et al. Secretion of nizatidine into human breast milk after single and multiple doses. Clin Pharmacol Ther 1990; 47: 724–30.

Oo CY, Kuhn RJ, Desai N et al. Active transport of cimetidine into human breast milk. Clin Pharmacol Ther 1995; 58: 548–55.

Pan H, Fleiss P, Moore L et al. Excretion of pravastatin, an HMG CoA reductase inhibitor, in breast milk of lactating women. J Clin Pharmacol 1988; 28: 942.

Plante L, Ferron GM, Unruh M et al. Excretion of pantoprazole in human breast. J Reprod Med 2004; 49: 825–7.

Silverman DA, Ford J, Shaw I et al. Is mesalazine really safe for use in breastfeeding mothers? Gut 2005; 54: 170–71.

Anti-infectives

Christof Schaefer

4.4

4.4.1   Antibiotics in general

With many antibiotics, a breastfed child receives less than 1% of the weight-related therapeutic dosage when the mother is being treated. Thus, in any case, only minimal concentrations are reached in the infant plasma, and in no case is a concentration reached that would inhibit bacterial growth.

The following risks have been discussed repeatedly in the literature:

- Effects on the intestinal flora (with diarrhea as a possible consequence)
- Effects on bacteriological studies which might be necessary in case the infant falls ill
- Development of bacterial resistance
- Sensitization.

None of these side effects has been proven as yet. The likeliest possibility – in rare cases – would be a temporary loosening of the stool consistency, which does not require any therapy (Ito 1993).

4.4.2   Penicillins, cephalosporins, and other β-lactam antibiotics

Experience

The M/P ratio of all commonly used *penicillin* derivatives is under 1. As a rule, the exclusively breastfed infant receives considerably less than 1% of a therapeutic dosage (survey in Bennett 1996).

This applies similarly to *cephalosporins*, which are, to some extent, inactivated in the intestine (survey in Bennett 1996). Benyamini and co-workers asked 67 mothers who were taking *amoxicillin* plus the enzyme inhibitor *clavulanic acid*, as well as 38 who were taking *cefuroxim*, about side effects in their breastfed children (Benyamini 2005). In the first group, symptoms were more frequent (22%), as with amoxicillin alone. The symptoms were dose-dependent, however, and did not require any intervention. With *cefuroxim* and *cefalexin*, only moderate side effects were reported and in scarcely 3% of cases.

In the case of *aztreonam*, a 0.2% relative dosage was reported for the baby in the next breastfeed after the mother had taken a single dose (Ito 1990).

In a Japanese study of *imipinem*, an average of 0.8% of a weight-related, intravenously administered dosage was measured (Ito 1988).

With *sulbactam*, the relative daily dosage transmitted was a maximum of 1% (Foulds 1985).

Aztreonam, imipinem, and sulbactam are hardly absorbed at all enterally. This provides additional support for limited bioavailability to the breastfed child.

Other β-lactam antibiotics have not as yet been shown to be toxic for the breastfed infant.

> **Recommendation.** Penicillin derivatives and cephalosporins are the antibiotics of choice during breastfeeding. As far as possible, substances that have been in use for a long time (e.g. second-generation cephalosporins) are preferable. When necessary, other β-lactam antibiotics and clavulanic acid can also be used.

4.4.3   Erythromycin and other macrolides

Experience

With *erythromycin*, which has an M/P ratio of about 0.5, the infant whose mother takes 2 g daily receives a maximum of 0.48 mg/kg daily – just 2% of a weight-related therapeutic infant dosage (Matsuda 1984, Knowles 1972). A connection between pyloric stenosis and erythromycin transmitted through the mother's milk was discussed (Soerensen 2003, Stang 1986), but a causal relationship has not been confirmed to date.

In a case report on 500 mg daily of *azithromycin*, a peak value of 2.8 mg/l of milk was cited. This represents 5% of the maternal dosage per kg of bodyweight (Kelsey 1994).

With 500 mg/daily of *clarithromycin*, used to treat a puerperal infection, a maximum of 1.5 mg of the active substance per liter of milk was measured (Sedlmayr 1993). This is 2.7% of the weight-related maternal dosage.

With *roxithromycin*, less than 0.05% is thought to pass into the milk (Lassman 1988).

There are no data on *spiramycin* and *telithromycin*.

There are no reports of specific intolerance during breastfeeding to any of the macrolides mentioned here. This also applies to *josamycin*.

> **Recommendation.** In addition to penicillin derivatives and cephalosporins, erythromycin and roxithromycin are the antibiotics of choice during breastfeeding. The macrolidic antibiotics, azithromycin, clarithromycin, josamycin, and spiramycin, are second-choice medications. Where there is already a noteworthy icterus in the first days of life, caution should be exercised if the mother receives high dosages of parenteral macrolides.

4   Lactation

4.4 Anti-infectives

4.4.4   Tetracyclines

Experience

Tetracyclines reach concentrations in the mother's milk that are significantly below the maternal plasma values. The calcium in mother's milk inactivates a part of the substance which is transmitted. Symptoms in the infants should not be expected, and have never been reported. In particular, there is no discoloration of the teeth as a result of exposure via mother's milk.

With 200 mg of *doxycycline* therapy followed 24 hours later by a 100-mg dose, a maximum of 1.4 mg/l was found in the milk. At most, 3–4% of the maternal weight-related dosage reaches the infant in this way. This is similar with *minocydine* and *tetracycline*.

With *chlortetracycline* therapy, the dosage transported by the milk is under 1% (survey by Bennett 1996).

> **Recommendation.** Tetracyclines, including doxycycline and minocycline, can be given when success using the antibiotics of choice (see above) cannot be expected.

4.4.5   Dapsone, nitrofurantoin, and other drugs for urinary tract infections

Experience

In the case of therapy with *dapsone*, 10–20% of the weight-related dosage can pass into the milk (Edstein 1986, Sanders 1982). In a case description, dapsone and its primary metabolite, *monoacetyl-dapsone*, were documented in the child's serum. The infant developed hemolytic anemia (Sanders 1982).

After a single dose of 100 mg *nitrofurantoin* to four women, an average of 1.3 μg/ml was measured in the milk; the maximal measurement (about 5 hours after administration) was 3.2 μg/ml. The M/P ratio was 6 (Gerk 2001). Based on these values, the relative dose for a fully breastfed child can reach 10%. Older investigations determined only 2.5% (Pons 1990). Haemolytic reaction of a baby with glucose-6-phosphate-dehydrogenase deficiency was described in an older report. Apart from such a constellation, threatening effects are not to be expected for a breastfed child – particularly one who is older than 4 weeks.

Sulfonamides pass into the mother's milk in various amounts. The percentage specifications, based on the weight-related maternal dosage, vary between 1% and over 50% (in the case of the old sulfonamid, *sulfanilamide*).

With *sulfamethoxazole*, the sulfonamide portion in *cotrimoxazole* is, on average, 2%.

For *trimethoprim*, an average of 4–5.5% of the relative dosage was calculated for the exclusively breastfed infant with a 5-day treatment with cotrimoxazole (survey by Bennett 1996).

There are no data on *fosfomycin* and *tetroxoprim*.

> **Recommendation.** Cotrimoxazole or trimethoprim alone (which is mostly just as effective as cotrimoxazole as monotherapy for urinary tract infections) can be used for appropriate indications. If actually indicated, nitrofurantoin and sulfonamides can also be prescribed. In the case of necessary treatment with dapsone, an individual decision must be made about limiting breastfeeding.

4

Lactation

4.4.6   Quinolones

Experience

Insofar as they have been studied at all, *nalidixic acid* (Traeger 1980) and the newer *quinolones* seem to accumulate in mother's milk.

With *ciprofloxacin*, it was calculated that between 2% and 7% of the weight-related maternal dosage reaches the infant (Gardner 1992, Cover 1990, Giamarellou 1989). However, no ciprofloxacin could be detected in the serum of a breastfed infant (maternal serum concentration 0.21 mg/l, detection limit 0.03 mg/l; Gardner 1992).

With *fleroxacin*, 10% of the maternal weight-related dosage was shown (Dan 1993).

Garenoxacin was given in a single dose of 600 mg to six women, who had already weaned. At maximum, 3 μg/ml was measured in the milk. The relative dose for a fully breastfed child was calculated to be 4.5%, and the M/P ratio 0.4 (Amsden 2004).

In the case of *levofloxacin*, a mother received 500 mg/day over 3 weeks, first parenterally and then orally. The maximum concentration in the milk was 8.2 μg/ml (5 hours after application). The relative dose reached a maximum of about 15%. In the available case, the child was not breastfed (Cahill 2005).

There are no data on the passage into the milk of *cinoxacin*, *enoxacin*, *gatifloxacin*, *grepafloxacin*, *levofloxacin*, *lomefloxacin*, *moxifloxacin*, *norfloxacin*, *ofloxacin*, *pefloxacin*, *rosoxacin*, and *sparfloxacin*.

In animal studies, quinolones damage the cartilage in the joints irreversibly during the growing years.

> **Recommendation.** Quinolones should not be used during breastfeeding. As a rule, a standard antibiotic with a lower potential for risk can easily be substituted for them. When a complicated infection (for example, of the urinary tract, or a pseudomonas infection) really requires a quinolone, whenever possible ciprofloxacin should be preferred and breastfeeding continued.

4.4.7   Other antibiotics and urinary tract antiseptics

Experience

With *clindamycin*, a maximum of 3.1 mg/l milk was measured. For the infant, this represents about 6% of the maternal weight-related dosage, or 15% of the daily dosage for an infant. In a case report, hemorrhagic enteritis was described in an infant whose mother had taken clindamycin and gentamicin. The symptoms improved spontaneously after breastfeeding was interrupted (survey by Bennett 1996).

With 1 g of *vancomycin* administered intravenously twice a day, 12.7 mg/l was found in milk (Reyes 1989). For the fully breastfed baby, such a concentration represents 5.8% of the weight-adjusted maternal dosage. However, significant amounts are not absorbed.

With *lincomycin*, a maximum of 1% of the maternal weight-related dosage was measured in the milk (Medina 1963).

Damage to the bone marrow has been attributed to *chloramphenicol*, but has not been observed as a result of exposure through the mother's milk. Peak values of up to 4 mg/kg daily, on average – only about 1% of the therapeutic infant dosage – pass into the milk (survey by Bennett 1996, Plomp 1983). Refusal of food and vomiting by the baby have been described in connection with maternal treatment (Havelka 1968).

There are no data on the use of *colistin* and *polymyxin B* during breastfeeding.

The urinary tract antiseptic *methenamine* has not been studied sufficiently. This also applies to the hydroquinone *arbutin* (in strawberry leaf extract).

> **Recommendation.** When it is unavoidable, clindamycin, vancomycin, and lincomycin, as well as colistin and polymyxin B, may be prescribed. However, clindamycin should not be routinely used after dental procedures. Chloramphenicol is contraindicated. Generally, an antibiotic with a lower risk potential can easily be substituted for it. Administration of a single dose does not require any limitation of breastfeeding. This also applies following short-term usage of the urinary tract antiseptic discussed.

4.4.8   Nitroimidazole antibiotics

Experience

In the newborn period, the half-life of *metronidazole* is extended – in premature babies it can be up to 35–74 hours. In adults it is up to 10 hours. Following a single oral dosage of 2 g for trichomoniasis, the highest concentration was found in the milk after 2–4 hours. This is on average around 21 mg/l; in a single case it reached 46 mg/l (Erickson 1981). On average, 12% (at most up to about 20%) of a weight-related therapeutic child's dosage (15 mg/kg per day) is calculated for a fully breastfed infant when the active metabolites in the milk are considered. In the plasma of breastfed children, 2 µg/ml each of metronidazole and its metabolite *hydroxymetronidazole* were detected. Comparable results were found with a 9-day course of 1200 mg/d (Passmore 1988, Heisterberg 1983, Erickson 1981). Specific toxicity via mother's milk has not been described among some 60 mother–child pairs published to date. Used therapeutically in prematures (i.e. for necrotizing enterocolitis), this drug is, in general, well-tolerated.

There has as yet been no indication of experimentally observed mutagenic and carcinogenic effects of metronidazole in human beings.

With *tinidazole*, transfer via mother's milk can reach a maximum of 10% of the weight-related maternal dosage administered intravenously (Mannisto 1983).

The use of *nimorazole* during breastfeeding has not been studied.

> **Recommendation.** With trichomoniasis, metronidazole should be used in preference to the other nitroimidazoles. A single oral dose of 2 g is preferable to vaginal application spread over several days. This is more effective therapeutically, and limits the exposure for the baby. Whenever possible, the administration of metronidazole should be in the evening after the last breastfeed in order to limit further the exposure during the nightly breastfeeding break.
>
> This also applies to intravenous administration spread over several days in cases where this really is urgently indicated. Weaning or interruption of breastfeeding with substitution of infant formula no longer seems justifiable based on the available experience.

4.4.9   Aminoglycoside antibiotics

Experience

With an intramuscular *gentamicin* dosage of 80 mg three times daily, a maximum of 0.78 mg/l of milk was measured (Celiloglu 1994).

4

Lactation

4.4 Anti-infectives

This is about 3% of the weight-related maternal dosage. However, in 5 of the 10 newborns included in this study, gentamicin concentrations equivalent to 10% of the maternal values were measured in the serum. This leads to the conclusion that newborns absorb aminoglycosides enterally, or accumulate them due to reduced excretion, at levels that cannot be ignored.

Kanamycin and *tobramycin* appear only in limited amounts (up to about 1%) in mother's milk (Takasa 1975).

The other aminoglycoside antibiotics *amikacin*, *neomycin*, *netilmicin, paromomycin, spectinomycin*, and *streptomycin* have been insufficiently documented in this respect. They may perhaps be evaluated in an analogous fashion. Apart from the newborn period, aminoglycosides are scarcely absorbed.

> **Recommendation.** When aminoglycosides are strongly indicated, they may be used during breastfeeding. Restricted use is particularly applicable to the early postnatal period, since both quantitative absorption and accumulation by the infant must be reckoned with and, at least in the case of streptomycin, an ototoxic effect cannot be ruled out.

4.4.10   Tuberculostatics

Experience

In two cases where women were treated with *ethambutol*, the quantities in the milk were 1.4 and 4.6 µg/ml respectively. In the first case, the maternal daily dosage was 15 mg/kg; in the second case, no dosage is given (Snider 1984). For the infant, this translates into 1.5% of the weight-related maternal dosage in the first case, and 0.7 mg/kg bodyweight in the second.

With *isoniazid*, with an M/P ratio of about 1, up to 2 mg/kg daily (i.e. 20% of a weight-related therapeutic dosage) is thought to reach the infant. However, no toxic effects have been described to date (Snider 1984, Berlin 1979).

In a report on *pyrazinamide*, the relative dosage is under 1%. The mother took 1 g daily (Holdiness 1984).

A maximum of 5% of a weight-related therapeutic dosage of *rifampicin* is transmitted to the infant (Snider 1984). The aminoglycoside *streptomycin* can be expected to appear only in limited amounts in the milk and, apart from during the newborn period, is not absorbed enterally in any noteworthy amount (see section 4.4.9).

There are no data on *protionamide*.

Recommendation. Tuberculostatics of choice during breastfeeding are isoniazid (in combination with 0.5–1 mg vitamin B_6 prophylaxis per day for the infant), rifampicin, and pyrazinamide. Ethambutol is also acceptable. Streptomycin is a second-choice drug. If possible, it should not be used in the newborn period. Protionamide should be avoided.

4.4.11   Malarial drugs

4

Lactation

Experience

M/P quotients of between 2 and 6 have been calculated for *chloroquine*. Following oral administration of 600 mg chloroquine base to breastfeeding mothers, peak values of 4.4 mg/l of milk were measured (Ogunbona 1987). However, the main metabolite, *desmethylchloroquine*, also needs to be considered. With the very long half-life, continuing high plasma/milk levels can be expected despite weekly intake of malaria prophylaxis. Assuming a weekly (prophylactic) dosage of 500 mg chloroquine phosphate (which equals approximately a 300-mg chloroquine base), a weight-related dosage of just 1 mg/kg daily is calculated for the mother. According to two studies (Ette 1987, Edstein 1986), an average of between 1 and 12%(!) of the maternal weight-related daily dosage is transmitted by the milk to the baby. With the prophylactic dosage common here, that would be up to 0.1 mg/kg daily. Chloroquine can be detected in the infant's urine (Witte 1990). However, despite the not insignificant transfer into the milk, symptoms have not yet been reported.

Quinine too, which has experienced a renaissance in malaria therapy because of increasing resistance, is well-tolerated during breastfeeding. With an M/P ratio of 0.2–0.5, a maximum of 1.2 mg/kg is transmitted to the baby via the milk when the mother has received intravenous therapy of 25 mg/kg per day. With oral therapy, the transfer to the baby is 0.5 mg/kg. This represents a relative dosage of about 5% or 2% (Phillips 1986).

Mefloquine has neurotoxic potential. There is one study on its use during breastfeeding in which an M/P ratio of 0.15 and a transfer of a maximum of 4% of the weight-related dosage were reported following a single dose of 250 mg of mefloquine base (Edstein 1988). The experience with mefloquine to date is insufficient for a differentiated risk assessment during breastfeeding.

Proguanil is well-tested and apparently well-tolerated during breastfeeding.

There is no experience with artemisinin derivatives (*arthemether*), *atovaquone, halofantrine primaquine*, and other antimalarials.

Anti-infectives

4.4   Anti-infectives

> **Recommendation.** Prophylaxis and therapy of malaria is primarily oriented to drug resistance in the specific region or country. Usually therapy is short, and is therefore no indication in itself to interrupt breastfeeding. In case of prophylaxis for several weeks, a decision on cessation of breast feeding must be taken individually. At least, chloroquine, proguanil, quinine and a combination of sulfadoxin/ pyrimethamine as well as mefloquine are acceptable because of sufficient experience.
>
> Chloroquine and quinine should not be used during breastfeeding for other indications requiring long-term daily administration (i.e. rheumatic or autoimmune illnesses).

4.4.12   Local antimycotics

Experience

Locally effective antimycotics include *nystatin* and *clotrimazole* For all practical purposes, they are not absorbed and are not available to the infant enterally. Extensive experience with their therapeutic use in infancy argues against any toxic potential. The same applies to *miconazole*, which is also, for all practical purposes, not absorbed.

Bifonazole, croconazole, econazole, fenticonazole, isoconazole, ketoconazole, omoconazole, oxiconazole, sertaconazole, and *tioconazole* are related to clotrimazole structurally and in their action but they have been studied less. There has been no experience with *amorolfin, ciclopiroxolamin, naftifin, terbinafine, tolcyclate,* and *tolnaftate,* or with the vaginally administered *chlorphenesin*.

> **Recommendation.** Local antimycotics of choice during breastfeeding are nystatin and clotrimazole. Miconazole is also acceptable. These three drugs are preferable to the other abovementioned locally effective antimycotics. If one of the other medications is urgently indicated, breastfeeding can continue with no limitation if its use is only temporary or if only small areas are being treated.

4.4.13   Systemic antimycotics

Experience

Today, *fluconazole, ketoconazole,* and *itraconazole* are the most commonly used systemic antimycotics.

In the case of *fluconazole*, following a single dosage of 150 mg orally, a maximum of 2.9 µg/ml was measured in the milk. Based on this, a fully breastfed infant would receive over 15% of the maternal weight-related dosage. A half-life of 30 hours was calculated for fluconazole in the milk (Force 1995). The good tolerance in infancy for fluconazole administered intravenously for therapeutic purposes was cited by many authors as grounds for clearing it for usage during breastfeeding.

In one case study on the systemic administration of *ketoconazole*, an average of 0.4% with a maximum of 1.4% of the weight-related maternal dosage was calculated for the infant (Moretti 1995).

There are insufficient data to evaluate *itraconazole* and other "conazole" antimycotics, as well as *amphotericin, flucytosine, griseofulvin*, and *terbinafine*.

4

Lactation

> **Recommendation.** When systemic therapy is unavoidable, fluconazole should be selected over ketoconazole because it is generally better tolerated. Fluconazole is not infrequently used to treat candida infection of the breast. However, diagnosis is not easy, and should be made with caution. It is estimated that 20% of lactating women complaining of breast pain have a candida infection. Local treatment is usually not sufficient, whereas oral therapy with fluconazole for 2–3 weeks, or for 2 weeks after symptoms have resolved, is recommended. The dosage should start with 400 mg on day 1, followed by 100–200 mg/d (Abou-Dakn 2006). The breastfed infant has also to be treated (for example, with local miconazole). When systemic treatment of the mother is unavoidable, it should, if possible, be taken at night after the last breastfeed. A longer interruption of breastfeeding with the substitution of infant formula is not justified.
>
> Systemic treatment with itraconazole or other "conazole" antimycotics, amphotericin, griseofulvin, flucytosine, and terbinafine should be avoided during breastfeeding.

4.4.14 Antihelminthics

Experience

Pyrviniumembonate, mebendazole, niclosamide, and *pyrantel* are, practically speaking, not absorbed, and seem to be tolerated during breastfeeding. This probably also applies to the echinococcus drug *albendazole. Praziquantel* appears in mother's milk in limited amounts (Pütter 1979).

By contrast, *ivermectin*, used to treat onchocerciasis, is well absorbed gastrointestinally; its half-life is 12 hours and the M/P

4.4 Anti-infectives

ratio is 0.5. Following a single dosage of 150 µg/kg to the mother, an average of 10 µg/l and a maximum of 23 µg/l was measured in the milk (Ogbuokiri 1994). Even considering the highest value, this is, mathematically speaking, only 2% of the weight-related maternal dosage for a fully breastfed baby.

> **Recommendation.** Pyrviniumembonate or mebendazole should be used to treat oxyuris (pin worms); niclosamide for band worms; and mebendazole for other worm infestations. With echinococcus, albendazole may also be used. Ivermectin may be used if necessary. If there is really no alternative to praziquantel, this may also be prescribed without any limitation of breastfeeding.

4.4.15   Acyclovir, antiretroviral drugs, and other virustatics

Experience

With *acyclovir*, with an M/P ratio of 2–4, the fully breastfed infant takes in 1% of an oral maternal weight-related dosage (Meyer 1988). When 900 mg daily is administered intravenously, this is on average 5% (Bork 1995). Toxic symptoms have not been observed (Taddio 1994, Meyer 1988). The risk of influencing the infant's immune system as a result of exposure via the mother's milk appears, in the light of current experience, to be simply theoretical.

Valaciclovir is the oral more easily available prodrug of aciclovir. In five mothers who received 500 mg twice daily, valaciclovir could not be detected either in the maternal serum or in the milk, because it is rapidly converted to aciclovir. The highest values (of aciclovir) in the milk were measured about 4 hours after administration; the M/P ratio was calculated as 3.4. Even considering the highest measured individual value in the milk, the relative dose for a fully breastfed child amounts to only 5.7%. Considering the limited oral availability and the therapeutically used dosages in neonatology, only 0.6% of a pediatric dose is transferred to the baby via the mother's milk. In the urine of the examined babies, on average 0.74 µg/ml aciclovir was found in steady-state conditions (Sheffield 2002).

For *oseltamivir* a maximum relative dose of 0.5% was calculated in a single patient with 75 mg bid at steady-state conditions (Wentge 2007, personal communication).

A study of 20 mother–child pairs with maternal antiretroviral therapy with *lamivudine, nevirapine*, and *zidovudine* calculated M/P ratios of 3.3, 0.7, and 3.2 respectively. There were high concentrations of nevirapine, with 971 ng/ml reaching therapeutic values usually achieved with a single pediatric dosage of 2 mg/kg. Therefore, the authors discussed both a preventive effect via the mother's milk, and potential toxicity or development of therapeutic resistance. For lamivudine, on average 28 ng/ml was measured in the infant's serum, which is about 5% of a therapeutic concentration. The transfer of zidovudine could not be investigated, because all infants received a therapeutic dosage to prevent infection (Shapiro 2005).

No statements regarding kinetics or tolerance during breastfeeding can be made for the other virustatics, *adefovir, amantadine, atazanavir, brivudine, cidofovir, famciclovir, fosamprenavir, sodium foscarnet, ganciclovir, ribavirin, valaciclovir*, and *zanamivir*, nor for the antiretroviral substances *abacavir, delavirdin, didanosine, efavirenz, indinavir, lopinavir, nelfinavir, ritonavir, saquinavir, stavudine, tipranavir*, and *zalcitabine*.

4

Lactation

> **Recommendation.** Breastfeeding may continue when acyclovir or valaciclovir are administered externally or systemically. The other virustatics and antiretroviral substances, if really indicated, require an individual decision about continuing breastfeeding. In the case of drugs developed for HIV infection, an additional consideration is the risk of virus transmission via the mother's milk (see Chapter 4.15); here, guidelines only clearly recommend exclusive breastfeeding in those regions where lack of clean water for preparing infant formula and feeding equipment would pose a greater risk for the infant. If chronic hepatitis B requires lamivudin therapy, breastfeeding might be tolerable after active plus passive vaccination of the child.

References

Abou-Dakn M. Stillen. In: F Kainer (eds), Facharzt Geburtsmedizin. München: Urban & Fischer, 2006, pp. 1091–111.

Amsden GW, Nicolau DP, Whitacker A-M et al. Characterization of the penetration of garenoxacin into the breast milk of lactating women. Pediatrics 2004; 44: 188–92.

Bennett PN (ed.). Drugs and Human Lactation, 2nd edn. Amsterdam: Elsevier, 1996.

Benyamini L, Merlob P, Stahl B et al. The safety of amoxicillin/clavulanic acid and cefuroxime during lactation. Ther Drug Monitor 2005; 27: 499–502.

Berlin CM, Lee C. Isoniazid and acetylisoniazid disposition in human milk, saliva and plasma. Fed Proc 1979; 38: 426.

Bork K, Benes P. Concentration and kinetic studies of intravenous acyclovir in serum and breast milk of a patient with eczema herpeticum. J Am Acad Dermatol 1995; 32: 1053–5.

Cahill JB Jr, Bailey EM, Chien S et al. Levofloxacin secretion in breast milk: a case report. Pharmacotherapy 2005; 25: 116–18.

4.4 Anti-infectives

Celiloglu M, Celiker S, Guven H et al. Gentamicin excretion and uptake from breast milk by nursing infants. Obstet Gynecol 1994; 84: 263–5.

Cover DL, Mueller BA. Ciprofloxacin penetration into human breast milk: a case report. DICP 1990; 24: 703–4.

Dan M, Weidekamm E, Sagiv R et al. Penetration of fleroxacin into breast milk and pharmacokinetics in lactating women. Antimicrob Agents Chemother 1993; 37: 293–6.

Edstein MD, Veenendaal JR, Newman K et al. Excretion of chloroquine, dapsone and pyri-methamine in human milk. Br J Clin Pharmacol 1986; 2: 733–5.

Edstein MD, Veenendaal JR, Hyslop R. Excretion of mefloquine in human breast milk. Chemotherapy 1988; 34: 165–9.

Erickson SH, Oppenheim GL, Smith GH. Metronidazole in breast milk. Obstet Gynecol 1981; 57: 48–50.

Ette EI, Essien E, Ogonor JI et al. Chloroquine in human milk. J Clin Pharmacol 1987; 27: 499–502.

Force RW. Fluconazole concentrations in breast milk. Pediatr Infect Dis J 1995; 14: 235–6.

Foulds G, Miller RD, Knirsch AK et al. Sulbactam kinetics and excretion into breast milk in postpartum women. Clin Pharmacol Ther 1985; 38: 692–6.

Gardner DK, Garbe SG, Harter C. Simultaneous concentrations of ciprofloxacin in breast milk and in serum in mother and breast-fed infant. Clin Pharm 1992; 11: 352–4.

Gerk PM, Kuhn RJ, Desai NS et al. Active transport of nitrofurantoin into human milk. Pharmacotherapy 2001; 21: 669–75.

Giamarellou H, Kolokythas E, Petrikkos G et al. Pharmacokinetics of three newer quinolones in pregnancy and lactating women. Am J Med 1989; 87(Suppl 5A): 49–51.

Havelka J, Hejzlar M, Popov V et al. Excretion of chloramphenicol in human milk. Chemotherapy 1968; 13: 204–11.

Heisterberg L, Branjeberg PE. Blood and milk concentrations of metronidazole in mothers and infants. J Perinatal Med 1983; 11: 114–29.

Holdiness MR. Antituberculous drugs and breastfeeding. Arch Int Med 1984; 144: 1888.

Ito K, Izumi K, Takagi H et al. Fundamental and clinical evaluation of inipenem/cilastatin sodium in the perinatal period. Jpn J Antibiot 1988; 11: 1778–85.

Ito K, Hirose R, Tamaya T et al. Pharmacokinetic and clinical studies on aztreonam in the perinatal period. Jpn J Antibiot 1990; 43: 719–26.

Ito S, Blajchman A, Stephenson M et al. Prospective follow-up of adverse reactions in breast-fed infants exposed to maternal medication. Am J Obstet Gynecol 1993; 168: 1393–9.

Kelsey JJ, Moser LR, Jennings JC et al. Presence of azithromycin breast milk concentrations: a case report. Am J Obstet Gynecol 1994; 170: 1375–6.

Knowles JA. Drugs in milk. Pediatr Curr 1972; 21: 28–32.

Lassmann HB, Puri SH, Ho I et al. Pharmacokinetics of roxithromycin (RU 965) J Clin Pharmacol 1988; 28: 141–52.

Mannisto PT, Karhunen K, Koskela O et al. Concentrations of tinidazole in breast milk. Acta Pharmacol Toxicol 1983; 53: 254–6.

Matsuda T. Transfer of antibiotics into maternal milk. Biol Res Preg 1984; 5: 57–60.

Medina A, Fiske N, Hjelt-Harvey I et al. Absorption, diffusion, and excretion of a new antibiotic, lincomycin. Antimicrob Agents Chemother 1963; 161: 189–96.

Meyer LJ, De Miranda P, Sheth N et al. Acyclovir in human breast milk. Am J Obstet Gynecol 1988; 158: 586–8.

Moretti ME, Ito S, Koren G. Disposition of maternal ketoconazole in breast milk. Am J Obstet Gynecol 1995; 173: 1625–6.

Ogbuokiri JE, Ozumba BC, Okonkwo PO. Ivermectin levels in human breast milk. Eur J Clin Pharmacol 1994; 46: 89–90.

Ogunbona FA, Onyeji CO, Bolaji O et al. Excretion of chloroquine and desethylchloroquine in human milk. Br J Clin Pharmacol 1987; 23: 473–6.

Passmore CM, McElnay JC, Rainey EA et al. Metronidazole excretion in human milk and its effects on the suckling neonate. Br J Clin Pharmacol 1988; 26: 45–51.

Phillips KE, Looareesuwan S, White NJ et al. Quinine pharmacokinetics and toxicity in pregnant and lactating women. Br J Clin Pharmacol 1986; 21: 677–83.

Plomp TA, Thiery M, Maes RAA. The passage of thiamphenicol and chloramphenicol into human milk after single and repeated oral administration. Vet Hum Toxicol 1983; 25: 167–72.

Pons G, Rey E, Richard M-O et al. Nitrofurantoin excretion in human milk. Dev Pharmacol Ther 1990; 14: 148–52.

Pütter J, Held E. Quantitative studies on the occurrence of praziquantel in milk and plasma of lactating women. Eur J Drug Metabol Pharmacokinet 1979; 4: 193–8.

Reyes MP, Ostrea EM Jr, Cabinian AE et al. Vancomycin during pregnancy. Does it cause hearing loss or nephrotoxicity in the infant? Am J Obstet Gynecol 1989; 161: 977–81.

Sanders SW, Zone JJ, Flotz RL et al. Haemolytic anemia induced by dapsone transmitted through breast milk. Ann Int Med 1982; 90: 465–6.

Sedlmayr Th, Peters F, Raasch W et al. Clarithromycin, a new macrolide antibiotic. Effectiveness in puerperal infections and pharmacokinetics in breast milk {in German}. Geburtsh Frauenheilk 1993; 53: 488–91.

Shapiro RL, Holland DT, Capparelli E et al. Antiretroviral concentrations in breastfeeding infants of women in Botswana receiving antiretroviral treatment. J Infect Dis 2005; 192: 720–27.

Sheffield JS, Fish DN, Hollier LM. Acyclovir concentrations in human breast milk after valaciclovir administration. Am J Obstet Gynecol 2002; 186: 100–102.

Snider DE Jr, Powell KE. Should women taking antituberculosis drugs breast-feed? Arch Intern Med 1984; 144: 589–90.

Soerensen HT, Skriver MV, Pedersen L et al. Risk of infantile hypertrophic pyloric stenosis after maternal postnatal use of macrolides. Scand J Infect Dis 2003; 35: 104–6.

Stang H. Pyloric stenosis associated with erythromycin ingested through breast milk. Minnesota Medicine 1986; 69: 669–70.

Taddio A, Klein J, Koren G. Acyclovir excretion in human breast milk. Ann Pharmacother 1994; 28: 585–7.

Takasa Z, Shirafuji H, Uchida M et al. Laboratory and clinical studies on tobramycin in the fields of obstetrics and gynecology. Chemotherapy (Tokyo) 1975; 23: 1399–1402.

Traeger A, Peiker G. Excretion of nalidixic acid via mother's milk. Arch Toxicol 1980; 4(Suppl): 388–90.

Witte AMC, Klever HJH, Brabin BJ et al. Field evaluation of the use of ELISA to detect chloroquine and ist metabolites in blood, urine and breast-milk. Trans R Soc Trop Med Hyg 1990; 84: 521–5.

4

Lactation

4.4 Anti-infectives

Vaccines and immunoglobulins

4.5

Ruth Lawrence and Christof Schaefer

4.5.1   Maternal immunization

A woman who has not received all the recommended immunizations before or during pregnancy may be immunized in the postpartum period even though she is breastfeeding. The presence of live viruses in the milk does not present a problem because the viruses have been attenuated. According to the statement of the American Academy of Pediatrics Committee on Infectious Diseases (2006), breastfeeding women may be immunized with both killed and live vaccines. All vaccines and *immunoglobulins* used for mothers are considered safe for the infant during breastfeeding. Lactating women can be immunized, using standard recommended doses for adults, against measles, mumps, rubella, tetanus, diphtheria, pertussis, influenza, streptococcus pneumoniae, neisseria meningitis, hepatitis A, hepatitis B, and varicella. Often it is the need to travel to endemic countries that raises the issue.

A lactating woman can be given inactivated poliovirus vaccine, for instance, if necessary. The administration of live vaccine (oral vaccine) should be delayed in the mother (or parents) of a young infant until the infant has been vaccinated with killed virus regardless of the feeding mode.

With some vaccines, i.e. against meningococcal or pneumococcal disease (Shahid 2002, 1995) and cholera, there is discussion on whether the relevant amounts of the maternal antibodies built up as a result of immunization appear in the milk.

4.5.2   Efficacy of immunization in breastfed infants

Many myths have circulated regarding the efficacy of immunization of the infant during breastfeeding. Actually, the immunogenicity of some vaccines is increased by breastfeeding, but long-range enhancement of efficacy has not been studied. In any case the response to vaccines while breastfeeding is not diminished, and the usual vaccination schedules should be followed.

4.5.3   Hepatitis A vaccine

Experience

Hepatitis A vaccine is available in two preparations which are prepared from cell culture-adapted hepatitis A virus which has in turn been cultured in human fibroblasts and inactivated. It has not been studied in breastfeeding or in children under 2 years of age.

> **Recommendation.** Hepatitis A vaccine is unlikely to present a problem during lactation and is not contraindicated.

4.5.4   Hepatitis B vaccine

Experience

Hepatitis B vaccine is a highly effective and safe vaccine which is produced by recombinant DNA technology. The vaccine is an inactivated non-infectious hepatitis B surface antigen vaccine, and contains between 10 and 40 µg of HB$_5$Ag protein per ml with apparently similar rates of seroconversion. Pediatric vaccines contain no thimerosal. The vaccine is given to newborns at birth. Hepatitis B vaccine is also combined with other vaccines, and can be given concurrently with other vaccines but via a separate syringe and at another site. A total of three injections is required in the first six months of life.

> **Recommendation.** Hepatitis B vaccines are considered safe during lactation.

4.5.5   Influenza vaccine

Experience

Influenza vaccines come in two forms. One is the traditional killed virus vaccine that is given by injection; the second is a live attenuated vaccine available in a mist package to be administered via the nasal passages. Both contain three virus strains, and typically one or two strains are given each year to anticipate the strains circulating in that particular year. Both are produced using embryonated hen eggs, and therefore cannot be given to individuals sensitive to eggs. The inactivated vaccine (TIV) is approved for individuals aged 6 months and older. The live attenuated vaccine (LAIV) is cold adapted, developed by passing tissue cultures through lower and lower temperatures. Thus, viral replication can only occur in the upper respiratory tract, where it is cool. It is licensed for individuals aged 5 years and older.

Both TIV and LAIV are considered safe during lactation. The live attenuated vaccine is heat sensitive and does not survive in the plasma or the milk. Whether the breastfed infant can be protected by maternal immunization by either TIV or LAIV has not been studied.

4.5.6   Polio vaccine

Experience

Oral polio vaccine (Sabin) is live attenuated vaccine combining three strains of the virus. The transfer of these vaccine viruses to an unvaccinated contact person, i.e. via a smear infection, can lead to a normal vaccination reaction and immunity against infection with the wild virus. However, it is also possible that the person will become ill with contact vaccine poliomyelitis. This complication – occurring once in 15.5 million immunizations – is very rare. In two cases, it has been reported in infants (Mertens 1983, Heyne 1977). When immunization is urgent for the mother, the killed virus vaccine can be given to her intramuscularly. In the immunized mother, polio antibodies are present in the milk at a level comparable to the mother's plasma levels. High concentrations of anti-polio virus antibody in the milk could theoretically interfere with the response of the breastfeeding infant to immunization, but no such outcome has ever been reported.

> **Recommendation.** Live oral vaccine should not be given to the mother until the infant has been immunized at 6 weeks or older.

4.5.7   Rabies vaccine

There are no breastfeeding data on rabies vaccine. Since it is an inactivated rabies virus, it would not be a threat to the infant if it were to appear in the milk.

4.5.8   Rubella vaccine

Experience

Rubella vaccine is a live virus of the RA 27/3 strain grown in human diploid cell cultures and attenuated. It can be given in a combination vaccine (MMR). The early postpartum period, when risk of pregnancy is lowest, is the best time to be immunized. The risk to the breastfeeding infant is minimal with the recent techniques for vaccine preparation. The original preparations in the 1970s were associated with several cases of rubella. While the virus may appear in the milk, as reported in several studies (Losonsky 1982, Isacson 1971), symptoms in these infants were rare (Landes 1980).

> **Recommendation.** Lactating mothers of normal full-term infants can receive rubella immunization during lactation.

4.5.9   Smallpox vaccine

A woman should not be vaccinated with smallpox vaccine while caring for an infant under 1 year of age unless she can be separated

4

Lactation

4.5 Vaccines and immunoglobulins

from the child until the site heals (at least 10 days). It is not known whether the virus passes into the milk.

> **Recommendation.** The killed-virus injectable form of the vaccine is recommended during lactation.

4.5.10   Typhoid vaccine

Protection is indicated when traveling to an endemic area. Typhoid vaccines are available with killed and with live attenuated viruses. The live attenuated vaccine is given orally. Although it has little potential for producing disease, there are no data about passage into milk. It is not recommended during lactation. The injectable form is a killed dried bacteria in a phenol inactivation preparation, and is preferable for a woman while lactating.

4.5.11   Immunoglobulins

Experience

Immunoglobulins are in general very large molecules and do not pass into milk. In addition, infants are given immunoglobulin directly. Immunoglobulins contain passive protective antibodies and are not contraindicated for newborns, and would not be contraindicated for a breastfeeding mother.

Immunoglobulin is used with specific immunoglobulins in high titer, such as immunoglobulin hepatitis B (Hepatitis B Immune Globulin) (HBIG), which is used when there is known exposure to hepatitis B. If the mother is hepatitis-positive, the recommended regime is to give the newborn immunoglobulin within 12 hours of birth, plus the first dose of hepatitis B vaccine. If a mother is exposed to hepatitis B while breastfeeding, HBIG would not put the child at any risk via the breast milk. If the child required HBIG at the same time, it would be necessary to medicate the child directly.

Varicella Zoster Immune Globulin (VZIG) is obtained from the plasma of adult volunteer blood donors. VZIG is given during pregnancy and is also given directly to infants, so should pose no risk to the breastfed infant. As above, if there is the risk of varicella, the infant should receive a dose directly.

> **Recommendation.** Immunoglobulins are given directly to infants and are not contraindicated during lactation.

References

American Academy of Pediatrics. 2006 Report of Committee on Infectious Diseases, 27 edn, p. 124. Am. Acad. Ped. Elkgrove Village, IL.

Heyne K. Paralytic poliomyelitis following vaccination contact in the 1st trimenon of an infant {in German). Med Welt 1977; 28: 1439–41.

Isacson P, Kehrer AF, Wilson H et al. Comparative study of life, attenuated rubella virus vaccines during the immediate puerperium. Obstet Gynecol 1971; 31: 332–7.

Landes RD, Bass JW, Millunchick EW et al. Neonatal rubella following postpartum maternal immunization. J Pediatr 1981; 98: 668–9.

Losonsky GA, Fishaut JM, Strussenberg J et al. Effect of immunization against rubella on lactation products. I. Development and characterization of specific immunologic reactivity in breast milk. J Infect Dis 1982; 145: 654–60.

Mertens T, Schürmann W, Gruppenbacher J et al. Problems of life virus vaccine associated poliomyelitis. Med Microbiol Immunol 1983; 172: 13–21.

Shahid NS, Steinhoff MC, Hogue SS et al. Serum, breast milk, and infant antibody after maternal immunisation with pneumococcal vaccine. Lancet 1995; 346: 1252–7.

Shahid NS, Steinhoff MC, Roy E et al. Placental and breast transfer of antibodies after maternal immunization with polysaccharide meningococcal vaccine: a randomized, controlled evaluation. Vaccine 2002; 20: 2404–9.

4

Lactation

4.5 Vaccines and immunoglobulins

Cardiovascular drugs and diuretics

4.6

Christof Schaefer

4.6.1   β-receptor blockers

Experience

Circulatory symptoms and hypoglycemia have been cited from time to time in connection with the intake of β-receptor blockers via mother's milk. In contrast to the experience with subpartu administration, such an effect is not very probable. Nevertheless, *acebutolol*, *atenolol*, and *sotalol* should be viewed critically because the low protein binding and primarily renal excretion allow for the possibility of a significant transfer to the baby and an accumulation in young (immature) infants.

Symptoms of β-blockade, such as hypotension, bradycardia, and transient tachypnea, were seen in connection with *acebutolol*. Mathematically speaking, the baby had received about 5–10% of the maternal dosage per kg of bodyweight (Boutroy 1986). The active metabolite, *diacetolol* in particular, accumulates in the mother's milk with unusually high M/P quotients of up to 25.

With 100 mg daily, up to 2.1 mg/l *atenolol* was measured in the mother's milk; the M/P quotients were calculated to be 1.1–6.8. Up to 19% of the adult weight-related dosage can be absorbed by the infant (survey by Bennett 1996). In one case, 3 mg/kg, equivalent to 180% of the adult dosage, was reported. The affected infant had to be hospitalized because of bradycardia, cyanosis, and hypothermia (Schimmel 1989). It is not clear whether, in this case, there had been an (accidental) direct administration of the medication.

The relative dosage of *betaxolol* transmitted by the milk reaches a maximum of 4.3% (Morselli 1990).

Following a single dose of 400 mg *dilevalol*, there was a maximum of 155 μg of the active ingredient (including the relevant metabolites) per liter of milk; this would represent 0.35% of the weight-related maternal dosage (Radwanski 1988).

Labetalol is both an α- and a β-receptor blocker. With ongoing treatment with 300–1200 mg daily, a maximum mother's milk concentration of 0.7 mg/l and an M/P ratio between 0.2 and 1.5 were reported. Thus, an infant would get, at most, 0.1 mg/kg daily. This represents 0.3% of the maternal dosage per kg bodyweight (survey by Bennett 1996).

The transfer of *mepindolol* can represent 5% of the maternal weight-related dosage (survey by Bennett 1996).

With long-term therapy using 100–200 mg *metoprolol*, a maximum of 0.7 mg/l in milk was measured. The M/P ratio is 3. Nevertheless, the daily dosage the infant takes in is, at most, 0.1 mg/kg. This represents 3.2% of the maternal weight-related dosage. About 10% of the northern European population is thought to metabolize metoprolol slowly. This could be the reason why a plasma concentration of 45 μg/l was measured in one (symptom-free) infant. Among the other breastfed infants, it was 0.5–3 μg/l (survey by Bennett 1996). The therapeutic level for adults is between 93 and 881 μg/l.

Up to 5% of the maternal weight-related dosage of *nadolol* can be transmitted to the baby (survey by Bennett 1996).

With *oxprenolol*, up to 1.5% of the maternal weight-related dosage is transmitted.

With *propranolol* treatment, this is 0.4% at most (survey by Bennett 1996).

Sotalol is described in section 4.6.10, on antiarrhythmics.

With oral use of *timolol*, the portion of the maternal weight-related dose that is transmitted is 3.3% (Fidler 1983). Timolol is also used as eye drops in glaucoma treatment. With this usage, concentrations in mother's milk are limited. If the mother takes 0.5 mg as eye drops daily, the infant receives a maximum of 0.8 μg/kg daily (Lustgarten 1983).

There are insufficient data on *alprenolol, bisoprolol, bopindolol, bupranolol, carteolol, carazolol, carvedilol, celiprolol, metipranolol, nebivolol, penbutolol, pindolol, talinolol*, and *tertatolol* to make a judgment.

> **Recommendation.** The following β-receptor blockers are preferred: metoprolol, oxprenolol, propranolol (mostly used for tachycardial arrhythmia), timolol (as eye drops), and labetalol. If another β-receptor blocker has been taken, there is no need to limit the breastfeeding, but the medication should be changed.

4.6.2   Hydralazine

Experience

With 150 mg daily of *hydralazine*, a maximum of 130 μg/l was measured in the milk – which is 20 μg/kg per day or 1% of the therapeutic dosage for an infant (Liedholm 1982). Following parenteral administration of 10–40 mg, an average of 47 μg/l, including the hydrazone metabolites, was measured in the mother's milk. The M/P ratio is 0.5. Up to 108 μg/l was found in the plasma of breastfed infants (Lamont 1986). By comparison, the plasma concentration in an infant being treated with 2 mg/kg was given as 1700 μg/l. No toxic symptoms have been observed while breastfeeding. *Dihydralazine* can be evaluated similarly.

> **Recommendation.** Hydralazine and dihydralazine are among the antihypertensives of choice during breastfeeding.

4.6.3   α-methyldopa

Experience

With daily treatment of 250–2000 mg α-*methyldopa*, up to 1.14 mg/l was measured in the milk. The M/P ratio is 0.2–0.5. This works out at a daily dosage of 0.17 mg/kg for the infant, which represents 3.2% of the maternal weight-related dosage (survey in Bennett 1996).

Only with one of three infants was the medication measurable in the plasma (90 µg/l). For the mother, it was 4250 µg/l. No toxic symptoms were observed in the infant. α-methyldopa can promote milk production as a result of increased prolactin secretion.

> **Recommendation.** α-methyldopa is among the antihypertensives of choice during breastfeeding.

4.6.4   Calcium antagonists

Experience

Among 11 mothers, only limited amounts of *nicardipine* were found in their milk under steady-state conditions (Jarreau 2000).

With *nifedipine* and its active pyridine metabolites, a maximum of 2–10 µg/kg daily is transmitted to the infant when the mother takes 30–90 mg a day. That is less than 5% of a weight-related child's dose. Average values of 2% and less are probably even more realistic (Murray 1992, Manninen 1991, Ehrenkranz 1989, Penny 1989). Nifedipin is also used successfully to treat Raynaud phenomenon of the breast nipple. Anderson (2004) reports on 12 breastfeeding women complaining of pain in the nipple, which was finally diagnosed as Raynaud phenomenon. Those choosing nifedipin therapy instantly improved. Of the 12 women, 8 had been treated with antimycotics previously because of suspected mycosis.

With 6 × 60 mg of *nimodipine*, maximum concentrations of 3.5 µg/l were described in the mother's milk (Tonks 1995). Mathematically, this would be only 0.01% of the weight-related maternal dosage. A further case study confirms this limited transfer of nimodipine (Carcas 1996).

With *nitrendipine*, a maximum relative dosage of 0.6%, including its metabolites, can reach the infant (White 1989).

Among breastfed infants, no intolerance to the calcium antagonists mentioned has been reported.

Verapamil and *diltiazem* are covered in section 4.6.10, on antiarrhythmics.

There is insufficient documented experience with *amlodipine, felodipine, flunarizine, gallopamil, isradipine, lacidipine, lercanidipine, nilvadipine,* and *nisoldipine.*

> **Recommendation.** Diltiazem, nifedipine, nitrendipine, and verapamil are the calcium antagonists of choice during breastfeeding. The results with nicardipine and nimodipine do not suggest any risk. Individual doses of other calcium antagonists do not require limitation of breastfeeding, but therapy should be changed.

4

Lactation

4.6 Cardiovascular drugs and diuretics

4.6.5   ACE inhibitors

Experience

With a daily dosage of 20 mg of *benazepril*, a maximum of 0.003 µg, including the active metabolite *benazeprilate*, was measured per liter of milk. For a breastfed baby, this represents 0.00014% of the maternal weight-related dosage (Kaiser 1989).

With 300 mg daily of *captopril*, 4.7 µg/l milk was found. The M/P ratio is 0.03. The infant received up to 0.7 µg/kg per day, which represents about 0.014% of the maternal weight-related dosage (Delvin 1981).

Enalapril can be evaluated similarly. The relative dosage for the baby is about 0.1% (Rush 1991, Redman 1990, Huttunen 1989). In contrast to the maternal serum, there was no lowering of the angiotensin-converting enzyme observed in milk samples (Huttunen 1989). No undesirable effects on the infant were described.

Quinapril could not be detected in the milk of six mothers. Based on the detection limit, a maximal relative dosage of 1.6% could have occurred (Begg 2001).

There are insufficient data on *cilazapril, fosinopril, imidapril, lisinopril, moexipril, perindopril, ramipril, spirapril*, and *trandolapril* to evaluate them.

Following the use of ACE inhibitors in late pregnancy, kidney function disturbances as extreme as anuria requiring dialysis were seen in the newborn (Schubiger 1988), but this was not seen during breastfeeding. Thus, the American Academy of Pediatrics considers the use of those ACE inhibitors that have been tested for a long time to be acceptable during breastfeeding.

> **Recommendation.** Those ACE inhibitors that have been in long use, such as captopril, enalapril, and benazepril, can be used during breastfeeding when the antihypertensives of first choice are not effective or not indicated. As a safety measure, attention should be paid to edema and a possible increase in the infant's weight as indicators for disturbed kidney function. Accidental prescribing of another ACE inhibitor does not require limiting breastfeeding, but the therapy should be changed.

4.6.6   Angiotensin-II receptor-antagonists

Experience

There is insufficient experience of the use of *candesartan, eprosartan, irbesartan, losartan, olmesartan, telmisartan*, and *valsartan* during breastfeeding.

> **Recommendation.** Angiotensin-II receptor-antagonists should be avoided during breastfeeding. The accidental administration of single dosages does not require weaning. However, therapy should be changed to those antihypertensives which have been better studied during breastfeeding.

4.6.7   Other antihypertensives

Experience

With long-term *clonidine* therapy using 240–290 µg/d, up to 2.8 µg/l of milk was measured. For the infant, this means a maximum of 8% of the weight-related maternal dosage. With 0.3–0.6 µg/l in the infant's plasma, a near-therapeutic concentration was reached (Hartikainen-Sorri 1987). In another study involving ongoing therapy with 75 µg daily, a maximum of 7% was measured for the fully breastfed infant in whose plasma no active ingredient could be detected (<0.096 µg/ml). There was 0.6 µg/l in the milk and 0.33 µg/l in the maternal plasma (Bunjes 1993). No undesirable effects, such as a drop in blood pressure, have been described in the cases documented to date.

Five percent of the weight-related dose of *minoxidil* can be transferred via breast milk. The affected infant showed no symptoms (Valdivieso 1985).

With *prazosin*, this was a maximum of 3% in the mother–child pair studied (manufacturer's report).

Following daily administration of 200 µg of *moxonidine* during the first postpartum days, a maximum of 2.7 µg/l was measured in the milk of five mothers. Mathematically, that was 12% of the maternal weight-related dosage for a fully breastfed infant. The M/P ratio was estimated at 1–2 (cited in Schaefer 1998).

There are no data on the passage of *reserpine* into the mother's milk. The half-life of several days encourages accumulation. Due to the sympatholytic action of this substance, the amount of milk may increase. Earlier reports of inhibited nasal breathing, bronchial hypersecretion, sedation, and diarrhea as the effects of resepine on breastfed infants could not be confirmed. For this reason, the American Academy of Pediatrics does not object to this preparation. Meanwhile, it has, for the most part, been displaced by other medications.

There is no experience with *bunazosin, cicletanine, diazoxide, diisopropylamine, doxazosin, guanabenz, guanethidin, guanfacine, indoramin, terazosin,* and *urapidil*.

> **Recommendation.** Those antihypertensives mentioned in this section should not be taken while breastfeeding. If treatment has begun then

4

Lactation

4.6 Cardiovascular drugs and diuretics

weaning is not necessary, but the therapy should be changed to the antihypertensives of choice, including an acceptable calcium antagonist or, if really indicated, an ACE inhibitor with low transfer dosage via breast milk.

4.6.8   Dihydroergotamine and other antihypotensives

Experience

Dihydroergotamine could not be detected in mother's milk. Generally speaking, ergotamine derivatives, as prolactin inhibitors, could inhibit the milk production. There is insufficient experience with the antihypotonics, *etilefrine* and *norfenefrine*, as well as with *amezinium*, *gepefrin*, *midodrin*, and *pholedrin*.

Recommendation. The use of dihydroergotamine during breastfeeding is considered safe. However, non-drug measures (sports, the use of cold water and brushes, moderate coffee consumption) should be the first choice for the treatment of hypotonia. Etilefrine and norfenefrine, as well as amezinium, gepefrin, midodrin, and pholedrin, should be avoided. However, accidental intake does not require interruption of breastfeeding.

4.6.9   Digitalis

Experience

With ongoing therapy of 250–750 µg of *digoxin* daily (half-life about 36 hours), the mother's milk concentrations of between 0.4 and 1.9 µg/l were measured. With an M/P ratio of about 0.8, the dosage transferred to the infant was at most 0.3 µg/kg per day (the therapeutic maintenance dosage in children is 10 µg/kg per day).

No digoxin was measurable in the infant's plasma when the mother took 250 µg a day regularly; with 750 µg daily there was 0.2 µg/l in the infant's plasma (therapeutic level 0.5–2 µg/l; survey by Bennett 1996).

There are no data on *digitoxin*.

Recommendation. Digoxin, acetyldigoxin, and methyldigoxin are no cause for concern during breastfeeding.

4.6.10   Antiarrhythmics

Experience

Antiarrhythmics, for which documented experience is available, will be discussed below according to their classification (see also Chapter 2.8).

Class IA

With daily administration of 1800 mg of *quinidine*, a maximum of 9 mg/l was measured in the milk. For a fully breastfed infant, this was up to 1.3 mg/kg daily, or about 4% of the maternal weight-related dosage. The M/P ratio is 0.9. Despite possible accumulation due to the infant's delayed metabolization, the American Academy of Pediatrics sees no cause for concern in using it during breastfeeding. There are no case reports on symptoms in breastfed children.

With *disopyramide*, apparently up to 15% of the maternal weight-related dosage can be taken in by the infant. Between 0.1 and 0.5 mg/l was measured in the plasma of one of the affected children; the therapeutic level for adults is above 3 mg/l. No symptoms were described in breastfed children (survey by Bennett 1996). After a single dose of 100 mg, 3% of the maternal weight-related dosage was calculated for the child (Wakaumi 2004).

With treatment using 2000 mg of *procainamide*, up to 10.2 mg/l as well as an additional 5.0 mg/l of the active metabolite *N-acetylprocainamide* were found in the milk. Based on this, a fully breastfed infant would get up to 1.5 mg/kg of procainamide and 0.75 mg/kg of acetylprocainamide (Pittard 1983). The active total ingredient would then represent 6.8% of the maternal dosage per kg bodyweight. With newborns, the half-life is extended to 13 hours. No symptoms were observed.

Class IB

Following intravenous administration of about 1000 mg *lidocaine*, and the resulting therapeutic plasma concentration in the mother of 5 μg/ml, a transfer of 1.8% of the weight-related dosage was observed (Zeisler 1986). A similar proportion was calculated following administration as a local anesthetic (Lebedevs 1993).

With long-term therapy using 600 mg *mexiletine* daily, a milk concentration of up to 0.96 mg/l was demonstrated among the mothers studied. This represents an exposure of 0.14 mg/kg daily, or 1.4% of the maternal weight-related dosage, for the infant. Mexiletine could not be detected in the infant's plasma (Lewis 1981). Another case study describes an infant, who had already been exposed prenatally, with growth disturbances and a questionable seizure 5 months after weaning; the development which followed was unremarkable (Lownes 1987). A causal association with exposure via mother's milk is not likely.

For *phenytoin*, see Chapter 4.8.

After a single dosage of 500 mg *pilsicainid*, 7% of the maternal weight-related dosage was calculated for the child (Wakaumi 2004).

Little is known about *tocainide*, with an M/P ratio of about 2 (Wilson 1988).

▶ **Class IC**

Flecainide was found in the milk of several test subjects in long-term treatment with 2×100 mg daily, at concentrations of 0.27–1.53 μg/ml (McQuinn 1990, Wagner 1990). Based on the highest value, an infant could get just about 7% of the maternal weight-related dosage. The American Academy of Pediatrics does not have any objection to the use of this drug (which is also used therapeutically in newborns) in breastfeeding.

Eighty-three percent of *propafenon* in maternal plasma is protein-bound. After a single dose of 150 mg *propafenon*, an M/P ratio of <1 and a weight-related dosage of 0.1% for the child were calculated (Wakaumi 2004).

▶ **Class II**

For β-receptor blockers, see section 4.6.1.

▶ **Class III**

Amiodarone has a very long half-life of 2–4 weeks. It consists of just about 40% iodide (see Chapter 4.11). With long-term therapy using 400 mg/daily, a maximum of 16.4 mg/l plus 6.5 mg/l of the metabolite *desethylamiodarone* (DA) was measured (survey by Bennett 1996). Based on this, the total amount of active substance, including the desethylamiodarone, that an infant could receive would be a maximum of 3.5 mg/kg daily, or 51.5% of the maternal weight-related dosage. Up to 0.4 mg/l was found in the infant's plasma (therapeutic level is 1.0–2.7 mg/l). In later studies, lower concentrations of amiodarone plus DA were measured in the mother's milk (up to 5 mg/l) and the infant's plasma (up to 0.15 mg/l) (Moretti 1995, Plomp 1992).

With *sotalol*, which has an M/P ratio of 3–5, an infant can get 20–40% of the maternal weight-related dosage – that is, up to 3 mg/kg daily (Hackett 1990, Wagner 1990).

There is one publication on *bretylium* treatment with an unremarkable infant (Gutgesell 1990).

4

Class IV

With ongoing treatment using 240–360 mg *verapamil* daily, up to 0.3 mg/l was measured in the milk. The M/P ratio lies between 0.2 and 0.9. The amount taken in by the infant daily was given as a maximum of 0.05 mg/kg. This represents about 1% of the maternal dosage per kg of bodyweight. A concentration of 2.1 μg/l was found in the plasma of one of the breastfed infants. No side effects were described (survey by Bennett 1996).

For *diltiazem*, the results were similar to those of verapamil (Okada 1985).

Adenosine cannot be classified in any of the classic antiarrhythmic groups. Because of its extremely short half-life, and the very brief time for which it is used, it should not be considered a cause for concern during breastfeeding.

Ajmaline, *aprindine*, *detajmium*, *ibutilide*, and *prajmalium* have not been sufficiently studied during breastfeeding to comment on their safety.

Lactation

Recommendation. In the class of IA antiarrhythmics, quinidine is preferable to ajmaline, detajmium, disopyramid, prajmalium, and procainamide.

Among the class IB drugs, lidocaine, mexiletine, tocainide, and, in some cases, phenytoin are acceptable.

In the class IC, flecainide is the drug of choice.

Within class II (β-receptor blockers), propranolol and metoprolol should be considered the drugs of choice (see section 4.6.1).

Within class III, if treatment is absolutely necessary, sotalol is preferable to the iodine-containing amiodarone.

The class IV drugs verapamil and diltiazem are well-tolerated during breastfeeding. The same can be assumed of adenosine.

If treatment has begun with an antiarrhythmic which is not recommended, weaning is not necessarily required. However, if possible, the therapy should be changed. Otherwise it must be decided on an individual basis whether exclusive breastfeeding can continue while observing the baby carefully, or whether breastfeeding should be limited.

4.6 Cardiovascular drugs and diuretics

4.6.11   Diuretics

Experience

With therapy using diuretics, milk production can decrease, especially if there was already some lactational deficiency. Displacement of bilirubin from the plasma protein binding in newborns was discussed for *furosemide* and the *thiazides*. A risk of kernicterus as a result should not, however, be considered a realistic possibility (see also section 3.6).

Chlorthalidone has a half-life of 44 hours or more. Long-term treatment with 50 mg daily leads to an accumulation with values of up to 0.86 mg/l of milk. However, because of the very high maternal plasma concentration, there is an M/P ratio of only about 0.06. The maximum dosage an infant would receive would be 0.13 mg/kg daily. This represents 15.5% of the maternal weight-related dosage. No symptoms have been observed as yet in breastfed children (Mulley 1982).

Furosemide has an M/P ratio of 0.5–0.8 (Wilson 1981). There are no indications of any special intolerance in breastfed infants.

With long-term treatment using 50 mg *hydrochlorothiazide* daily, there was, at most, 0.12 mg/l milk. The dosage taken in by the infant would be 0.02 mg/kg daily – that is, 2.2% of the maternal weight-related dosage (Miller 1982).

Spironolactone is a potassium-saving diuretic. As soon as it is absorbed it is changed into the active metabolite, *canrenone*, which is up to 98% bound to plasma protein. In animal studies, canrenone is carcinogenic in very high doses; no such effect has been observed in human beings. The M/P ratio lies between 0.5 and 0.7. With ongoing treatment of 100 mg daily, a maximum milk concentration of 0.1 mg/l was found. For the infant, this would mean a daily intake of 0.016 mg/kg – 1.2% of the maternal weight-related dosage (Phelps 1977).

The carbonic anhydrase inhibitor *acetazolamide*, which is related to the thiazides and is prescribed for glaucoma therapy per os as well as in eye drops, plays a special role. Therapeutic doses of 1000 mg/daily per os led to peak values of 2.1 mg/l milk. Mathematically, this translated into 1.9% of the maternal weight-related dosage for the symptom-free infant described, in whose blood 0.2–0.6 mg/l of the active ingredient was measured (maternal plasma 5.8 mg/l) (Södermann 1984). Similar characteristics can be assumed for the eye drops *brinzolamide* and *dorzolamide*.

There are insufficient data to make a judgment on *amiloride*, *azosemide*, *bendroflumethiazide*, *bumetanide*, *butizide*, *chlorazanil*, *clopamide*, *ethacrynic acid*, *etozolin*, *indapamide*, *mefruside*, *metolazone*, *piretanide*, *polythiazide*, *torasemide*, *triamterene*, *trichlormethiazide*, and *xipamide*.

Recommendation. During breastfeeding, diuretics should not be used primarily for treating hypertonia. However, when such a drug is urgently needed, moderately dosed treatment with hydrochlorothiazide can be undertaken, with attention to the side effects described. If furosemide is indicated, this may also be prescribed. Spironolactone should be used only for special indications, such as primary hyperaldosteronism, ascites, nephrotic syndrome, and the like.

Carbonic anhydrase inhibitors for glaucoma are acceptable. Chlortalidone is contraindicated because of its accumulation, and the other drugs mentioned should not be used because of insufficient experience during breastfeeding. Single doses do not require limitation of breastfeeding, but the therapy should be changed.

4.6.12   Circulatory drugs and vasodilators

Experience

A hearing loss, or so-called sudden deafness, occasionally appears in the weeks after the birth. Therapeutically, intravenous *hydroxy ethyl starch* and other medications are prescribed that are said to promote circulation in the inner ear. None of these therapeutic measures have, as yet, been proven effective.

Naftidrofuryl and its primary metabolite *LS74* appear only in traces in the milk. Within 72 hours, only about 300 μg of the total administered 3500 mg had been excreted in the milk. With this, the infant received 0.1% of the maternal weight-related dosage per kg daily (report of the manufacturer, Lipha). There are no known toxic effects on the infant.

Pentoxifylline is a methylxanthine derivate with a more limited central stimulation and indirect sympathicomimetic action on the heart than, for instance, theophylline. Following a single oral administration of 400 mg, a maximum concentration of 1 mg/l milk, including the active metabolites, was measured (Witter 1985). Based on this, an infant would get 0.5% of the weight-related adult dosage per feed. No toxic effects have been described as yet.

There is no information on the passage into the milk of *buflomedil*, *gingko biloba*, and other drugs which are said to promote circulation. On the other hand, we have observed no toxic symptoms in the infant as a result of *gingko biloba* – a medication that is not infrequently also used during breastfeeding.

Isosorbide mononitrates, *isosorbide dinitrate*, and *glyceryl trinitrate* have been insufficiently studied with respect to breastfeeding. The short half-lives and the usually brief use argue against a toxic risk for the breastfed infant.

For low-dose *acetylsalicylic acid*, see Chapter 4.7.

There are no data on the other cardiac medications such as *amrinon*, *dipyridamole*, and *molsidomin*.

> **Recommendation.** In cases where a therapeutic effect is, in fact, expected with pentoxifyllin, naftidrofuryl, or temporary gingko biloba therapy, these seem to be acceptable. Hydroxyethyl starch, nitrate, and low-dose acetylsalicylic acid are acceptable for the appropriate indications. Other so-called circulatory stimulants should be avoided.

References

American Academy of Pediatrics, Committee on Drugs. The transfer of drugs and other chemicals into human breast milk. Pediatrics 2001; 108: 776–89.

Anderson JE, Held N, Wright K. Raynaud's phenomenon of the nipple: a treatable cause of painful breastfeeding. Pediatrics 2004; 113: 360–64.

Begg EJ, Robson RA, Gardiner SJ et al. Quinapril and its metabolite quinaprilat in human milk. Br J Clin Pharmacol 2001; 51: 478–81.

Bennett PN (ed.). Drugs and Human Lactation, 2nd edn. Amsterdam: Elsevier, 1996.

Boutroy MJ, Bianchetti G, Dubruc C et al. To nurse when receiving acebutolol: is it dangerous for the neonate? Eur J Clin Pharmacol 1986; 30: 137–9.

Bunjes R, Schaefer C. Clonidine and breast-feeding. Clin Pharm 1993; 12: 178–9.

Carcas AJ, Abad-Santos F, de Rosendo JM et al. Nimodipine transfer into human breast milk and cerebrospinal fluid. Ann Pharmacother 1996; 30: 148–50.

Devlin RG, Fleiss PN. Captopril in human blood and breast milk. J Clin Pharmacol 1981; 21: 110–13.

Ehrenkranz RA, Ackermann BA, Hulse JD. Nifedipine transfer into human milk. J Pediatr 1989; 114: 478–80.

Fidler J, Smith V, de Sweet M. Excretion of oxprenolol and timolol in breast milk. Br J Obstet Gynaecol 1983; 90: 961–5.

Gutgesell M, Overholt E, Boyle R. Oral bretylium tosylate use during pregnancy and subsequent breastfeeding: a case report. Am J Perinatol 1990; 7: 144–5.

Hackett LP, Wojnar-Horton RE, Dusci LJ et al. Excretion of sotalol in breast milk. Br J Clin Pharmacol 1990; 29: 277–8.

Hartikainen-Sorri AL, Heikkinen JE, Koivisto M. Pharmacokinetics of clonidine during pregnancy and nursing. Obstet Gynecol 1987; 69: 598–600.

Huttunen K, Gronhagen-Riska C, Fyhrquist F. Enalapril treatment of a nursing mother with slightly impaired renal function. Clin Nephrol 1989; 31: 278.

Jarreau PH, le Beller C, Guillonneau M et al. Excretion of nicardipine in human milk. Paediatr Perinat Drug Ther 2000; 4: 28–30.

Kaiser G, Ackermann R, Dieterle W et al. Benazepril and benazeprilat in human plasma and breast milk. IV World Conference on Clinical Pharmacology and Therapeutics, July 1989.

Lamont RE, Elder MG. Transfer of hydralazine across the placenta and into breast milk. J Obstet Gynaecol 1986; 7: 47–8.

Lebedevs TH, Wojnar-Horton RE, Yapp P et al. Excretion of lignocaine and its metabolite monoethylglgly-cinexylidide in breast milk following its use in a dental procedure. A case report. J Clin Periodontol 1993; 20: 606–8.

Lewis AM, Johnston A, Patel L et al. Mexiletine in human blood and breast milk. Postgrad Med J 1981; 57: 546–7.

Liedholm H, Wahlin-Boll E, Hansson A et al. Transplacental passage and breast milk concentrations of hydralazine. Eur J Clin Pharmacol 1982; 21: 417–19.

Lownes HE, Ives TJ. Mexiletine use in pregnancy and lactation. Am J Obstet Gynecol 1987; 157: 446–7.

Lustgarten JS, Podos SM. Topical timolol and the nursing mother. Arch Ophthalmol 1983; 101: 1381–2.

Manninen AK, Juhakoski A. Nifedipine concentrations in maternal and umbilical serum, amniotic fluid, breast milk and urine of mothers and offspring. Intl J Clin Pharmacol Res 1991; 11: 231–6.

McQuinn RL, Pisani A, Wafa S et al. Flecainide excretion in human breast milk. Clin Pharmacol Ther 1990; 48: 262–7.

Miller ME, Cohn RD, Burghart PH. Hydrochlorothiazide disposition in a mother and her breast-fed infant. J Pediatr 1982; 101: 789–91.

Moretti M. Presentation of the 8th International Conference of the Organisation of Teratogen Information Specialists (OTIS) 1995, San Diego, USA.

Morselli PL, Boutroy MJ, Bianchetti G et al. Placental transfer and perinatal pharmacokinetics of betaxolol. Eur J Clin Pharmacol 1990; 38: 477–83.

Mulley BA, Parr GD, Pau WK et al. Placental transfer of chlortalidone and its elimination in maternal milk. Eur J Clin Pharmacol 1982; 13: 129–31.

Murray C, Haverkamp AD, Orleans M et al. Nifedipine for treatment of preterm labor: a historic prospective study. Am J Obstet Gynecol 1992; 167: 52–6.

Okada M, Inoue H, Nakamura Y et al. Excretion of diltiazem in human milk. N Engl J Med 1985; 312: 992–3.

Penny WJ, Lewis MJ. Nifedipine is excreted in human milk. Eur J Clin Pharmacol 1989; 36: 427–8.

Phelps DL, Karim A. Spironolactone: relationship between concentrations of dethioacetylated metabolite in human serum and milk. J Pharm Sci 1977; 66: 1203.

Pittard WB III, Glazier H. Procainamide excretion in human milk. J Pediatr 1983; 102: 631–3.

Plomp TA, Vulsma T, de Vijlder JJM. Use of amiodarone during pregnancy. Eur J Obstet Gynecol Reprod Biol 1992; 43: 201–7.

Radwanski E, Nagabhushan N, Affrime MB et al. Secretion of dilevalol in breast milk. J Clin Pharmacol 1988; 28: 448–53.

Redman CW, Kelly JG, Cooper WD. The excretion of enalapril and enalaprilat in human breast milk. Eur J Clin Pharmacol 1990; 38: 99.

Rush JE, Snyder BA, Barrish A et al. Comment Clin Nephrol 1991; 35: 234.

Schaefer HG, Toublanc N, Weimann HJ. The pharmacokinetics of moxonidine. Rev Contemp Pharmacother 1998; 9: 481–90.

Schimmel MS, Wilschanski MA, Shaw Jr D et al. Toxic effects of atenolol consumed during breast feeding. J Pediatr 1989; 114: 476–8.

Schubiger G, Flury G, Nussberger J. Enalapril for pregnancy induced hypertension: acute renal failure in a neonate. Ann Int Med 1988; 108: 215–16.

Södermann P, Hartvig P, Fagerlund C. Acetazolamide excretion into human breast milk. Br J Clin Pharmacol 1984; 17: 599–600.

Tonks AM. Nimodipine levels in breast milk. Aust NZ J Surg 1995; 65: 693–4.

Valdivieso A, Valdes G, Spiro TE et al. Minoxidil in breast milk. Ann Int Med 1985; 102: 135.

4

Lactation

4.6 Cardiovascular drugs and diuretics

Wagner X, Jouglard J, Moulin M et al. Coadministration of flecainide acetate and soltalol during pregnancy: lack of teratogenic effects, passage across the placenta, and excretion into human breast milk. Am Heart J 1990; 119: 700–702.

Wakaumi M, Tsuruoka S, Sakamoto K et al. Pilsicainide in breast milk from a mother: comparison with disopyramide and propafenone. Br J Clin Pharmacol 2004; 59: 120–22.

White WB, Yeh SC, Krol GJ. Nitrendipine in human plasma and breast milk. Eur J Clin Pharmacol 1989; 36: 531–4.

Wilson JT. Drugs in Breast Milk. New York: ADIS Health Science Press, 1981.

Wilson JH. Breast milk tocainide levels. J Cardiovasc Pharmacol 1988; 12: 497.

Witter FR, Smith RV. The excretion of pentoxyfylline and its metabolites into human breast milk. Am J Obstet Gynecol 1985; 151: 1094–7.

Zeisler JA, Gaarder TD, de Mesquita SA. Lidocaine excretion in breast milk. Drug Intell Clin Pharmacol 1986; 20: 691–3.

Anticoagulants and fibrinolytics

4.7

Christof Schaefer

4.7.1   Heparin

Experience

Due to its molecular mass, heparin is not detectable in mother's milk. Furthermore, it is not absorbed in relevant quantities in the gastrointestinal tract. This would also be expected for the low molecular-weight preparations *certoparin, dalteparin, enoxaparin, nadroparin, reviparin*, and *tinzaparin*. Fifteen women who received 2500 IU dalteparin daily after cesarean section were studied with respect to factor anti-Xa activity in serum and milk as indicators for heparin effects. The M/P ratio for factor anti-Xa activity was calculated as < 0.025–0.2. Based on the peak value in milk (0.037 IU/ml) the authors found that, at maximum, 5% of the weight-adjusted anti-Xa activity is transferred via breastmilk, on day 5, to a child that drinks 250 ml. However, because there is no quantitative resorption via the intestine, an anticoagulative effect is not expected (Richter 2001).

Recommendation. Breastfeeding may continue during treatment with heparins, including low molecular-weight heparins.

4.7.2   Vitamin K antagonists (coumarin derivatives and indanediones)

Experience

Acenocoumarol, phenprocoumon, and *warfarin* are the coumarin derivatives used as oral anticoagulants; *fluindione* and *phenindione* belong to the group of *indanediones* with vitamin K antagonistic effects. The most widely used substances (warfarin, phenprocoumon, and acenocoumarol) have a very high protein binding (>95%), and thus only very small amounts would be expected in the mother's milk.

Acenocoumarol and *warfarin* could not be detected in the milk at all (survey in Bennett 1996). In women who were treated with phenprocoumon, $33\,\mu g/l$ of milk was measured and an intake of $5-6\,\mu g/kg$ per day was calculated for the infant (von Kries 1993). This is about 10% of an adult maintenance dosage.

No changes in the coagulation parameters have as yet been detected in infants who were being breastfed during their mothers' treatment with these oral anticoagulants (Bennett 1996, Fondevila 1989, personal observations), nor would this be expected.

In contrast, only about 70% of *phenindione* is protein-bound, and a higher transfer with a therapeutic dosage for an infant has been shown. A case description refers to a breastfed baby with pathological coagulation parameters and hematomas during the mother's treatment (survey in Bennett 1996).

Recommendation. During treatment with the oral anticoagulants aceno-coumarol, phenprocoumon, and warfarin, breastfeeding may continue. To be on the safe side, the infant should receive 1 mg vitamin K orally, two to three times a week, in the first 4 weeks of life. To avoid any possible complications, the coagulation status should be determined after about 10–14 days, at least with premature infants. Fluindone and phenidone are contraindicated.

4.7.3   Other anticoagulants

Experience

Low-dose *acetylsalicylic acid* (80–300 mg daily) is widely used to inhibit thrombocyte aggregation, and is well-tolerated during breastfeeding.

There was no factor anti-Xa activity identified in three milk samples while the mother was on *danaparoid* treatment (Lindhoff-Last

2005, Myers 2003). There are no data on the other hirudin derivative, *desirudin*. These medications are used when heparin is not tolerated – for example, in cases of heparin-induced thrombocytopenia
(HIT). Theoretically, no problems for the breastfed infant should be
expected.

There is a case study on *lepirudine* in which a breastfeeding mother
who could not tolerate heparin received 50 mg of this *hirudin* derivative subcutaneously, twice a day, for 3 months. The maternal plasma
showed 0.73 mg/l, a therapeutic concentration, and virtually no
hirudin was detected in the milk (<0.1 mg/l). The breastfed child had
no symptoms (Lindhoff-Last 2000).

The direct thrombin inhibitor *ximelagatran* was studied in seven
mothers who received 36 mg as a single dose. Only 0.0009% of the
total dose (no ximelagatran, but the active metabolite *melagatran*)
was found in the milk within 72 hours (Hellgren 2004). Based on
the peak concentrations 2 hours after administration, a relative
dose of less than 1% is calculated for the fully breastfed child.

There is insufficient experience for *argatroban, clopidogrel*, and
ticlopidine during breastfeeding.

> **Recommendation.** Low-dose acetylsalicylic acid is the thrombocyte
> aggregation inhibitor of choice. In cases where danaparoid, desirudin, lep-
> irudin or ximelagatran are indicated, weaning does not seem to be justified.

4.7.4   Fibrinolytics

Experience

Streptokinase is neither detectable in the mother's milk, nor
absorbed in relevant quantities from the gastrointestinal tract. This
can also be assumed for the other direct and indirect fibrinolytics,
alteplase, reteplase, and *urokinase*.

> **Recommendation.** Breastfeeding may continue after using fibrinolytics.

References

Bennett PN (ed.). Drugs and Human Lactation, 2nd edn. Amsterdam: Elsevier, 1996.
Fondevila CG, Meschengieser S, Blanco A et al. Effect of acenocoumarine on the
  breastfed infant. Thromb Res 1989; 56: 29–36.

Hellgren M, Johansson S, Eriksson UG et al. The oral direct thrombin inhibitor, xime-lagatran, an alternative for anticoagulant treatment during the puerperium and lactation. Br J Obstet Gynaecol 2004; 112: 579–83.

Lindhoff-Last E, Willeke A, Thalhammer C et al. Hirudin treatment in a breastfeeding woman. Lancet 2000; 355: 467.

Lindhoff-Last E, Kreutzenbeck HJ, Magnani HN. Treatment of 51 pregnancies with danaparoid because of heparin intolerance. Thromb Haemost 2005; 93: 63–9.

Myers B, Westby J, Strong J. Prophylactic use of danaparoid in high-risk pregnancy with heparin-induced thrombocytopaenia-positive skin reaction. Blood Coagul Fibrinolysis 2003; 14: 485–7.

Richter C, Sitzmann J, Lang P et al. Excretion of low molecular weight heparin in human milk. Br J Clin Pharmacol 2001; 52: 708–10.

von Kries R, Nöcker D, Schmitz-Kummer E et al. Transfer of phenprocoumon in breast milk. Is oral anticoagulation with phenprocoumon a contraindication for breastfeeding? [in German]. Monatsschr Kinderheilkd 1993; 141: 505–7.

Antiepileptics

Christof Schaefer

4.8

All anticonvulsants pass into the milk, albeit in differing amounts. With monotherapy, breastfeeding is, in most cases, acceptable. In principle, the lower protein binding of newer antiepileptics may facilitate drug transfer to the breast milk.

If treatment with more than one anticonvulsant is required, supplementation or weaning may be necessary to limit the exposure. This must be decided individually.

For a discussion of expanded vitamin-K prophylaxis in the newborn period, see Chapter 2.10.

In this chapter, sections 4.8.1–7 discuss the classical antiepileptic drugs, while sections 4.8.8–15 concentrate on the newer antiepileptics.

4.8.1 Carbamazepine

Carbamazepine has a half-life of 15–35 hours in both adults and newborns, and 75% is protein bound. Studies on more than 50 milk samples show M/P quotients of about 0.5. Including the metabolite *carbamazepinepoxide*, a relative dosage of not more than 3–8% should be expected. However, in one case with a maternal dosage of only 250 mg daily, the relative dosage was about 15% (Shimoyama 2000). Serum concentrations of between 0.5 and 1.5 µg/ml were measured in breastfed children; however, in one case this reached 4.7 µg/ml (therapeutic range 5–10 µg/ml) (survey in Hägg 2000, Shimoyama 2000, Brent 1998, Wisner 1998). Some case reports describe transient toxic liver changes in infants exposed prenatally and via mother's milk (Frey 2002, Merlob 1992). Another case report describes an infant, whose mother was taking not only carbamazepine but also flouxetine and buspirone, who suffered a questionable seizure and a cyanotic attack. Further development of the baby was normal through to the end of the first year of life. The authors, quite correctly, hesitate to make a connection between the medication and the symptoms (Brent 1998). Another infant had feeding difficulties and was sedated. Its mother took an anticonvulsive combination therapy with carbamazepine plus phenytoin and barbiturates (survey in Hägg 2000). Further symptoms have not been published, as yet.

For recommendations, see section 4.8.7.

4.8.2 Clobazam and clonazepam

For *clobazam*, see Chapter 4.9. The half-life of *clonazepam* is 20–40 hours. Only 60% is protein-bound. In the serum of one child, 4.7 µg/l could be measured; in the mother it was between 15 and 30 µg/l

(Söderman 1988). The serum of a premature infant whose mother had continuous therapy was found to contain 13 µg/l. In another study, apnea occurred repeatedly in a premature baby; this was viewed as being related to previous exposure *in utero* (survey in Hägg 2000). In a further instance, the mother regularly took 6 mg daily (plus 1400 mg carbamazepine); a level of 20 µg/l was found in the infant's serum, while the mother's serum contained 50 µg/l and her milk 12 µg/l. The baby was described as "somewhat lazy at the breast" and tired (personal observation).

For recommendations, see section 4.8.7.

4.8.3   Ethosuximide and mesuximide

Ethosuximide has a half-life of 55 hours. For the newborn it is between 32 and 38 hours. Only a limited amount is protein-bound. The M/P ratio is just under 1. An infant can get well over 50% of a child's dosage or the maternal weight-related dosage. This has been shown in studies on more than 10 mothers. The concentrations in the child's serum can reach 10–40 mg/l (the therapeutic range is 40–100 mg/l). Symptoms such as irritability, weak suck, and sedation have been described in individual cases (survey in Hägg 2000, Bennett 1996).

There are no data on *mesuximide*.

For recommendations, see section 4.8.7.

4.8.4   Phenobarbitone (phenobarbital), primidone, and barbexaclone

Primidone and *barbexaclone* are metabolized to *phenobarbitone*. The half-life of phenobarbitone can be up to 100 hours in both adults and mature newborns. Only 50% of the medication is bound to protein; in infants it is even less. Among more than 160 milk samples analyzed, the M/P ratio for phenobarbitone was about 0.5 and for primidone around 0.8. A fully breastfed infant could receive a significant portion of the substance – for phenobarbitone, 50% to well over 100% of the maternal weight-related dosage was calculated; for primidone up to 38%! (Pote 2004, survey in Hägg 2000, Sugawara 1999, Bennett 1996). Up to 50% of the maternal concentration can be reached in the infant's serum. Thus, sedation and resultant feeding problems seem possible, and have been described repeatedly. Among these descriptions is one of the oldest publications on toxicity via mother's milk (Frensdorf 1926). In a single mother, phenobarbitone concentrations were more or less stable around 5 µg/ml in milk specimens taken just before medication and 2.5 hours afterwards on days 6 and 19 after delivery (Pote 2004). Maternal serum concentration was also stable. The child was temporarily lethargic and needed intravenous fluid therapy. In the infant's serum, the phenobarbitone level reached 55 µg/ml – twice the mother's value. The death of a child was also discussed in connection with maternal phenobarbitone plus primidone therapy; here, 8.3 mg/l phenobarbitone, a therapeutic concentration, was found in the baby's serum (cited in Hägg 2000).

Other barbiturates should be similarly evaluated. Depending on the half-life and the dosage administered, symptoms in the infant should be expected, especially when there has been more than a single dosage and in combination with other anticonvulsants.

For recommendations, see section 4.8.7.

4.8.5   Phenytoin

Phenytoin has an M/P ratio of about 0.3. Studies of more than 80 milk samples have shown that a fully breastfed infant can get between 0.5 and 5%, with a maximum of 10%, of the maternal weight-related dosage via the mother's milk. This is normally less than 5% of a pediatric phenytoin dosage (10 mg/kg) (survey in Hägg 2000). The phenytoin concentration in the serum of affected children was, at most 1.5% of the maternal value. The half-life of 10–40 hours does not appear to be extended in infants when they have already been exposed *in utero* (Shimoyama 1998, survey in Bennett 1996). With the exception of two case observations, side effects in breastfed babies have not been reported. These two observations described swallowing difficulties and methemoglobinemia, as well as feeding problems and sedation, with anticonvulsive combination therapy using phenytoin plus barbiturates or with carbamazepine in addition (survey in Hägg 2000).

For recommendations, see section 4.8.7.

4.8.6   Valproic acid

Of all the anticonvulsants studied to date, *valproic acid* passes least into the mother's milk, with an M/P ratio of about 0.05 and a relative dosage of around 1% on average (maximum value 7%). This has been shown in more than 40 mothers studied (survey in Hägg 2000). Even so, as a result of the decidedly longer half-life of around

47 hours, a "steady state" can develop in the breastfed infant with a serum concentration of 7% (or even more) of the maternal value. However, a more recent study of six children found 0.7–1.5 µg/ml, or only 0.9–2.3% of the maternal concentrations, which were between 39 and 79 µg/ml (Piontek 2000). No symptoms have ever been observed.

For recommendations, see section 4.8.7.

4.8.7   Recommendations: classical anticonvulsants

Recommendations. Monotherapy with phenytoin, valproate or carbamazepine is compatible with breastfeeding. With carbamazepine, however, the baby should be observed for symptoms such as weak suck, vomiting, and tiredness. If these symptoms occur, the concentration of carbamazepine in the infant's serum should be measured. In suspicious cases, liver values should also be measured.

Antiepileptic therapy with the barbiturates, clonazepam and ethosuximide should be considered problematic during breastfeeding. If treatment is unavoidable, the decision to breastfeed should be made individually, and the infant should be observed for symptoms such as weak suck, vomiting, and tiredness. Where there is a suspicion of side effects, the concentration in the infant's serum should be determined and a decision taken regarding whether formula should be added to reduce drug transfer via mother's milk, or the baby should be weaned.

Anticonvulsive combination therapy with barbiturates, clonazepam or ethosuximide is not compatible with breastfeeding.

Sections 4.8.8–15 discuss the newer antiepileptic drugs (add-on antiepileptics).

4.8.8   Gabapentin

For *gabapentin*, there is published experience with more than 10 lactating mothers (Öhman 2005, Hägg 2000). The average M/P ratio is 1. Based on five mothers, Öhman (2005) calculated a relative dosage of 1.3–3.8% for the fully breastfed child. As the milk specimens were taken before drug administration, these relative dosages do not represent the maximum values. Concentrations in the infant's serum were around 12% of maternal values; no adverse effects were reported.

For recommendations, see section 4.8.15.

4.8.9   Lamotrigine

Two case reports (Rambeck 1997, Tomson 1997) and a study of
lamotrigine among nine mothers (Öhman 2000) showed an M/P
ratio of about 0.6. According to the two case reports, lamotrigine
appears to pass into the milk in significant quantities. Up to 6.5 mg/l
was found in the milk of a woman who took 300 mg daily as monotherapy. This represents a maximum relative dosage of 20%.
Concentrations of up to 2.8 mg/l were measured in the serum of the
unremarkable baby. This is not far from the lower range of the
maternal serum concentrations (3.6–9.6 mg/l). In the serum of four
children whose mothers took between 200 and 800 mg daily, levels
of <1–$2\,\mu g/ml$ were found 10 days after birth. Maternal serum concentrations were 4.6–$9.2\,\mu g/ml$. Based on three children, 20–43%
of the maternal serum concentration was reached in the infant's
blood; 2 months after birth it was 23% (Liporace 2004).

For recommendations, see section 4.8.15.

4.8.10   Levetiracetam

Substantial amounts of *levetiracetam* were measured in the milk of
a single mother ($99\,\mu g/ml$); the M/P ratio was 3 (Kramer 2002).
Based on seven mothers taking between 1500 and 3500 mg daily,
Johannessen (2005) calculated an M/P ratio of 1, which remained
stable until 10 months after birth. The relative dosage for the
infants was 7.8% at maximum. No side effects were observed in the
infants. The drug was detected in only one of the exposed children.

For recommendations, see section 4.8.15.

4.8.11   Oxcarbazepine

With long-term therapy with *oxcarbazepine* (1200 mg/d) plus *topiramate* (150 mg/d), neither oxcarbazepine nor its metabolite were
found in the blood of an unremarkable fully breastfed 2-month-old
child (detection limits 0.1 and $1.0\,\mu g/ml$, respectively) (personal
observation). In a 5-day-old fully breastfed newborn, oxcarbazepine
and its metabolite 10-hydroxy-carbazepin were measured. Compared
to the values measured directly after birth, which represented cord
blood transfer, only 12% of the drug and 7% of the metabolite were
detected on day 5 (cited in Pennell 2003).

For recommendations, see section 4.8.15.

4.8.12   Topiramate

No *topiramate*, or only a low concentration, was detected in the serum of three infants aged 2–3 weeks. At maximum, 20–30% of the maternal serum concentration was reached in the infants. No side effects were observed. The M/P ratio was 0.7–0.9, the relative dosage 3–23% (Öhman 2002).

For recommendations, see section 4.8.15.

4.8.13   Vigabatrin

Only minimal amounts of *vigabatrin* (M/P ratio about 0.3) are protein-bound in plasma. For this reason, and as a result of its limited distribution volume, a quantitatively significant transfer into the mother's milk could be expected. Nevertheless, in a study on two women who received 2000 mg daily, only about 1% of the pharmacologically active substance was shown as a relative dosage for the infant (Tran 1998).

For recommendations, see section 4.8.15.

4.8.14   Zonisamide

With 300 mg *zonisamide* daily, an average of 10.1 mg/l was measured in the maternal plasma and 9.4 mg/l in the milk. This represents an M/P ratio of just under 1. From this, an average relative dosage of 28% can be calculated (Sugawara 1999)! In a later follow-up study, three breastfed children had developed normally (Kawada 2002, Shimoyama 1999).

There is insufficient experience with the use of *felbamate*, *pregabalin*, *sultiame*, and *tiagabine* during breastfeeding.

For recommendations, see section 4.8.15.

4.8.15   Recommendations: newer antiepileptics

Recommendation. As monotherapy, new antiepileptics are compatible with breastfeeding. However, close observation of the infant is recommended regarding drugs where there has been little experience or where substantial transfer has been documented. If there are any symptoms that could be associated with maternal drug therapy, the serum concentration in the child should be measured. To limit exposure, it may be necessary to supplement with formula or cease breastfeeding. In cases of prematurity, other risks and/or antiepileptic combination therapy, an individual decision on breastfeeding must be taken.

4.8 Antiepileptics

References

Bennett PN (ed.). Drugs and Human Lactation, 2nd edn. Amsterdam: Elsevier, 1996.

Brent NB, Wisner KL. Fluoxetine and carbamazepine concentrations in a nursing mother/infant pair. Clin Pediatr (Phila) 1998; 37: 41–4.

Frensdorf W. Übergang von Luminal in die Milch. Münch Med Wschr 1926; 73: 322–3.

Frey B, Braegger CP, Ghelfi D. Neonatal cholestatic hepatitis from carbamazepine exposure during pregnancy and breast feeding. Ann Pharmacother 2002; 36: 644–7.

Hägg S, Spigset O. Anticonvulsant use during lactation. Drug Saf 2000; 22: 425–40.

Johannessen SI, Helde G, Brodtkorb E. Levetiracetam concentrations in serum and in breast milk at birth and during lactation. Epilepsia 2005; 46: 775–7.

Kawada K, Itoh S, Kusaka T et al. Pharmacokinetics of zonisamide in perinatal period. Brain Dev 2002; 24: 95–7.

Kramer G, Hosli I, Glanzmann R et al. Levetiracetam accumulation in breast milk. Epilepsia 2002; 43(Suppl 7): 105.

Liporace J, Kao A, d'Abreu A. Concerns regarding lamotrigine and breast-feeding. Epilepsy Behav 2004; 5: 102–5.

Merlob P, Mor N, Litwin A. Transient hepatic dysfunction in an infant of an epileptic mother treated with carbamazepine during pregnancy and breastfeeding. Ann Pharmacother 1992; 26: 1563–5.

Öhman I, Vitols S, Tomson T. Lamotrigine in pregnancy: pharmacokinetics during delivery, in the neonate, and during lactation. Epilepsia 2000; 41: 709–13.

Öhman I, Vitols S, Luef G et al. Topiramate kinetics during delivery, lactation, and in the neonate: preliminary observations. Epilepsia 2002; 43: 1157–60.

Öhman I, Vitols S, Tomson T. Pharmacokinetics of gabapentin during delivery, in the neonatal period, and lactation: does a fetal accumulation occur during pregnancy? Epilepsia 2005; 46: 1621–4.

Pennell PB. Antiepileptic drug pharmacokinetics during pregnancy and lactation. Neurology 2003; 61(Suppl 2): 35–42.

Piontek CM, Baab S, Peindl KS et al. Serum valproate levels in 6 breastfeeding mother-infant pairs. J Clin Psychiatry 2000; 61: 170–72.

Pote M, Kulkarni R, Agarwal M. Phenobarbital toxic levels in a nursing neonate. Indian Pediatrics 2004; 41: 963–4.

Rambeck B, Kurlemann G, Stodieck SRG et al. Concentrations of lamotrigine in a mother on lamotrigine treatment and her newborn child. Eur J Clin Pharmacol 1997; 51: 481–4.

Shimoyama R, Ohkubo T, Sugawara K et al. Monitoring of phenytoin in human breast milk, maternal plasma and cord blood plasma by solid-phase extraction and liquid chromatography. J Pharm Biomed Anal 1998; 17: 863–9.

Shimoyama R, Ohkubo T, Sugawara K. Monitoring of carbamazepine and carbamazepine 10,11-epoxide in breast milk and plasma by high-performance liquid chromatography. Ann Clin Biochem 2000; 37: 210–15.

Söderman P, Matheson I. Clonazepam in breast milk. Eur J Ped 1988; 147: 212–13.

Sugawara K, Shimoyama R, Ohkubo T. Determinations of psychotropic drugs and antiepileptic drugs by high-performance liquid chromatography and its monitoring in human breast milk. Hirosaki Med J 1999; 51(Suppl): S81–6.

Tomson T, Öhman I, Vitols S. Lamotrigine in pregnancy and lactation: a case report. Epilepsia 1997; 38: 1039–41.

Tran A, O'Mahoney T, Rey E et al. Vigabatrin: placental transfer in vivo and excretion into breast milk of the enantiomers. Br J Clin Pharmacol 1998; 45: 409–11.

Wisner KL, Perel JM. Serum levels of valproate and carbamazepine in breastfeeding mother-infant pairs. J Clin Psychopharmacol 1998; 18: 167–9.

Psychotropic drugs

Christof Schaefer

4.9

4.9.1   Antidepressants in general

Occurring with a frequency of approximately 10–15%, depression represents a significant problem after delivery. Women delivering their first child are overrepresented. The symptomatology ranges from slight depression as a reaction to the new situation and pressures after delivery, to deep depression with melancholic characteristics – or even to psychotic depression. Untreated pronounced depression can lead, just like other psychiatric illness, to a disturbance in the early mother–child relationship, and impairment of early behavioral development.

Under such circumstances, psychotherapeutic and (if necessary) psychopharmacological therapy should be considered. Apart from tricyclic antidepressants, selective serotonin reuptake inhibitors (SSRI) are predominantly used. Among tricyclics, tertiary amines with pronounced anticholinergic and sedating characteristics (*amitriptylin, imipramine, clomipramin, doxepin*) are distinguished from secondary (*desipramin, nortriptylin*) and primary (*amoxapin*) amines, where these properties are less strong. Recently, 95 women with postpartum depression were treated with either tricyclic *nortriptyline* or the SSRI *sertraline*. The proportions of women who responded and remitted did not differ between the drugs at 4, 8 or 24 weeks. The total side-effect burden of each drug was similar, although side-effect profiles differed between agents. Breastfed infant serum levels were near or below the level of quantifiability for both agents (Wisner 2006).

In so far as they have been studied, the M/P ratios of antidepressants lie between 1 and 2. However, there are considerable individual variations. For most antidepressants, only traces were detected in the serum of breastfed children. Toxic symptoms (mostly moderate) have only been observed in breastfed infants whose mothers were being treated with *citalopram, doxepin*, and *fluoxetin* (overview in Weissman 2004).

With SSRIs in particular, the highest drug concentration in the milk can be expected up to 8 hours after intake – and thus brief interruptions of breastfeeding for a few hours do not necessarily limit the baby's exposure. However, it might be advisable to take the medication after the last feed at night.

Combination therapy using several psychoactive drugs should be viewed very critically while breastfeeding. When combination therapy is unavoidable, decisions about possible limitations on breastfeeding need to be made on a case-by-case basis. Basically, accumulation in young infants under 8 weeks of age, especially in those born prematurely, cannot be ruled out under long-term medication.

Long-term effects of antidepressants used during breastfeeding have barely been studied. The WHO Working Group on Drugs and Human Lactation (Bennett 1996) classifies most of the tricyclic antidepressants and some of the SSRI as "probably safe", as does the American Academy of Pediatrics (2001).

4.9.2 Tri- and tetracyclic antidepressants

Amitriptyline

Up to 95% of *amitriptyline* is protein-bound and is rapidly metabolized to *nortriptyline*, which is also pharmacologically active. Six

4

Lactation

4.9 Psychotropic drugs

breastfeeding women taking 75–175 mg amitriptyline a day were studied (survey in Weissman 2004). The M/P ratio was 1; the relative dosage for a fully breastfed baby, including the active metabolites, should not, in light of current experience, exceed 2.5%. Amitriptyline and nortriptyline could not be detected in the infants' serum. The children had no acute clinical symptoms. Among the 10 infants breastfed while their mothers were taking tricyclic antidepressants, development in the first year of life did not differ from that of the artificially fed infants in a control group (Yoshida 1997A).

▶ **Amoxapine**

Galactorrhea was reported with a daily intake of 250 mg *amoxapine*. The patient was neither pregnant nor breastfeeding. Less than 20 μg/l amoxapine plus 140 μg/l of the metabolite *8-hydroxy-amoxapine* were excreted in the milk. An M/P ratio of about 0.3 and a relative dosage of 0.7% can be calculated with the available data (cited in Spigset 1998).

▶ **Clomipramine**

Clomipramine, half-life 32 hours, increases the prolactin levels and can stimulate lactation. The pharmacologically active metabolites are *N-desmethylclomipramine* and two hydroxy-metabolites – *8-OH-clomipramine* and *8-OH-desmethylclomipramine*. Based on seven published mother–child pairs, the average relative dosage is 1.3% (overview in Weissman 2004). After birth, 267 μg/l were measured in the plasma of an infant who had been exposed prenatally (the mother took 125 mg clomipramine a day). From the seventh day postpartum, the dosage was increased to 150 mg daily. The maternal plasma concentration rose from 355 μg/l on day 10 to 510 μg/l on day 35. The milk concentration was between 270 and 624 μg/l. In the same period of time, concentrations decreasing from 45 μg/l to 9.8 μg/l were measured in the infant's serum (this was due to the breakdown of the drug transferred prenatally). Assuming the highest value reported in the milk, the dosage for a fully breastfed baby – without considering the metabolites – would seem to be 4% of the maternal weight-related dosage (Schimmell 1991).

   In a further study, four mother–child pairs were studied. The mothers took between 75 mg and 125 mg of clomipramine daily. Milk samples were not studied. Neither clomipramine nor its metabolites (detection level 10 μg/l) could be detected in the infants' serum (Wisner 1995). A newer study showed concentrations in the milk of wo women, that were similar to those reported by Schimmell in 1991 (Yoshida 1997A). The infants did not show any signs of effects from the medication.

Desipramine

Desipramine, with a half-life ranging from 12 to 54 hours, is the pharmacologically active metabolite of *imipramine*. Up to 95% is bound to plasma protein.

On the basis of five published mother–child pairs, an average relative dose of 1.6% can be expected (overview in Weissman 2004).

In a case report, 381 µg/l were measured in the milk with a dosage of 300 mg/day. An infant would get up to 2.4% of the maternal weight-adjusted dose, when the metabolite *2-hydroxydesipramine* is included (Stancer 1986). Only slight traces (if any) of imipramine could be measured in the serum of four further examined children. The babies did not show symptoms.

Dosulepine

Dosulepine (= *dothiepin*), half-life 9 hours, is metabolized in the liver into the three pharmacologically active metabolites *nordosulepine, dosulepine sulfoxide*, and *nordosulepine sulfoxide*. One study examined eight women (Ilett 1993). In a further study, 20 breastfeeding mothers received dosulepine (Buist 1993A). The M/P ratio of dosulepine is about 1. With treatment of up to 225 mg daily, a maximum of 475 µg/l dosulepine plus 1200 µg/l of the metabolites was measured. The highest values on the same order of magnitude were reported in another study of two women (Yoshida 1997A). Based on these data, a maximum of 7% of the maternal weight-related dosage is calculated for the infant when the metabolites are included. However, on average it is below 1% (survey in Weissman 2004). For one child, only traces of the active ingredient (4 µg/l) were detected in the serum; the maternal serum level was 2623 µg/l (Yoshida 1997A). No effects were observed in the newborns. In a further study, prenatally exposed children aged 3 and 5 years were followed up. There was nothing remarkable about them compared to a non-exposed control group (Buist 1995).

Doxepin

Up to 80% of *doxepin* and its active metabolite *N-desmethyldoxepin* is bound to the plasma protein. The half-life of doxepin ranges

4

Lactation

4.9 Psychotropic drugs

from 8 to 25 hours; that of N-desmethyldoxepin is 33–81 hours. In a study of two breastfeeding mothers, one of whom received 150 mg and the other 75 mg of doxepin daily, an average of 0.3–1% of the maternal weight-related dosage (including the metabolite N-desmethyldoxepin) was reported for the infant (Kemp 1985). One of the infants had to be treated for depressed breathing and sedation. Values of 2.2 µg/l doxepin and – corresponding to the maternal concentration – 66 µg/l N-desmethyldoxepin – were measured in his serum (Matheson 1985). Symptoms improved after changing to artificial feeding. It would seem that accumulation must be expected in an infant. A further case report describes a 9-day-old boy with a weak suck, muscular hypotonia, and vomiting. His mother took 35 mg doxepin a day. Doxepin was found in the infant's serum just at detection level (10 µg/l); the metabolite could not be detected. The symptoms disappeared 48 hours after changing to artificial feeding (Frey 1999).

▶ Imipramine

Imipramine has a half-life of 6–20 hours. Up to 95% is bound to plasma protein. With a dose of 200 mg *imipramine* a day, a maximum of 29 µg/l of imipramine and 35 µg/l of desipramine (metabolite) were measured in the milk (Sovner 1979). By contrast, in four mothers in a newer study taking 75–150 mg daily, active ingredient concentrations of up to 600 µg/l were measured in the milk. Most of the values, however, were significantly under 300 µg/l (Yoshida 1997A). Based on these data, a maximum of 90 µg/kg per day, or 7% of the maternal weight-related dosage, could be calculated for the baby. However, on average, it is below 2% (survey in Weissman 2004).

▶ Maprotiline

Following treatment with 100–150 mg daily of *maprotiline*, a tetracyclic antidepressant, a relative dosage of 1.6% was reported in an older study; however, this did not take into account active metabolites (survey in Bennett 1996).

▶ Mianserin

Mianserin is also a tetracyclic antidepressant. Up to about 90% of it is bound to plasma protein, and it has a half-life of around 22 hours. The primary active metabolite is *desmethylmianserin*. Two breastfeeding women, one of whom took 40 mg and the other 60 mg of mianserin daily, were studied; levels of 20 µg/l and 80 µg/

respectively, of mianserin were measured in the milk. For desmethylmianserin, these figures were $20\,\mu g/l$ and $10\,\mu g/l$ respectively. Including the metabolites, a maximum of 1.5% of a weight-related dosage for an infant was calculated. No medication could be detected in the serum of the first baby; when the urine of the second baby was examined, $12\,\mu g/l$ of mianserin and $14\,\mu g/l$ of desmethylmianserin were reported (Buist 1993B).

Nortriptyline

Nortriptyline, half-life 37 hours, is the active metabolite of *amitriptyline*. Experience with a total of 27 mother–infant pairs, where the mothers were taking 50–175 mg *nortriptyline* a day, indicated that no acute toxic symptoms would be expected among the breastfed infants. The M/P ratio (about 1) and the relative dosage (not over 2–3%) correspond to the experience with amitriptyline mentioned above (survey in Weissman 2004, Spigset 1998). Only in the case of a 4-week-old baby, whose mother took 60 mg a day and had a serum concentration of just $42\,\mu g/l$, could $10\,\mu g/l$ nortriptyline be detected in the infant's serum. In other studies, infant serum levels were near or below the level of quantifiability (Wisner 2006). With some of the other children, only very minute amounts of nortriptyline's 10-hydroxy-metabolite were found.

Opipramol

There is an older study of 10 women on *opipramol*, which indicates an M/P ratio of 0.1 and a relative dosage of only 0.3% (Herrmann 1970).

There are either no or insufficient data on the substances *dibenzepin, lofepramine*, and *trimipramine*.

> **Recommendation.** When drug treatment for depression is urgently needed, monotherapy with amitriptyline, clomipramine, nortriptyline, imipramine, desipramine or dosulepine is the treatment of choice during breastfeeding. With compelling indications, other tricyclics are also acceptable. Doxepin should be avoided. In cases of symptoms potentially associated with drug therapy, a pediatrician and a teratology information center should be contacted to decide individually upon measuring drug values in the infant's serum, supplementary formula feeding, weaning, and/or changing therapy. There is insufficient information on the long-term effects of antidepressant medication taken during breastfeeding.

4

Lactation

4.9 Psychotropic drugs

4.9.3   Selective serotonin reuptake inhibitors

▶ Citalopram

Citalopram has a half-life of approximately 35 hours. The activity
of the metabolites *norcitalopram* and *desmethylcitalopram* amounts
to 13%. On the basis of over 65 mother–child pairs (Lee 2004A,
Weissman 2004, Heikkinen 2002), it can be summarized that the relative dose a fully breastfed child receives, including active metabolites, is on average 3–5% (maximum about 10%). Citalopram could
be detected only in traces in the child's serum, if at all (Berle 2004).
The maximum values amounted to approximately one-fifteenth of
the therapeutic maternal concentration. Restless sleep was noted in
one baby aged about 6 weeks whose mother received 40 mg a day.
With steady-state conditions, a level of 205 µg/l was found in the
milk and 12.7 µg/l in the baby's serum. A relative dosage of 5.4% was
calculated. Following a reduction of the maternal dosage by half, and
two feeds of infant formula, the baby's sleep pattern was normal
(Schmidt 2000). Of 31 examined children (Lee 2004A), 3 showed
insignificant and non-specific symptoms – for example, restlessness
in a 2-month-old child, whose symptoms resolved after weaning.
Few case reports present breastfed children with somnolence. For
the remaining children described in the literature, toxic symptoms
are not mentioned. Also, the further development up to the age of
1 year was predominantly unremarkable (Weissman 2004, Heikkinen
2002, Rampono 2000).

▶ Escitalopram

Escitalopram is an active isomer of citalopram with a molecular
mass of 414. At 56%, the protein binding is lower than that of citalopram (80%) and could facilitate a transfer to the milk. Data are
insufficient with respect to lactation. A case report describes a child
aged 3 weeks, whose weight gain was insufficient from the beginning of the maternal therapy and up to the age of 4 months. In addition, slightly elevated liver enzymes, moderate muscle hypertonia of
the upper extremities, irritability, and frequent crying were observed.
The symptoms resolved after adding formula feeding in the fifth
month (Merlob 2005). A similar observation was documented by
the current author and colleagues. A hyperirritable newborn started
high-pitched crying 2 hours after breastfeeding (5–6 hours after escitalopram intake by the mother), every afternoon. When the mother
took her tablet in the morning instead, her child's symptoms
appeared at the same time interval after breastfeeding. After adding

formula, symptoms improved, and resolved completely after weaning on day 11.

Fluoxetine

Up to 94% of *fluoxetine* and its active metabolite *norfluoxetine* is bound to plasma protein. The half-life of fluoxetine is 4 days; that of norfluoxetine is 7 days. The M/P ratio is 0.25. Experience with 16 mother–baby pairs in two studies showed that the relative dosage of fluoxetine plus norfluoxetine taken in by the breastfed baby was, on average, 6.5%, with a maximum of 17%. The children were unremarkable (Yoshida 1998A, Taddio 1996, Burch 1992). Another case report described an infant with screaming attacks, watery stools, and increasing vomiting, whose symptoms disappeared when he changed to artificial feeding. When he was put to breast again, the symptoms reappeared (Lester 1993). The mother took 20 mg fluoxetine daily. A relative dosage of around 8%, including norfluoxetine, was calculated. Therapeutic concentrations (340 µg/l fluoxetine and 208 µg/l norfluoxetine), such as would be expected in an adult taking 20 mg, were found in the serum of the 10-week-old baby. In an additional case, there were indications of increased irritability in the baby during the first 2 weeks of his mother's therapy with 20 mg fluoxetine daily; 28.8 µg/l fluoxetine and 41.6 µg/l norfluoxetine were measured in the milk (Isenberg 1990). From this, a dosage for the child of about 11 µg/kg/daily – corresponding to 3.2% of the maternal weight-related dosage – was calculated. A case report describes an infant with questionable convulsive-like symptoms and a cyanotic attack, whose mother took carbamazepine and buspirone in addition to fluoxetine. Further development of the baby through to the end of the first year of life was normal. The authors were, with justification, hesitant to conclude that there was a connection between the medication and the symptoms (Brent 1998). Four additional children, who were followed up neurologically until age of 1, were unremarkable (Yoshida 1998A).

Chambers (1998) found a statistically significant lower weight gain of about 9% in a group of 28 breastfed children whose mothers were taking fluoxetine, compared to a control group of 34 breastfed children who were not exposed to psychoactive medication. However, no other symptoms were observed.

Epperson (2003) studied the potential effects of maternal fluoxetine on the serotonin metabolism in five newborns. All but one infant experienced little or no decline in whole-blood (platelet) 5-hydroxytryptamine (5-HT) concentrations after exposure to fluoxetine through breast milk. The substantial reduction in platelet 5-HT seen in one infant, and the coupling of this drop with a measurable plasma fluoxetine level, raises some concern. Possible reasons for the infant's measurable plasma fluoxetine level include his mother's high plasma drug level and his being breastfed exclusively. However, the observations may be coincidental, and the infant experienced no discernible adverse effects.

All in all, of 80 published mother–child pairs (Weissman 2004), only 5 infants showed symptoms. The majority of children did not show any side effects of maternal fluoxetine therapy during lactation. However, the rate of symptomatic children is greater than that of the other SSRIs, possibly because fluoxetine's relative dose is higher and its half-life is longer.

▶ Fluvoxamine

Fluvoxamine has a half-life of 16 hours. Levels of 310 µg/l *fluvoxamine* in the serum and 90 µg/l in the milk of a breastfeeding mother taking 200 mg daily have been reported. Based on this, an M/P ratio of 0.3 can be calculated; thus the infant would get 13.5 µg/kg daily, which represents 0.5% of the maternal weight-related dosage (Wright 1991). A second case report observed proportionally lower concentrations when the dosage was 100 mg daily. Mathematically, this too represents a relative dosage of 0.5%. Cognitive and motor development of this baby, who was breastfed for 5 months, tested at 4 months and again at 21 months, was unremarkable (Yoshida 1997B).

In a third mother–child pair, where the mother was taking 200 mg fluvoxamine daily, a level of 48 µg/kg a day was calculated, representing a relative dosage of 1.6% for the clinically unremarkable baby (Hägg 2000A). A further group of authors reported on the determination of fluvoxamine levels in the serum of a 10-week-old breastfed baby, which, based on the maximum active ingredient concentration in the milk, indicated a relative dosage of only 0.6% for the baby. Nevertheless, 45% of the maternal serum concentration was found in his serum. During the period of observation (up to the age of 4 months), the baby's development was unremarkable (Arnold 2000). No substance was detected in the serum of five additional children without symptoms (Weissman 2004, Hendrick 2001A).

▶ Paroxetine

Based on about 110 mother–child pairs, the average relative dose of *paroxetine* (half-life 22 hours) for a fully breastfed child is 1%. In almost all infants, paroxetine could not be detected in blood and no side effects were observed, apart from one child with lethargy possibly associated with prenatal exposure (Berle 2004, Merlob 2004, Weissman 2004, Hendrick 2001A). Peak values in the milk correlated with the dosage. The highest level was 101 µg/l, with a daily maternal dosage of 50 mg. This represents a relative dosage of less than 2% (Stowe 2000). Another woman took 20 mg *paroxetine* daily, and 7.6 µg of the medication were detected per liter of the mother's milk. Thus, the baby received 1.14 µg/kg paroxetine daily, which represents about 0.4% of the maternal weight-related dosage (Spigset 1996). With respect to serum concentrations and symptoms in the neonatal period, there has been one recorded exception, in a 5-day-old newborn who had 31.4 µg/l in the blood. Although the milk value (153 µg/l) was also five times higher than the average level found in other studies, lethargy, poor weight gain, and hypotonia persisting through the first 4–6 weeks of life could also be attributed to the prenatal exposure (cited in Weissman 2004).

Sertraline

Sertraline has a half-life of 26 hours. Based on about 110 mother–child pairs, the average relative dose for a fully breastfed child is almost 2% (Merlob 2004, Weissman 2004, Hendrick 2001A). In 1997, Stowe analyzed 148 milk samples from 12 mothers. The highest concentrations for sertraline were around 173 µg/l; for *desmethylsertraline*, which has a significantly lower psychopharmacological action, it was 294 µg/l. Maternal dosages ranged from 25 to 200 mg daily. There were traces of sertraline in the serum of some children, and in three of them a level of about 10 µg/l desmethylsertraline was measured (Merlob 2004, Weissman 2004, Hendrick 2001A). In other infants either no substance was found or the levels were near or below the level of quantifiability (Wisner 2006, Berle 2004). In only one breastfed baby were serum levels equal to 50% of the maternal values found (Wisner 1998). The authors of the study could not understand this, and suggested direct administration of the medication to the baby as the cause. None of the babies was remarkable. Decreasing serum values of desmethylsertraline with age were observed among 30 breastfed children (Hendrick 2001A). A maternal dosage of above 100 mg/day was significantly correlated with the detection of sertraline in the infant's serum. Breastfed infants showed little or no change in platelet 5-hydroxytryptamine (5-HT) levels after exposure through breastfeeding. According to the authors of this study, the observations suggest that peripheral or central 5-HT transport in these infants is not affected by sertraline therapy of their mothers.

4

Lactation

4.9 Psychotropic drugs

Recommendation. Sertraline, paroxetin, citalopram, and fluvoxamin are the drugs of choice among SSRIs for breastfeeding mothers. In case of fluoxetin or escitalopram therapy, special attention should be paid to potential side effects in the breastfed child. In general, monotherapy should be the goal. If symptoms appear that are potentially associated with SSRI therapy, a pediatrician and a teratology information center should be contacted to decide individually upon measuring drug values in the infant's serum, supplementary formula feeding, weaning, and/or changing therapy. As with all psychoactive drugs, there is insufficient experience on the long-term effects on breastfed children as a result of ongoing therapy to their mothers.

4.9.4   Other antidepressants

▶ **Bupropion**

A case report describes *bupropion* (= *amfebutamon*; half-life 21 hours), a drug with a serotonin, noradrenaline, and dopamine blocking action, which is also used for weaning from cigarette smoking. An M/P ratio of up to 8, and a relative dosage (including the 50% effective metabolites *erythrohydrobupropion, hydroxybupropion*, and *threohydrobupropion*) of less than 1% on average and 3% at maximum, have been calculated (Weissman 2004). Neither in this nor in two other cases was the drug detected in the infant's serum (Baab 2002). A more recent study of 10 mothers receiving 150 mg/d for 3 days and then 300 mg/d for 4 days calculated, on average, 6.75 µg/kg per day bupropion plus 10.8, 15.75, and 68.9 µg/kg per day of the respective metabolites (see above) for a fully breastfed child. Considering bupropion only, the relative dose is 0.14%; including its metabolites, this is about 2% (Haas 2004).

▶ **Hypericin (St John's wort)**

St John's wort or *hypericin* preparations can inhibit prolactin secretion. Therefore, they have the potential to reduce milk production (Franklin 1999). Traces of hyperforin were found in the milk of a mother on long-term therapy of 900 mg/d; hypericin, however, was not detectable (detection limit < 0.2 ng/ml). There was no drug in the infant's serum (Klier 2006). Based on five mothers taking a similar dose, an M/P ratio of 0.04–0.3 and a relative dosage of 0.9–2.5% were calculated. In the blood of two of the children the substance was measured at the detection limit (0.1 ng/ml). Another study involving 33 mother–child pairs observed moderate symptoms, such as colic and lethargy, in 5 of the exposed infants. Although the number of symptomatic children was significantly higher than in the two control groups, no child required therapy. The authors could not exclude additional psychotropic drugs as a confounding factor (Lee 2003). The weight gain of these children was not compromised, and neither was the milk production. This speaks against a clinically relevant inhibitory effect on prolactin.

Mirtazapine

Mirtazapine has a protein binding of 85% and a half-life of 20–40 hours. Three weeks after delivery, a mother was switched from sertraline to mirtazapine 30 mg/d. After reaching steady state, a level of 25 µg/l was measured in her serum; 34 µg/l was the peak value in the milk, and 0.2 µg/l was found in the infant's serum. A relative dose of up to 1% was calculated. The breastfed child was normally developed at the age of 6 weeks (Aichhorn 2004).

Moclobemide

The reversible MAO inhibitor *moclobemide* was studied in six mother–child pairs. An M/P ratio of 0.7 and a relative dosage of 1.2% were reported (Pons 1990).

Nefazodone

Nefazodone, a 5-HT_2-receptor antagonist, was studied in three samples with two patients. With a daily dosage of between 100 and 400 mg, concentrations of the active ingredient, including the active metabolite *hydroxynefazodone*, of 57–700 µg/l were found in the milk. However, the sampling was done before the patients took the tablets (two single doses daily). The patients had been in treatment for at least 3 weeks (Dodd 1999). From these measurements, a relative dosage of between <1% and 7% can be calculated for the fully breastfed baby. A further case report describes a premature infant who, mathematically, received only 0.5% of the weight-related maternal dosage (daily dosage 300 mg), and still had to be hospitalized because of lethargy, weak suck, and problems with temperature regulation. These symptoms improved within 72 hours after weaning (Yapp 2000).

4 Lactation

4.9 Psychotropic drugs

▶ **Trazodone**

Among six women who took single doses of 50 mg of *trazodone*, an M/P ratio of 0.14 and a child's dosage of 15 μg/kg trazodone daily were calculated. This represents just under 2% of the weight-related dosage. However, it should be noted that the pharmacologically active metabolite 1-m-chlorophenylpiperazine was not included in the calculations (Verbeek 1986).

▶ **Venlafaxine**

The half-life of *venlafaxine*, a serotonin and noradrenaline reuptake inhibitor, is 26 hours. Based on eight mother–child pairs, an M/P ratio of about 4 was reported. When the active metabolite *O-desmethyl-venlafaxine* is included the breastfed baby receives on average 6% (a maximum of 9%) of the maternal weight-related dosage. The metabolite, but not venlafaxine itself, was measured at levels of 3–38 μg/l in the serum of the breastfed infants, who developed uneventfully. These serum values correspond to 10% of the maternal concentrations (Berle 2004, Weissman 2004, Ilett 2002, Hendrick 2001B).

There are either no or insufficient data on the use of *amineptine, amoxapine, atomoxetine, duloxetine, iprindole, medifoxamine, oxitriptan, reboxetine, tranylcypromine, L-tryptophan*, and *viloxazine* during breastfeeding.

> **Recommendation.** Due to the quantity and the results of documented experience, St. John's wort or hypericin preparations and mirtazapine are acceptable during breastfeeding. If compellingly indicated, moclobemid, venlafaxine, and bupropion are also tolerable. Whenever possible, the drugs of choice among tricyclic antidepressants or SSRIs are preferable. In general, monotherapy should be the goal. In cases of symptoms potentially associated with the drug therapy, a pediatrician and a teratology information center should be contacted to decide individually upon measuring drug values in the infant's serum, supplementary formula feeding, weaning, and/or changing the therapy. As with all psychoactive drugs, there is insufficient experience on the long-term effects on breastfed children of ongoing maternal therapy.

4.9.5   Phenothiazine and thioxanthene neuroleptics

Although this group of neuroleptics has been used for a long time, there are only very few publications with a small number of cases regarding therapy during breastfeeding. In none of these reports, which have been published over a period of 40 years, is there any mention of serious or permanent effects on the child breastfed while his mother was being treated with this group of drugs (McElhatton 1992). The American Academy of Pediatrics considers phenothiazines compatible with breastfeeding because only very limited concentrations have been found in all the mothers' milk samples measured up to now, due to the high plasma protein binding. At the same time, however, it has been pointed out that long-term effects cannot be judged definitively. This, of course, also applies to all the other drugs with a central nervous system action. There was speculation recently that sudden infant death syndrome (SIDS) and sleep apnea could be induced by phenothiazines. Atypical neuroleptics were discussed as a therapeutic alternative (Hale 2004).

Chlorpromazine

Chlorpromazine, with a half-life of 30 hours, is absorbed at a very individual rate after oral administration. According to an older study, 2 hours after a single dose of 1200 mg chlorpromazine (20 mg/kg), levels of 750 µg/l and 290 µg/l were measured in the mother's serum and in the milk, respectively. An M/P ratio of less than 0.5 was calculated. With a dosage of 600 mg, no medication could be detected in the milk (Blacker 1962). In another study, concentrations in the milk of between 7 and 98 µg/l (maternal serum: 16–52 µg/l) were found in four women. The maternal dosages are unknown. Two of the children were breastfed. The one whose mother's milk had a concentration of 7 µg/l was unremarkable; the second, whose mother's milk had a concentration of up to 98 µg/l, was lethargic after breastfeeding, which the authors were unable to explain, considering the low relative dosage of considerably less than 1% (Wiles 1978). Other publications confirm that a very low amount is transmitted (i.e. Sugawara 1999, Yoshida 1998B). In one of these studies on five women, a maximum of 0.7 ng/ml of the active ingredient was found in the serum of breastfed babies. No acute symptoms were observed. However, in three of these children, whose mothers were also treated with haloperidol, a mental or psychomotor developmental delay was observed in the second year of life. A connection with the medication was discussed by the authors (Yoshida 1998B).

Chlorprothixene

The primary metabolite of *chlorprothixene* is *chlorprothixene sulfoxide*, which has no neuroleptic action but possibly has an

4

Lactation

4.9 Psychotropic drugs

anticholinergic action. Two women were studied; one took 200 mg of chlorprothixene a day, the second 200–400 mg a day. From the concentrations reported in the mother's milk, a child's chlorprothixene dosage was calculated to be an average of 2.4 µg/kg daily (with a maximum of 4.7 µg/kg daily) and the chlorprothixene sulfoxide dosage 3.5–4.5 µg/kg daily. Thus, a fully breastfed infant would take in 0.2% of the maternal weight-related dose of the active ingredient. The babies studied were unremarkable (Matheson 1984).

▶ Flupenthixol

Flupenthixol is taken orally or administered intramuscularly as a depot preparation. In the cases of three mothers who received 2 mg flupenthixol a day, or 40 mg every 2 weeks, or 60 mg every 3 weeks, the concentration of the drug in the milk was the same – 1.8 µg/l (maternal serum 1.3–1.5 µg/l). On this basis, it is calculated that the infant would receive 0.27 µg/kg daily. This represents a maximum of 0.8% of the maternal weight-related flupenthixol dosage (Kirk 1980). In another case, the same amount was reported to be transferred with oral therapy of 4 mg a day (Matheson 1988). Clinical examination of the exposed children did not reveal anything remarkable. They developed normally for their ages.

▶ Levomepromazine

A case report on *levomepromazine* reported a relative dose of 0.8% (Ohkubo 1993).

▶ Perazin

The current author and colleagues measured 30–34 µg/l *perazin* in the milk of a mother treated with 25 mg/d. The concentration remained stable over 24 hours, and corresponds to a relative dose of 1% for a fully breastfed infant.

▶ Perphenazine

There is only one study on *perphenazine*. The mother received 24 mg of perphenazine a day at first and then 16 mg/daily. The level in milk was initially 3.2 µg/l; at the lower dosage it was 2.1 µg/l.

In the maternal serum, concentrations of perphenazine were between 4.9 and 2.0 µg/l. Mathematically, the infant was therefore getting 0.48 or 0.32 µg/kg daily. In both cases, this is 0.1% of the maternal weight-related dosage. The affected child was breastfed over 3 months while his mother was taking the medication, and was unremarkable (Olesen 1990).

Trifluoperazine

In a study of two women taking 5 or 10 mg *trifluoperazine* a day, an immunoassay (EIA) of the milk showed a concentration of 359 µg/l in one case. By comparison, the value was beneath detection level in a chromatographic control study. No active ingredient was found in the serum of the asymptomatic children with either method (Yoshida 1998B).

Zuclopenthixol

Among eight women who received 4–50 mg *zuclopenthixol* daily, an average M/P ratio of 0.5 was found. The portion transferred with the milk was under 1% of the maternal weight-related dosage (Matheson 1988, Aaes-Jørgensen 1986). None of the exposed children was remarkable.

There is insufficient experience on the use of *alimemazine, clopenthixol, dixyrazine, fluphenazine, metofenazate, promazine, promethazine, prothipendyl, thioridazine, triflupromazine*, and *zotepine* during breastfeeding.

> **Recommendation.** When neuroleptic or phenothiazine therapy is urgently needed, levomepromazine (among those neuroleptics with weak action) and perphenazine or triflupromazine (among those with moderately strong action) are preferable. The appearance of acute toxic symptoms as a result of phenothiazine in the milk is unlikely. Basically, monotherapy should be the goal. In cases of symptoms potentially associated with the drug therapy, a pediatrician and a teratology information center should be contacted to decide individually upon measuring drug values in the infant's serum, supplementary formula feeding, weaning, and/or changing therapy. As with all psychoactive drugs, there is insufficient experience on the long-term effects on breastfed children as a result of ongoing therapy to their mothers.

4

Lactation

4.9 Psychotropic drugs

4.9.6   Butyrophenones

Experience

Among a total of 16 women who received between 1 and 40 mg of *haloperidol* daily, a relative dosage of 0.2–2.1% – with 10% in an extreme case – was calculated for their infants (Yoshida 1998B, survey in Bennett 1996). In so far as there was follow-up, the breastfed children whose mothers had had monotherapy developed normally. However, Yoshida (1998B) observed mental or psychomotor development delays during the second year of life in three of the children whose mothers were also treated with chlorpromazine. The authors could not rule out a connection with the medication.

There are no data on the other butyrophenones, such as, for instance, *bromperidol, droperidol, melperone, pipamperone,* and *trifluperidol,* or on the structurally related neuroleptics, *pimozide* and *fluspirilene.*

> **Recommendation.** If indicated, haloperidol may be used during lactation. Uncritical use of fluspirilene (as a depot injection) should, in particular, be avoided for non-psychotic indications. Basically, monotherapy is the goal. In cases of symptoms potentially associated with the drug therapy, a pediatrician and a teratology information center should be contacted to decide individually upon measuring drug values in the infant's serum, supplementary formula feeding, weaning, and/or changing therapy. As with all psychoactive drugs, there is insufficient experience on the long-term effects on breastfed children as a result of ongoing therapy to their mothers.

4.9.7   Atypical neuroleptics

Clozapine

Clozapine has a half-life of up to 25 hours. With a daily dosage of 50 mg *clozapine,* a concentration of 63.5 μg/l was reported in the colostrum on the day after birth; the maternal serum level was 14.7 μg/l. One week later, with a dosage of 100 mg daily, the concentration of the drug in the milk had risen to 115.6 μg/l; the maternal serum level was 41.4 μg/l (Barnas 1994). This represents an M/P ratio of 2.8. Based on this, an infant would take in 17.3 μg/kg daily, or about 1% of the maternal weight-related dosage. In two of the case studies collected by the manufacturer, sleepiness in the breastfed babies of mothers using clozapine was reported. One of the mothers took 150 mg a day; the other took 12.5 mg plus 3 mg of flupenthixol. Agranulocytosis has also been discussed (Gentile 2004); however, the risk is remote, considering the low dose to the infant via breast milk.

Olanzapine

Olanzapine has a rather long half-life of up to 54 hours. Based on the data of seven mother–child pairs, the median infant dose of olanzapine ingested via milk was 1% of the maternal dose; the median milk/plasma ratio was 0.4 for the six patients with data collected over the dose interval. Corresponding values in the patient with single-point data were 1.1% and 0.8. Olanzapine was not detected in the plasma of the six infants with an evaluable plasma sample. All the infants were healthy and experienced no side effects (Gardiner 2003). In another child whose mother has already been treated during pregnancy with 10 mg/d, after delivery the plasma level of olanzapine in the infant was one-third of the maternal plasma level, and during breastfeeding it decreased to an undetectable limit (Kirchheiner 2000). In a study with five mother–child pairs, the median relative infant dose was 1.6% (range 0–2.5%) of the weight-adjusted maternal dose. During the study period, there were no apparent ill effects on the infant as a consequence of exposure to these doses of olanzapine (Croke 2002). Icterus and sedation were observed in two other children; however, these symptoms were attributed to other factors (Goldstein 2000). Symptoms like sedation and feeding problems were observed in 4 of 20 infants reported to the drug company. A causal association has not been confirmed, but cannot be excluded, at least in very young infants, due to the long half-life (cited in Ernst 2002). However, if such symptoms appear in the early neonatal period they are probably related to the prenatal exposure. We observed a symptomatic newborn with therapeutic olanzapine values (0.01 µg/ml) on day 3 (maternal dosage 7.5 mg/d). Milk levels of 0.01 µg/ml corresponded to a relative dose of 1.5%. The continuously breastfed child improved, and was normally developed at the age of 6 weeks.

Quetiapine

Quetiapine has a half-life of 7 hours. A case report on quetiapine, 200 mg/d, measured peak values of 62 µg/l milk 1 hour after drug

4

Lactation

4.9 Psychotropic drugs

intake. Levels rapidly fell to almost pre-dose levels by 2 hours. A relative dose of on average 0.1%, and at maximum 0.4%, was calculated. The child was fully breastfed from 8 weeks after birth, and was normally developed at 4.5 months (Lee 2004B).

▶ Risperidon

Risperidon has a half-life of 3 hours, its metabolites up to 24 hours. A relative dose of 4% (including active metabolites) was calculated, and no symptoms were observed in the child (Hill 2000). Two other children developed normallly until the age of 9 months (Ratnayake 2002). Traces or no substances at all were detected in the serum of three other infants. Galactorrhea was observed in one woman. The relative dose calculated with the data in these publications is 2% with a peak value of 6% (Aichhorn 2005, Ilett 2004). No symptoms were observed in the fully breastfed infants.

▶ Sulpiride

Sulpiride is a dopamine antagonist that stimulates the secretion of prolactin, and thus may increase the amount of milk. Its half-life is about 8 hours. In two studies, the mothers received 100 mg daily. Concentrations of, on average, 0.97 mg/l and 0.83 mg/l, with maximums of 1.97 and 1.46 mg/l respectively, were measured in the mothers' milk. Based on this, an infant would take in an average of 0.135 mg/kg daily. This is 8.7% (at maximum 17.7%) of the maternal weight-related dosage. No information on the babies was published (survey in Bennett 1996).

There are no data on *amisulpride, aripiprazole, sertindole* (half-life 72 hours!), and *ziprasidone*.

> **Recommendation.** Clozapine, olanzapine, quetiapine, and risperidone are acceptable during lactation. The other atypical neuroleptics should, if possible, not be used, due to lack of data or to higher drug transfer into the milk. Basically, monotherapy is the goal. In cases of symptoms potentially associated with the drug therapy, a pediatrician and a teratology information center should be contacted to decide individually upon measuring drug values in the infant's serum, supplementary formula feeding, weaning, and/or changing therapy. As with all psychoactive drugs, there is insufficient experience on the long-term effects on breastfed children as a result of ongoing therapy to their mothers.

4.9.8   Antimanic drugs

Experience

Lithium is the standard therapeutic for treating manic-depressive illnesses, between episodes. The half-life in adults is 8–45 hours. The therapeutic range is, at 0.8–1.5 mmol/l, very narrow. Toxic symptoms may occur during treatment with as little as 2 mmol/l. The M/P ratio varies, with the dosage, between 0.3 and (with high doses) 1.7. Based on 11 mother–child pairs, the relative dose to a fully breastfed child is up to 30%, but in half of the cases it was less than 10% (Moretti 2003). Older publications report that up to 80% of the maternal weight-related dosage can be transmitted to the baby via the mother's milk. After the very high immediate postpartum levels have dropped, significantly lower concentrations are found in the infant's serum. Seldom do they exceed a third of the maternal levels, and frequently they are even lower. None of the 11 infants observed by Moretti (2003) was symptomatic. However, one publication reported on a 2-month-old infant with a tremor and abnormal pattern of movement. The lithium levels in his serum were twice as high as those in his mother (overview in Llewellyn 1998, Spigset 1998, Bennett 1996).

Anticonvulsants are also used prophylactically against manic-depressive episodes, especially when there are contraindications for lithium. See Chapter 4.8 regarding their use during breastfeeding.

> **Recommendation.** Breastfeeding may be permitted when the baby is carefully observed (muscle tone, tremor, involuntary movements, cyanosis, dehydration) and the maternal lithium dosage is kept as low as possible. In cases of symptoms potentially associated with the drug therapy, a pediatrician and a teratology information center should be contacted to decide individually upon measuring drug values in the infant's serum, supplementary formula feeding, weaning, and/or changing therapy. As with all psychoactive drugs, there is insufficient experience on the long-term effects on breastfed children as a result of ongoing therapy to their mothers.

4.9.9   Benzodiazepines

Experience

In the last 30 years, a number of benzodiazepines have been introduced into therapy. Structurally, they are related to each other. Primarily medium- and long-acting benzodiazepines are used as

4

Lactation

4.9 Psychotropic drugs

anxiolytics and sedatives; the shorter-acting substances are available for the induction of anesthesia and as hypnotics. Among full-term newborns, the elimination capacity for benzodiazepines develops within the first week of life.

Shorter-acting benzodiazepines (<6 hours) are *brotizolam, flurazepam, midazolam,* and *triazolam.*

Benzodiazepines with medium to long action (6–24 hours) are *alprazolam, bromazepam, clotiazepam, flunitrazepam, loprazolam, lorazepam, lormetazepam, metaclazepam, nitrazepam, oxazepam,* and *temazepam.*

Long-acting benzodiazepines (>24 hours) are *chlordiazepoxide, clobazam, diazepam, dikaliumclorazepat, medazepam, nordazepam,* and *prazepam.*

In the following sections, each of the benzodiazepines for which there is experience during breastfeeding will be discussed in alphabetical order.

With *alprazolam* (half-life 12–15 hours, M/P ratio 0.4), a fully breastfed baby would, according to a study of eight women, receive on average 3% (maximum 6.7%) of the maternal weight-related dosage (Oo 1995). Metabolites could not be detected in the milk. In another publication, sleepiness in the infant was discussed in connection with maternal therapy. However, despite continued breastfeeding, the symptoms disappeared (Anderson 1989).

Clobazam (half-life about 20 hours, M/P ratio 0.3) was measured in the milk of six women who had been treated with 30 mg a day for 2 or 5 days. The maximum concentration in the milk was 330 µg/l (cited in Bennett 1996). This would lead to a relative dosage of 10%.

Over 97% of *diazepam* is bound to plasma protein. The half-life is 24–48 hours; that of its active metabolite, *desmethyldiazepam,* is 30–90 hours. Among 11 women who took 10–40 mg/d, 3% (maximum 13%), including the metabolites, was calculated for a fully breastfed infant (survey in Hägg 2000B, Bennett 1996). This represents up to about 4% of an infant's therapeutic dosage of 0.5 mg/kg daily. The M/P ratio for diazepam and desmethyldiazepam is between 0.1 and 0.3. Only traces of diazepam were detected in the serum of the breastfed babies. However, levels of up to 46 µg/l desmethyldiazepam were detected. These values are significantly higher in the first days of life if the mother has already taken diazepam repeatedly before the birth, and the newborn has not yet excreted the transplacentally acquired agent. The very few case descriptions on symptoms in the breastfed baby whose mother is being treated with diazepam (such as lethargy, lack of interest in sucking, sleepiness or remarkable EEG) give the impression that only repeated high doses of at least 30 mg a day, or treatment begun before birth, lead to clinical symptoms. Single maternal doses do not appear to have any effect on the infant.

Flunitrazepam (half-life 29 hours, M/P ratio 0.5) was studied in 10 women who took a single oral or intravenous dose (survey in Bennett 1996). Since the active metabolites were not included and the concentration under steady-state conditions are unknown, the relative dosage of a maximum of 2.5% reported here should be viewed with caution.

For *lorazepam* (half-life 15 hours, M/P ratio 0.2), a relative dosage of about 5% was calculated for the infant when the mother received 2.5–3.5 mg/d (8–12 μg/l lorazepam in the milk; survey in Bennett 1996). No symptoms were observed in the baby.

Up to 88% of *lormetazepam* is bound to plasma protein and conjugated to pharmacologically inactive glucuronide. Its half-life is 10 hours, and the M/P ratio is 0.05. In a study of five mothers who received 2 mg daily, 0.4% of the maternal weight-related dosage was calculated for the baby. Only the inactive lormetazepam-glucuronide was detected in the serum of the children studied. The babies were clinically unremarkable (Hümpel 1982).

Among 10 women who took a single dose of 20 mg, *metaclazepam* or its metabolite, *desmethylmetaclazepam* (half-life 11 hours, M/P ratio about 0.3), led to a maximum relative dosage of 5.5% via the milk (Schotter 1989).

Midazolam, a widely used short-acting hypnotic for induction of diagnostic and surgical procedures, has, with its active metabolite *hydroxymidazolam*, a short half-life of 1.5–5 hours. The M/P ratio is significantly below 0.5. Among 12 women who either took 15 mg for 5 days or received it as a single dose, a maximum of 12 μg/l of the agent was found in the milk (Matheson 1990A). This converts, at most, to 0.7% of the weight-related maternal dosage. In an additional case report involving intravenous administration of 6 mg, the highest concentration of 25 μg/l was measured after 30 minutes, followed within 4 hours by a rapid fall-off below the detection level (Koitabashi 1997). Five lactating women underwent premedication with midazolam (Nitsun 2006). Plasma midazolam pharmacokinetics were consistent with reports of others. In a 24-hour milk collection, averages of 0.005% (range 0.002%–0.013%) of the maternal midazolam dose were collected in the milk – i.e. the relative dose for a fully breastfed child is below 1%. As expected, no symptoms were observed in the breastfed babies.

Nitrazepam has a half-life of just under 30 hours and an M/P ratio of 0.3. Among nine women, a maximum transfer dosage of 2.6% was calculated. During 5 days of treatment with 5 mg nitrazepam, an increase in the concentration in the milk from 8.4 to 13.5 μg/l was measured (Matheson 1990A).

Oxazepam breaks down into inactive metabolites. It has a half-life of 9 hours in adults; in newborns this is 20 hours. Based on the experience with three mothers, the M/P ratio is 0.2 and the maximum relative dosage is 0.9% (survey in Bennett 1996).

4

Lactation

4.9 Psychotropic drugs

Prazepam is a prodrug of *desmethyldiazepam*, thus a half-life of up to 90 hours must be expected. The available data argue for an evaluation similar to that for *diazepam*. The same applies to *pinazepam*.

For *quazepam*, where the half-life of its metabolite is up to 72 hours, there is experience with four women taking a single dose of 15 mg. The M/P ratio is about 6. Including active metabolites, a maximum of 263 µg/l was found in the milk (Hilbert 1984). This means that a fully breastfed baby could, in an extreme case, receive active ingredients in the range of more than 10% of the maternal weight-related dosage. Since the mothers under study did not breastfeed, there is no comment on the condition of the infants.

In a study of 10 mothers who took 10–20 mg *temazepam* at least twice a day (half-life 5–13 hours), only in the milk of one mother was 28 µg/l temazepam detected, 15 hours after a second administration (detection limit 5 µg/l). The active metabolite *oxazepam* could not be found in any of the samples. Based on this, a relative dosage of just under 2% is calculated. No active ingredient was found in the serum of two babies studied. The breastfed babies were unremarkable (Lebedevs 1992).

> **Recommendation.** For sleep disturbances, the drug of choice is the antihistamine diphenhydramine (see Chapter 4.2). If a benzodiazepine is urgently needed for this purpose, lormetazepam or temazepam should be chosen. Oxazepam and diazepam are acceptable as tranquilizers, but these substances should also be prescribed in low dosage and for a short time only. Single doses of the other benzodiazepines do not require any limitation of breastfeeding. Fundamentally, monotherapy should be the goal. In cases of symptoms potentially associated with the drug therapy, a pediatrician and a teratology information center should be contacted to decide individually upon measuring drug values in the infant's serum, supplementary formula feeding, weaning, and/or changing therapy. As with all psychoactive drugs, there is insufficient experience on the long-term effects on breastfed children as a result of ongoing therapy to their mothers.

4.9.10   Other anxiolytics

Experience

With *meprobamate*, concentrations in the milk of two to four times those in the maternal serum were measured (Wilson 1980). There are no clinical observations available for babies who were breastfed while their mothers were treated with meprobamate.

For *buspirone, hydroxyzine*, and *kavain*, there are either no or insufficient data on their use during breastfeeding. Like the other older antihistamines, hydroxyzine can lead to sedation or irritability in the infant.

Recommendation. Hydroxyzine may be used if it is really indicated. The other drugs should be avoided. Basically, monotherapy is the goal. As with all psychoactive drugs, there is insufficient experience on the long-term effects on breastfed children of ongoing maternal therapy.

4.9.11   Other hypnotics

Experience

Clomethiazole has a short half-life of about 5 hours. An M/P ratio of 0.9 has been reported. A relative dosage of, on average, 0.1% (maximum 1.6%) has been reported for five mother–baby pairs where the mother took up to 4000 mg a day. Only in a few infant serum samples was it detectable, with a level up to 0.018 mg/l (18 μg/l) (Tunstall 1979).

According to an older study, following a single dose of *glutethimide* there is a transfer to the infant of less than 1% (cited in Bennett 1996).

Only traces of *zaleplon* are transferred to the breast milk (Darwish 1999).

Zolpidem has a short half-life (about 2 hours). The metabolites do not appear to be active. An M/P ratio of 0.1 was reported with five women (Pons 1989). The relative dosage for a fully breastfed baby would not be expected to exceed 1.5%.

The half-life of *zopiclone* is about 5 hours. In a study in which 12 breastfeeding women received a single dose of 7.5 mg, levels of 80 μg/l and 34 μg/l were found in the maternal serum and in the milk, respectively. A maximum of 4% of the maternal weight-related dosage was calculated for the infant (Matheson 1990B). Another study involving three mothers showed similar results (Gaillot 1983).

There are either no or insufficient data on the use of *chloral hydrate, doxylamine*, and *eszopiclone*, the S-enantiomere of zopiclone during breastfeeding.

For phenobarbital, see Chapter 4.8.

There is no indication that *valerian* products are not well-tolerated by the breastfeeding baby.

4 Lactation

4.9 Psychotropic drugs

> **Recommendation.** Valerian poses no problem during breastfeeding; however, if it is taken repeatedly, then preparations without alcohol or with only a modest alcohol content are preferable. Single doses of doxylamine, phenobarbital, and zopiclone are tolerable during breastfeeding. With clomethiazole treatment for alcoholism, the alcoholism is the actual problem for the baby.
>
> Basically, monotherapy should be the goal. In case of symptoms potentially associated with the drug therapy, a pediatrician and a teratology information center should be contacted to decide individually upon measuring drug values in the infant's serum, supplementary formula feeding, weaning, and/or changing therapy. As with all psychoactive drugs, there is insufficient experience on the long-term effects on breastfed children as a result of ongoing therapy to their mothers.

4.9.12   Psychoanaleptics

Experience

There is no experience regarding the use of *amfetaminil, fenetyllin, methylphenidate, pemoline*, and *modafinil* during breastfeeding.

> **Recommendation.** Repeated use of psychoanaleptics should be avoided during breastfeeding. When therapy is urgently needed, the decision on limiting breastfeeding should be made on a case-by-case basis.

4.9.13   Parkinson drugs

Experience

Apart from the more widely used ergotamine derivatives, *bromocriptine* and *cabergoline*, there is little experience regarding the use of Parkinson drugs in breastfeeding. There is insufficient experience on the use of *amantadine, benserazide, benzatropine, biperiden, bornaprine, budipin, carbidopa, α-dihydroergocryptine, entacapon, levodopa, lisurid, metixen, pergolide, pridinol, pramipexol, procyclidine, ropinirol, tiaprid, trihexyphenidyl*, and the monoaminooxydase-B (MAO-B) *inhibitors selegilin* and *rasagilin* during breastfeeding. There has not been, as yet, any noteworthy toxic risk indicated for the infant as a result of the occasional combination of neuroleptics or haloperidol with *biperiden*.

> **Recommendation.** A case-by-case decision on breastfeeding must be made when therapy is urgently needed. Biperiden treatment during breast-feeding is probably tolerable.

References

Aaes-Jørgensen T, Bjørndal F, Bartels U. Zuclopenthixol levels in serum and breast milk. Psychopharmacology 1986; 90: 417–18.

Aichhorn W, Whitworth AB, Weiss U et al. Mirtazapine and breast-feeding. Am J Psychiatry 2004; 161: 2325.

Aichhorn W, Stuppaeck C, Whitworth AB. Risperidone and breast-feeding. J Psychopharmacol 2005; 19: 211–13.

American Academy of Pediatrics, Committee on Drugs. The transfer of drugs and other chemicals into human breast milk. Pediatrics 2001; 108: 776–89.

Anderson PO, McGuire G. Neonatal alprazolam withdrawal; possible effects on breast-feeding. Drug Intelligence Clin Pharm 1989; 23: 614.

Arnold LM, Lichtenstein PK, Suckow RF. Fluvoxamine concentrations in breast milk and in maternal and infant sera. J Clin Psychopharmacol 2000; 20: 491–3.

Baab SB, Peindl KS, Piontek CM et al. Serum bupropion levels in 2 breastfeeding mother-infant pairs. J Clin Psychiatry 2002; 63: 910–11.

Barnas C, Bergant A, Hummer M et al. Clozapine concentration in maternal and fetal plasma, amniotic fluid, and breast milk. Am J Psychiatry 1994; 151(6): 945.

Bennett PN (ed.). Drugs and Human Lactation, 2nd edn. Amsterdam: Elsevier, 1996.

Berle JO, Steen VM, Aamo TO et al. Breastfeeding during maternal antidepressant treatment with serotonin reuptake inhibitors: infant exposure, clinical symptoms, and cytochrome p450 genotypes. J Clin Psychiatry 2004; 65: 1228–34.

Blacker KH, Weinstein BJ, Ellman GL. Mothers' milk and chlorpromazine. Am J Psychol 1962; 114: 178–9.

Brent NB, Wisner KL. Fluoxetine and carbamazepine concentrations in a nursing mother/infant pair. Clin Pediatr 1998; 37: 41–4.

Buist A (A), Norman TR, Dennerstein L. Plasma and breast milk concentrations of dothiepin and northiaden in lactating women. Hum Psychopharmacol 1993; 8: 29–33.

Buist A (B), Norman TR, Dennerstein L. Mianserin in breast milk. Br J Clin Pharmacol 1993; 36: 133–4.

Buist A, Janson H. Effect of exposure to dothiepin and northiaden in breast milk and children's development. Br J Psychiatry 1995; 167: 370–73.

Burch KJ, Wells BG. Fluoxetine/norfluoxetine concentrations in human milk. Pediatrics 1992; 89(4): 676–7.

Chambers CD, Anderson PO, Dick LM et al. Weight gain in infants breastfed by mothers who take fluoxetine. Teratology 1998; 57: 188.

Croke S, Buist A, Hackett LP et al. Olanzapine excretion in human breast milk; estimation of infant exposure. Intl J Neuropsychopharmacol 2002; 5: 243–7.

Darwish M, Martin PT, Cevallos WH et al. Rapid disappearance of zaleplon from breast milk after oral administration to lactating women. J Clin Pharmacol 1999; 39: 670–74.

4

Lactation

4.9 Psychotropic drugs

Dodd S, Buist A, Burrows GD et al. Determination of nefazodone and ist pharmacologically active metabolites in human blood plasma and breast milk by high-performance liquid chromatography. J Chromatogr B 1999; 730: 249–55.

Epperson CN, Jatlow PI, Czarkowski K et al. Maternal fluoxetine treatment in the postpartum period: effects on platelet serotonin and plasma drug levels in breast-feeding mother–infant pairs. Pediatrics 2003; 112: 425–9.

Ernst LC, Goldberg JF. The reproductive safety profile of mood stabilizers, atypical antipsychotics, and broad-spectrum psychotropics. J Clin Psychiatry 2002 63(Suppl 4): 42–55.

Franklin M, Chi J, McGavin C et al. Neuroendocrine evidence for dopaminergic actions of hypericum extract (LI 160) in healthy volunteers. Biol Psychiatry 1999; 46: 581–4

Frey OR, Scheidt P, von Brenndorff AI. Adverse effects in a newborn infant breast-fed by a mother treated with doxepin. Ann Pharmacother 1999; 33: 690–93.

Gaillot J, Heusse D, Hougton GW et al. Pharmacokinetics and metabolism of zopiclone. Pharmacology 1983; 27(Suppl 2): 76–91.

Gardiner SJ, Kristensen J, Begg EJ et al. Transfer of olanzapine into breast milk, calculation of infant drug dose, and effect on breast-fed infants. Am J Psychiatry 2003; 160: 1428–31.

Gentile S. Clinical utilization of atypical antipsychotics in pregnancy and lactation Ann Pharmacother 2004; 38: 1265–71.

Goldstein DJ, Corbin LA, Fung MC. Olanzapine-exposed pregnancies and lactation early experience. J Clin Psychopharmacol 2000; 20: 399–403.

Haas JS, Kaplan CP, Barenboim D et al. Bupropion in breast milk: an exposure assessment for potential treatment to prevent post-partum tobacco use. Tobacco Control 2004; 13: 52–6.

Hägg S (A), Granberg K, Carleborg L. Excretion of fluvoxamine into breast milk Br J Clin Pharmacol 2000; 49: 283–8.

Hägg S (B), Spigset O. Anticonvulsant use during lactation. Drug Saf 2000; 22: 425–40

Hale TW. Presentation Annual meeting of the Organization of Teratogen Information Services (OTIS) 2004.

Heikkinen T, Ekblad U, Kero P et al. Citalopram in pregnancy and lactation Clin Pharmacol Ther 2002; 72: 184–91.

Hendrick V (A), Fukuchi A, Altshuler L et al. Use of sertraline, paroxetine and fluvoxamine by nursing women. Br J Psych 2001; 179: 163–6.

Hendrick V (B), Altshuler L, Wertheimer A et al. Venlafaxine and breast-feeding Am J Psychiatry 2001; 158: 2089–90.

Herrmann B, von Kobyletzki D. Opipramol in human milk? {in German}. Med Welt 1970; 7: 267–9.

Hilbert JM, Gural RP, Symchowicz S et al. Excretion of quazepam into human milk J Clin Pharmacol 1984; 24: 457–62.

Hill RC, McIvor RJ, Wojnar-Horton RE et al. Risperidone distribution and excretion into human milk: case report and estimated infant exposure during breast feeding. J Clin Psychopharmacol 2000; 20: 285–6.

Hümpel M, Stoppeli I, Milia S et al. Pharmacokinetics and biotransformation of the new ben-zodiazepine, lormetazepam, in man. III. Repeated administration and transfer to neonates via breast milk. Eur J Clin Pharmacol 1982; 21: 421–5.

Ilett KF, Lebedevs TH, Wojnar-Horton RE et al. The excretion of dothiepin and it primary metabolites in breast milk. Br J Clin Pharmacol 1993; 33: 635–9.

Ilett KF, Kristensen JH, Hackett LP et al. Distribution and excretion of venlafaxine and its O-desmethyl metabolite in human milk and their effects in breast fed infants. Br J Clin Pharmacol 2002; 53: 17–22.

Ilett KF, Hackett LP, Kristensen JH et al. Transfer of risperidone and 9-hydroxyrisperidone into human milk. Ann Pharmacother 2004; 38: 273–6.

Isenberg KE. Excretion of fluoxetine in human breast milk. J Clin Psychiatry 1990; 51(4): 169.

Kemp J, Ilett KF, Booth J et al. Excretion of doxepin and N-desmethyldoxepin in human milk. Br J Clin Pharmacol 1985; 20: 497–9.

Kirchheiner J, Berghofer A, Bolk-Weischedel D. Healthy outcome under olanzapine treatment in a pregnant woman. Pharmacopsychiatry 2000; 33: 78–80.

Kirk L, Jörgensen A. Concentrations of Cis(Z)-flupenthixol in maternal serum, amniotic fluid, umbilical cord serum, and milk. Psychopharmacology 1980; 72: 107–8.

Klier CM, Schmid-Siegel B, Schäfer MR et al. St. John's wort (Hypericum perforatum) and breastfeeding: plasma and breast milk concentrations of hyperforin for 5 mothers and 2 infants. J Clin Psychiatry 2006; 67: 305–9.

Koitabashi T, Satoh N, Takino Y. Intravenous midazolam passage into breast milk. J Anesth 1997; 11: 242–3.

Lebedevs TH, Wojnar-Horton RE, Tapp P et al. Excretion of temazepam in breast milk. Br J Clin Pharmacol 1992; 33: 204–6.

Lee A, Minhas R, Matsuda N. The safety of St. John's Wort (Hypericum perforatum) during breastfeeding. J Clin Psychiatry 2003; 64: 966–8.

Lee A (A), Woo J, Ito S. Frequency of infant adverse events that are associated with citalopram use during breast-feeding. Am J Obstet Gynecol 2004; 190: 218–21.

Lee A (B), Giesbrecht E, Dunn E et al. Excretion of quetiapine in breast milk. Am J Psychiatry 2004; 161: 1715–16.

Lester BM, Cucca J, Andreozzi L et al. Possible association between fluoxetine hydrochloride and colic in an infant. J Am Acad Child Adolesc Psychiatry 1993; 32: 1253–5.

Llewellyn A, Stowe ZN, Strader JR. The use of lithium and management of women with bipolar disorder during pregnancy and lactation. J Clin Psychiatry 1998; 59(Suppl 6): 57–64.

Matheson I, Evang A, Fredricson Overoe K et al. Presence of chlorprothixene and its metabolites in breast milk. Eur J Clin Pharmacol 1984; 27: 611–13.

Matheson I, Pande H, Altersen AR. Respiratory depression caused by N-desmethyldoxepin in breast milk. Lancet 1985; 2: 1124.

Matheson I, Skjaeraasen J. Milk concentrations of flupenthixol, nortriptyline and zuclopenthixol and between-breast differences in two patients. Eur J Clin Pharmacol 1988; 35: 217–20.

Matheson I (A), Lunde PKM, Bredesen JE. Midazolam and nitrazepam in the maternity ward: milk concentrations and clinical effects. Br J Clin Pharmacol 1990; 30: 787–93.

Matheson I (B), Sande HA, Gaillot J. The excretion of zopiclone into breast milk. Br J Clin Pharmacol 1990; 30: 267–71.

McElhatton PR. The use of phenothiazines during pregnancy and lactation. Reprod Toxicol 1992; 6: 475–90.

Merlob P, Stahl B, Sulkes J. Paroxetine during breast-feeding: infant weight gain and maternal adherence to counsel. Eur J Pediatr 2004; 163: 135–9.

Merlob P. Use of escitalopram during lactation. 13. BELTIS-Newsletter June 2005: 40–43.

Moretti ME, Koren G, Verjee Z et al. Monitoring lithium in breast milk: an individualized approach for breast-feeding mothers. Ther Drug Monit 2003; 25: 364–6.

Nitsun M, Szokol JW, Saleh HJ et al. Pharmacokinetics of midazolam, propofol, and fentanyl transfer to human breast milk. Clin Pharmacol Ther 2006; 79: 549–57.

4

Lactation

4.9 Psychotropic drugs

Ohkubo T, Shimoyama R, Sugawara K. High performance liquid chromatographic determination of levomepromazine in human breast milk and serum using solid phase extraction. Biomed Chromatogr 1993; 7: 227–8.

Olesen OV, Bartels U, Poulsen JH. Perphenazin in breast milk and serum. Am J Psychiatry 1990; 147, 10: 1378–9.

Oo CY, Kuhn RJ, Desai N et al. Pharmacokinetics in lactating women: prediction of alprazolam transfer into milk. Br J Clin Pharmacol 1995; 40: 231–6.

Pons G, Francoual C, Guillet PH et al. Zolpidem excretion in breast milk. Eur J Clin Pharmacol 1989; 37: 245–8.

Pons G, Schoerlin MP, Tarn YK et al. Moclobemide excretion in human breast milk. Br J Clin Pharmacol 1990; 29: 27–31.

Rampono J, Kristensen JH, Hackett LP et al. Citalopram and demethylcitalopram in human milk; distribution, excretion and effects in breast fed infants. Br J Clin Pharmacol 2000; 50: 263–8.

Ratnayake T, Libretto SE. No complications with risperidone treatment before and throughout pregnancy and during the nursing period. J Clin Psychiatry 2002 63: 76–7.

Schimmell MS, Katz EZ, Shaag Y et al. Toxic neonatal effects following maternal clomipramin therapy. J Toxicol Clin Toxicol 1991; 29: 479–84.

Schmidt K, Olesen OV, Jensen PN. Citalopram and breast-feeding: serum concentration and side effects in the infant. Biol Psychiatry 2000; 47: 164–5.

Schotter A, Müller R, Günther C et al. Transfer of metaclazepam and its metabolites into breast milk. Arzneimittelforschung 1989; 39: 1468–70.

Sovner R, Orsulak PJ. Excretion of imipramine and desipramine in human breast milk. Am J Psychiatry 1979; 136: 451–2.

Spigset O, Carleborg L, Norstrom A et al. Paroxetine level in breast milk. J Clin Psychiatry 1996; 57: 39.

Spigset O, Hägg S. Excretion of psychotropic drugs into breastmilk. Pharmacokinetic overview and therapeutic implications. CNS Drugs 1998; 9: 111–34.

Stancer HC, Reed KL. Desipramine and 2-hydroxydesipramine in human breast milk and the nursing infant's serum. Am J Psychiatry 1986; 143(12): 1597–600.

Stowe ZN, Owens MJ, Landry JC et al. Sertraline and des-methylsertraline in human breastmilk and nursing infants. Am J Psych 1997; 154: 1255–60.

Stowe ZN, Cohen LS, Hostetter A et al. Paroxetine in human breast milk and nursing infants. Am J Psychiatry 2000; 157: 185–9.

Sugawara K, Shimoyama R, Ohkubo T. Determinations of psychotropic drugs and antiepileptic drugs by high-performance liquid chromatography and ist monitoring in human breast milk. Hirosaki Med J 1999; 51(Suppl): S81–6.

Taddio A, Ito S, Koren G. Excretion of fluoxetine and its metabolite norfluoxetine in human breast milk. J Clin Pharmacol 1996; 36: 42–7.

Tunstall ME, Campbell DM, Dawson BM et al. Clomethiazole treatment and breast-feeding. Br J Obstet Gynaecol 1979; 86: 793–8.

Verbeek RK, Ross SG, McKenna EA. Excretion of trazodone in breast milk. Br J Clin Pharmacol 1986; 22: 367–70.

Weissman AM, Levy BT, Hartz AJ et al. Pooled analysis of antidepressant levels in lactating mothers, breast milk, and nursing infants. Am J Psychiatry 2004; 161: 1066–78.

Wiles DH, Orr MW, Kolakowska T. Chlorpromazine levels in plasma and milk of nursing mothers. Br J Clin Pharmacol 1978; 5: 272.

Wilson JT, Brown RD, Cherek DR et al. Drug excretion in human breast milk: principles, pharmacokinetics and projected consequences. Clin Pharmacokinet 1980 5: 1–66.

Wisner KL, Perel JM, Foglia JP. Serum clomipramine and metabolite levels in four nursing mother-infant pairs. J Clin Psychiatry 1995; 56(1): 17–20.

Wisner KL, Perel JM, Blumer JB. Serum sertraline and N-desmethylsertraline levels in breastfeeding mother-infant pairs. Am J Psychiatry 1998; 155: 690–92.

Wisner KL, Hanusa BH, Perel JM et al. Postpartum depression: a randomized trial of sertraline versus nortriptyline. J Clin Psychopharmacol 2006; 26: 353–60.

Wright S, Dawling S, Ashford JJ. Excretion of fluvoxamine in breast milk. Br J Clin Pharmacol 1991; 31: 209.

Yapp P, Llett KF, Kristensen JH et al. Drowsiness and poor feeding in a breast-fed infant: association with nefazodone and its metabolites. Ann Pharmacother 2000; 34: 1269–72.

Yoshida K (A), Smith B, Craggs M et al. Investigation of pharmacokinetics and of possible adverse effects in infants exposed to tricyclic antidepressants in breast-milk. J Affect Disord 1997; 43: 225–37.

Yoshida K (B), Smith B, Kumar RC. Fluvoxamine in breast-milk and infant development. Br J Clin Pharmacol 1997; 44: 210–11.

Yoshida K (A), Smith B, Craggs M et al. Fluoxetine in breastmilk and developmental outcome of breast-fed infants. Br J Psychiatry 1998; 172: 175–9.

Yoshida K (B), Smith B, Craggs M et al. Neuroleptic drugs in breast-milk: a study of pharmacokinetics and of possible adverse effects in breastfed infants. Psychological Med 1998; 28: 81–91.

Immunomodulating and antineoplastic agents 4.10

Ruth Lawrence and Christof Schaefer

At one time immunomodulating and antineoplastic agents were automatically considered a contraindication to breastfeeding, because any amount of antimetabolic drug was contraindicated in a newborn or young infant. Some of the newer compounds have relatively short half-lives and thus much shorter total clearance times (usually calculated as 5 × half-life). It is possible, therefore, for a woman determined to breastfeed her infant to pump and discard her milk right after a dose of medication, continuing until it has totally cleared. She then resumes breastfeeding until she receives another dose 2 or 3 weeks later.

4.10.1   Immunosuppressive and immune antineoplastic agents

Experience

Azathioprine and *cyclosporine* have been given to lactating women, and levels in the mother and in the milk have been reported. *Azathioprine*, which metabolizes to *6-mercaptopurine* (6-MP), was measured in the milk of two mothers and varied from 3.5 µg/l to 18 µg/l, which were peak levels done at 2 hours post-dose (Grekas 1984). These levels would represent 0.1% of the maternal dose. Since peak plasma time is 1–2 hours and azathioprine is poorly orally bioavailable (only 41–44%), the simple procedure of avoiding feeding for at least 2 hours post-dose would further decrease the amount available to the infant and maintain a level below 0.1% of the maternal dose. Among six breastfed children, one developed temporary symptoms of bone marrow dysfunction (Khare 2003). Considering the low relative dose, a causal association is remote. However, infants with the rare deficiency of thiopurine-methyltransferase (TPMT) could be sensitive to maternal long-term therapy while being breastfed. Even considering this case report, regular blood cell counts in breastfed children are not recommended.

Cyclosporine use in lactating women has been reported in several studies. Levels in maternal plasma studied in 15 mother–child pairs (Moretti 2003, Munoz-Flores-Thiagarajan 2001, Merlob 2000, Nyberg 1998, Thiru 1997) varied from 55 to 903 ng/ml. Corresponding milk levels were 14–1016 ng/ml, which works out at (at maximum) 2% of the weight-adjusted maternal dose. In another case, where the mother received 3 mg/kg per day, milk levels averaged 596 μg/l but infant trough blood levels remained under 3 μg/l when mother's were 260 μg/l. In a series of five patients receiving cyclosporine, however, one clinically unremarkable infant had trough blood levels (131 μg/l) near therapeutic levels (Moretti 2003). The other four infants had levels below 25 μg/l. Another 17 unremarkable breastfed infants were reported by Armenti (2003). The peak time for maternal blood level is 3.5 hours post-dose, so this would mean not breastfeeding for at least 4 hours to avoid peak milk levels. It is poorly absorbed orally (less than 30%).

Interferons are large molecules, and do not pass into the milk. They are not absorbed orally, and are given by injection. They are not contraindicated during lactation (Kumar 2000).

Tacrolimus is used for immunosuppression after liver transplant, and is reported on in 25 full-term pregnancies. The first milk samples after birth were measured at 0.6 μg/l, which suggests that the infant would receive less than 0.1 μg/kg daily. This represents a relative dosage of about 0.1%. Because the babies were not breastfed, there are no observations of any possible effects available (Jain 1997). A single case is reported where the mother received 0.1 mg/kg per day throughout pregnancy. Milk levels were measured sequentially. The maximum was measured at 1 hour post-dose, at 0.57 μg/l. This was estimated to be 0.06% of the maternal dose, or 0.02% absorbed by the infant based on the poor oral bioavailability (14–32%) (French 2003). A 29-year-old woman was exclusively breastfeeding her healthy 3-month-old infant while on tacrolimus 4 mg daily plus other drugs relevant to her transplant. The milk-to-blood ratio was 0.23, and average tacrolimus concentrations in milk were 1.8 g/l. The baby ingested approximately 0.5% of the maternal weight-adjusted dose (Gardiner 2006). Armenti (2003) reported on the normal development of seven breastfed children.

There are no data on *sirolimus*, *everolimus*, and *glatiramer* during lactation. Glatiramer has a molecular mass of 4700–11 000, which makes transfer to the milk almost impossible.

4

Lactation

4.10 Immunomodulating and antineoplastic agents

In a mother receiving 25 mg *etanercept* twice weekly, the maximum measured in her milk was 75 ng/ml (Ostensen 2004), resulting in a weight-adjusted dose of <3%. As a protein, etanercept is scarcely absorbed in an active form via the intestine.

There are insufficient data on monoclonal antibodies, for example the tumor necrosis factor-α (TNF-α), *infliximab*, which has a half-life of 9.5 days, or the substances *adalimumab, basiliximab* (half-life 7 days), *daclizumab*, and *muronomab-CD3*.

This also applies for the immunosuppressive *mycophenolate mofetil*, with a half-life of 6 hours, and for the cytokines *interleukin-10* and *interleukin-11*, for antibodies against CD4-positive lymphocytes, and for antibodies against *interleukin-12*, etc, whose immune modulator effect in practice is still being studied.

Boswellia serrata preparations (Indian incense tree), which are among the phytopharmaceuticals, are said to inhibit 5-lipoxygenesis. Used for chronic inflammatory bowel diseases and rheumatoid illnesses, they too have not been studied sufficiently with respect to breastfeeding.

> **Recommendation.** Azathioprine, mercaptopurine, cyclosporine A, and interferons should not, considering these data, be obstacles to breastfeeding. Tacrolimus, etanercept, and glatiramer are probably also very acceptable. Caution is advised with others, pending specific information.

4.10.2 Antineoplastics

Experience

There are only a few case reports on antineoplastics during lactation. The results of three reports on *cisplatin* are controversial: Egan (1985) could not detect cisplatin in breast milk, while de Vries (1989) found identical levels in milk and maternal blood. Ben-Baruch (1992) measured 10-fold lower concentrations in the milk compared to maternal plasma. *Cyclophosphamide* passes into mother's milk in large quantities, and thus acute toxic effects on the breastfed infant are possible. Relative dosages of under 5% have been reported for *hydroxyurea, doxorubicin*, and *methotrexate* (survey in Bennett 1996). A mother treated with *etoposid* for promyelocytic leukemia in remission initially had high levels in her milk, but there was no substance detectable 24 hours later. Concomitant *mitoxantrone* was measured at 129 µg/l in milk, and persisted in high concentrations 4 weeks later (Azuno 1995). There are no specific data on the other antineoplastics. This also applies to the mistletoe preparation *viscum album*.

Table 4.10.1 Antineoplastics during breastfeeding

Compound	Indication	Peak plasma time	Half-life	Recommendation
Altretamine	Ovarian, breast, cervical, pancreatic	0.5–3.0 hours	4.7–10.5 hours	Withhold breastfeeding for 72 hours
Anastrozole	Suppresses estrogen, ovarian and breast cancers		40–50 hours	One dose, withhold breastfeeding for 10 days; if taken daily, lactation is contraindicated
Asparaginase	Leukemia	14–24 hours	39–49 hours	Withhold breastfeeding for at least 7 days, total clearance = $50 \times 5 = 250$ hours ≈ 10 days
Bleomycin sulfate	Cervical, Hodgkins and non-Hodgkins		2–4 hours	Poor oral bioavailability, large molecular weight; withhold breastfeeding for 20 hours
Capecitabine	Colon cancer		0.5–0.75 hours, rapidly metabolized	Withhold breastfeeding for 6 hours
Carmustine – BCNU	Brain tumor, Hodgkins, gastric		1.5 ± 2 hours	Withhold breastfeeding for at least 24 hours, especially if side effects are still present
Cetuximab			70–100 hours	55 days to clear, makes breastfeeding impractical
Chlorambucil	Chronic leukemia, malignant lymphoma		1–2 hours	Withhold breastfeeding for 10 hours
Cisplatin	Affinity for plasma proteins		58–90 hours	Clearance is > 56 days; follow platinum levels in milk or discontinue breastfeeding

(Continued)

4.10 Immunomodulating and antineoplastic agents

4

Lactation

Table 4.10.1 (Continued)

Compound	Indication	Peak plasma time	Half-life	Recommendation
Cladribine	Leukemia, multiple sclerois		3–22 hours	Clearance in 14 hours, withhold breastfeeding
Cyclophosphamide	Breast cancer		4–8 hours	Breastfed infants have had effects on their bone marrow; withhold breastfeeding for 48 hours
Cytosine arabinoside	Acute lymphoid leukemia	20% overall absorbed from GI tract	1–3 hours	Withhold breastfeeding 15 hours
Dactinomycin	Wilm's tumor, Ewing's sarcoma		36 hours	Withhold breastfeeding for at least 7 days
Daunorubicin	Acute myelogenous and lymphocytic leukemias		20–40 hours	Withhold breastfeeding for a minimum of 7–10 days
Docetaxel			11 hours	Withhold breastfeeding for 48 hours
Doxorubicin		Peak 24 hours	24–36 hours	Withhold breastfeeding for at least 7 days
Epirubicin	Breast, lung, and bladder cancer		35 hours	Withhold breastfeeding for at least 7 days
Erlotinib		Peak 4 hours	36 hours	Withhold breastfeeding for a minimum of 7–10 days
Etoposide	Testicular and lung cancers, bone marrow transplant		4–11 hours	Withhold breastfeeding for 24–36 hours
Exemestane			24 hours	Discontinue breastfeeding if using multiple dosing; withhold for at least 5 days after last dose
Fluorouracil	Actinic keratosis, breast cancer, colorectal cancer, condylomata acuminata		8–20 minutes, 52 minutes (metabolites)	Mothers receiving injections of 5-FU should withhold breastfeeding for a minimum of 8 hours; mothers receiving topical therapy

Gemcitabine	Metastatic breast cancer, non-small cell lung cancer, pancreatic cancer	49 minutes (short infusions); 345–638 minutes (long infusions)	do not need to discontinue if the surface area is minimal Withhold breastfeeding for a minimum of 6 hours with short infusion and 7 days for long infusions
Ifosfamide	Breast cancer	4–8 hours	Withhold breastfeeding for at least 48 hours
Letrozole	Estrogen-dependent tumors, particularly breast cancer	Given daily for 2–6 weeks	2 days	Long treatment period of weeks usually precludes breastfeeding
Melphalan	Multiple myeloma, rhabdomyosarcoma, carcinoma of the ovary	1.5 hours	Withhold breastfeeding for 8 hours
Methotrexate		8–15 hours	Withhold breastfeeding for 4 days (96 hours)
Mitomycin	Stomach, breast, pancreas	23–78 minutes	Withhold breastfeeding for 8 hours
Mitoxantrone	Cancers and multiple sclerosis	23–215 hours, median 75 hours, still found in milk at 28 days	Withhold breastfeeding for a minimum of 31 days
Oxaliplatin	Platinum compound	39 hours	Either test breast milk for platinum levels and don't use if levels are measurable, or permanently interrupt breastfeeding without measuring
Paclitaxel	Kaposi's sarcoma, metastatic breast cancer	27 hours	Withhold breastfeeding for at least 6 days

(Continued)

4.10 Immunomodulating and antineoplastic agents

Table 4.10.1 (*Continued*)

Compound	Indication	Peak plasma time	Half-life	Recommendation
Pentostatin	Hairy cell leukemia		3–18 hours (mean = 5.7 hours)	Withhold breastfeeding for 4 days or longer if renal function is poor
Tamoxifen	Breast cancer	Usually taken daily	3–21 days	Mothers receiving tamoxifen should not breastfeed
Teniposide	Hematologic malignancies		5.4 hours	Withhold breastfeeding for 30–48 hours
Toremifene	Binds estrogen receptors		5 days	Withhold breastfeeding for a minimum of 25–30 days
Trastuzumab	Metastatic breast cancer		5.8 days	Low risk, but unknown; mothers should probably not breastfeed
Vinblastine	Breast cancer, Kaposi's sarcoma, Hodgkin's choriocarcinoma		24.8 (range = 3–29, depending on dose)	Withhold breastfeeding for a minimum of 7 days
Vincristine	Breast cancer, Kaposi's sarcoma, non-Hodgkin's, lymphoma	19–155 hours		Withhold breastfeeding for a minimum of 35 days
Vinorelbine	Advanced breast cancer, non-small cell lung cancer, non-Hodgkin's lymphoma, Hodgkin's disease, ovarian carcinoma		31.2–80 hours	Withhold breastfeeding for a minimum of 30 days

Information is obtained from multiple sources, including Hale 2006, Sweetman 2006, Briggs 2005.

> **Recommendation.** Table 4.10.1 lists many of these compounds, with an estimation of pump and discard times when appropriate. Others substances take so long to clear (4 weeks) that it is impractical to breastfeed. Some (such as tamoxifen) are given daily for long periods of time, so breastfeeding is not feasible.

References

Armenti VT, Radomski JS, Moritz MJ et al. Report from the national transplantation registry (NTPR): outcomes of pregnancy after transplantation. Clin Transpl 2003; 131–43.

Azuno Y, Kaku K, Fujita N. Mitoxantrone and etoposide in breast milk. Am J Hematol 1995; 48: 131–2.

Ben-Baruch G, Menczer J, Goshen R et al. Cisplatin excretion in human milk. J Natl Cancer Inst 1992; 84: 451–2.

Bennett PN (ed.). Drugs and Human Lactation, 2nd edn. Amsterdam: Elsevier, 1996.

Briggs, GG, Freeman RK, Yaffe SJ. Drugs in Pregnancy and Lactation, 7th edn. Philadelphia, PA: Lippincott Williams & Wilkins, 2005.

de Vries EGE, van der Zee AGJ, Uges DRA et al. Excretion of platinum into breast milk. Lancet 1989; 1: 497–8.

Egan PC, Costanza ME, Dodion P et al. Doxorubicin and cisplatin excretion into human milk. Cancer Treat Rep 1985: 69: 1387–9.

French AE, Soldin SW, Soldin OP et al. Milk transfer and neonatal safety of tacrolimus. Ann Pharmacother 2003; 37: 815–18.

Gardiner SJ, Begg EJ. Breastfeeding during tacrolimus therapy. Obstet Gynecol 2006; 107: 453–5.

Grekas DM, Vasiliou SS, Lazarides AN. Immunosuppressive therapy and breast-feeding after renal transplantation. Nephron 1984; 37: 68.

Hale TW Jr. Medications and Mother's Milk, 12th edn. Amarillo, TX: Hale Publishing, 2006.

Jain A, Venkataramanan R, Fung JJ et al. Pregnancy after liver transplantation under tacrolimus. Transplantation 1997; 64: 559–65.

Khare MM, Lott J, Currie A et al. Is it safe to continue azathioprine in breast feeding mothers? J Obstet Gynaecol 2003; 23(Suppl 1): S48.

Kumar AR, Hale TW, Mock RE. Transfer of interferon alpha into human breast milk. J Hum Lactation 2000; 16(3): 226–8.

Merlob P. Cyclosporine during lactation. BELTIS-Newsletter, 2000; 67–73.

Moretti ME, Sgro M, Johnson DW et al. Cyclosporin excretion into breast milk. Transplantation 2003; 75(12): 2144–6.

Munoz-Flores-Thiagarajan KD, Easterling T, Davis C et al. Breast-feeding by a cyclosporine-treated mother. Obstet Gynecol 2001; 97: 816–18.

Nyberg G, Haljamäe U, Frisenette-Fich C et al. Breast-feeding during treatment with cyclosporine. Transplantation 1998; 65: 253–5.

Ostensen M, Eigenmann GO. Etanercept in breast milk. J Rheumatol 2004; 31: 1017–18.

Sweetman SC (ed.). Martindale. The Complete Drug Reference, 34th edn. London: Pharmaceutical Press, 2006.

Thiru Y, Bateman DN, Coulthard MG. Successful breastfeeding while mother was taking cyclosporine. Br Med J 1997; 315(7106): 463.

4

Lactation

4.10 Immunomodulating and antineoplastic agents

Hormones and hormone antagonists

4.11

Christof Schaefer

4.11.1   Pituitary and hypothalamic hormones

Experience

There are only a few publications that discuss tolerance of hypothalamic and pituitary hormones during breastfeeding.

In a series of studies on the contraceptive effect of 600 µg of *buserelin*, a luteinizing hormone-releasing hormone (LRH) antagonist, administered nasally, a dosage of 1–2 µg was reported for the fully breastfed infant. Oral bioavailability is poor, so a toxic effect on a breastfed child would not be expected (Fraser 1989).

The thyrotrophin-releasing hormone (TRH) *protirelin* releases *prolactin*. Its lactation-promoting use has been discussed (Peters 1991). Toxic effects on a breastfed infant would not be expected; however, there have been no studies.

Desmopressin is found in mother's milk only in limited amounts.

Oxytocin, which has long been used to induce labor and for postpartum uterine involution, promotes the milk ejection reflex, and has not been shown to be toxic for the infant.

Carbetocin is a synthetic analog of oxytocin which is used intravenously and intramuscularly. It is effective for longer than oxytocin, and appears in the mother's milk in minimal amounts (0.00005% of the maternal weight-related dosage) (Silox 1993).

There are no data on the use during breastfeeding of the other hypothalamic and pituitary hormones, or their synthetic analogs *corticorelin, sermorelin, somatorelin, cetrorelix, chorionic gonadotrophin, gonadorelin, goserelin, leuprolide acetate, menotropin, nafarelin, triptorelin, urogonadotropin, octreotide, somatostatin, tetracosactid, somatropin* (growth hormone), *follitrophin-α, follitrophin-β, urofollitrophin, argipressin, lypressin, ornipressin, lanreotide*, and *terlipressin*. This also holds true for the oxytocin-antagonist *atosiban* and the somatropin-receptor antagonist *pegvisomant*.

> **Recommendation.** With the exception of oxytocin, hypothalamic and pituitary hormones are seldom indicated during breastfeeding. No toxic effect on the infant has been demonstrated as yet, nor, due to its limited oral bioavailability, is this to be expected. Usage for appropriate indications during breastfeeding is allowed.

4.11.2   Methylergometrine (methylergonovine)

Experience

With therapy using 2×0.125 mg *methylergometrine* up to 1.1 µg/l was measured in the milk. This is a maximum of 0.16 µg/kg of the infant's bodyweight, or 3.1% of the maternal weight-related dosage. In a more recent study on 20 women with postpartum uterine atony, either 250 µg methylergometrine or 200 µg *misoprostol* were applied orally (see also section 4.11.13). The maximum methylergometrine concentration in milk was reached at 2 hours. It has a half-life of 1.9 hours. Considering the maximum concentration in milk, the relative dose was 2.4%. The median M/P ratio was 0.2 (Vogel 2004).

A potentially negative influence on milk production due to prolactin antagonism is known. For breastfed infants themselves, the preparation seems to be tolerated in the overwhelming majority of cases. It should, however, be mentioned that the author has received to date 15 case descriptions involving ergotism-like symptoms in breastfed children (particularly restlessness, vomiting, and diarrhea). This cannot be explained in light of the above-mentioned limited transfer. Experiences with accidental direct administration of methylergometrine, owing to a mix-up of the medication in the delivery room, also argue against a toxic risk via the mother's milk. In such cases, ergotism-like symptoms were first observed after a dosage that was 150–200 times above that transferred through mother's milk (Hoffmann-Walbeck 2001, Poison Control Center Berlin, unpublished observations). However, hypersensitivity, or the transfer of individual higher doses via breast milk, cannot be ruled out. In this connection, those studies on the pharmacological effects of ergotamine residue in mothers' milk carried out in the 1930s are of at least historical interest (Fomina 1933).

> **Recommendation.** Single parenteral administration of methylergometrine in the delivery room is apparently unproblematic for the breastfed infant, and may be used if it is really indicated. Postpartum oral treatment with methylergometrine over several days, or even weeks, is rarely indicated in modern obstetrics. It should be considered that this agent counteracts the natural uterine involution, which normally occurs during breastfeeding via prolactin secretion. Oxytocin, which promotes the milk ejection reflex, is preferable as a medical support for uterine involution. If, however, there are sound grounds to use methylergometrine for a protracted time, there is no need for breastfeeding to be limited.

4.11.3 Bromocriptine and other prolactin inhibitors

Experience

Bromocriptine is an ergotamine derivative. As a prolactin inhibitor, it reduces the milk production and is used to treat prolactinoma. Because of the possible cardiovascular side effects in the mother, particularly the threat of cerebral angiopathy (Hopp 1996, Iffy 1996), it has a very limited use in stopping lactation (see also section 3.7).

The American Food and Drug Administration (FDA) has withdrawn permission to use bromocriptine for this purpose (Herings 1995). Following a dosage of 2.5 mg, less than 0.1 μg/l can be expected to appear in the mother's milk; this represents 0.04% of the maternal weight-related dosage (reported by manufacturer Sandoz).

Intolerance in the breastfed baby, even with prolactinoma treatment, has not been observed (Canales 1981). Even after an intake of 5 or 10 mg daily, no side effects via the mother's milk are to be expected in the infant.

The effect of breastfeeding on the growth of the prolactinoma appears to be more limited than that of the pregnancy, so an interruption of dopamine agonist treatment with bromocriptine during breastfeeding can be considered (Rau 1996).

Cabergoline is taken less often (e.g. once a week) because of its considerably longer half-life and period of effectiveness. In addition, there seem to be fewer side effects. With respect to the other prolactin inhibitors, *lisuride, metergoline,* and *quinagolide,* experience during breastfeeding is insufficient.

Recommendation. Because of maternal risks, routine prescription of bromocriptine to stop lactation is not indicated. If physical measures (and, in cases of mastitis, antibiotic treatment) are insufficient, cabergoline should be preferred (see also Chapter 3.7). If therapy with prolactin inhibitors for mastitis is unavoidable, the briefest and lowest dosage should be used so that milk production will not diminish. As long as milk is being produced, breastfeeding may continue, even when cabergoline is being given. In so far as other experience is available, this also applies to the other prolactin inhibitors. If the milk supply has diminished during antiprolactin treatment, relactation may be undertaken if desired.

4.11.4   Thyroid hormones and thyroid receptor antibodies

Experience

L-thyroxine is used as a substitute in cases of hypothyroidism (at least 1 μg/kg daily for adults), and, for this reason, is not problematic. The normal thyroid content of mother's milk is approximately 1 μg/l. An infant takes in about 0.15 μg/kg in 24 hours; this represents about 1% of a substitution dosage at this age (10 μg/kg daily). This amount does not influence the thyroid function of a healthy infant. The same applies for treatment (substitution) of a maternal hypoparathyroidism.

4

Lactation

4.11 Hormones and hormone antagonists

Of course, this also means it has no therapeutic effect in case of a congenital hypo- or athyroidism. This has to be taken into account in case of extremely premature newborns with a higher risk for hypothyroidism. Neither breast milk nor formula contains enough thyroxine for substitution (van Wassenaer 2002).

Thyroid receptor antibodies (TRAb) can result in transient neonatal thyroid disease by transfer through milk from mothers treated for thyrotoxicosis. Serum TRAb concentration in neonates decrease continuously with time after birth. The calculated half-life for offspring-serum and breast-milk TRAb was calculated as approximately 3 weeks and 2 months, respectively. Transient neonatal thyroid disease may be worse and more prolonged during breastfeeding as a consequence of TRAb in breast milk (Törnhage 2006).

> **Recommendation.** Substitution of thyroid and parathyroid hormones establishes a physiological state, and, thus should be continued during breastfeeding if necessary. Thyroid hormones should not be given together with thyrostatics, because higher dosages of thyrostatics would then be necessary.

4.11.5   Thyrostatics

Experience

The thyrostatics include *carbimazole, propylthiouracil, thiamazol (= methimazol)*, and *sodium perchlorate*. Carbimazole is metabolized to thiamazol as the active metabolite.

The M/P quotients of *carbimazole* and *thiamazol* are about 1. With 40 mg *carbimazole* daily, peak methimazole values of 0.72 mg/l of milk were measured (Cooper 1984). A maximum relative dosage of 27% carbimazole is calculated for the breastfed infant. On average, however, 2–10% of the weight-related dosage is more likely (survey by Bennett 1996).

With 5 mg *thiamazol* per day, up to 65 μg/l milk could be measured. Accordingly, an infant would receive up to 9.8 μg/kg daily. This represents about 12% of the maternal dosage per kg bodyweight. In the plasma of breastfed twins, 45 and 53 μg/l – subtherapeutic levels – of thiamazol were found. The children had no symptoms, and their thyroid status was unremarkable (Rylance 1987).

A study of 46 children whose mothers received 20 mg *methimazole* daily for 1 month, and 42 children whose mothers started with 30 mg daily and subsequently reduced to 5–10 mg, reported normal T_3, T_4 and TSH values (Azizi 2002). Psychomotor development was normal at the age of 49–86 months (Azizi 2003).

With treatment using 400 mg *propylthiouracil*, a maximum of 0.7 mg/l was found in the mother's milk. For the infant this is at most 0.1 mg/kg, i.e. 1.5% of the maternal weight-related dosage in 24 hours. The M/P ratio is 0.1 (Kampmann 1980). In older studies in which the methodology was insufficient, M/P values of 12 were calculated. In a newer study of 11 children whose mothers took 300–750 mg daily, elevated TSH values were seen in 2 children 7 days after birth. However, these normalized over the course of time, although the maternal dosage remained stable or was even increased. No correlation was found between the maternal dosage or the maternal thyroid hormone FT4 on the one hand, and the infant's TSH on the other. Even with the highest daily dosage, there appears to be no risk for the breastfed baby (Momotani 2000).

Sodium perchlorate is a reserve thyrostatic. It blocks the thyroid by replacing iodine, and is used during scintigraphic studies of other organs with radioactive iodine. Sodium perchlorate blocks also the transport to the breast, where iodine accumulates (Janssen 2001). There is no experience of its use during breastfeeding.

> **Recommendation.** Propylthiouracil is the thyrostatic of choice during breastfeeding, and should be used in preference to thiamazol and carbimazole, especially when more than 10 mg daily of either of these substances is required regularly. If the breastfeeding mother has been or still is being treated with a dosage in the upper therapeutic range, the thyroid parameter of the infant should be tested after about 3 weeks just to be safe. This also applies for propylthiouracil. Sodium perchlorate should not be used during breastfeeding. Thyroid hormones should not be given together with thyrostatics, because a higher thyrostatic dosage would be necessary.

4.11.6   Iodine

Experience

While breastfeeding, the mother's iodine requirement is 260 μg/daily. For infants aged up to 4 months, a daily intake of 50 μg *iodine* is recommended; for prematures this should be 30 μg. Iodine supplementation must be ensured during breastfeeding in areas where iodine is deficient. This can be difficult to achieve by diet with iodized salt and weekly salt-water fish meals if the level of iodine in iodized salt is only 15–25 μg/g and below the amount needed, if iodized foods are still the exception, and if regular consumption of saltwater fish does not appeal. In these cases, supplemental iodine tablets must be taken to cover the above-mentioned requirements. A newer study confirms that this supplementation significantly increases the iodine content in mother's milk, which tends to be too low. However, it does not always achieve this on a scale that is desirable. With prematures, the amount of iodine transferred with the milk every day could only be increased to 12 μg/kg (Seibold-Weiger 1999).

Iodine accumulates more significantly in mother's milk than any other medication studied to date. Different authors report M/P quotients between 15 and 65 with iodine products such as *povidone iodine* or the radioactive isotope *iodine[131]*. Up to 49% of the total maternal iodine[131] dosage is excreted in the milk within 24 hours!

Inhibition of the infant's thyroid function (Wolff–Chaikoff effect) caused by high iodine dosage is possible if the child takes in 100 μg/kg daily, or has a plasma concentration of 250 μg/l (Schönberger 1982). The use of iodine-containing disinfectants such as *povidone iodine* over wide areas (Chanoine 1988), or *potassium iodine* as an expectorant, could lead to a relatively high dosage of free iodine in the mother's milk and cause inhibition of the infant's thyroid function. In a healthy, term, fully breastfed newborn, hypothyroid parameters were diagnosed on day 17. The mother was treated with iodoform gauze because of a rectal abscess. The laboratory findings normalized after the treatment was stopped. The clinically normal infant was temporarily treated with thyroxin supplementation (l'Italien 2004).

Recommendation. Sufficient iodine supplementation (about 260 μg daily) should be attempted in the interests of both mother and child. A risk of iodine overload for the infant via the mother's milk should not be expected at this dosage level.

Iodine-containing disinfectants should only be used on small wounds. Iodine-containing expectorants are contraindicated.

4.11.7   Corticosteroids

Experience

Corticosteroids are of practical significance during breastfeeding. Those that are used therapeutically include the non-fluorinated *prednisone, prednisolone*, and *methylprednisolone*, as well as *deflazacort, hydrocortisone* and *prednyliden*; and the fluoridated substances *amcinonide, beclomethasone, betamethasone, budesonide, cloprednol, dexamethasone, flunisolide, flumetasone, fluocortolone, fluticasone, mometasone*, and *triamcinolone*. Some preparations are used exclusively as inhalants for treating obstructive respiratory illnesses.

The M/P ratio of prednisone and prednisolone varies between 0.05 and 0.25.

One hour after parenteral administration of a single dose of 110 mg of *prednisolone*, a level of 760 µg/l was measured in the milk. Four hours later it was 260 µg/l, and about 9 hours after administration the level was still 60 µg/l. Following an intravenous injection of 1 g of prednisolone, a nine-fold higher value was measured in the milk, reflecting the nine-fold higher dosage. Twenty-four hours after administration, it could no longer be detected in the milk (unpublished observation of the author).

Other authors have reported proportional or even lower transfer amounts with a lower daily dosage of 10–80 mg (survey by Bennett 1996, Greenberger 1993). All in all, an average of 1–2% of the maternal weight-related dosage can be expected for the infant. In the case of the 1-g dose described above, the infant received 0.2 mg of prednisolone per kg bodyweight with the first breastfeed an hour after the injection. Over 24 hours, it was 0.32 mg/kg. Even this highest maternal dosage provides only about a sixth of a therapeutic child's dosage, which is usually well-tolerated (2 mg/kg per day). There is no risk for the infant from the usual short-term high-dose treatment, even when breastfed right after the injection.

Even with longer-term treatment using 80 mg daily, only a small amount of prednisolone, which does not equal 10% of the body's own cortisol production, is transferred into the milk. There are insufficient documented data on transfer with the other corticoids.

> **Recommendation.** Prednisolone, prednisone, and methylprednisolone are the corticoids of choice for systemic treatment during breastfeeding. Even high doses of up to 1 g administered once or for a few consecutive days – for example, for an asthma attack or multiple sclerosis – do not require any limitation of breastfeeding. When such high doses are given repeatedly, there should be a 3–4-hour wait for breastfeeding if that can be arranged. Other corticoids are probably also tolerated. Routine inhalation of a corticoid for asthma is no cause for concern.

4.11.8   Adrenaline

Experience

Adrenaline and *noradrenaline* are reserved for emergency situations, when breastfeeding is not permitted in any case. No toxic effect on the infant should be expected from the limited amount of adrenaline which is added to local anesthesia.

4 Lactation

4.11 Hormones and hormone antagonists

> **Recommendation.** If adrenaline, noradrenaline or similar catecholamines must be administered during breastfeeding, this does not require weaning.

4.11.9   Insulin and oral antidiabetics

Experience

Insulin as a proteohormone does not reach the mother's milk, and is not absorbed intestinally. Any effect on the infant can therefore be ruled out.

Neither *glibenclamide* nor *glipizide* were detected in the breast-milk of three mothers. Hypoglycemia was not observed in any of the children. In another eight women receiving a single dosage of gliben-clamide, no substance was found in milk. A high protein-binding of 98% could explain these results (Feig 2005).

Only small amounts of *metformin* are found in mothers' milk; the weight-adjusted dose for a fully breastfed child is 0.1–0.7% (Briggs 2005, Gardiner 2003, Hale 2002). Hypoglycemia was not reported in breastfed infants. Metformin concentrations in breast milk remained stable over the time of observation. Growth, motor-social development, and illness requiring a pediatrician's visit were assessed in 61 nursing infants (21 male, 40 female) and 50 formula-fed infants (19 male, 31 female) born to 92 mothers with polycystic ovary syndrome (PCOS) taking a median of 2.55 g metformin per day throughout pregnancy and lactation. At 3 and 6 months of age, the weight, height, and motor-social development did not differ between breast- and formula-fed infants. No infants had retardation of growth, or of motor or social development. Intercurrent illnesses did not differ (Glueck 2006).

Up to 16.2% of the weight-related dosage of *tolbutamide* can pass into the milk (Moiel 1967).

There are no data on the other oral antidiabetics, *acarbose, glibornuride, gliclazide, glimepiride, gliquidone, glisoxepide, miglitol, pioglitazone, repaglinide,* and *rosiglitazone*.

There is also insufficient experience on the antihypoglycemics *glucagon* and *diazoxide*.

> **Recommendation.** Insulin and metformin are not problems during breastfeeding. Glibenclamide may also be taken; however, the infant should be observed for symptoms of hypoglycemia after the start of therapy. Other oral antidiabetics should not be taken, but single doses do not require any limitation of breastfeeding.

4.11.10 Estrogens, gestagens, and hormonal contraceptives

Effect on milk production

The amount of milk produced can decrease as a result of the influence of *estrogen*. With the older, higher-dosage contraceptives, a reduction of up to 40% was described. Changes in the calorie, protein, nitrogen, and lipid content were also observed, and are apparently dependent on the starting point. With normally nourished women, the alterations stay within the physiological bounds. However, when there is a prior milk-supply problem, the influence on the milk production can be unfortunate; when the mother is poorly nourished, it can be dramatic. In follow-up studies, including those on the new low-dosage preparations, the slight reductions observed in the average length of breastfeeding and in milk production, as well as the temporarily slightly reduced weight gain of the infants, did not have any effect on the physical or cognitive development (survey in Bennett 1996).

Gestagens (*norethisterone, levonorgestrel, medroxyprogesterone*) as an ingredient of a mini- or combination pill or as a "3-month shot", have little or no effect on the milk supply, and only a very limited effect on the composition. In fact, many researchers observed a longer period of breastfeeding with mothers with depot-*medroxyprogesterone* as compared to those mothers without hormonal contraception (survey in Bennett 1996).

Hormonal transfer to the infant via the mother's milk

With a daily intake of 50 μg, *ethinylestradiol* cannot be detected in the mother's milk. Only after oral administration of 500 μg can an infant's dose be calculated, at 0.026 μg/kg daily. This is about 0.2% of the maternal dosage per kg bodyweight.

Vaginal administration of 50 or 100 mg of *estradiol* also leads to negligible amounts in the mother's milk – less than 0.1% of the maternal weight-related dosage (survey by Bennett 1996).

The other estrogens, *chlorotrianisen, epimestrol, estriol, fosfestrole, mestranol*, and *polyestradiol*, have not been studied during lactation. For most of them, there is no indication for use during breastfeeding.

The gestagen intake of the infant lies between 1 and 2% of the weight-related maternal dosage in a contraceptive preparation. This has been shown for "pills" with *desogestrel, megestrol, norethisterone acetate, norethynodrel*, and *norgestrel* (survey by Bennett 1996, Shaaban 1991).

With 3 mg/d *drospirenon* in combination with ethinylestradiol, there was, on average, 3.7 ng/ml milk in six breastfeeding women.

4

Lactation

4.11 Hormones and hormone antagonists

A fully breastfed infant would therefore receive 0.6 μg/kg per day, i.e. 1% of the weight-adjusted maternal dosage. No symptoms were observed in any of the children (Blode 2001).

With *lynestrenol*, a relative dosage of less than 1% was reported. The transferred portion for the infant directly after injection of 150 mg depot-*medroxyprogesterone* acetate as a "3-month shot" was 7.5 μg/kg daily (survey by Bennett 1996).

Elcometrin, with an effectiveness of 6 months, is administered in a subdermal capsule. A maximum of 674 pmol of the active ingredient was found in the maternal serum. In the milk this was up to 640 pmol, and in the serum of individual children up to 55 pmol, while in others the serum concentration was beneath the detection limit of 13 pmol. The samples were taken 75 days following implantation. Up to the end of the first year of life, the development of the 66 children participating did not differ from those in a control group in which the mothers had copper IUDs as contraception devices (Coutinho 1999).

Centchroman, a new nonsteroid oral contraceptive which is initially taken twice a week and later only once a week, has been studied in 13 women. With doses of 30 mg, a maximum of 122 μg/l was found in the milk. On average, however, the values were more likely to be about 50 μg/l or less. Mathematically speaking, a fully breastfed baby would receive up to 11% of a maternal weight-related dosage. The M/P ratio is between 1 and 2 (Gupta 1995).

There is no special information on milk transfer with *chlormadinon, dydrogestone, gestonorone, gestoden, hydroxyprogesterone, levonorgestrel, medrogestone*, and *norgestimate*.

When used in oral contraceptive preparations, in gestagen-containing intrauterine pessaries, and in the "morning-after pill", these substances can probably be evaluated similarly to the above-mentioned contraceptives. Higher-dosed gestagen preparations used for other indications have not been studied with respect to their kinetics, but there are unlikely to be many indications for their use during breastfeeding.

▶ **Long-term effects of hormonal contraception**

The hormonal transfer from contraceptive gestagen monopreparations (the mini-pill or depot injection) and low-dosage combination "pills" into the milk does not affect the development of the infant's sexual organs. In his literature review, Truitt (2003) could not find any differences between gestagene monotherapy and combination pills regarding the amount and quality of milk production. However, he underlined methodological problems in many of the evaluated studies that limited his conclusions. Another study compared long-term development between 220 breastfed infants of mothers with lev-onorgestrel therapy and 222 infants whose mothers used copper IUDs for contraception. Children with levonorgestrel had slightly more mild respiratory tract infections, eye infections, and skin problems during the first year of life. Children whose mothers used copper IUDs more frequently showed slight psychomotor development retardation (Schiappacasse 2002). These observations should also be interpreted with caution.

Up to 6 months postpartum and in the presence of ongoing amenorrhea, the contraceptive protection from exclusive breastfeeding should be similar to that of an intrauterine pessary (IUP) or hormonal contraception (Kennedy 1992). In the so-called developing world, much more "birth control" is attributed to breastfeeding than to the other family planning measures (Hanson 1994).

> **Recommendation.** Pure gestagen preparations (mini-pills) are the oral contraceptive of choice during breastfeeding. If the mother does not tolerate them, then the low-dosage combination "pills" (ethinylestradiol plus gestagen), or gestagen depot preparations, are acceptable. If necessary, they can be started about 6–8 weeks after birth. There is no preparation among the well-established hormonal contraceptives which requires an interruption of breastfeeding.

4.11.11   Androgens and anabolics

Experience

There is no experience with the available androgens, *mesterolone, testolactone*, and *testosterone*. The same applies to the anabolics, *clostebol, metenolone*, and *nandrolone*.

> **Recommendation.** Androgens and anabolics are contraindicated during breastfeeding. Accidental intake of a single dose does not require an interruption in breastfeeding.

4.11.12   Cyproterone acetate and other sex-hormone inhibitors

Experience

Following a dosage of 50 mg of *cyproterone acetate*, peak values of $260\,\mu g/l$ were measured in the milk. The infant's exposure would be

39 µg/kg/daily. That is just about 5% of the maternal weight-related dosage (Stoppeli 1980). The more common daily intake of 2 mg of cyproterone acetate for acne therapy has not yet been studied.

Other antiandrogens, such as *bicalutamide* and *flutamide*, and antiestrogen-acting substances, such as *aminoglutethimide, anastrozole, formestan, raloxifene,* and *tamoxifen*, as well as the sex-hormone inhibitors *danazol* and *tibolone*, have practically no role during breastfeeding and have also not been studied.

There are also no data on *clomiphene* and the progesterone antagonist *mifepristone*. In so far as its (accidental) use during breastfeeding happens at all, a toxic effect on the infant should not be expected due to the brief exposure.

> **Recommendation.** Antiandrogens and antiestrogens are contraindicated during breastfeeding. Accidental intake of a single dose does not require an interruption of breastfeeding. However, treatment should not be continued.

4.11.13 Prostaglandins

Experience

Prostaglandins are, for the most part, used in obstetrics for priming and inducing labor. After birth, other pharmaceuticals are used for uterine involution so that therapy during breastfeeding for obstetrical indications is not common. *Latanoprost* is administered as eye drops for glaucoma.

Prostaglandin derivatives have short half-lives ranging from a few seconds to 20–40 minutes at maximum. Both milk-promoting and milk-inhibiting effects have been noted with the various prostaglandins. In a study of 20 women with postpartum uterine atony, either 200 µg *misoprostol* or 250 µg *methylergometrine* were administered orally. The maximum misoprostol concentration in milk was reached at 1 hour, with a half-life of 0.6 hours on average, whereas methylergometrine reached the maximum at 2 hours with a half-life of 1.9 hours. Considering the maximum concentration in milk, the relative dose for misoprostol was 0.04% and that of methylergometrine 2.4%. The median M/P ratios were 0.04 and 0.2, respectively (Vogel 2004).

There is no indication yet of negative effects of prostaglandins in the breastfed infant. However, documented experience is still insufficient.

> **Recommendation.** Prostaglandins should only be used for compelling treatment indications during breastfeeding. If severe glaucoma requires local treatment with latanoprost, breastfeeding can continue provided there is careful observation of the baby. Single doses of other prostaglandins, such as misoprostol for uterine atony, do not require any limitation of breastfeeding.

References

Azizi F, Hedavati M. Thyroid function in breast-fed infants whose mothers take high doses of methimazole. J Endocrinol Invest 2002; 25: 493–6.

Azizi F, Bahrainian M, Khamseh ME et al. Intellectual development and thyroid function in children who were breast-fed by thyrotoxic mothers taking methimazole. J Pediatr Endocr Metab 2003; 16: 1239–43.

Bennett PN (ed.). Drugs and Human Lactation, 2nd edn. Amsterdam: Elsevier, 1996.

Blode H, Foidart JM, Heithecker R. Transfer of drospirenone to breast milk after a single oral administration of 3 mg drospirenone + 30 microg ethinylestradiol to healthy lactating women. Eur J Contracep Reprod Health Care 2001; 6: 167–71.

Briggs GG, Ambrose PJ, Nageotte MP et al. Excretion of metformin into breast milk and the effect on nursing infants. Obstet Gynecol 2005; 105: 1437–41.

Canales ES, Garcia IC, Ruiz JE et al. Bromocriptine as prophylactic therapy in prolactinoma during pregnancy. Fertil Steril 1981; 36: 524–6.

Chanoine JP, Boulvain M, Bourdoux P et al. Increased recall rate at screening for congenital hypothyroidism in breast fed infants born to iodine overloaded mothers. Arch Dis Child 1988; 63: 1207–10.

Cooper DS, Bode HH, Nath B et al. Methimazole pharmacology in man: studies using a newly developed radioimmunoassay for methimazole. J Clin Endocrinol Metab 1984; 58: 473–9.

Coutinho EM, Athayde C, Dantas C et al. Use of a single implant of elcometrine (ST-1435), a non-orally active progestin, as a long acting contraceptive for postpartum nursing women. Contraception 1999; 59: 115–22.

Feig DS, Briggs GG, Kraemer JM et al. Transfer of glyburide and glipizide into breast milk. Diabetes Care 2005; 28: 1851–5.

Fomina PI. Untersuchungen über den Übergang des aktiven Agens des Mutterkorns in die Milch stillender Mütter. Archiv f Gynäkologie 1933; 157: 275–85.

Fraser HM, Dewart PJ, Smith SK et al. Luteinizing hormone releasing hormone agonist for contraception in breast-feeding women. J Clin Endocrinol Metab 1989; 69: 996–1002.

Gardiner SJ, Kirkpatrick CMJ, Begg EJ et al. Transfer of metformin into human milk. Clin Pharmacol Ther 2003; 73: 71–7.

Glueck CJ, Salehi M, Sieve L et al. Growth, motor, and social development in breast- and formula-fed infants of metformin-treated women with polycystic ovary syndrome. J Pediatr 2006; 148: 628–32.

Greenberger PA, Odeh YK, Frederiksen MC et al. Pharmacokinetics of prednisolone transfer to breast milk. Clin Pharmacol Ther 1993; 53: 324–8.

Gupta RC, Paliwal JK, Nityanand S et al. Centchroman: a new non-steroidal oral contraceptive in human milk. Contraception 1995; 52: 301–5.

4

Lactation

4.11 Hormones and hormone antagonists

Hale TW, Kristensen JH, Hackett LP et al. Transfer of metformin into human milk. Diabetologia 2002; 45: 1509–14.

Hanson LA, Ashraf R, Zaman S et al. Breast feeding is a natural contraceptive and prevents disease and death in infants, linking infant mortality and birth rates. Acta Paediatr 1994; 83: 3–6.

Herings RM, Strieker BH. Bromocriptine and suppression of postpartum lactation. Pharm World Sci 1995; 17: 133–7.

Hopp L, Haider B, Iffy L. Myocardial infarction post-partum in patients taking bromocriptine for the prevention of breast engorgement. Intl J Cardiology 1996; 57: 227–32.

Iffy L, McArdle JJ, Ganesh V. Intracerebral hemorrhage in normotensive mothers using bromocriptine postpartum. Zentralbl Gynäkol 1996; 118: 392–6.

Janssen OE, Heufelder AE, Mann K. Schilddrüsenerkrankungen. In: D Ganten (ed.), Molekulargenetische Grundlagen von Endokrinopathien. Berlin Heidelberg Springer Verlag, 2001, pp. 47–8.

Kampmann JP, Hansen JM, Johansen K et al. Propylthiouracil in human milk. Lancet 1980; 1: 736–8.

Kennedy KI, Visness CM. Contraceptive efficacy of lactational amenorrhoea. Lancet 1992; 339: 227–30.

l'Italien A, Starceski PJ, Dixit NM. Transient hypothyroidism in a breastfed infant after maternal use of iodoform gauze. J Pediatr Endocrinol Metab 2004; 17: 665–7.

Moiel RH, Ryan RJ. Tolbutamide orinase in human breast milk. Clin Pediatr 1967; 6: 480.

Momotani N, Yamashita R, Makino F et al. Thyroid function in wholly breastfeeding infants whose mothers take high doses of propylthiouracil. Clin Endocrinol 2000; 53: 177–81.

Peters F, Schulze-Tollert J, Schuth W. Thyrotropin-releasing hormone – a lactation-promoting agent? Br J Obstet Gynecol 1991; 98: 880–85.

Rau H, Badenhoop K, Usadel KH. The treatment of prolactinomas during pregnancy and the lactation period {in German}. Dtsch Med Wschr 1996; 121: 28–32.

Rylance RY, Woods CG, Donnelly MC et al. Carbimazole and breast feeding. Lancet 1987; i: 928.

Schiappacasse V, Diaz S, Zepeda A et al. Health and growth of infants breastfed by Norplant contraceptive implants users: a six-year follow-up study. Contraception 2002; 66: 57–65.

Schönberger W, Grimm W. Transient hypothyroidism caused by iodine-containing disinfectants in the newborn {in German; author's transl}. Dtsch Med Wochenschr 1982; 107: 1222–7.

Seibold-Weiger K, Wollmann H, Rendl J et al. Iodine concentration in the breast milk of mothers of premature infants {in German}. Z Geburtsh Neonatol 1999; 203: 81–5.

Shaaban MM. Contraception with progestogens and progesterone during lactation. J Steroid Biochem Mol Biol 1991; 40: 705–10.

Silox J, Schulz P, Horbay GLA et al. Transfer of carbetocin into human breast milk. Obstet Gynecol 1993; 83: 456–9.

Stoppeli I, Rainer E, Humpel M. Transfer of cyproterone acetate to the milk of lactating women. Contraception 1980; 22: 485–93.

Törnhage CJ, Grankvist K. Acquired neonatal thyroid disease due to TSH receptor antibodies in breast milk. J Pediatr Endocrinol Metab 2006; 19: 787–94.

Truitt ST, Fraser AB, Grimes DA et al. Hormonal contraception during lactation. Systematic review of randomized controlled trials. Contraception 2003; 68: 233–8.

van Wassenaer AG, Stulp MR, Valianpour F et al. The quantity of thyroid hormone in human milk is too low to influence plasma thyroid hormone levels in the very preterm infant. Clin Endocrinol (Oxf) 2002; 56: 621–7.

Vogel D, Burkhardt T, Rentsch K et al. Misoprostol versus methylergometrine: pharmacokinetics in human milk. Am J Obstet Gynecol 2004; 191: 2168–73.

Dermatological drugs and local therapeutics

4.12

Ruth Lawrence and Christof Schaefer

4.12.1 General aspects of external applications: cosmetics, hair products, sunscreens

Experience

The skin is a portal of entry for pharmacologically active compounds; however, most skin preparations are intended to soften, lubricate, and beautify. Oils, emollients, creams, and beauty lotions generally act locally on the skin, and do not contain active principles. There are, however, skin preparations that contain potent active chemicals, including liniments and treatments for acne, psoriasis, and other skin diseases. It then becomes a matter of dose, including the concentration of the active ingredient, the surface area covered, the thickness of skin in the area treated, and the treatment interval. In the following section, a selection of products will be discussed. For substances not mentioned here, those recommendations in Chapter 2.17 can serve as orientation. If treatment involves a large area of the skin over a long period, then the absorption and effects of the individual substances must be considered. Here, the advice on systemic use can serve as orientation (see, for instance, iodine and salicylates).

When the breast needs to be treated externally, it should be cleaned before the baby is fed. In principle, the absorption and transfer of substances into the mother's milk (see, for example, moschus derivatives – Chapter 4.18), as well as an allergic sensitization in the breastfed baby, cannot be ruled out. However, hypersensitization as well as toxic symptoms have not been demonstrated as yet. This does not change the obligation to reduce dermal applications to those that are absolutely essential.

Hair preparations require some care in applying. It is recommended that bleaching, dying, straightening or curling be done by a professional to reduce the exposure of the lactating woman. The scalp is thick and absorbs poorly, so these chemicals can be used carefully if the hair is rinsed thoroughly. The application should be done wearing protective gloves. No studies have been done to measure the chemicals in the milk, but it is highly unlikely that much is absorbed and that any reaches the milk. Having the procedure done while lactating is considered safe.

Sunscreens have become universal at the urging of dermatologists. The absorption is considered minimal. Para-amino benzoic acid (PABA) is being removed from most preparations because of concern regarding absorption and a possible link to cancer. Current preparations can contain octocrylene 8% w/w, octyl methoxycinnamate 7.5% w/w, oxyenzone 4 w/w, octyl salicylate 5% w/w, ethylhexyl P-methoxycinnamate 7.5% w/w, 2-ethylhexyl salicylate 3% w/w, titanium dioxide 1.64% w/w, benzophenone-3, and octocrylene.

Preparations that can be applied directly to an infant's skin in the form of baby sunscreen contain oxybenzone 5% ethylhexyl P-methoxycinnamate 7.5%, and 2-ethylhexyl salicylate 3%. There are no data regarding measurement of these chemicals in milk.

Maternal use of sunscreen while lactating is considered safe when mother relies on shading to minimize direct sun exposure as well.

Recommendation. Hair preparations, cosmetics, and sunscreens can be used with caution while lactating.

4.12.2 Medications for lice and scabies

Experience

Lice

Medications for lice include over-the-counter preparations containing 1% *pyrethrum*, a natural insecticide. This is relatively non-toxic, and application can be repeated. Herbal preparations which also contain *chrysanthemums* can cause allergic reaction in individuals who are allergic to this family of plants (chrysanthemums, ragweed, and Echinacea are all members of the Composite family). *Permethrin* and *allethrin* are synthetic *pyrethroids*, and are used similarly. These are rapidly metabolized and well-tolerated. No human milk data are available.

In difficult cases which no longer respond to permethrin, a prescription for *lindane* 1% may be given; this must be rinsed off within 4 minutes. It is highly toxic to the central nervous system and is contraindicated in children weighing under 50 kg. It does appear in breast milk, although levels are not published. Oral absorption is more rapid than dermal, so application is contraindicated during lactation.

Malathion (0.5%) is an organophosphate available by prescription as a lotion, and is highly effective; however, there is the risk of absorption. It can cause respiratory depression, and should not be used in a child under 2 years of age. Oral absorption is high but dermal absorption from the scalp is low. There are no breast-milk data. Used carefully and following the instructions for rinsing, this should be safe during lactation as long as the mother develops no symptoms (lacrimation, salivation, shortness of breath) and the infant is not exposed directly.

Crotamiton (10%) is not approved by the FDA for lice, although it is reportedly effective if left on the scalp for 24 hours. There are no breastfeeding data.

Oral *ivermectin* is not approved by the FDA as a pediculicide, and does cross the blood–brain barrier with the potential to block neural transmission. It is also used successfully with onchocerciasis (see Chapter 4.4).

Suffocation of lice by application of occlusive agents such as coconut oil, petroleum jelly, olive oil, or full-fat mayonnaise is reported to be successful, and carries no toxicity or risk during lactation.

Scabies

Medications for scabies include the preparations for lice, but they must be applied over a wide area of skin (usually the entire body). *Permethrin* cream (5%) is recommended, including during pregnancy and lactation, in spite of the large amount required, but not for use in children under 2 months of age. It is removed by bathing after 8–14 hours. *Benzylbenzoate* and *allethrin*, a synthetic pyrethroid, are also effective and are not absorbed intradermally. They are considered safe during lactation as a second choice to *pyrethrum*.

Lindane, as mentioned previously, poses a theoretical risk which is amplified when the compound is used for scabies, based on the area exposed (dose). Concentrations in the milk after ingesting the agent from treated foods range from 0–113 ppb. Lindane is found in the environment, and has been found in maternal milk in environmental screenings. Approximately 10% of the chemical is absorbed through the skin. In a single case reported by Senger (1989), a 3-day treatment for scabies with 0.25% lindane, 0.9 mg/kg was found in milk fat and 2.0 mg/kg after a repeat application. This is 60 times greater than the baseline measured from environmental contamination.

> **Recommendation.** Lice infestation should be treated with coconut oil or pyrethrum extract/permethrin, and scabies with crotamiton or benzyl benzoate. Synthetic pyrethroids are drugs of second choice. Lindane is not appropriate for use while lactating.

4.12.3   Treatments for acne and psoriasis

Experience

Over-the-counter applications and scrubs for acne (*benzoyl peroxide, sulfur regorcinol*) are not absorbed and do not present a hazard during lactation. *Tretinoin* is a vitamin A congener that is used topically and is poorly absorbed through the skin. The risk of use during lactation has not been reported, but will be low because of lack of absorption. It is applied once daily at bedtime and then removed. Blood concentrations measured up to 48 hours after application are zero. The retinoid *isotretinoin*, however, which is taken orally, could appear in the milk as it is absorbed orally, has a small volume of distribution, and is lipid-soluble. With *acitretin*, which has supplanted *etretinate* in psoriasis therapy, about 1% of the maternal weight-related dosage is passed to the fully breastfed infant. This was reported for a patient who received 40 mg daily (Rollman 1990).

Minocycline, now available in an extended-release oral preparation (Saladyn), is effective in moderate to severe acne (Shalita 2006). The extended-release form reduces the incidence of vestibular side effects and allows the lowest possible effective dose (1 mg/kg). Minocycline is a broad-spectrum tetracycline antibiotic capable of causing dental staining and reduced bone growth in children, though. It binds to milk calcium and is more effectively absorbed than previous tetracyclines. In the short term (less than 2 weeks) it is probably tolerable, but chronic use would be contraindicated during lactation. Minocycline has been measured in human milk, although it was not found in the plasma of breastfeeding infants whose mothers took 500 mg orally four times a day. For other anti-infectives, see Chapter 4.4.

4

Lactation

4.12 Dermatological drugs and local therapeutics

There are no reports of toxic symptoms. There is no published experience with the external use of *tazarotene, calcipotriol, dithranol* (sometimes with salicylic acid), *urea*, and *coal tar* preparations.

> **Recommendation.** Systemic therapy with retinoids should not be undertaken during breastfeeding because of the toxic potential and the long half-life. This also applies to external use of coal tar preparations because of their mutagenic and carcinogenic potential. Individual doses do not require any limitation of breastfeeding. Minocycline for less than 2 weeks is probably tolerated. The other medications mentioned are acceptable unless significant absorption must be assumed due to a large area of application and regular use, and/or with application under occlusive bandages.

4.12.4   Other dermatological medications

Immune-modulating substances such as *tacrolimus* and *pimecrolimos* are used externally for atopical dermatitis. There are no studies regarding the lactation period. However, pimecrolimos treatment is well-tolerated in young infants from 2 months (Kapp 2002). From tacrolimos, only 0.1% of the weight-adjusted dosage was calculated for a fully breastfed child (Jain 1997). There were no symptoms observed in the breastfed infants of seven treated mothers (Armanti 2003). Therefore, immune-modulating medicines may be used during lactation. However, direct contact of the child with the drug should be avoided – i.e. treated breasts should be washed before suckling the infant.

Essential oils may be used externally during lactation, when direct contact of the child with the oil is avoided – again, treated breasts should be washed before suckling the infant.

4.12.5   Eye, ear, and nose drops

Experience

Chloramphenicol, quinolones, and *streptomycin* are usually contraindicated. However, the total dose of active principal could be calculated and may well be below the level of concern when given by drops to the eye or ear.

Eye treatments include dilators, constrictors, antibiotics, anti-inflammatories, and artificial tears. Most of these are in small doses and work only locally.

Atropine (*belladonna*) drops have the potential for systemic absorption, but do not pose a problem unless the dose is taken too frequently, which tends to be an issue with the elderly rather than with women in their childbearing years. Atropine is absorbed from the eye quickly, peaks systemically within an hour and clears in less than 24 hours (half-life 4 hours). Atropine does dry secretions, so continued use has the potential for reducing milk production.

Anti-inflammatories that are used in the eye are usually *corticosteroids*. The dose that is absorbed systemically is minimal, and well below the acceptable daily intake for a lactating woman. There were no symptoms observed in a breastfed infant whose mother was treated with eye drops containing *timolol, dipivefrin,* and *dorzolamid,* and who occasionally took *acetazolamid* orally (Johnson 2001). *Acetazolamid* and *timolol* have been categorized as acceptable during lactation by the American Academy of Pediatrics (2001), as no side effects have been reported.

Other pharmacologically active compounds may be administered via these routes, and may be an issue.

The safest therapy for an acute upper respiratory infection (URI or cold) is not with systemic vasoconstrictors or *decongestants*, which can decrease milk production, but with local treatment. Nose drops which shrink mucous membranes (*pseudoephedrine*) are given in small doses and provide relief locally, and do not interrupt breastfeeding.

Ear drops work locally in the ear canal, and do not represent a problem as they are not absorbed. Most are antibiotics or antifungals.

> **Recommendation.** Medication by drops in the eye, ear, and nose are usually compatible with breastfeeding. Ophthalmic atropine can be an issue if used chronically, as it may decrease milk production. Preparations for the eyes or ears that contain chloramphenicol, quinolines, and streptomycin should be avoided.

4.12.6 Vaginal therapeutics

Experience

The vaginal mucosa absorbs pharmacologically active compounds readily. Antibiotics and antifungals are commonly used in the form of suppositories and douches. If the compound can be used systematically for other infections, it is safe via the vagina. Trichomoniasis is usually treated with *metronidazole*, vaginally or orally. In general, anti-infective treatment is more effective systemically than locally.

Of considerable concern is the use of iodine preparations, including *providone-iodine* suppositories or douching. These compounds are used as antiseptics or antimicrobials. Iodine is absorbed via the skin and mucous membranes and moves into milk via a positive pump, so milk levels far exceed maternal plasma levels (see Chapter 4.11). A high intake of iodine suppresses the infant's thyroid activity.

Other douche treatments containing disinfectants such as *dequalinium salts*, *hexetedine*, and *policresulen* are probably safe. *Hexachlorophene* is an antibacterial that inhibits gram-positive organisms. It was used freely 20 years ago, until cases of toxicity in burn cases and in premature infants were reported, particularly where the lotion was not rinsed off. Occasional vaginal use with adequate rinsing minimizes any absorption. No levels have been reported in human milk, but it is known to be well-absorbed orally. Little is known about the absorption of other disinfectants.

Spermicides such as *nonoxynol-9* and *octoxynol-9* inactivate sperm on contact. Although human data are lacking, nonoxynol-9 is rapidly excreted into the milk of lactating rats (Briggs 2005).

> **Recommendation.** Medications administered vaginally are probably safe during lactation, except for those containing iodine. However, good therapeutic practice should be the goal, and the old and questionably effective medications, especially among the disinfectants, should be avoided. Vaginal anti-infective therapy with metronidazole for trichomoniasis or with the nitrofurans *furazolidone* and *nifuratel*, as well as the antimycotic, *chlorphenesin*, should be evaluated critically. Hexachlorophene is acceptable if followed by thorough rinsing. In cases of proven bacterial infection, systemic (oral) therapy should be considered. Vaginally administered spermicide contraceptives, such as nonoxinol-9, are as unproblematic for the breastfed baby as the various intrauterine pessaries (IUP).

4.12.7 Vein therapeutics and other local therapeutics

Experience

Local sclerosing therapy to treat varicose veins usually involves *sodium tetradecyl sulfate* or *polidocanol*, which irritates the intima of the vein. It is injected into the empty vein and compression bandages are applied, keeping the leg elevated. It takes about 3 weeks for the vein to sclerose. The chemical is removed from the vein within a few hours. It is not circulated or absorbed, and is safe during lactation (Beers 1999).

Aescein preparations (horse-chestnut extract) are insufficiently studied. Use of the crude unprocessed forms are highly toxic. Horse-chestnut cream is applied to the legs for varicose veins. A well-manufactured product is standardized to contain 16–20% aescin. Venastat is a delay-release capsule that is also used. No side effects are reported. It is approved for lactation by the German Commission.

Hemorrhoid medications commonly contain local analgesics or anesthetics, and anti-inflammatory agents. To relieve local pain, *lidocaine* 1–2% is often used. Lidocaine has been measured in human milk, where it is calculated to be 40% of the maternal plasma level. When lidocaine was given intravenously for maternal ventricular arrhythmia, the breastfeeding infant received an estimated 2 mg/day. Lidocaine is poorly absorbed orally (35%), so little would be absorbed via the milk. Thus the local use of preparation by the lactating women would have negligible effect on the infant (Giuliani 2001). When used for dental block and other local procedures, the dose is usually less than a total of 40 mg. On the other hand, the dose used for local liposuction is quite large.

Common *wart removal medications* usually contain a collodion solution with 10–20% *salicylic acid* and *lactic acid*. The dose is small, depending on the size and number of the lesions. There is minimal absorption from these lesions. Although milk levels have not been reported, acetylsalicylic acid has been evaluated and is considered safe during lactation (see Chapter 4.1). Salicylic acid does not bind to platelets or cause Reye's syndrome.

Genital or veneral warts are *condylomata acuminata* caused by the human papilloma virus (HPV) of several types, especially 6 and 11. Treatment is usually by electrocautery, laser, cryotherapy, or surgical excision. Chemical abalation can be used, and involves the use of topical antimitotics such as *podophyllotoxin, podophyllin*, or *5-fluorouracil*, or caustics such as *trichloroacetic acid*. Interferon-inducers such as *imiquimode* are also used, and again require multiple applications. Information about these chemicals while breastfeeding is not available, but both the area treated and the dosage are small. *Interferon* is known to be a large molecule that does not pass into milk even during systemic treatment. The development of the HPV vaccine has shown a decrease in the incidence of these lesions, and will perhaps decrease the need for these medications.

Recommendation. Most agents used topically to remove small growths are acceptable. Treatments utilizing lidocaine are safe in small doses (i.e. for hemorrhoids) during lactation. Sclerotherapy is considered safe during lactation. Horse chestnuts are toxic, and their products should be avoided during lactation.

4

Lactation

4.12 Dermatological drugs and local therapeutics

References

American Academy of Pediatrics, Committee on Drugs. The transfer of drugs and other chemicals into human milk. Pediatrics 2001; 108: 776–89.

Armenti VT, Radomski JS, Moritz MJ et al. Report from the national transplantation registry (NTPR): outcomes of pregnancy after transplantation. Clin Transpl 2003; 131–41.

Beers MH, Berkow R (eds). Peripheral vascular disorders. In: Merck Manual, 17th edn. Whitehouse Station, NJ: Merck Research Laboratories, 1999, pp. 1786–96.

Briggs GG, Freeman RK, Yaffe SJ. Drugs in Pregnancy and Lactation, 7th edn. Philadelphia, PA: Lippincott Williams & Wilkins, 2005.

Giuliani M, Grossi GB, Pileri M et al. Could local anesthesia while breastfeeding be harmful to infants? J Pediatr Gastroenterol Nutr 2001; 32: 142–4.

Jain A, Venkataramanan R, Fung JJ et al. Pregnancy after liver transplantation under tacrolimus. Transplantation 1997; 64: 559–65.

Johnson SM, Martinez M, Freedman S. Management of glaucoma in pregnancy and lactation. Survey Ophthalmol 2001; 45: 449–54.

Kapp A, Papp K, Bingham A et al. Long-term management of atopic dermatitis in infants with topical pimecrolimus, a nonsteroid anti-inflammatory drug. J Allergy Clin Immunol 2002; 110: 277–84.

Rollman O, Phil-Lundin I. Acitretin excretion into human breastmilk. Acta Derm Venerol (Stockh) 1990; 70: 487–90.

Senger E, Menzel I, Holzmann H. Therapy-induced lindane concentration in breast milk {in German}. Dermatosen 1989; 37: 167–70.

Shalita AR, Paller AS. Weight-based dosing of a novel antibiotic for moderate-to-severe acne vulgaris – redefining minocycline. www.millennium.com. Dermatology Education Initiative, Millennium Medical Communications, 10 July 2006.

Ruth Lawrence and Christof Schaefer

4.13.1 Alternative remedies and phytotherapeutics

Experience

The interest in and experimentation with alternative remedies has increased in the last decades. Just as in pregnancy, there are minimal evidenced-based safety data for the use of alternative remedies and herbs in lactation; however, also as in pregnancy, history and traditional data in general support their safe use. There have, though, been case reports of unfortunate outcomes. In the United States, the Food and Drug Administration (FDA) has no jurisdiction if the material is labeled with the following statement: "This product is not intended to diagnose, treat, cure or prevent any disease."

Plant preparations (in high doses) are not always harmless; contamination with pesticides and heavy metals (e.g. lead in Ayurvedic medicine or traditional Chinese herbs) has been observed (see Chapter 4.18). There are many herbs which may be used by the nursing mother for a variety of ailments, and there are very few studies regarding their efficacy. The most serious concern (beyond the obvious purity, toxicity, and efficacy) is the problem of self-diagnosis and failing to get the proper medical diagnosis and treatment. Herbs that are used particularly commonly include *valerian, hops*, and *kavain* (*kava-pyrone* from the *kava-kava root*), for nervousness and sleep disturbances; *echinacea* as an immunostimulant; *ginko biloba* to improve general circulation; *ginseng* to improve performance; *aescin* preparations (horse-chestnut extract) for vein problems; *agnus castus (monk's pepper)* for gynecological indications; and *hypericin (St John's wort)* for depression. Systematic studies on these drugs during breastfeeding are lacking, but no damage to the infant via the mother's milk has been described, as yet.

An example of a preparation that has now been banned in many countries is *comfrey* (*Symphytum officinale*), which is available both as the leaf or the root. Root preparations in general are more potent. It has the potential for causing venocclusive disease, liver failure, and death. Two neonatal deaths were reported in Canada after mothers used comfrey as a cream on the nipples; after this it was banned in Canada.

Although ethnobotanists have studied specific plant species in depth and noted some of their pharmacological properties, there are no studies, regarding herbals used during lactation, that meet pharmaceutical standards. Most of the information is derived from hearsay and experience without controls. These plants and herbals are being used, and it is important to be aware of possible side effects or even toxicities.

Ginkgo, Echinacea, and *ginseng* have been studied in blinded placebo controlled studies which failed to show a therapeutic effect. There are no known studies during lactation. Because of the disclaimer on the container, there is no guarantee that the contents are the real plant, and not a mixture or contaminated. It is unwise to experiment during lactation. There are many chemicals in one plant.

St John's wort (*Hypericum perfortum*) has been shown to be effective against mild depression. It contains 26 identifiable chemicals, one of which is 10% *hypercin*, a red dye originally credited for the therapeutic effect. For its use during lactation, see Chapter 4.9.

There is no systematic study of homeopathy as it relates to lactation. The doses of active principles in homeopathy, however, are minute.

Recommendation. The most common standardized preparations containing well-known phytotherapeutics (e.g. St John's wort for mild depression) are probably tolerable during lactation. Herbals and herbal products, at least those of unknown dosage and contamination, should be used with caution and obtained from a reliable source. Many plants, and especially roots, appear to be similar. Herbals should only be used with an expert herbalist's guidance. In general, therapeutic doses should be adhered to, and herbal teas should not be used excessively. If there is a choice, non-alcoholic preparations are preferable. Sensory changes in the milk can lead to feeding problems.

4.13.2   Herbal galactogogues and anti-galactogogues

Experience

Dozens of herbals are used as *galactogogues*, and these are the most frequently used herbals during lactation, to improve milk supply. They are usually ingested as teas, where several seeds, leaves, flowers or roots are steeped in a cup of boiling water. Taken in large quantities, some are anticoagulants and others can cause veno-occlusive disease, as with comfrey.

The best known of the herbal galactogogues is *fenugreek* (*Trigonella foenum-graecum*), also known as *greek hayseed*. It is a member of the Leguminosac family of plants, which includes peanuts, soy, and chickpeas. It has the odor of maple syrup, and is used as artificial maple flavoring. When the mother takes the usual dose (1–4 capsules 580–610 mg, three to four times daily), her milk, sweat, tears, and urine, and even her baby, smell of maple syrup. Fenugreek has been known for centuries to help some women but not all. It can cause colic in the infant, which is believed to be an allergic response. It can aggravate asthmatic symptoms. It has also been documented to lower blood sugar, and is used as a natural treatment for diabetics. In pregnancy, it can cause uterine cramps. It is available in capsule form or as seeds for teas and decoctions. It probably appears in the milk, as this usually smells of maple syrup. It is given a rating of C (moderate potential for toxicity), which is dose-related, by herbalists (Humphrey 2006).

Goat's rue (*Galega officinalis*) is another plant credited as a galactogogue, but is rarely used alone. The only studies were in cows in 1900, when it was added to their feed. *Raspberry leaf* (*Rubus idaeus*) is mentioned in several mixtures, but it is astringent and may, over time, decrease milk supply. *Red clover* (*Trifolium pretense*) is also used, but often contains coumadin, which can cause bleeding. *Fennel* (*Foeniculum vulgare*) is a common constituent of galactogogue teas, and appears in the milk. The dried ripe fruit or seeds have some estrogenic effects, which have been demonstrated by increasing menses and increasing libido, and could actually decrease milk. The oil is toxic.

Alfalfa (*Medicago sativa*, a member of the pea family), which comes in tablet form, is also credited with being a galactogogue. It can cause diarrhea in both mother and baby, although it is otherwise non-toxic and increases milk production. The plant is benign, but the seeds have a potential for toxicity (Humphrey 2006).

Blessed thistle (*Cnicus benedictus*) is different from *milk thistle* (*Sitybum marianum*). It has an unjustified reputation as a galactogogue, but is not known to be toxic except for some reported gastrointestinal symptoms and allergic reactions. It contains many chemicals and volatile oils. It has many "uses", including bacteriostatic and antiseptic, and for dyspepsia. Experiments show antibacterial effects against a number of bacteria.

Borage (*Borage officinalis*) is a powerfully active plant that has been used to treat pain. It contains amabiline, which is a hepatotoxic *pyrrolizidine alkaloid* that can cause veno-occlusive disease. It should not be used in pregnancy or lactation, or as a galactogogue.

There are several herbs recommended for their effect in decreasing milk supply in cases of over-abundance or when weaning is desired. Occasionally, they are used inadvertently for other reasons and result in a decreased milk supply. These are *peppermint, sage, parsley*, and *agnus castus* (*monk's pepper*) (Conover 2004). *Peppermint oil* (*Menthax pierita*) contains menthol, which is the active ingredient. The oil should not be used on or near the infant. *Sage* (*Salvia officinalis*) should not be used as an essential oil, as it is concentrated thujone, which can cause seizures. Use of the cut or powdered leaves available as an herb for cooking, in small amounts, is safe, and does reduce milk supply. In larger amounts, it can cause tachycardia, dizziness, and hot flashes.

Parsley (*Petroselinium crispum*) will also lower milk supply when taken as leaves or juice in large amounts. The oil is toxic, as are the seeds. The popular tabbouleh salad is half parsley, and can affect milk supply.

Bromelain/trypsin complex was found to improve significantly the symptoms of painful breast engorgement during lactation (Snowden 2001).

Recommendation. The galactogogues fenugreek, goat's rue, alfalfa, and blessed thistle are safe in modest doses in lactation. Sage, peppermint oil, and parsley can be used to reduce milk supply in modest doses. In general, therapeutic doses should be adhered to and herbal teas should not be used excessively. If there is a choice, non-alcoholic preparations are preferable. Flavor changes in the milk can lead to feeding problems.

4.13.3 Topical treatment for breast problems

Experience

There are some herbs that have been used safely for topical application for breast problems in lactating women. The evidence again is historical and traditional. These include the following:

- *Green tea* – tea bags are applied four times a day for sore or cracked nipples
- *Calendula* ointment – this is applied topically to encourage healing and retain moisture in chafed nipples
- *Cabbage leaf* – fresh, cool, dry cabbage leaves are applied to the breasts three to four hours after nursing to reduce breast engorgement
- *Jasmine* – topical application of jasmine flowers is used to suppress lactation.

Recommendation. In any case of topical treatment, washing the breast after the application and before breastfeeding is recommended.

4.13.4 Vitamins, minerals, and trace elements

Experience

A balanced nutritious diet should normally provide a good supply of vitamins, minerals, and trace elements unless the mother has a malabsorption syndrome or other nutritional deficiency. There are circumstances that require some attention, however. Mothers who wish to diet need to consume at least 1500 kilocalories per day. Vegetarians may have marginal intakes of the B vitamins, which are found in higher amounts in animal proteins. Strict "vegans" or macrobiotic vegetarians who exclude milk, eggs, and dairy products are at significant risk of being deficient in B vitamins, especially B_{12}. There are cases reported in the literature of megaloblastic anemia in breastfed infants whose mothers are vegans, due to B_{12} deficiency. Vegetarians are also at risk for inadequate mineral intake, especially iron and zinc (O'Connor 1994, Higginbottom 1978).

The issue of vitamin D has become significant because pregnant and lactating women have been noted to have reduced levels of vitamin D in their serum. With the use of sunscreen and the avoidance of sunlight, all women are converting less substrate to vitamin D because of lack of stimulation by sunshine. Cases of rickets in breastfed infants, even in sunny climates, have precipitated the recommendation of, for example, the American Academy of Pediatrics, to give

200–400 iu vitamin D daily to breastfed infants (Collier 2004, Holli
2004). Even when large doses of vitamin D (4000 iu daily) were given
to the mother for 3 months, no ill effects were observed in the infant
(Hollis 2004). Wagner (2006) discussed the option of maternal supplementation instead of giving vitamin D to the infant. Substitution of
vitamins B_1, B_6, and B_{12} was also well-tolerated by the breastfed
infant (American Academy 2001).

> **Recommendation.** Vitamins, minerals, and trace elements can and should
> be used when the mother has real deficiencies. This also applies to iron and to
> vitamin D preparations. Such usage – and this also applies to *fluoride* for den-
> tal prophylaxis (Koparal 2000) – does not require lowering the infant's dosage
> in cases where he or she is also being treated directly. However, routine pre-
> scription of vitamin and mineral preparations during breastfeeding is not nec-
> essary if nutrition is balanced. In the interest of the future diet of the child who
> is still being breastfed, the mother should be made aware of the special
> importance of healthy nutrition, which, in the long run, can prevent the need
> for both her and her child to take not only substitutes but also therapeutic
> tablets. For iodine, see Chapter 4.11. Postpartum *hair loss*, which is frequently
> bemoaned and can be observed for many months, is physiologic and almost
> always improves spontaneously. The effectiveness of using mineral nutrients
> (for this condition) is no better proven than is the local use of estrogens.

4.13.5   Biphosphonates

Experience

Biphosphonates (*alendronate, clodronate, etidronate, ibandronate,
pamidronate*, and *tiludronate*) are a group of chemicals that alter
bone turnover and are used for various forms of osteoporosis.

Each one acts slightly differently. Inactivated by calcium ions,
biphosphonates are poorly absorbed orally (between <1 and <5%)
and would not be absorbed from the milk. Furthermore, in the few
studies carried out, the chemical is almost undetectable in the milk
(Siminoski 2000). Biphosphonates are considered to be safe during
lactation (Lawrence 2005).

> **Recommendation.** Even though a direct, harmful effect on the breastfed
> child would not be expected, these medications should, if possible, not be
> used during breastfeeding. If alendronate is required during lactation, the

infant should not be breastfed for 2 hours after dosing. The present forms of drug require dosing only once a week. If etidronate is necessary during lactation, breastfeeding should be delayed for more than 2 hours to avoid the peak plasma time. Pamidronate is poorly absorbed orally, so it is not considered to be a problem for the breastfed infant.

4.13.6   Exercise

Experience

Exercise studies have been conducted by a number of investigators. Lactic acid production as a result of serious exercise has been carefully studied. Lactic acid is bitter or sour in taste, and may, as a result, lead in some cases to temporary rejection of the breast milk (Wallace 1992). The levels of lactic acid in the milk rose from baseline before exercise (0.61 ± 0.14 mM) to 1.06 ± 33 mM after typical moderate exercise, and to 2.88 ± 0.80 mM after maximal effort, in these same women. This is above the adult taste level of 1.6 mM. The effect lasted for 90 minutes. The impact of regular exercise on the volume and composition of breast milk as well as prolactin levels was studied. No difference was found between exercising and sedentary women (Dewey 1994). Moderate exercise sufficient to improve cardiovascular fitness without marked changes in energy expenditure, dietary intake, and bodyweight and composition does not jeopardize lactation performance (Prentice 1994).

Recommendation. There are no contraindications to moderate exercise while lactating.

4.13.7   Glucose 6-phosphate-dehydrogenase deficiency

Experience

Infants with glucose 6-phosphate-dehydrogenase deficiency (G 6-PD deficiency) may develop hemolytic crisis when exposed to *primaquine, salicylates, sulfonamides, nitrofurans, phenacetin, naphthalene,* some *vitamin K* derivatives (although usual neonatal vitamin K prophylaxis seems to be well tolerated), and certain foodstuffs (e.g. *fava beans*). G 6-PD deficiency is found in 10% of the black population, and in those from the Mediterranean basin (Italians, Greeks, Arabs, and Sephardic Jews). There are no data available regarding the reaction to these drugs when present in breast milk. Apparently, the dosage of the medications involved and the nutritional components in the milk are too low.

References

American Academy of Pediatrics, Committee on Drugs. The transfer of drugs and other chemicals into human milk. Pediatrics 2001; 108: 776–89.

Collier S, Fulhan J, Duggan C. Nutrition for the pediatric office: update on vitamins infant feeding and food allergies. Curr Opin Pediatr 2004; 16: 314–20.

Conover E, Buehler BA. Use of herbal agents by breastfeeding women may affect infants. Pediatr Ann 2004; 33: 235–40.

Dewey KG, Lovelady CA, Nommsen-Rivers LA et al. Randomized study of the effects of aerobic exercise by lactating women on breast-milk volume and composition N Engl J Med 1994; 330: 449–53.

Higginbottom MC, Sweetman L, Nyhan WL. A syndrome of methylmalonic aciduria homocystinuria, megaloblastic anemia and neurologic abnormalities in a vitamin B12-deficient breastfed infant of a strict vegetarian. New Engl J Med 1978; 299: 317–23.

Hollis BW, Wagner CL. Vitamin D requirements during lactation: high-dose maternal supplementation as therapy to prevent hypovitaminosis D for both the mother and the nursing infant. Am J Clin Nutr 2004; 80: 1752–8.

Humphrey S. The Nursing Mother's Herbal. Minneapolis, MN: Fairview Press, 2001.

Koparal E, Ertugrul F, Oztekin K. Fluoride levels in breast milk and infants food. J Clin Pediatr Dent 2000; 24: 299–302.

Lawrence RA, Lawrence RM. Breastfeeding: A Guide for the Medical Profession, 6th edn. Philadelphia, PA: Elsevier, 2005.

O'Connor DL. Folate status during pregnancy and lactation. Adv Exp Med Biol 1994; 352: 157.

Prentice A. Should lactating women exercise? Nutr Rev 1994; 52: 358.

Siminoski K, Fitzgerald AA, Flesch G et al. Intravenous pamidronate for treatment of reflex sympathetic dystrophy during breastfeeding. J Bone Miner Res 2000; 15: 2052–5.

Snowden HM, Renfrew MJ, Woolridge MW. Treatments for breast engorgement during lactation. Cochrane Database Syst Rev 2001; (2): CD000046.

Wagner CL, Hulsey TC, Fanning D et al. High-dose vitamin D3 supplementation in a cohort of breastfeeding mothers and their infants: a 6-month follow-up pilot study. Breastfeeding Medicine 2006; 1: 59–70.

Wallace JP, Inbar G, Ernsthausen K. Infant acceptance of postexercise breast milk. Pediatrics 1992; 89: 1245–7.

4.14.1   X-ray studies, ultrasound, and magnetic resonance

Experience

X-ray, ultrasound, and magnetic resonance imaging (MRI) are forms of imagery that use ionizing radiations, sound waves, and magnetic fields, respectively, to produce images, and do not leave residual energy in the tissues. These examinations can be performed on any part of the body, including the breasts, without interfering with lactation. It is not necessary to wean the infant and stop lactation to carry out satisfactory mammography. An experienced mammographer can interpret the films very well. Mammography does compress the breast with considerable force, so it is recommended the infant be fed and/or the breasts be pumped immediately prior to the examination.

The issues with imagery involve the use of contrast materials. Most contrast materials are poorly orally bioavailable, so they would not be absorbed from the milk in any appreciable amount by the infant.

The half-life and clearance times are also well documented. The ultrasound contrast agent *D-galactose* may be used. The contrast materials that are of concern contain some form of iodine, especially radioactive iodine and other radioactive compounds. Their clearance is well studied, as technically it is easy to do.

4.14.2   Iodine-containing contrast media

Experience

The water-soluble iodine-containing contrast media, *meglumine amidotrizoate* and *sodium amidotrizoate*, *iodamide*, *iohexol*, and *metrizamide*, appear in the milk of a fully breastfed infant in a relative dose considerably under 1% (Nielsen 1987, Texier 1983, Fitzjohn 1982, Ilett 1981).The portion of free iodine in contrast media is under 0.1% of the total amount of the contrast medium, although this can increase during storage. Once administered, more free iodine may be released as a result of the activity of the de-iodizing enzymes in the mother's or the child's body. The effect of free iodide on the infant's thyroid depends on the iodine saturation before the study began. If there is a latent deficiency status, flooding with iodine is more likely to lead to an effect on function than it would if the iodine supply were well adjusted.

The implication of the iodine transfer to the baby, following an examination of the breastfeeding mother using a contrast agent, cannot be adequately determined simply by measuring the iodine in the infant's urine. It is only with an examination of the infant's iodine uptake and thyroid function that the individual situation can be described precisely.

In cases of direct use of iodine-containing contrast media, particularly in infants under 3 months of age, transient hypothyroidism has been described. There are no known cases of gross impairment to breastfed infants following administration to the mother. However, discrete effects on the sensitive central nervous system differentiation in infancy cannot be ruled out when there has been maternal exposure with subsequent iodine transfer via breast milk.

In the case of *iohexol* and *metrizoate*, Nielsen and colleagues concluded that a noteworthy exposure which would be a barrier to breastfeeding should not be expected (Nielsen 1987). However, this seems questionable, since one of the four subjects in his study, with ongoing high iodine concentrations of up to 141 mg/l milk, was not considered when his study results were summarized. The authors calculated half-lives in the milk of 15–108 hours for *iohexol* and *metrizoate*. In the serum, by contrast, the half-lives of the water-soluble contrast media are, at 2 hours, considerably shorter.

In the case of the fat-soluble *iopanoic acid* used for biliary duct examination, 7% of the maternal weight-related dosage was calculated for the breastfed infant in an older study (Holmdahl 1956).

There is no published experience on the other iodine-containing contrast media, such as *iobitridol, iodixanol, iomeprol, iopamidol, iopentol, iopodate, iopromide, iotalaminic acid, iotrolan, iotroxine acid, ioversol, ioxaglinic acid, ioxitalaminic acid, lysine amido-trizoate,* and *sodium iodine* (with and without *indocyanin green*).

> **Recommendation.** When a mother is given an iodine-containing contrast agent, the possibility that the infant will absorb a significantly higher quantity of free iodide than would be necessary for supplementation cannot be ruled out (see Chapter 4.11). The need for such an examination should be very critically considered. With the extensive choice of other procedures, such as ultrasound, computer tomography, and magnetic resonance imaging, there are safer options. If the use of an iodine-containing contrast agent is unavoidable, breastfeeding should be interrupted for 24–48 hours, at least for the young, fully breastfed infant. This period can be bridged with milk that has been pumped ahead of time.

4.14.3 Radionuclides

Experience

Iodine[131] (^{131}I) accumulates in mother's milk at the same levels as "normal" iodine (see Chapter 4.11). Among 31 radionuclides studied for their appearance in mother's milk, ^{131}I had the highest transfer (with 30% of the maternal dose), followed by [45]Ca and [137]Cs (both 20%) and [90]Sr (10%) (Harrison 2003). In their review on ^{131}I, Simon and co-workers (2002) found a median half-life in milk of 12 hours. When the mother received stable iodine to block her thyroid before administration of ^{131}I, the median half-life was 8.5 hours. Peak values were measured after 9 hours. Stable iodine blocks also the ^{131}I uptake of the breast and the infant's thyroid. In 1996, Bennett summarized the kinetics of many radiopharmaceuticals during breastfeeding, among them iodine and technetium isotopes. It is difficult to decide what dosage of radioactivity is tolerable for the breastfed infant; most authors accept 1 mSv. In the context of the radioiodine contamination after Chernobyl, the German Radiation Protection Commission recommended 500 Bq/l as a threshold value for infant nutrition and cow's milk (Strahlenschutzkommission 1986). For comparison, about 48 hours after administration of 0.37 MBq sodium-iodide[131] for medical purposes, a level of 27 kBq/l was measured in the breast milk – which is still 50 times of the threshold value mentioned above.

The scintillation scans that are done today, primarily with *technetium* (^{99m}Tc), are considered much less problematic compared to iodine isotopes. An acceptable residual dosage of 1 mSv is normally reached with pumping and discarding the milk for 12 hours (Prince 2004, Bennett 1996).

Other radioactive compounds are used for various specific indications. *Gallium-67* is used for bone scanning, and whole body scans show an affinity for the breast. With a half-life of 78 hours for the radiation and 9 days for the gallium ion, interruption of breastfeeding is suggested based on the initial dose. Thus, a dose of 0.2 mCi (7.4 MBq) would require a week's cessation of breastfeeding, and 4 mCi (148 MBq) would require a month.

Thallium-201 is unique in its affinity for the ischemic myocardium, and is used to delineate this lesion; 85% appears in the heart muscle on the first pass, and only 5% is left in the plasma in 5 minutes. The radioactive half-life is 73 hours; however, it takes 10 days to clear the thallium ion. It has been studied in a lactating woman given 3 mCi (11 mBq) for a brain scan. In 4 hours the milk level was 8.8 mCi (326 Bq/ml), and in 72 hours it was 2.4 mCi (87 Bq/ml). If the infant had consumed the milk, the dose would have been less than the NCRP radiation safety guidelines (Stabin 2000).

^{18}FDG (*2-fluoro-2-deoxy-D-glucose*) is used for positron-emission-tomography (PET), and appears in the lactating breast (Shor 2002).

Recommendation. The diagnostic or therapeutic use of radiopharmaceuticals, mostly technetium or iodine isotopes, should be postponed until breastfeeding has come to an end. With indications that cannot be postponed, breastfeeding should be interrupted depending on the isotope used and its dosage. If the radioactivity of the milk can be measured simply, then a decision regarding the length of time for which pumped milk is required can be made based on the clearance of radiation from the milk and specifics of the case.

4.14.4   Magnetic resonance contrast agents

Experience

Compounds containing the *gadolinium* ion as the opaque entity are used as radiocontrast agents in magnetic resonance studies (Table 4.14.1). These compounds are administered intravenously, absorbed orally poorly or not at all, and penetrate peripheral compartments poorly (including in the breast), remaining in extracellular water. They are used to follow excretion pathways, especially

Table 4.14.1 Gadolinium compounds used as contrast agents

Name	Half-life	Route	Oral bioavailability	Transfer into milk
Gadodiamide	77 min	i.v.	Nil	<0.04% maternal dose
Gadopentetate	96 min	i.v.	0.8%	<0.04% maternal dose
Gadoteridol	96 min	i.v.	Poor to nil	Not available
Gadoversetamide	102 min	i.v.	Nil	Does appear in maternal milk when doses are excessive

the kidney. They are non-tonic, non-iodinated, water-soluble compounds. Gadolinium compounds peak in the blood immediately, and their half-life values are an hour to an hour and a half. Total clearance is calculated to be less than 8 hours. The estimated total dose of drug absorbed from 24 hours of breastfeeding would be less than 1% of intravenous dose (Kubik-Huch 2000, Rofsky 1993).

There are no published data on *gadobene acid* and *gadoxetic acid* during lactation.

Theoretically, *ferristen*, from a toxicological viewpoint, is harmless for the breastfed infant.

Due to insufficient experience, no risk assessment is possible with the manganese-containing *mangafodipir*. On the other hand, the advice of the manufacturer to interrupt breastfeeding for 14 days does not seem to make sense.

> **Recommendation.** There is no indication to interrupt breastfeeding when gadolinium compounds or ferristen are used. Mangafodipir should be avoided.

4.14.5 Fluorescein

Fluorescein (fluorescein sodium) has yellow coloring, and is used as a diagnostic agent as topical, ophthalmic and intravenous solutions. It is excreted into breast milk. Fluorescein is photosensitive and there is a risk of phototoxicity, especially in neonates who may require phototherapy (i.e. extensive light exposure). There is a case reported of a premature infant who received the compound directly, and had a skin reaction (Kearns 1985). A woman was given 5 ml intravenous dose of a 10% solution for diagnostic angiography shortly after birth,

4

Lactation

4.14 Diagnostics

and had seven milk samples collected between 6 and 76 hours afterwards. Levels were 772 ng/ml at 6 hours and 170 ng/ml at 72 hours (half-life 62 hours) (Maguire 1985). Even when considering the peak values, a weight-adjusted dosage of <1% is calculated for a fully breastfed child, which should not carry a risk of phototoxicity. Furthermore, there are no data regarding absorption orally with food. When given to a woman 3 months' postpartum as a 2% topical solution to both eyes, levels in the plasma were 30 and 40 ng/ml at 45 and 75 minutes respectively. Corresponding milk samples at 30, 60, and 90 minutes had levels of 20, 22, and 15 ng/ml respectively, suggesting a half-life of 60 minutes and a probable calculated clearance time of 5 hours (Mattern 1990).

> **Recommendation.** Breastfeeding may continue after diagnostic administration of fluorescein.

4.14.6   Other diagnostics

Skin tests such as a *tuberculin test* or *allergy test* are considered harmless during breastfeeding. Allergy injections for diagnostic purposes consist of proteins and carbohydrates from plants and/or animals. There have been no reported reactions in breastfed infants. It is not anticipated that much would be absorbed from these intradermal injections. *Enzyme tests* such as *secretin* are also considered acceptable during lactation.

References

Bennett PN (ed.). Drugs and Human Lactation, 2nd edn. Amsterdam: Elsevier, 1996.

Fitzjohn TP, Williams GD, Laker MF et al. Intravenous urography during lactation. Br J Radiol 1982; 55: 603–5.

Harrison JD, Smith TJ, Phipps AW. Infant doses from the transfer of radionuclides in mothers' milk. Radiat Prot Dosimetry 2003; 105: 251–6.

Holmdahl KH. Cholecystography during lactation. Acta Radiol 1956; 45: 305–7.

Ilett KF, Hackett LP, Paterson JW. Excretion of metrizamide in milk. Br J Radiol 1981; 54: 537–8.

Kearns GL, Williams BJ, Timmons OD. Fluorescein phototoxicity in a premature infant. J Pediatr 1985; 107: 796–8.

Kubik-Huch RA, Gottstein-Aalame NM et al. Excretion of gadopentetate dimeglumine into human breast milk during lactation. Radiology 2000; 216: 555–8.

Maguire AM, Bennett J. Fluorescein elimination in human breast milk. Arch Ophthalmol 1985; 106: 718–19.

Mattern J, Mayer PR. Excretion of fluorescein into breast milk. Am J Ophthalmol 1990; 109: 598–9.

Nielsen ST, Matheson I, Rasmussen JN et al. Excretion of iodohexol and metrizoate in human breast milk. Acta Radiol 1987; 28: 523–6.

Prince JR, Rose MR. Measurement of radioactivity in breast milk following 99mTc-Leukoscan injection. Nucl Med Commun 2004; 25: 963–6.

Rofsky NM, Weinreb JC, Litt AW. Quantitative analysis of gadopentetate dimeglumine excreted in breast milk. J Magn Reson Imaging 1993; 3: 131–2.

Shor M, Dave N, Reddy M et al. Asymmetric FDG uptake in the lactating breast. Clin Nuclear Med 2002; 27: 536.

Simon SL, Luckyanov N, Bouville A et al. Transfer of ^{131}I into human breast milk and transfer coefficients for radiological dose assessments. Health Phys 2002; 82: 796–806.

Stabin MG, Breitz HB. Breast milk excretion of radiopharmaceuticals: mechanisms, findings, and radiation dosimetry. J Nucl Med 2000; 41: 836–73.

Strahlenschutzkommission beim Bundesministerium des Inneren. Drei Wochen nach Tschernobyl: 3. Empfehlung der Strahlenschutzkommission beim Bundesministerium des Inneren zu den möglichen Auswirkungen des Reaktorunfalls in der U.d.S.S.R. auf die Bundesrepublik Deutschland. Dtsch Ärzteblatt 1986; 83: 1704–6.

Texier E, Roque O, D'Orbcastel OR et al. Teneur en iode stable du lait humain apres une angiographie pulmonaire. La Presse Medicale 1983; 12: 769.

4

Lactation

Infections

4.15

Ruth Lawrence and Christof Schaefer

There are very few situations where a mother who is breastfeeding and develops an infection puts her infant at risk because the infection might be transmitted through the milk. Vertical transmission after birth mainly occurs via close contact between mother and child. Pathogens discussed in context with breast milk transmission are HIV, human cytomegaly virus (HCMV), and – limited to tropical regions – Human T cell lymphotropic virus (HTLV), with the potential for leukemia, myelopathies, and neurological diseases (Biggar 2006, Lawrence 2004). The following sections discuss the most important infections. The issue of anti-infectious drug therapies has been covered in Chapter 4.4.

4.15.1 Simple infections

The most common questions arise because the mother has developed a fever of unknown origin in the immediate postpartum period. The most likely is a urinary tract infection, an upper respiratory infection or a wound infection. Modest engorgement also may cause a fever. Breastfeeding does not need to be interrupted while the work-up is completed. Treatment may be initiated or found unnecessary. An infection with β-hemolytic strep requires aggressive therapy for both mother and infant, interrupting breastfeeding until the mother has received 24 hours of antibiotics. Illness in the infant requires neither interruption of breastfeeding, nor separation of mother and infant. For viral infections, breastfeeding is not interrupted and can be therapeutic, as mother provides her antibodies through the milk to her infant.

4.15.2   Mastitis

Mastitis is not a contraindication to breastfeeding; in fact, it is important to continue to empty the breast on the usual schedule. Even when an abscess has to be surgically drained, breastfeeding should continue unless the incision for drainage is on the areola. An undiagnosed abscess that ruptures spontaneously into a duct would require interruption of breastfeeding on that breast, and the breast would require routine pumping on schedule to hasten the healing. Direct breastfeeding on that breast should resume as soon as drainage stops and antibiotic therapy has been in place at least 24 hours. Most common causes are staphylococcus and *E. coli*. If streptococcus is suspected by culture or because mastitis is bilateral, the infant should also be treated vigorously. The diagnosis is made when a tender, warm, red swollen area appears on the breast, usually in a wedge shape, and the mother has a temperature and 'flu-like symptoms. In contrast, plugged ducts are not red and warm, and the mother is well. Plugged ducts can be relieved with warm compresses and massage to remove the plug. Continued breastfeeding to help this is very important.

> **Recommendation.** When mastitis is suspected, the mother should be seen immediately, the diagnosis confirmed, and antibiotics initiated. Antibiotic treatment must be maintained for 2 full weeks to avoid relapse. Relapsing mastitis is extremely difficult to clear. It is easier to prevent it than to cure it. Continued breastfeeding is essential (antibiotics are discussed in Chapter 4.4).

4.15.3   Hepatitis A

> **Recommendation.** If the mother has hepatitis A at the time of delivery or develops hepatitis A while breastfeeding, the infant should promptly receive immunoglobulin. In either case, breastfeeding need not be interrupted. No

cases of hepatitis A transmitted to the breastfed infant have been reported. Since a vaccine is now available, at-risk individuals and all children and adolescents will eventually be vaccinated and the risk of the disease should diminish (Lawrence 2005).

4.15.4   Hepatitis B

Experience

Hepatitis B is only rarely transmitted via the placenta. In contrast, there is a great risk of infection during the birth. For this reason, newborns whose mothers carry hepatitis antigens (HBs-Ag and HBe-Ag), which indicate the possibility of infection, are simultaneously vaccinated immediately after birth. HBs-Ag has also been detected in mothers' milk (Boxall 1974). However, various studies have shown that there is no increased risk of illness for infants when their mothers are only HBs-Ag carriers (González 1995, Tseng 1988, Beasley 1975). No infection via breast milk was observed in the infants of 100 mothers with chronic hepatitis B. The infants had received simultaneous vaccination, and 11 mothers were HBe-Ag positive (Hill 2002). Nevertheless, the authors interpret their data with caution because of the small cohort of HBe-Ag-positive mothers with potentially higher infection risk.

Recommendation. Regardless of how the infant will be fed, every child born to a hepatitis-B-positive mother should receive hepatitis B-immunoglobulin (HBIG) within 12 hours of birth. The infant should then also receive the first of three doses of hepatitis B vaccine. As soon as the HBIG has been given, the infant may begin breastfeeding (American Academy 2005, Lawrence 2005).

4.15.5   Hepatitis C

Experience

Hepatitis C is transmitted in a similar way to hepatitis B. Contaminated syringes and blood products are the most critical sources of infection, although the latter has become significantly less of a risk factor since 1993 due to mandatory testing of all blood donations. Hepatitis C infection is typically asymptomatic or mild. Drug addicts are not infrequently infected simultaneously with HIV, hepatitis B, and hepatitis C. Concomitant HIV infection is linked with higher risk of vertical (perinatal) HCV infection.

Anti-HCV antibodies and HCV-RNA have been found in colostrum and breast milk (Grayson 1995, Ogasawara 1993). Transmission rates are similar between breastfed and non-breastfed infants; however, many factors are uncontrolled (Zanetti 1995). A risk of infection for infants whose mothers are ill with only hepatitis C has not been observed as yet. The virus load in the mother's milk appears to be too low to transmit the illness (Lin 1995). In a further study, viruses were only detected in the mother's milk when there were very high concentrations of anti-HCV antibodies in the mother's serum. In these cases (about 10% of the women studied), the mothers were advised not to breastfeed (Zimmermann 1995). In a newer study of 97 milk samples from 95 mothers chronically infected with HCV, no PCR-reactive HCV-RNA results were found. Just under 68% of the mothers had PCR-positive blood samples. The virus load was between 10^2 and 10^7 – on average, 10^4 RNA-copies/ml. Only one of these children was infected with HCV. Transmission apparently took place during the birth. The authors concluded from their findings that there is no contraindication to breastfeeding (Laufs 2000, Polywka 1999). It must be noted, however, that a cohort of 76 breastfed babies is in no way sufficient to rule out transmission of the infection via the mother's milk. Furthermore, another study with 73 infants found HCV-RNA-positive breast milk samples among 20% of the viremic mothers. The rate of (perinatal) HCV transmission was higher for infants of mothers with higher HCV viremia, and also for infants whose mothers were HCV-RNA positive in breast milk. However, seven of the eight infected children had spontaneous clearance of the virus without developing antibodies (Ruiz-Extremera 2000). The European Association for the Study of the Liver also sees no risk of hepatitis C infection through breastfeeding (EASL 1999). The current position of the Center for Disease Control (CDC) is that there are no data to indicate that HCV is transmitted through breast milk. They conclude that breastfeeding by an HCV-positive but HIV-negative mother is not contraindicated.

Recommendation. The available experience does not, in principle, argue against breastfeeding when the mother is infected with hepatitis C. Whether the decision not to breastfeed should be taken when there is a high viral load (i.e. of more than 10^6 copies/ml) in the mother's serum remains to be seen. At the start of teething, with the possible resulting injury to the nipples, mothers with hepatitis C should not continue breastfeeding.

4

Lactation

4.15 Infections

4.15.6   Hepatitis E

Experience

A study covering 93 pregnant women with hepatitis E (36 anti-HEV positive and 57 HEV-RNA positive) infection was confirmed in a colostrum specimen. However, parameters were significantly lower compared to maternal blood (Chibber 2004). Some of the infants of mothers with acute infection also developed liver symptoms. There was no indication that transmission occurred via breast milk. The authors concluded that breast feeding is probably safe, but stress the need to confirm their results by other studies, and the possibility that close contact between mother and child may facilitate transmission.

> **Recommendation.** There is no evidence yet that breastfeeding should be prohibited in cases of hepatitis E. However, experience is insufficient definitely to exclude any risk.

4.15.7   Herpes simplex

Experience

Perinatal herpes infections are transmitted during birth because of the presence of the virus in the birth canal. When lesions are present near the anticipated time of delivery, a cesarian section is performed immediately when labor starts or the membranes rupture to avoid infection of the infant. With the exception of one case (Dunkle 1979), no herpes simplex virus has been detected in mother's milk. This is as would be expected, because the infection in adults is usually a local one that does not involve viremia. All infant deaths that have been reported have been subsequent to suckling at a breast with a herpetic lesion (Sullivan-Bolyai 1983).

> **Recommendation.** Any local herpetic lesion should be covered, and strict hand-washing employed. Individuals with lesions on the face and mouth should not kiss or fondle infants. Lesions on the breast require temporary interruption of breastfeeding until the lesion has completely dried. Treatment of the breast lesion with topical, oral or even i.v. antiviral preparations may hasten recovery and decrease the period of viral shedding.

4.15.8 Herpes zoster (shingles), chickenpox

Experience

Perinatal varicella infection can lead to severe infection in the infant if the maternal rash develops 5 days or less before delivery, or within 2 days after delivery. Illness in the infant usually develops before 10 days of age, and is more severe because of lack of maternal antibodies. The infant should receive varicella zoster immunoglobulin (VZIG). The infant can be infected by aerosolized virus from lesions or the maternal respiratory track. Postnatal varicella can develop from non-maternal sources, and is usually mild if the mother has had varicella or the vaccination.

Varicella zoster virus (VZV) has not been cultured from the milk with either herpes zoster or chickenpox (Frederick 1986), but VZV-DNA has been identified in breast milk (Yoshida 1992). One case of suspected transfer of VZV to an infant via breastfeeding has been reported, but the virus may have been transmitted by droplet or exposure to the rash.

Recommendation. When the mother develops chickenpox 2–4 days after the birth, the baby is given varicella immunoglobulin and perhaps prophylactic acyclovir. The milk can be expressed and fed to the baby. If the mother becomes ill after this point, prophylactic measures are not needed and the baby can be breastfed. If the baby becomes ill, varicella infections normally proceed without complications. With herpes zoster, the baby may continue to be breastfed, but direct contact with the affected part of the skin should be avoided. With the readily available vaccine to prevent chickenpox and the approval of the varicella vaccine for adults to prevent zoster, these cases should be greatly reduced.

4.15.9 HIV infection

Experience

The overwhelming majority of HIV-positive children are infected during the birth. Postpartum infection via breastfeeding has also been described. The virus has been detected in the mother's milk, especially among women with mastitis and infected infants (Pillay 2000, Semba 1999). On the other hand, the protective effect of substances in the mother's milk, such as maternal anti-HIV antibodies, lactoferrin, and secretory leukocyte protease inhibitors on a vertical transmission, has

4

Lactation

4.15 Infections

been discussed for a long time (Becquart 2000, van de Perre 1999). A South African study of 549 HIV-1 infected women showed that babies who were exclusively breastfed for 3 months did not have a higher transmission rate than non-breastfed babies (14.6% versus 18.8%). The highest rate of infection was among those babies who were partially breastfed and partially artificially fed (24.1%) (Coutsoudis 1999). Based on 4085 infants, the Breastfeeding and HIV International Transmission Study Group (Coutsoudis 2004) has found out that, in contrast with earlier findings, the transmission risk remains stable during the whole lactation period. The cumulative probability of infection via breast milk after the neonatal period and up to the age of 18 months (late postnatal transmission) is 9.3%. This risk is similar to the early perinatal and neonatal infection risk. The authors summarize an overall risk of 8.9 per 100 infant years for becoming infected via breast milk. The infection risk is increased with lower counts of maternal CD4+ lymphocytes probably indicating a higher virus load. Male newborns were found to have a higher risk too. Mixed feeding is associated with a higher infection risk than is exclusive breastfeeding (Coovadia 2007). Therefore it has been suggested that exclusive breastfeeding be recommended for 4–6 months, followed by abrupt weaning, in regions where a lack of clean water presents a risk for the preparation of infant formula. No schedule has been agreed upon yet.

There are several studies comparing antiretroviral medication regimens (*nevirapine* versus *zidovudine* plus *lamivudine*) with various treatment intervals for the prevention of mother-to-child transmission (Gaillard 2004). However, antiretroviral drugs have a rather short half-life, carry the risk of side effects and resistance, and are expensive. Therefore, research has focused on vaccines and specific immunoglobulins to protect infants (Safrit 2004). In addition, simple measures are needed to pasteurize breast milk with adapted techniques, e.g. the so-called Pretoria pasteurization. Apart from providing appropriate technical equipment, social acceptance of such measures is not always easy to achieve (Rollins 2004).

A randomized trial in Kenya covering 425 HIV-1-positive pregnant women found a relative risk of death of 3.2 for breastfeeding mothers versus formula-feeding mothers. There was an association between maternal death and subsequent infant death, even after HIV-1 infection status was controlled for. The metabolic burden of breastfeeding in women with inadequate nutrition intake was, among others, discussed as a causal factor (Nduati 2001).

There has been no change of the WHO/UNICEF recommendations of 1992 that the newborns of HIV-infected mothers in industrialized countries should not be breastfed because safe artificial feeding is available, and thus a postpartum HIV infection via mother's milk can be avoided (World Health Organization 1992). In regions where infant mortality due to the lack of clean water is above 40/1000, however, the advantage of preventing infections by using formula feeding would be neutralized. Conversely, breastfeeding is the more dangerous form of nutrition only in those countries where infant mortality due to deficient hygiene is below 40/1000 (Kuhn 2004).

> **Recommendation.** Newborns of HIV-infected mothers should not be breastfed. Exceptions are in those regions in developing countries in which the preparation of infant formula with a lack of clean water presents a greater risk. In such areas, babies should be exclusively breastfed for at least 3 months but not longer than 6 months wherever possible.

4.15.10   Human cytomegalovirus

Experience

Human cytomegalovirus (HCMV) infection is the most frequent congenital infection, affecting 1–3% of newborns. Even more relevant is the postnatal infection, transmitted mainly via breast milk. Of seropositive mothers, 40–96% shed the virus with their milk, reaching a peak 1 month after delivery (survey in Meier 2005, Hamprecht 2001). A reactivated infection in the lactating breast probably explains the frequent detection of HCMV in milk, leading to an infection rate of 10–60% of the infants. Postnatal infection via the breast milk in term infants does not cause illness. Very premature infants, however, develop bronchopulmonary dysplasia and other problems. Approximately 10% of premature infants become severely ill. In up to 50% of the typical problems of premature newborns, such as respiratory distress syndrome, HCMV infection was causative. The virus is killed by pasteurization. Recommendations vary regarding from when (gestational week 28 or week 32, or below a birth weight of 1500 g?) and for how long (until 6 weeks of age, or less than 1500 g bodyweight?) pasteurization of breast milk should be carried out. Freezing of the milk has not been shown to be totally protective for the premature infant (Curtis 2005).

> **Recommendation.** Full-term infants may be breastfed by HCMV seropositive mothers. In premature infants, HCMV-positive milk (donor or mother's milk) should be pasteurized. From which stage and for how long milk should be pasteurized should follow updated recommendations.

4.15.11   Tuberculosis

Experience

Transmission of tuberculosis in the newborn period is via respiratory droplets from the mother or another family member. An infection via the mother's milk is considered to be extremely rare. Tuberculus mastitis does occur, although rarely in developed countries. It must be considered if a woman with tuberculosis develops mastitis or a lump in the breast.

> **Recommendation.** A mother may breastfeed with closed tuberculosis. If the mother has open tuberculosis in the lungs, direct contact with the infant should be avoided at first, and the infant should receive chemoprophylaxis (e.g. isoniazid plus vitamin B_6) in accordance with the currently valid pediatric plan.

4.15.12   Other infectious diseases

Although there is no evidence of transmission via breast milk, the following infections require preventive measures (Lawrence 2004)

- *Haemophilus influenza* infection requires 24 hours' treatment of the mother before breastfeeding
- In cases of *gonorrhoea*, breastfeeding can continue if the mother is efficiently treated with antibiotics, e.g. ceftriaxon
- In cases of *streptococcal B* infection during the neonatal period for example as endometritis, separation of the child for 24 hours along with feeding of pumped milk is recommended
- A mother with *syphilis* should be treated for 24 hours before breastfeeding or pumping and feeding her milk.

References

American Academy of Pediatrics Section on Breastfeeding. Breastfeeding and the use of human milk. Pediatrics 2005; 115: 496–506.

Beasley RP, Stevens CE, Shiao IS et al. Evidence against breast-feeding as a mechanism for vertical transmission of hepatitis B. Lancet 1975; 2: 740–41.

Becquart P, Hocini H, Levy M et al. Secretory anti-human immunodeficiency virus (HIV) antibodies in colostrum and breast milk are not a major determinant of the protection of early postnatal transmission of HIV. J Infect Dis 2000; 181: 532–9.

Biggar RJ, Ng J, Kim N et al. Human leukocyte antigen concordance and the transmission risk via breast-feeding of human T cell lymphotropic virus type I. J Infect Dis 2006; 193: 277–82.

Boxall EH, Flewett TH, Dane DS et al. Hepatitis B surface antigen in breast milk. Lancet 1974; 2: 1007–8.

Chibber RM, Usmani MA, al-Sibai MH. Should HEV infected mothers breast feed? Arch Gynecol Obstet 2004; 270: 15–20.

Coovadia HM, Rollins NC, Bland RM et al. Mother-to-child transmission of HIV-1 infection during exclusive breastfeeding in the first 6 months of life: an intervention cohort study. Lancet 2007; 369: 1107–16.

Coutsoudis A, Pillay K, Spooner E et al. for the South African Vitamin A Study Group. Influence of infant-feeding patterns on early mother-to-child transmission of HIV-1 in Durban, South Africa: a prospective cohort study. Lancet 1999; 354: 471–6.

Coutsoudis A, Dabis F, Fawzi W et al. Breastfeeding and HIV International Transmission Study Group. Late postnatal transmission of HIV-1 in breast-fed children: an individual patient data meta-analysis. J Infect Dis 2004; 189: 2154–66.

Curtis N, Chau L, Garland S et al. Cytomegalovirus remains viable in naturally infected breast milk despite being frozen for 10 days. Arch Dis Child Fetal Neonatal Ed 2005; 90: F529–30.

Dunkle LM, Schmidt RR, O'Connor DM. Neonatal herpes simplex infection possibly acquired via maternal breast milk. Pediatrics 1979; 63: 250–51.

EASL International Consensus Conference on Hepatitis C. Consensus statement. J Hepatol 1999; 30: 956–61.

Frederick IB, White RJ, Braddock SW. Excretion of varicella-herpes zoster virus in breastmilk. Am J Obstet Gynecol 1986; 154: 1161–7.

Gaillard P, Fowler MG, Dabis F et al. Ghent IAS Working Group on HIV in Women and Children. Use of antiretroviral drugs to prevent HIV-1 transmission through breast-feeding: from animal studies to randomized clinical trials. J Acquir Immune Defic Syndr 2004; 35: 178–87.

González ML, Viela Sala C, Salvá Armengod F et al. Should we recommend breastfeeding to newborns of HBsAg carrier-mothers. An Esp Pediatr 1995; 43: 115–19.

Grayson ML, Braniff KM, Bowden DS et al. Breast-feeding and the risk of vertical transmission of hepatitis C virus. Med J Austr 1995; 163: 107.

Hamprecht K, Maschmann J, Vochem M et al. Epidemiology of transmission of cytomegalovirus from mother to preterm infant by breastfeeding. Lancet 2001; 357: 513–18.

Hill JB, Sheffield JS, Kim MJ et al. Risk of hepatitis B transmission in breast-fed infants of chronic hepatitis B carriers. Obstet Gynecol 2002; 99: 1049–52.

Kuhn L, Stein Z, Susser M. Preventing mother-to-child HIV transmission in the new millennium: the challenge of breast feeding. Paediatr Perinat Epidemiol 2004; 18: 10–16.

Laufs R, Polywka S. Breast-feeding and perinatal hepatitis C transmission (in German). Dtsch Ärztebl 2000; 97: C1863–4.

Lawrence RM, Lawrence RA. Breast milk and infection. Clin Perinatol 2004; 31: 501–28.

Lawrence RM. Transmission of infectious diseases through breast milk and breastfeeding. In: RA Lawrence and RM Lawrence (eds), Breastfeeding: A Guide for the Medical Profession, 6th edn. Philadelphia, PA: Elsevier, 2005, pp. 629–94.

Lin HH, Kao JH, Hsu HY et al. Absence of infection in breast-fed infants to hepatitis C virus-infected mothers. J Pediatr 1995; 126: 589–91.

Meier J, Lienicke U, Tschirch E et al. Human cytomegalovirus reactivation during lactation and mother-to-child transmission in preterm infants. J Clin Microbiol 2005; 43: 1318–24.

4

Lactation

4.15 Infections

Nduati R, Richardson BA, John G et al. Effect of breastfeeding on mortality among HIV-1 infected women: a randomized trial. Lancet 2001; 357: 1651–5.

Ogasawara S, Kage M, Kosai K et al. Hepatitis C virus RNA in saliva and breastmilk of hepatitis C carrier mothers. Lancet 1993; 341: 561.

Pillay K, Coutsoudis A, York D et al. Cell-free virus in breastmilk of HIV-1-seropositive women. J Acquir Immune Defic Syndr 2000; 24: 330–6.

Polywka S, Laufs R. Vertical transmission of the hepatitis-C-virus from infected mothers to their children {in German}. Bundesgesundheitsbl Gesundheitsforsch Gesundheitsschutz 1999; 42: 562–8.

Rollins N, Meda N, Becquet R et al. Ghent IAS Working Group on HIV in Women and Children. Preventing postnatal transmission of HIV-1 through breast-feeding: modifying infant feeding practices. J Acquir Immune Defic Syndr 2004; 35: 188–95.

Ruiz-Extremera A, Salmeron J, Torres C et al. Follow-up of transmission of hepatitis C to babies of human immunodeficiency virus-negative women: the role of breast feeding in transmission. Ped Infect Dis J 2000; 19: 511–16.

Safrit JT, Ruprecht R, Ferrantelli F et al. Ghent IAS Working Group on HIV in Women Children. Immunoprophylaxis to prevent mother-to-child transmission of HIV-1. J Acquir Immune Defic Syndr 2004; 35: 169–77.

Semba RD, Kumwenda N, Hoover DR et al. Human immunodeficiency virus load in breast milk, mastitis, and mother-to-child transmission of human immunodeficiency virus type 1. J Infect Dis 1999; 180: 93–8.

Sullivan-Bolyai JZ, Fife KH, Jacobs RF et al. Disseminated neonatal herpes simplex virus type I from a maternal breast lesion. Pediatrics 1983; 71: 455.

Tseng RYM, Lam CWK, Tam J. Breast-feeding babies of HBsAG-positive-mothers. Lancet 1988; 1: 1032.

van de Perre P. Transmission of human immunodeficiency virus type I through breast-feeding: how can it be prevented. J Infect Dis 1999; 179(Suppl 3): S405–7.

World Health Organization. Global Programme on AIDS. Consensus statement from the WHO/UNICEF consultation on HIV transmission and breast-feeding. Geneva: WHO, 1992.

Yoshida M, Yamagami N, Tezuka T et al. Case report: detection of varicella-zoster virus DNA in maternal breast milk. J Med Virol 1992; 38: 108–10.

Zanetti AR, Tanzi E, Paccagiuni S et al. Mother-to-infant transmission of hepatitis C virus. Lancet 1995; 345: 289–91.

Zimmerman R, Perucchini D, Fauchere JC. Hepatitis C virus in breast milk. Lancet 1995; 345: 928.

Recreational drugs

Ruth Lawrence and Christof Schaefer

4.16

4.16.1 Alcohol

Experience

The concentration of alcohol in the breast milk is about the same as in maternal plasma at a given time (M/P = 1.0). As a result, the fully breastfed infant gets about 10% of the weight-related amount of alcohol that is taken in by the mother (survey in Bennett 1996). The milk levels drop parallel to the plasma levels. The peak plasma time varies depending on the rate at which the drink is consumed (immediate consumption versus sipping over an hour or so). The breast does not store alcohol.

Most of the studies have been done by laboratory protocol. Mothers serving as their own controls were given vodka in orange juice, which they had to consume in 10 minutes. Except in the case of alcoholics, this is not generally how alcohol is consumed. Blood and milk levels were drawn and the infants fed promptly. The infants receiving alcohol sucked less well. Vodka, which is tasteless and odorless, was reportedly detected by smell in the milk by adult volunteers (Mennella 1991). Alcohol can change the taste of the milk and, as a result, lead to feeding problems.

Infants who received alcohol via the breast milk consumed less milk in that 4-hour time period compared to the 8–12 hours when no alcohol was in the milk. Despite the limited activity of alcohol dehydrogenase in early infancy, and an elimination rate only half as rapid as that of an adult, the alcohol that is transmitted to the infant as a result of occasional and limited consumption of alcohol (e.g. a glass of champagne once or twice a week) does not, as far as we know today, cause any damage. However, according to a study on 1-year-old children, a statistically significant increased rate of mild delay in psychomotor development was observed when the mother regularly had two drinks a day during both pregnancy and lactation (Little 1989). However, these findings could not be confirmed at the age of 18 months (Little 2002). Beer – both alcoholic and non-alcoholic – has been credited with stimulating prolactin levels and milk production; whether this is because of the barley or the hops is the question. Excessive alcohol has been shown to reduce let-down (Cobo 1973). Assuming a regular, massive use of alcohol, damage to the baby is conceivable. In one case, a reversible pseudo-Cushing syndrome was attributed to the mother's massive intake of alcohol (survey in Bennett 1996).

> **Recommendation.** Occasionally consuming a glass of wine (8 oz) or beer (12 oz), or 2 oz of hard liquor, is thought to be safe by the Institute of Medicine. Mothers should be counseled that excessive use is contraindicated. Furthermore, they should consume a drink over a period of time (more than 30 minutes), and refrain from nursing for 2 hours thereafter to avoid any alcohol reaching the infant. When alcohol use is excessive or chronic, the baby should be weaned.

4.16.2   Caffeine

Experience

Methyl xanthines, which include not only *theophylline* but also *caffeine, theobromine*, and *paraxanthin*, are part of the "normal" components of milk and come from sources in the diet or in recreational drugs. In an extreme case, a fully breastfed infant can take in 3 mg/kg of methyl xanthine daily (Blanchard 1992). In a random sampling in Switzerland, 80% of the milk samples contained caffeine; in half of these there was over 1 μg/ml (Bucher 1985).

Caffeine levels in a cup of coffee depend on the method of preparation (percolated, filtered, instant, etc.) and the source of the coffee beans; the average is 100–150 mg per cup. Tea, cola, many carbonated beverages, herbal teas, and chocolate all contain varying amounts of caffeine, depending upon the method of preparation. Even some innocent drinks such as orange soda may have caffeine added to them. Caffeine is absorbed quickly and reaches maximum serum time at 60 minutes and readily enters the milk. The milk/plasma ratio (M/P) for caffeine is around 0.6.

When mothers were given one dose of 100 mg of caffeine p.o., peak levels in maternal serum occurred 30–60 minutes afterwards and it remained in the milk for 95–120 minute. The average concentration of caffeine in the milk was 2.5 µg/ml at 60 minutes. The dose to the infant was calculated to be 1.8–3.1 mg/d after this 100-mg dose (Stavchansky 1988). Caffeine levels in mothers who consumed 35–336 mg of caffeine daily ranged from 2.1–7.2 µg/ml, and the dose to the infant was 0.01–1.6 mg/d – which translates to 20% of the weight-adjusted maternal intake. Due to the immature cytochrom-P450-monooxygenasis system in the liver, which is responsible for metabolizing caffeine, the elimination half-life of caffeine is greatly prolonged in the newborn compared to an adult. Instead of 3.5 hours, it can be over 80 hours. The usual amounts of coffee, drunk socially, are well-tolerated by the infant. Much has been learned about caffeine clearance in the neonate since the advent of caffeine use for apnea in newborns. Because the metabolism is so slow, caffeine tends to accumulate over time. Thus, a breastfed infant who appears to tolerate maternal caffeine the first few days subsequently becomes irritable and jittery by 7–10 days, feeding frequently but never being satisfied. The mother then interprets this as failure of her milk supply. Some breastfed infants have been readmitted for a neurologic work-up and found to have caffeine levels above the therapeutic level. It usually takes weeks for a premature infant to clear caffeine. The half-life decreases with age to 14 hours at 3–5 months, and 2–6 hours at 6 months and older (Hale 2006).

A review of caffeine intake in infants (Nehlig 1994) reported that chronic maternal use can be associated with irritability and sleeplessness in infants. The association of chronic coffee drinking and reduction of iron in the milk has also been reported (Nehlig 1994).

Recommendation. Caffeine intake should be monitored by lactating women, who should be aware of the many sources of caffeine and the range of volume of the containers of beverages available. "Normal" caffeine intake, i.e. a maximum of three cups of coffee or six cups of tea (24 ounces of caffeine-containing beverage or 300 mg of caffeine in 24 hours, is not considered to be of concern during breastfeeding. Exceeding this amount does not necessarily require interruption of breastfeeding, but symptoms of over-excitability may be expected. In the early weeks of life, the newborn is especially at risk for accumulating caffeine and the resultant irritability until about 3 months of age. In such cases, consumption should be reduced.

4.16.3   Cannabis

Experience

Cannabis, commonly referred to as marijuana or hashish, contains *tetrahydrocannabinol* as the primary active ingredient. It is found in mothers' milk. It is also rapidly distributed into the brain and fat where it is stored. In heavy users, the milk/plasma ratio is as high as 8 (Perez-Reyes 1982). The half-life is up to 57 hours, and oral absorption is 100%. In a study of 68 infants exposed via mothers' milk, compared with unexposed infants the motor development of the exposed infants was reported to be delayed (Astley 1990).

Recommendation. Hashish should not be used during lactation. Regular use would require weaning the infant.

4.16.4   Cocaine

Experience

Cocaine is found in mothers' milk (Winecker 2001). It is completely orally bioavailable, and appears in the plasma within 15 minutes. The half-life is less than an hour, and total clearance is less than 5 hours. Urine samples, however, can be positive for 7 days or longer because of the slow excretion of the metabolites. The impact on the nursing infant is known only by case reports (Shannon 1989, Chaney 1988, Chasnoff 1987) describing tachycardia, hypertonia, trembling, and excitation.

Recommendation. If a mother takes cocaine, she should pump and discard her milk for 24 hours to assure clearance. A mother who is habituated should not breastfeed.

4.16.5 Nicotine

In Europe, about every third or fourth breastfeeding mother smokes. *Nicotine* has been shown to interfere with the let-down reflex. Although it does not appear to interrupt lactation once it has been initiated, smoking has clearly been associated with poor milk supply. Production has been shown to slowly diminish over the 6 weeks postpartum in smokers with prematures compared with non-smokers with prematures (Hopkinson 1992). Restlessness, poor suck, vomiting, and reduced weight gain have been observed in the infants of heavy smokers (survey in Lawrence 2005). Of course, more frequent respiratory illnesses are seen in connection with smoke inhalation. As yet, no permanent damage – with respect to either growth or functional development – as a result of being breastfed by a mother who smokes has been documented. Many studies indicate that mothers who smoke breastfeed their babies for less time. Here, social and psychological as well as physiological reasons (i.e. the antiprolactinergic effect of nicotine) play a role (Amir 2002, Letson 2002). Mothers who resume smoking regularly after the birth tend to stop breastfeeding early up to four times as frequently as those who do not smoke at all or who only smoke occasionally (Ratner 1999, Edwards 1998, Haug 1998). The father's smoking is also negatively correlated with the length of breastfeeding (Haug 1998).

Nicotine is present in passive smoke, and is better absorbed via the respiratory tract than orally. *Cotinine*, the major metabolite, is well-absorbed orally and less so by secondhand smoke. Both breast- and bottle-fed infants of smokers have nicotine in their urine. Women who smoke 10–20 cigarettes a day have 0.4–0.5 mg/l nicotine in their milk.

A direct correlation exists between the mother's plasma level and her milk level. Nicotine passes into milk quickly, as does cotinine. The half-life of nicotine is 90 minutes, but for cotinine is 24 hours (Bennett 1996). The levels increase with the number of cigarettes smoked (Schwartz-Bickenbach 1987). Newborn infants nursed by smoking mothers but kept in the newborn nursery to avoid passive smoke had concentrations of nicotine of 0.2 ng/ml and cotinine of 5–30 ng/ml (Counsilman 1985). Cotinine concentrations are 5–10 times as high in the urine of breastfed babies as they are in the urine of non-breastfed babies of smokers (Becker 1999, Mascola 1998).

As well as nicotine and cotinine, other toxic and carcinogenic chemicals and cadmium (Radisch 1987) also appear in the milk of smokers (Radisch 1987). Among 50 smoking mothers, a lower iodine content of the milk was found compared to a control group of 90 non-smokers. According to the authors, this could cause iodine deficiency in the infants requiring supplementation (Laurberg 2004).

Mothers who wish to stop smoking often seek help from nicotine therapies. Nicotine gum contains 2 mg nicotine per piece in the

Lactation

4.16 Recreational drugs

USA and 4 mg per piece in Canada and Europe. Nicotine is rapidly and completely absorbed through the oral mucosa. One hour of chewing a 2-mg piece produces a nicotine plasma concentration of 11.8 ng/ml, and an hour of chewing a 4-mg piece produces a concentration of 23.2 ng/ml. A study was conducted in Sweden during pregnancy to measure the Doppler effect on the fetus using a 4-mg dose compared with 1 cigarette, which contains a 1.6 mg dose (Lindblad 1987). It did not appear to affect the fetus (by Doppler). The nicotine patch provides nicotine transdermally. Up to 114 mg of nicotine can be contained in a high-dose patch, which has a delivery rate of 21–22 mg/h. A low-dose patch delivers only 7 mg/d. Serum levels vary accordingly. It was shown that similar amounts of nicotine reach the milk as with smoking cigarettes (Ilett 2003). Even higher levels were measured in the milk of 2 snuff-taking mothers compared to a group of 18 smokers (Dahlström 2004). These authors measured the nicotine transfer via milk, and found peak values of 51 μg/l milk 0.6 hours after nicotine exposure and 21 μg/l after 7 hours. Based on the mean level of 44 μg/l, a fully breastfed child would ingest 7 μg/kg per day.

The impact of passive smoking during lactation has been discussed intensively. Groner (2004) found similar cotinine levels in the hair of children up to 3 years and in their smoking mothers. In non-smoking mothers, contamination of hair was even stronger in the children compared to their mothers. Dahlström (2004) still measured half of the concentration in the milk of passively exposed mothers compared to that of smoking mothers.

Some vegetables contain measurable amounts of nicotine, especially eggplants, green tomatoes, and cauliflower (10 g of eggplant contains 1 μg of nicotine).

Recommendation. Smoking mothers should be encouraged to stop smoking or attempt to keep the number of cigarettes to a minimum. The environment for the infant should be smoke-free, so no-one should smoke inside the home. There are no studies that show definitively at which point the advantages of breastfeeding are outweighed by the disadvantages of smoking. Although infants of smokers are at greater risk for SIDS and respiratory illness and asthma, it was shown that infants of smoking mothers who are breastfed have a lesser risk of SIDS, respiratory illness, asthma, and infections than do those who are bottle fed. Thus, smoking women should be encouraged to breastfeed and to continue for as long as possible. Mothers who can't stop smoking should be encouraged to schedule cigarettes right after a feed so there is the longest time possible after smoking until the next feed.

4.16.6 Opiates, including methadone

Experience

All opiates can be found in the breastfed infant, having been transferred via the milk. Recreational use is of concern because of excessive doses, contaminated material, and the mode of use – i.e., smoking and intravenous injection.

Heroin is rapidly converted to 6-acetylmorphine and then slowly to morphine. Heroin is poorly absorbed orally, but morphine is absorbed. *Methadone* and *levomethadone* have pharmacological properties similar to morphine. The main use of methadone is for prevention of withdrawal in patients with opiate addiction. The protein binding is 85%, and the plasma half-life for adults is given as 25 hours. A number of studies have documented the presence of methadone in the milk. Doses varying from 10 to 105 mg/d have resulted in breast milk levels of 0.02–0.57 µg/ml (review in Jansson 2004). A fully breastfed infant would therefore receive up to 85 µg/kg daily, but on average levels of only 17.4 µg/kg were calculated (Wojnar-Horton 1997). The relative infant dose was estimated to be 1–6% (Begg 2001, survey in Bennett 1996). The M/P quotient ratio varies between 0.2 and 0.8.

A case report describes the death of an infant, allegedly caused by methadone in the mother's milk (Smialek 1977). However, the concentration of 400 µg/l found in the infant's serum in this case suggests that the methadone may have been administered directly.

All other experience suggests that methadone is well-tolerated during breastfeeding, even with high maternal daily dosages of up to 130 mg (McCarthy 2000, Malpas 1999, Geraghty 1997, Wojnar-Horton 1997). Among eight children studied, whose mothers took between 0.3 and 1.1 mg/kg methadone base daily, the methadone could only be detected in the plasma of one baby who had a level of 5.5 µg/l (Wojnar-Horton 1997). Two infants who had not needed any therapy up until that point first showed withdrawal symptoms following sudden weaning. Such observations lead to the discussion of breastfeeding as a preventive measure (Arlettaz 2005, Ballard 2002, 2001, Begg 2001, Malpas 1999).

The American Academy of Pediatrics has changed its recommendations regarding methadone so it has become a drug that is usually compatible with breastfeeding. The range of acceptable maternal dose has increased from 50 mg/d to 80 mg/d or higher (Philipp 2003).

During recent years, *buprenorphine* was discussed as being superior to methadone because of its shorter half-life and a lower risk of withdrawal symptoms in the neonate. For studies during lactation, see Chapter 4.1.3.

Intranasal application of *hydromorphone* was studied in eight lactating mothers. An M/P ratio of 2.5 and a relative infant dose of

0.7% were calculated (Edwards 2003). During delivery, hydromorphone is used to enhance epidural anesthesia. Experience is insufficient with its use for substitution in opioid-addicted mothers.

The long-term effects of opioids on breastfed children cannot be
easily separated from the effects of the opiate exposure prenatally.

Recommendation. Heroin as a street drug is a contraindication to breastfeeding because the ingredients, dosage, and possible contamination of ille-
gally produced products cannot be properly calculated. When methadone
substitution is continued, a fully breastfed child who has already been
exposed *in utero* to opiates or methadone is likely to develop fewer withdrawal symptoms after birth than one who is not breastfed. For this reason,
the baby can or should be breastfed if there is maternal methadone substitution when it is certain that there are no other drugs involved, and no maternal
infection, such as HIV, that would argue against it. The daily methadone
dosage that can be tolerated by the breastfed baby should be decided individually, considering the therapy up to the birth and any symptoms in the infant.
Each individual case must be reviewed individually, including social services in
the discussions, to be sure the mother has been stable with her therapy.
Abrupt weaning after hospital discharge is a risk, and follow-up is essential.

4.16.7   Other drugs

Experience

With a 20-mg intake of *amphetamines* daily, levels of 55–138 µg/l
were detected in breast milk. An M/P ratio ranging from 2.8 to 7.5
was calculated (Steiner 1984). A relative infant dose of up to 3%
would result from these values. Another study could not find any
symptoms among 103 infants whose mothers took various amounts
of amphetamines (Ayd 1973).

Two publications report on *phencyclidine* in breast milk
(Kaufman 1983, Nicholas 1982). However, these data are insufficient to assess its risk. There is insufficient experience with other
drugs of abuse during breastfeeding.

Recommendation. If a mother regularly takes amphetamines or abuses
other drugs, she should not breastfeed.

References

Amir LH, Donath SM. Does maternal smoking have a negative physiological effect on breastfeeding? The epidemiological evidence. Birth 2002; 29: 112–23.

Arlettaz R, Kashiwagi M, das Kundu S et al. Methadone maintenance in a Swiss perinatal denter: II. Neonatal outcome and social resources. Acta Obstet Gynecol Scand 2005; 84: 145–50.

Astley S, Little RE. Maternal marijuana use during lactation and infant development at one year. Neurotoxicol Tetratol 1990; 12: 161–8.

Ayd FJ. Excretion of psychotropic drugs in human milk. Intl Drug Ther News Bull 1973; 8: 33–40.

Ballard JL, d'Apolito K. Shortened length of stay for neonatal abstinence syndrome from methadone using mother's milk as therapy. Pediatr Res 2001; 49: 354.

Ballard JL. Treatment of neonatal abstinence syndrome with breast milk containing methadone. J Perinat Neonatal Nurs 2002; 15: 76–85.

Becker AB, Manfreda J, Ferguson AC et al. Breastfeeding and environmental tobacco smoke exposure. Arch Pediatr Adolesc Med 1999; 153: 689–91.

Begg EJ, Malpas TJ, Hackett LP et al. Distribution of R- and S- methadone into human milk during multiple, medium to high oral dosing. Br J Clin Pharmacol 2001; 52: 681–5.

Bennett PN (ed.). Drugs and Human Lactation, 2nd edn. Amsterdam: Elsevier, 1996.

Blanchard J, Weber CW, Shearer L-E. Methylxanthine levels in breast milk of lactating women of different ethnic and socioeconomic classes. Biopharm Drug Dispos 1992; 13: 187–96.

Bucher HU, Gautschi K. Detection of caffeine, theophylline and theobrome in the umbilical cord blood and breast milk. Helv Paediatr Acta 1985; 40(2–3): 163–7.

Chaney NE, Franke J, Wadlington WB. Cocaine convulsions in a breastfed baby. J Pediatr 1988; 112: 134–5.

Chasnoff IJ, Lewis DE, Squires L. Cocaine intoxication in a breast-fed infant. Pediatrics 1987; 80: 836–4.

Cobo E. Effect of different doses of ethanol on the milk-ejecting reflex in lactating women. Am J Obstet Gynecol 1973; 115: 817–21.

Counsilman JJ, MacKay EV. Cigarette smoking by pregnant women with particular reference to their past and subsequent breastfeeding behavior. Aust NZ Obstet Gynecol 1985; 25: 101.

Dahlström A, Ebersjö C, Lundell B. Nicotine exposure in breastfed infants. Acta Paediatr 2004; 93: 810–16.

Edwards J, Rudy A, Wermeling D et al. Hydromophone transfer into breast milk after intranasal administration. Pharmacotherapy 2003; 23: 153–8.

Edwards N, Sims-Jones N, Breithaupt K. Smoking in pregnancy and postpartum: relationship to mother's choices concerning infant nutrition. Can J Nurs Res 1998; 30: 83–98.

Geraghty B, Graham EA, Logan B et al. Methadone levels in breastmilk. J Hum Lact 1997; 13: 227–30.

Groner J, Wadwa P, Hoshaw-Woodard S et al. Active and passive tobacco smoke: a comparison of maternal and child hair cotinine levels. Nicotine Tob Res 2004; 6: 789–95.

Hale TW Jr. Medications and Mother's Milk, 12th edn. Amarillo, TX: Hale Publishing, 2006.

Haug K, Irgens LM, Baste V et al. Secular trends in breastfeeding and parental smoking. Acta Paediatr 1998; 87: 1023–7.

Hopkinson JM, Schanler RJ, Fraley JK et al. Milk production by mothers of premature infants: influence of cigarette smoking. Pediatrics 1992; 90: 934–8.

Ilett KF, Hale TW, Page-Sharp M et al. Use of nicotine patches in breast-feeding mothers: transfer of nicotine and cotinine into human milk. Clin Pharmacol Ther 2003; 74: 516–24.

Jansson L, Velez M, Harrow C. Methadone maintenance and lactation: a review of the literature and current management guidelines. J Hum Lact 2004; 20: 62–71.

Kaufman KR, Petrucha RA, Pitts FN Jr et al. PCP in amniotic fluid and breast milk: case report. J Clin Psychiatr 1983; 44: 269–70.

Laurberg P, Nohr SB, Pedersen KM et al. Iodine nutrition in breast-fed infants is impaired by maternal smoking. J Clin Endocrinol Metab 2004; 89: 181–7.

Lawrence RA, Lawrence RM. Breastfeeding: A Guide for the Medical Profession, 6th edn. Philadelphia, PA: Elsevier, 2005.

Letson GW, Rosenberg KD, Wu L. Association between smoking during pregnancy and breastfeeding at about 2 weeks of age. J Hum Lact 2002; 18: 368–72.

Lindblad A, Marsal K. Influence of nicotine chewing gum on fetal blood flow. J Perinatal Med 1987; 15: 13.

Little RE, Anderson KW, Ervin CH et al. Maternal alcohol use during breastfeeding and infant mental and motor development at one year. New Eng J Med 1989; 321: 425–30.

Little RE, Northstone K, Golding J. ALSPAC Study Team. Alcohol, breastfeeding, and development at 18 months. Pediatrics 2002; 109: 72.

Malpas TJ, Darlow MD. Neonatal abstinence syndrome following abrupt cessation of breastfeeding. NZ Med J 1999; 112: 12–13.

Mascola MA, van Vunakis H, Tager IB et al. Exposure of young infants to environmental tobacco smoke: breast feeding among smoking mothers. Am J Publ Health 1998; 88: 893–6.

McCarthy JJ, Posey BL. Methadone levels in human milk. J Hum Lact 2000; 16: 115–20.

Mennella JA, Beauchamp GK. The transfer of alcohol to human milk. Effects of flavor and the infant's behavior. N Engl J Med 1991; 325: 981–5.

Nehlig A, Debry G. Consequences on the newborn of chronic maternal consumption of coffee during gestation and lactation: a review. J Am Coll Nutr 1994; 13: 6–21.

Nicholas JM, Lipshitz J, Schreiber EC. Phencyclidine: its transfer across the placenta as well as into breast milk. Am J Obstet Gynecol 1982; 143: 143–6.

Perez-Reyes M, Wall ME. Presence of delta 9-tetrahydrocannabinol in human milk. N Eng J Med 1982; 307: 819–20.

Philipp B, Merewood A, O'Brien S. Methadone and breastfeeding: new horizons. Pediatrics 2003; 111: 1429–30.

Radisch B, Luck W, Nau H. Cadmium concentrations in milk and blood of smoking mothers. Toxicol Letts 1987; 36: 147–52.

Ratner PA, Johnson JL, Bottorff JL. Smoking relapse and early weaning among postpartum women: is there an association? Birth 1999; 26: 76–82.

Schwartz-Bickenbach D, Schulte-Hobein B, Abt S et al. Smoking and passive smoking during pregnancy and early infancy. Toxicol Letts 1987; 35: 73–81.

Shannon M, Lacouture PG, Roa J et al. Cocaine exposure among children seen at a pediatric hospital. Pediatrics 1989; 83: 337–42.

Smialek JE, Monforte JK, Aronow R et al. Methadone deaths in children. J Am Med Assoc 1977; 238: 2156–7.

Stavchansky S, Combs A, Sagraves R et al. Pharmacokinetics of caffeine in breast milk and plasma after single oral administration of caffeine to lactating mothers. Biopharm Drug Dispos 1988; 9: 285–99.

Steiner E, Villen T, Hallberg M et al. Amphetamine secretion in breast milk. Eur J Clin Pharmacol 1984; 27: 123–4.

Winecker RE, Goldberger BA, Tebbett IR et al. Detection of cocaine and its metabolites in breast milk. J Forensic Sci 2001; 46: 1221–3.

Wojnar-Horton RE, Kristensen JH, Ilett KF et al. Methadone distribution and excretion into breast milk of clients in a methadone maintenance programme. Br J Clin Pharmacol 1997; 44: 543–7.

Plant toxins

Ruth Lawrence and Christof Schaefer

4.17

Not much is known about the damage to an infant via breast milk as a result of maternal exposure to animal or plant poisons or toxins, or via the "physiological" parts of plants. There is one report (Hallebach 1985) in which an infant was harmed via his mother's milk after she had suffered *Amanita* poisoning. In another case report (Kautek 1988), it was presumed that a hemolytic crisis in an infant with congenital glucose 6-phosphate-dehydrogenase deficiency might have been caused when the mother ate *fava beans* (favism). However, this supposition is not very realistic and has not been confirmed by other publications.

Currently there can only be speculation about the meaning of the relatively high amounts of *aflatoxin* detected in many samples of mother's milk. In countries such as the Sudan or Thailand food is more highly contaminated with aflatoxins, and significant concentrations, which would exceed levels permitted in our foods, are sometimes detected in mothers' milk (Coulter 1984). However, a study in West Africa found a substantially greater contamination of infant nutrition after weaning. Their finding that children who were breastfed for longer grew better was discussed as being due to a toxic effect on children with artificial nutrition (Gong 2003). Another study also found aflatoxin M1 in the mother's milk in a population in Australia supposed to have little exposure to contaminated food (El-Nezami 1995). High concentrations of aflatoxin B1 in mother's milk have also been discussed in connection with the development of Kwashiorkor in breastfed children (Hendrickse 1997).

Recommendation. If a breastfeeding mother has symptoms caused by poisons or toxins, breastfeeding should be interrupted until symptoms have improved.

References

Coulter JBS, Lamplugh SM, Suliman GI et al. Aflatoxins in human breast milk. Ann Trop Pediatr 1984; 4: 61–6.

El-Nezami HS, Nicoletti G, Neal GE et al. Aflatoxin M1 in human breast milk samples from Victoria, Australia and Thailand. Food Chem Toxicol 1995; 33: 173–9.

Gong YY, Egal S, Hounsa A et al. Determinants of aflatoxin exposure in young children from Benin and Togo, West Africa: the critical role of weaning. Int J Epidemiol 2003; 32: 556–62.

Hallebach M, Kurze G, Springer S et al. Knollenblätterpilzvergiftung über Muttermilch. Z Klin Med 1985; 40: 943–5.

Hendrickse RG. Of sick turkeys, kwashiorkor, malaria, perinatal mortality, heroin addicts and food poisoning: research on the influence of aflatoxins on child health in the tropics. Ann Trop Med Parasit 1997; 91: 787–93.

Kautek L, Solem E, Böhler H. Hämolytische Krise nach Stillen! Der Kinderarzt 1988; 19: 808.

4

Lactation

4.17 Plant toxins

Industrial chemicals and environmental contaminants

4.18

Christof Schaefer

The same rules as those described in Chapter 3.2 for the transfer of medication into mother's milk apply to chemicals. Lipophilia, acidity, limited protein binding and low molecular mass enhance the transfer into the milk. The intake of contaminants occurs primarily via contaminated foods that cannot necessarily be avoided. Theoretically, absorption via the skin and respiration can also lead to measurable plasma concentrations, and thereby to exposure of the infant via the mother's milk.

Unlike the situation with medications, the lengthy persistence in nature of some toxicologically important industrial and environmental contaminants, as a result of limited photochemical or bacteriological decomposition and accumulation in the food chain, plays a significant role. There is virtually no way these compounds can be detoxified or decomposed in the human body.

4.18.1 Persistent organochlorine compounds (pesticides, polychlorinated biphenyls and dioxins)

Experience

Within this group are the classic pesticides *dichlordiphenyl-trichlorethan (DDT)*, *hexachlorbenzene (HCB)*, *dieldrin*, *hexachlorcyclohexan (HCH)*, and "synthetic oils" made from *polychlorinated biphenyls (PCBs)* as well as the *polychlorinated dioxins* and *furans*.

Of the organochlorine pesticides, only the short-lived χ-HCH *(lindane)* is still produced today (see Chapter 4.12). Other organochlorine pesticides such as DDT have been produced since the 1970s for export only to developing countries – at present there is a DDT "renaissance" for malaria prevention in Africa. For the most part, however, organochlorine pesticides have been replaced by *carbamates*, *organophosphates*, and *pyrethroids*. These substances are, to some extent, significantly more toxic, but they have a lesser tendency towards persistence and accumulation in nature.

Polychlorinated biphenyls were used as softeners and color additives. Since the 1970s they may only be used in closed systems, such as hydraulic fluid and transformer or condenser filling. Since the end of the 1980s the use of polychlorinated biphenyls has been banned in most countries, but the machines installed earlier still contain large quantities of these congeners.

Polychlorinated dibenzodioxins and *-furans*, among which group is the quadruply-chlorinated "seveso toxin" *2,3,7,8-TCDD*, occur in connection with technical activities as by-products or impurities during the synthesis of organochlorine compounds, and when they are recycled and burned. Trash dumps and chlorinated additives in automobile fuel are among the most significant sources of dioxin in our environment.

Toxic symptoms in the infant as a result of organochlorine compounds in the mother's milk have been described only after extreme exposure. The *Turkish porphyria (Pemba–Yarda syndrome)* occurred after consumption of seed grain treated with *hexachlorbenzene*. Apart from skin rash and weight loss, there were also lethal consequences for breastfed babies (Peters 1982). *Yusho disease* was caused by *polychlorinated biphenyls* in contaminated cooking oil. It caused muscular hypotonia, hyperexcitability, and apathy in the infants. The illness continued for many years (Miller 1977).

Concentrations in mothers' milk

Safety levels for organochlorine compounds in mothers' milk are aligned with the "no adverse effect level" (NOAEL) determined in

4

Lactation

4.18 Industrial chemicals and environmental contaminants

animal studies. This is understood to be the amount of a contaminant per kg bodyweight, taken in daily, that no longer causes any toxic effect (for example, a weight increase of the liver with a rise in enzyme activity in the rat). Based on the NOAEL, and taking into consideration a safety factor (SF), the acceptable daily intake (ADI) of the contaminant involved is calculated for a human being (adult or infant). The safety factor should actually be of the magnitude of 100–1000, but in practice, for PCBs in mothers' milk, a factor of only 10 was occasionally calculated. This means that beyond a level 10 times the amount ingested by a breastfed infant per kg bodyweight daily, toxic effects can be expected in animal studies. Contamination of human milk with polychlorinated biphenyls is very much greater than in cows' milk. The term *PCB* covers some 200 congeners, among which the congeners 138, 153, and 180 predominate, and are frequently presented as a proxy for the entirety of PCB contamination.

The average dioxin load in mother's milk is usually expressed in I-TEQ (International TCDD-equivalent) – i.e. the equivalent amount of seveso toxin 3,4,7,8-tetrachlordibenzodioxin that corresponds to the total amount of all dioxin- and furan-congeners in the analyzed specimen. According to the WHO (1989), the acceptable daily intake is 1–4 pg I-TEQ/kg bodyweight per day; the American Environmental Protection Agency (EPA) allows 0.1 pg/kg per day. These values are exceeded by nursing infants by up to 100-fold or more – for example, in Germany a fully breastfed infant receives on average 55 pg I-TEQ/kg per day. However, the acceptable dosages were defined for lifelong intake and not limited to the lactation period.

Regional differences in milk contamination

The different analytical methods used in different countries must be considered when comparing contamination in mothers' milk. In general, significantly higher contamination with DDT and DDE can be observed in many so-called "developing countries" (Kunisue 2004, Minh 2004), while PCBs and dioxins are found at higher levels in industrialized countries. Corresponding differences were found between Eastern and Western Europe, with more PCBs in the West (Mehler 1994, Hesse 1981). Regional differences may also be explained by differences in nutrition of the studied cohorts (Nadal 2004).

During the 1980s, DDT/DDE concentrations of, on average, 45 mg/kg milk fat were reported in Indonesia. Levels in South Africa, Kenya, Hong Kong, and India were between 10 and 20 mg/kg; in Europe, the USA, and Australia, levels were between 1 and 2 mg/kg. Depending on the analytical methodology, the average results for PCBs in Europe, Israel, and the USA were between 0.5 and 2.5 mg/kg milk fat (survey in Bennett 1996). In industrial nations, dioxins in human milk fat were between 15 and 25 ng I-TEQ/kg milk fat. Up to 1991, some authors still observed a rise in the average contamination in mothers' milk (Mehler 1994).

Since the early 1990s, a tendency towards declining levels of persistent organochlorine compounds has been noted in the milk. Today, PCB contamination has reduced to one-third of the values measured in Europe in the 1980s – in Germany, for example, more than 30 000 samples of human milk have been analyzed (BgVV 2000) to come to this conclusion. The current data on dioxin contamination in mothers' milk show that here, too, there has been a decline, from 37 pg/g fat in 1988 to 12 pg/g fat in 2002. Nevertheless, contamination levels in the Netherlands (18 pg/g fat) and Germany are still among the highest in Europe. Lower levels have been reported in Croatia and Spain, and also in Taiwan (Chao 2004, Schuhmacher 2004).

In another German publication on the development of contamination in mothers' milk in Baden-Württemberg, it was reported that in 1988 a total of 14% of the milk samples contained at least one of the studied substances at levels above 10% of the NOAEL (mostly PCBs). In accordance with the recommendations that were in effect until 1996, mothers with such levels were advised not to breastfeed beyond 4 months. By 1996, only 2% of the milk samples exceeded this so-called SF-10 value. The number of milk samples studied every year was initially over 1000; by 1990 it reached its peak, with 1983 samples studied. By 1996, the number had declined to 280 (Seidel 1998).

Persistently high PCB levels in mother's milk were found in the Faro islands – the level was 2300 ng/g fat in 1987, and by 1999 it was still 1800 ng/g (Fängström 2005).

Polybrominated diphenyl ethers

Increasing levels of *polybrominated diphenyl ethers* (PBDE) were observed in mothers' milk on the Faro islands (rising from 2 ng/g fat in 1987 to 8 ng/g in 1999; Fängström 2005). PBDE contamination of breast milk was also found in other countries. PBDEs are a group of more than 200 structurally similar congeners that are used as flame-retardants in electrical appliances such as television sets and computers, as well as in carpets and furniture upholstery. Because these compounds can accumulate in human tissues and, in adequate concentrations, alter metabolic and physiologic functions, the European Union (EU) banned the production, use, and import of *pentabromodiphenyl* ether and *octabromodiphenyl* ether products in 2004. *Decabromodiphenylether* is still in use, and its main congener, deca-BDE 209, can be detected in breast milk. A German study of 89 lactating women found, on average, 1.65 ng/g milk fat among vegetarians and a significantly higher level (2.47 ng/g) among women eating a varied diet that included meat. As with organochlorines, the levels were lower in women who had

4

Lactation

4.18 Industrial chemicals and environmental contaminants

breastfed many infants. However, no significant decrease was observed between the neonatal period and 3 months after birth. A fully breastfed child ingests, on average, 10 ng/kg bodyweight and, at maximum, 50 ng/kg. Considering the NOAEL for PBDE, this corresponds to a margin of safety (MOS) of $>10^4$. Therefore, health problems are not to be expected (Vieth 2005). PBDE contamination in North America is one order of magnitude higher than that measured in Germany.

Levels measured in breastfed infants

It is estimated that breastfed infants receive one to two magnitudes more dioxines than adults. Teufel (1990) found the highest plasma concentrations after birth. At 6 months, regardless of the type of feeding, the lowest values were measured. Although the absolute amount of polychlorinated biphenyls and dioxins transferred with the milk is greater than that transferred by the placenta during pregnancy, the "dilution effect" that occurs as a result of the infant's rapidly increasing fatty tissue appears to decrease the concentration in the infant's plasma.

For dioxin, the elimination half-life of 4 months in newborns is significantly shorter than that in adults (5 years). This too contributes to the fact that although fully breastfed children have significantly higher TCDD concentrations in the blood and fatty tissue than do non-breastfed babies, the differences have completely leveled out after a few years (Kreuzer 1997). A detailed model to predict dioxin levels in the body fat of infants, dependent on the duration of breastfeeding (no breastfeeding; and after 6 weeks, 6 months, 1 year, and 2 years), was presented by Lorber (2002). According to this model that was validated with data from the study cohort of Abraham (1998), breastfed infants reach peak values during their first months of life. Up to the age of 7–10 years, however, these levels approach those found in children who were not breastfed. For PCBs, Heudorf (2002) observed no difference between breastfed and formula-fed children at the age of 12 years.

Effects of average contamination on infant development

Among the numerous studies on persistent organochlorines in the "normal" environment, some present levels in maternal and infant blood and in breast milk (Fängström 2005, Lackmann 2005, Chao 2004, Kunisue 2004, Minh 2004, Nadal 2004, Schuhmacher 2004, Heudorf 2002). Others focus on somatic and mental development (survey in LaKind 2004). There are mainly four larger research projects which have led to several publications, i.e. the studies in North Carolina, Michigan, The Netherlands, and Germany. In North Carolina, 865 infants were enrolled in around 1980 to investigate their development until the age of 5 and at puberty (Gladen 2000, 1991, 1988). Illnesses during childhood were not associated with exposure to PCB and DDE via breast milk. Furthermore, there was no significant correlation with mental and psychomotor development, or with somatic development and puberty.

The so-called Michigan study covered 240 children whose mothers regularly consumed PCB-contaminated fish from the Great Lakes (>11.8 kg over 6 years). The control group consisted of 71 children of mothers who did not consume such fish. Visual recognition at the age of 7 months was not affected. However, subtle differences of development were observed at the age of 4 years. These were more pronounced in children who had been breastfed for at least 1 year. Intelligence was not affected, at least up to the age of 11 years (Jacobson 2002, 1996, 1990).

A Dutch study with 100 breastfed and 100 formula-fed children focused on PCB and dioxins (Koopman-Esseboom 1996). Higher levels in milk were associated with elevated TSH values at birth and at 3 months, indicating disturbance of thyroid function. Neurological examinations of 400 newborns and psychomotor and cognitive tests up to the age of 4 years revealed no persisting effects of PCBs or dioxins (survey in LaKind 2002).

A German study on mental and motor development found a negative association between PCB levels in milk and performance of the Kaufman score at the age of 42 months. Other outcome parameters were uneventful in this study, which covered in total 171 mother–child-pairs (Walkowiak 2001).

Other studies with smaller cohorts observed associations between dioxins, furans, and PCB in breast milk with lower levels of thyroid hormones, increased CD4+ lymphocytes, reduced CD8+ lymphocytes (T suppressor cells), slightly elevated liver enzymes, and lower platelet counts. In general, development was normal up to 6 months of age (survey in LaKind 2004). Even considering moderate contamination of breast milk, some authors suggest an overall positive effect of breastfeeding on psychomotor and cognitive development that compensates for potential impairments due to toxic contaminants (Vreugdenhil 2004, Ribas-Fito 2003, Boersma 2000).

Recommendation. Average contamination of breast milk with persistent organochlorines does not seem to have detrimental effects on children's development. If it is assumed that any toxic effect of organochlorines is associated with their plasma level, prenatal exposure would be more relevant than intake through breast milk. All in all, breastfeeding has a positive, and probably compensatory, effect on psychomotor and cognitive development that outweighs potential toxic effects before birth and via breast milk.

4

Lactation

4.18 Industrial chemicals and environmental contaminants

4.18.2   Mercury

Experience

Elemental or *metallic mercury* is used in mercury thermometers and (in combination with silver and other metals) in dental amalgam. In China, dental amalgam was used to fill teeth over 1000 years ago (cited in Drexler 1998). *Inorganic mercury*, e.g. *mercury chloride*, has been used as a disinfectant. *Organic mercury* (*ethyl mercury*) is used for the preservation of vaccines, and is accumulated in contaminated seafood (*methyl mercury*). Apart from high doses elemental mercury is hardly absorbed via intestine (<0.01%), but 80% may reach the circulation via inhalation. Inorganic mercury (<10%) and, even more so, organic mercury (up to 95%) are orally available. The liver, kidneys, and CNS are target organs of mercury poisoning. Elemental and inorganic mercury are excreted via the kidneys, whereas organic mercury is excreted through the colon. Mercury accumulates; its half-life ranges from 6 months to several years. The mercury content in mother's milk does not reach toxic levels under normal nutritional conditions, or even in the presence of a great many amalgam fillings. Other conditions have prevailed, though – for instance, as a result of an environmental scandal in Japan, industrial waste water containing mercury heavily contaminated the fish and led to an outbreak of Minamata disease among those who had eaten the fish and also, via their milk, among their children. The result was a spate of neurological developmental disorders, including some serious cerebral damage with spasticity. In other cases, it was mercury-contaminated seed grain, used for food (in Iran and the USSR), that caused toxic damage (Wolff 1983). In such cases, concentrations of up to 540 µg/l were measured in mothers' milk.

The average mercury concentrations in Europe are 1 µg/l in the blood or 1 µg/g creatinine in the urine. In Scandinavia and Japan (Sakamoto 2002), significantly higher "normal" levels have been reported. Due to the regular intake of contaminated seafood, levels of between 16 µg/l and 40 µg/l were measured among the Inuit. Methyl mercury from contaminated seafood is measured in erythrocytes. In general, prenatal mercury exposure is more relevant than that via breast milk. Cord blood levels exceed those in maternal blood by 50–100% (Björnberg 2005, Sakamoto 2002).

Concentration in mothers' milk

In a German study of 116 women, an average of 0.9 µg/l milk (ranging from <0.25 to 20.3) was reported after birth. After 2 months of breastfeeding it was, on average, below 0.25 µg/l (ranging from <0.25 to 11.7). In the first sample, the individual value correlated with the number of fillings in the teeth and the frequency of fish meals (there was no differentiation between fresh- and salt-water fish, and no particular information on contamination). With the second sample, which involved 84 of the 116 women in the study, there was a positive association only with the consumption of fish (Drexler 1998).

According to a study of mothers' milk samples in East Germany, more than 80% of the mercury values found were under the detection limit of 0.5 µg/l milk (Henke 1994). Similar results were found in other European countries – for example, in a recent study of 20 mother–child-pairs in Sweden, total mercury was 0.2–0.3 µg/l at 4 days, and 6 and 13 weeks after delivery (Björnberg 2005).

Ten years earlier a Swedish study of 30 women found a correlation, about 6 weeks after birth, between the number of amalgam fillings and the mercury concentration (total value and inorganic portion) both in the blood (mean value 2.3 µg/l) and in the milk (mean 0.6 µg/l). According to the authors, each filling increased the total concentration in the mother's blood by about 0.1 µg/kg and in the milk by about 0.05 µg/kg. The level of fish consumption (methyl mercury) was significantly reflected only in the contamination of the mother's blood, but not in the milk (Oskarsson 1996). A recent study from Taiwan investigated 68 healthy urban mothers, and mothers married to fishermen, in relation to fish intake (Chien 2006A). The breast milk mercury geometric mean concentration was 2.02 µg/l (0.24–9.45) in the urban group, and comparable values were found for the fishermen's group.

Based on the milk levels presented above, a fully breastfed baby would ingest up to 0.3 µg of mercury per kg daily. The ADI value set by WHO is 0.715 µg/kg bodyweight.

According to a study of 583 children on the Faro Islands, the mercury concentration in hair samples of 1-year-old babies is correlated with the length of breastfeeding (Grandjean 1994).

Recommendation. Mercury contamination from dental amalgam does not lead to dramatic increases in heavy metal concentrations that would demand consequences such as weaning. Detoxification treatment is not indicated. In addition, chelating agents may mobilize heavy metals and in this way increase contamination of the mother's milk. On the other hand, amalgam fillings should only be removed in case of dental problems. Extensive restoration should be postponed until after the breastfeeding period. Wherever possible, amalgam should be avoided. However, at an individual level, the amalgam issue should not be stirred up into a "toxicological crisis" that puts an unjustifiable strain on the mother–child relationship.

Consumption of fish highly contaminated with mercury is not recommended during pregnancy and breastfeeding. Among such fish are shark, true eel, sturgeon, ocean perch, swordfish, perch, halibut, pike, ray, monkfish, and tuna.

4

Lactation

4.18 Industrial chemicals and environmental contaminants

4.18.3   Lead

Experience

Inorganic lead (e.g. *lead oxide*) is distinguished from *organic lead* (e.g. *tetraethyl lead*). Lead salts are absorbed via the intestine and inhalation. Sources are glazes, paints, additives in leaded fuel, lead pipes, and occupational exposure. Mainly due to the ban of leaded fuel, average lead levels in blood have substantially declined to concentrations below 10 or even $5 \mu g/dl$ during the past two decades. With a half-life of approximately 30 years in adults, >90% of lead is stored in bones.

The current authors observed a case of lead poisoning due to acid spring water (pH 5.5) which was carried through a 300-m lead pipe, resulting in tap water contaminated with $4000 \mu g/l$ lead. At the age of 3 months, the fully breastfed infant developed serious cerebral palsy. The level in the mother's milk was $80 \mu g/l$. It cannot be determined to what extents the prenatal exposure *in utero* and the postnatal exposure through the mother's milk caused the lead poisoning.

Concentration in mothers' milk

According to a study in West Germany in the 1980s, the average lead concentrations in mothers' milk were between 9 and $13 \mu g/l$ (Sternowsky 1985). Another study in Eastern Germany produced similar results. Interestingly, the content in mother's milk did not necessarily correlate with the industrial contaminant load in the respective region (Henke 1994). Levels were 20–50% of the ADI value of $5 \mu g/kg$ bodyweight recommended by the WHO. Significantly higher lead concentrations were found in mothers' milk in the 1980s in Tyrol ($29 \mu g/l$) and in Singapore ($46 \mu g/l$) (cited in Henke 1994), while $62 \mu g/l$ milk was measured in one worker in a factory producing storage batteries (Wolff 1983).

Corresponding to the lead levels in blood, contamination of milk has also decreased. Average levels below $5 \mu g/l$ are measured today. Even a recent report from a poor region in Ecuador where lead glazes are manufactured found mean lead levels of $4.6 \mu g/l$ (range 0.4–$20.5 \mu g/l$) as a consequence of improved working conditions (Counter 2004). Among 310 women in Mexico City, $1.1 \mu g/l$ milk was measured 1 month after delivery (Ettinger 2004). A Greek study analyzed 180 specimen of colostrum for lead and found, on average, $0.5 \mu g/l$ (Leotsinidis 2005). In Croatia, 158 women had a mean contamination of $4.7 \mu g/l$ milk 4 days after birth (Ursinyova 2005).

In a Chinese study, mothers who consumed traditional Chinese herbs were compared to a control group of mothers who did not

(Chien 2006B). The geometric mean of lead concentrations in all colostrum samples ($n = 72$) was $7.68 \pm 8.24\,\mu g/l$. The concentration of lead in the breast milk of the consumption group was $8.59 \pm 10.95\,\mu g/l$, a level significantly higher than that of $6.84 \pm 2.68\,\mu g/l$ found in the control group. Sixteen of the mothers provided breast milk weekly at 1–60 days postpartum. In the group that had consumed herbs ($n = 9$) the mean concentration of lead in the breast milk decreased, within days postpartum, from $9.94\,\mu g/l$ in the colostrum to $2.34\,\mu g/l$ in mature milk.

All these data are well below the ADI for infants recommended by the WHO. However, several studies have indicated that there is no safe threshold for lead in infant's blood with respect to neurological development (e.g. reaction time, motor skills, attention, and intelligence). Even with very low blood levels of $<3\,\mu g/l$, subtle correlations can be found between lead concentration and neurological test performance (Chiodo 2004).

> **Recommendation.** Apart from extreme exposure such as that described above, lead in a mother's milk would not be expected to pose a substantial risk to her infant. Nevertheless, every unnecessary exposure to high levels of lead should be avoided (for example, ceramic vessels with lead glazing, traditional herbal medicines; see also Chapter 2.23) in order to prevent even discrete effects on the development of the central nervous system.

4.18.4   Cadmium

Experience

Moderate *cadmium* concentrations of $6–12\,\mu g/l$ were measured in mothers' milk in a German study (Henke 1994), but there were also concentrations two to three times as high, as well as those below $1\,\mu g/l$. Low concentrations (average $0.09\,\mu g/l$, range $0.02–0.73\,\mu g/l$) were also measured in a recent Austrian study that enrolled 124 women (Gundacker 2005, personal communication). A Greek study of 180 colostrum samples found $0.19\,\mu g/l$ (Leotsinidis 2005), and a Croatian study of 158 women found $0.43\,\mu g/l$ on day 4 postpartum (Ursinyova 2005). Smoking, including passive smoking, has a significant influence on the cadmium level (Gundacker 2005, personal communication; Radisch 1987).

The WHO ADI value for adults is $1\,\mu g$ cadmium/kg bodyweight. This was exceeded by the findings in Germany (Henke 1994, cited above).

> **Recommendation.** Toxic effects of cadmium via the mothers' milk have not, as yet, been described, and are unlikely under normal circumstances.

4.18.5   Other contaminants

Experience

A case report describes obstructive icteric liver disease in a breastfed baby after exposure to the volatile organochlorine *tetrachloroethene (PER)*, which is used as a cleaning agent. The mother had visited her husband every day at his workplace, which was apparently strongly contaminated. This also led to neurological symptoms in the mother (Bagnell 1977). A milk sample given an hour after maternal exposure had 10 mg tetrachloroethene/l. After 24 hours, the level was still 3 mg/l. The baby's condition returned to normal after weaning. A follow-up examination at 10 years of age showed nothing remarkable. Other groups of authors have demonstrated *volatile chlorhydrocarbons* – on average 6.2 µg/l – in the milk of mothers whose exposure was not occupational. It can be 4–8 weeks after exposure before the concentration in milk of the lipophilic tetrachloroethene "normalizes" (Schreiber 1993). However, this should in no way be a basis for recommending weaning after "trivial" exposure. Ongoing exposure at the workplace, on the other hand, should be looked at critically during breastfeeding.

Various other contaminants, such as the organic solvents *benzene* and *toluene* (Fabietti 2004), and the bactericide *triclosan* (Adolfsson-Erici 2002), have been detected in breast milk.

Synthetic musk compounds, such as *musk xylol*, *musk ketone*, *musk ambrette*, and others, are among the nitroaromatics. These substances have a limited acute toxicity, but, like the organochlorine compounds, they seem to accumulate in the fatty tissue and persist in the environment. Current analyses of mothers' milk have indicated a mean of about 0.1 mg/kg milk fat for musk xylol. The other compounds have levels two to three times lower. Synthetic musk compounds are added to detergents and cosmetics because of their fragrance, and thus dermal absorption is a likely path for their intake. There are no indications of toxic effects as a result of intake via mothers' milk. The studies to date on general toxicity and on mutagenic and carcinogenic potential do not permit a conclusive judgment (Liebl 2000, Rimkus 1994). Since 1993, contamination of mother's milk with musk xylol has declined in Germany to about 0.02 mg/kg milk fat, following a recommendation that this substance be avoided in detergents and other cleaning agents. Since the beginning of the 1990s, musk ketone levels have remained relatively constant at 0.02 mg/kg milk fat.

There are insufficient data on the polycyclic musk compounds such as *galaxolide* and *tonalide*. These substances are also added to detergents and other cleaning agents.

In addition to these aromatics, *UV-filtering* substances (sunlight protection factors and sun block) are detectable in the milk (BgVV 2000).

According to a small study, *silicon* from breast implants was said to lead to disturbances of motility in the lower esophageal tract of breastfed infants, caused by scleroderma-like changes (Levine 1994). A definitive judgment on this hypothesis is not yet possible. A corresponding suspicion that silicon implants could cause collagenoses in the women themselves has not been confirmed in a meta-analysis (Janowsky 2000). Silicon compounds are used in many common medications, and exposure from these is more common than from implants.

4.18.6   Breastfeeding despite environmental contaminants?

Breast milk is a bioindicator for environmental contaminants accumulating in fat tissues (Fenton 2005). In recent years, laboratory findings in breast milk samples, combined with public pressure, have led to a declining tendency in the concentrations of contaminants. This was impressively confirmed in, for instance, the evaluation of the measurements collected over many years by the Human Milk and Dioxin Data Bank at the German Federal Institute for Consumer Health Protection and Veterinary Medicine (BgVV 2000).

Persistent organochlorine compounds are stored in the fatty tissue for life, and are only mobilized by losing weight and breastfeeding. For this reason, a low-calorie diet should be avoided while breastfeeding. Apart from a marked intake of animal fat and contaminated seafood (especially shellfish), the current dietary habits of the mother have little influence on the contamination levels in the milk. However, a primarily vegetarian diet of products having low pesticide residues does lead to a lower level of contaminants in the mother's milk.

Every breastfed child reduces the contaminant load in the fatty tissue of the mother and in the milk by about 10–20%. It could be said, somewhat cynically, that breastfeeding is the most effective detoxification technique for the mother.

Not enough is known about the long-term effect of the contaminants discussed in this chapter. There are indications that polychlorinated dioxins and furans may inhibit the immune system and promote tumor development (WHO 1989, Knutsen 1984), but not yet in connection with average exposure via the mother's milk.

4

Lactation

4.18 Industrial chemicals and environmental contaminants

There is speculation as to whether so-called endocrine disruptors, i.e. contaminants with estrogenic properties (some PCBs, dioxins, phthalates), taken in via the mother's milk, may impair an infant's development (Massart 2005, Borgert 2003). What must be considered in the discussion as to whether or not to breastfeed is that the contaminants stored by the mother have already been transferred to the embryo and fetus during pregnancy.

The positive effects of breastfeeding are well documented. Poisoning of the breastfed child is mainly documented in association with severe environmental pollution (e.g. methyl mercury in Minamata) or individual intoxication of the mother. From a global standpoint, the WHO estimates that 1.3 million infant deaths below the age of 5 years can be prevented annually by breastfeeding (Jones 2003). No adverse effect on the infant as a result of the "normal" contamination of the mother's milk has been shown as yet. The recommendation, issued some years ago, of a limit on breastfeeding because of general environmental contamination, is no longer justifiable.

Due to the newer contaminant data, a contaminant analysis is no longer recommended as an aid to an individual decision on the length of breastfeeding, except in particularly contaminated regions.

Nevertheless, it is important not to rely only on what has been achieved already. In the future, monitoring programs should continue to oversee efforts to further reduce the toxic contamination of mother's milk.

4.18.7   Breastfeeding and the workplace

The motto for the World Breastfeeding Week 2000 ("Breastfeeding: It's Your Right"), coined by the World Alliance for Breastfeeding Action (WABA), raised awareness that it is the responsibility of both political bodies and society at large to make it possible for women to breastfeed. Part of this responsibility is creating conditions that permit a mother to breastfeed for as long as she and her baby want to, despite her being employed outside the home. At the same time, the motto emphasized the "right" of the child to be nourished optimally – and that means the right to be breastfed.

The revised International Labor Organization Convention (ILO Convention No. 183), passed in June 2000, codifies the mother's right to retain her job, protection from being dismissed, and the adaptation of both the work and the working hours to suit the situation of the pregnant or breastfeeding mother.

Some countries have gone beyond the convention and passed legislation which provides that pregnant or breastfeeding mothers who return to their jobs after the statutory (paid) maternity leave, or at the end of their child-rearing leave, may not be required to perform certain tasks that might compromise their health or the health of their babies. Among these are regular lifting of heavy burdens, constant squatting or bending over, extreme stretching or bending, continuous standing or sitting without a break, and contact with poisonous or infectious materials, or with openly radioactive substances.

In some cases, the total working hours per day or per week are limited. Ideally, if a transfer to another workplace is necessary for any health reason, this should not involve any financial disadvantage for the pregnant or breastfeeding woman.

The ILO convention provides for paid breastfeeding breaks – at least two half-hour sessions per day. Breastfeeding breaks are not a substitute for the general breaks required by law, and nor should breastfeeding mothers be required to make up this time.

References

Abraham K, Papke O, Gross A et al. Time course of PCDD/PCDF/PCB concentrations in breast-feeding mothers and their infants. Chemosphere 1998; 37: 1731–41.

Adolfsson-Erici M, Pettersson M, Parkkonen J et al. Triclosan, a commonly used bactericide found in human milk and in the aquatic environment in Sweden. Chemosphere 2002; 46: 1485–9.

Bagnell PC, Ellenberger HA. Obstructive jaundice due to a chlorinated hydrocarbon in breast milk. Can Med J 1977; 117: 1047–8.

Bennett PN (ed.). Drugs and Human Lactation, 2nd edn. Amsterdam: Elsevier, 1996.

BgVV. Belastung der Bevölkerung mit Dioxinen und anderen unerwünschten Stoffen in Deutschland deutlich zurückgegangen. Trends der Rückstandsgehalte in Frauenmilch der Bundesrepublik Deutschland – Aufbau der Frauenmilch- und Dioxin-Humandatenbank am BgVV. BgVV-Pressedienst 15, 2000.

Björnberg KA, Vahter M, Berglund B et al. Transport of methylmercury and inorganic mercury to the fetus and breast-fed infant. Environ Health Perspect 2005; 113: 1381–5.

Boersma ER, Lanting CI. Environmental exposure to polychlorinated biphenyls (PCBs) and dioxins. Consequences for longterm neurological and cognitive development of the child lactation. Adv Exp Med Biol 2000; 478: 271–87.

Borgert CJ, LaKind JS, Witorsch RJ. A critical review of methods for comparing estrogenic activity of endogenous and exogenous chemicals in human milk and infant formula. Environ Health Perspect 2003; 111: 1020–36.

Chao HR, Wang SL, Lee CC et al. Level of polychlorinated dibenzo-p-dioxins, dibenzofurans and biphenyls (PCDD/Fs, PCBs) in human milk and the input to infant body burden. Food Chem Toxicol 2004; 42: 1299–308.

Chien LC (A), Han BC, Hsu CS et al. Analysis of the health risk of exposure to breast milk mercury in infants in Taiwan. Chemosphere 2006; 64: 79–85.

Chien LC (B), Yeh CY, Lee HC et al. Effect of the mother's consumption of traditional Chinese herbs on estimated infant daily intake of lead from breast milk. Sci Total Environ 2006; 354: 120–26.

4

Lactation

4.18 Industrial chemicals and environmental contaminants

Chiodo LM, Jacobson SW, Jacobson JL. Neurodevelopmental effects of postnatal lead exposure at very low levels. Neurotoxicol Teratol 2004; 26: 359–71.

Counter SA, Buchanan LH, Ortega F. Current pediatric and maternal lead levels in blood and breast milk in Andean inhabitants of a lead-glazing enclave. J Occup Environ Med 2004; 46: 967–73.

Drexler H, Schaller KH. The mercury concentration in breast milk resulting from amalgam fillings and dietary habits. Environ Res A 1998; 77: 124–9.

Ettinger AS, Tellez-Rojo MM, Amarasiriwardena C et al. Levels of lead in breast milk and their relation to maternal blood and bone lead levels at one month post-partum. Environ Health Perspect 2004; 112: 926–31.

Fabietti F, Ambruzzi A, Delise M et al. Monitoring of the benzene and toluene contents in human milk. Environ Intl 2004; 30: 397–401.

Fängström B, Strid A, Grandjean P et al. A retrospective study of PBDEs and PCBs in human milk from the Faroe Islands. Environ Health 2005; 4: 12.

Fenton SE, Condon M, Ettinger AS et al. Collection and use of exposure data from human milk biomonitoring in the United States. J Toxicol Environ Health A 2005; 68: 1691–712.

Gladen BC, Rogan WJ, Hardy P et al. Development after exposure to polychlorinated biphenyls and dichlordiphenyldichlorethene transplacentally and through human milk. J Pediatr 1988; 113: 991–5.

Gladen BC, Rogan WJ. Effects of perinatal polychlorinated biphenyls and dichlorodiphenyldichloroethene on later development. J Pediatr 1991; 119: 58–63.

Gladen BC, Ragan NB, Rogan WJ. Pubertal growth and development and prenatal and lactational exposure to polychlorinated biphenyls and dichlorodiphenyl dichloroethene. J Pediatr 2000; 136: 490–96.

Grandjean P, Jørgensen PJ, Weihe P. Human milk as a source of methyl mercury exposure in infants. Environ Health Perspect 1994; 102: 74–7.

Henke J, Großer B, Ruick G. Konzentration von toxischen Schwermetallen in der Frauenmilch. Sozialpädiatrie 1994; 16: 544–6.

Hesse V, Gabrio T, Kirst E et al. Untersuchungen zur Kontamination von Frauenmilch, Kuhmilch und Butter in der DDR mit chlorierten Kohlenwasserstoffen. Kinderärztliche Praxis 1981; 49: 292–303.

Heudorf U, Angerer J, Drexler H. Polychlorinated biphenyls in the blood plasma: current exposure of the population in Germany. Rev Environ Health 2002; 17: 123–34.

Jacobson JL, Jacobson SW, Humphrey HEB. Effects of in utero exposure to polychlorinated biphenyls and related contaminants on cognitive functions in young children. J Pediatr 1990; 116: 38–45.

Jacobson JL, Jacobson SW. Intellectual impairment in children exposed to polychlorinated biphenyls in utero. N Engl J Med 1996; 335: 783–9.

Jacobson JL, Jacobson SW. Association of prenatal exposure to an environmental contaminant with intellectual function in childhood. J Toxicol Clin Toxicol 2002; 40: 467–75.

Janowsky E, Kupper LL, Hulka BS. Meta-analysis of the relation between silicone breast implants and the risk of connective-tissue diseases. N Engl J Med 2000; 342: 781–90.

Jones G, Steketee RW, Black RE et al. Bellagio Child Survival Study Group. How many child deaths can we prevent this year? Lancet 2003; 362: 65–71.

Knutsen AP. Immunologic effects of TCDD exposure in humans. Bull Environ Contam Toxicol 1984; 33: 673–81.

Koopman-Esseboom C, Weisglas-Kuperus N, de Ridder MAJ et al. Effects of poly-chlorinated biphenyl/dioxin exposure and feeding type on infants mental and psy-chomotor development. Pediatrics 1996; 97: 700–706.

Kreuzer PE, Csanády GyA, Baur C et al. 2,3,7,8-Tetrachlordibenzo-p-dioxin (TCDD) and congeners in infants. A toxicokinetic model of human lifetime body burden by TCDD with special emphasis on its uptake by nutrition. Arch Toxicol 1997; 71: 383–400.

Kunisue T, Someya M, Monirith I et al. Occurrence of PCBs, organochlorine insecticides, tris(4-chlorophenyl)methane, and tris(4-chlorophenyl)methanol in human breast milk collected from Cambodia. Arch Environ Contam Toxicol 2004; 46: 405–12.

Lackmann GM, Schaller KH, Angerer J. Lactational transfer of presumed carcinogenic and teratogenic organochlorine compounds within the first six months of life {in German}. Z Geburtshilfe Neonatol 2005; 209: 186–91.

LaKind JS, Amina Wilkins A, Berlin CM Jr. Environmental chemicals in human milk: a review of levels, infant exposures and health, and guidance for future research. Toxicol Appl Pharmacol 2004; 198: 184–208.

Leotsinidis M, Alexopoulos A, Kostopoulou-Farri E. Toxic and essential trace elements in human milk from Greek lactating women: association with dietary habits and other factors. Chemosphere 2005; 61: 238–47.

Levine JJ, Ilowite NT. Sclerodermalike esophageal disease in children breast-fed by mothers with silicone breast implants. J Am Med Assoc 1994; 271: 213–16.

Liebl B, Mayer R, Ommer S et al. Transition of nitro musks and polycyclic musks into human milk. Adv Exp Med Biol 2000; 478: 289–305.

Lorber M, Phillips L. Infant exposure to dioxin-like compounds in breast milk. Environ Health Perspect 2002; 110: A325–32, Figure 3.

Massart F, Harrell JC, Federico G et al. Human breast milk and xenoestrogen exposure: a possible impact on human health. J Perinatol 2005; 25: 282–8.

Mehler HJ, Henke J, Scherbaum E et al. Pestizide, polychlorierte Biphenyle und Dioxine in Humanmilch. Sozialpädiatrie 1994; 16: 490–2.

Miller RW. Pollutants in breast milk. J Pediatr 1977; 90: 510–12.

Minh NH, Someya M, Minh TB et al. Persistent organochlorine residues in human breast milk from Hanoi and Hochiminh City, Vietnam: contamination, accumulation kinetics and risk assessment for infants. Environ Pollut 2004; 129: 431–41.

Nadal M, Espinosa G, Schuhmacher M et al. Patterns of PCDDs and PCDFs in human milk and food and their characterization by artificial neural networks. Chemosphere 2004; 54: 1375–82.

Oskarsson A, Schütz A, Skerfving S et al. Total and inorganic mercury in breast milk and blood in relation to fish consumption and amalgam fillings in lactating women. Arch Environ Health 1996; 51: 234–41.

Peters HA, Gocmen A, Cripps DJ et al. Epidemiology of hexachlorobenzene-induced porphyria in Turkey: clinical and laboratory follow-up after 25 years. Arch Neurol 1982; 39: 744–9.

Radisch B, Luck W, Nau H. Cadmium concentrations in milk and blood of smoking mothers. Toxicol Letts 1987; 36: 147–52.

Ribas-Fito N, Cardo E, Sala M et al. Breastfeeding, exposure to organochlorine compounds, and neurodevelopment in infants. Pediatrics 2003; 111: 580–85.

Rimkus G, Rimkus B, Wolf M. Nitro musks in human adipose tissue and -breast milk. Chemosphere 1994; 28: 421–32.

Sakamoto M, Kubota M, Matsumoto S et al. Declining risk of methylmercury exposure to infants during lactation. Environ Res 2002; 90: 185–9.

Schreiber JS. Predicted infant exposure to tetrachloroethene in human breast milk. Risk Analysis 1993; 13: 515–24.

Schuhmacher M, Domingo JL, Kiviranta H et al. Monitoring dioxins and furans in a population living near a hazardous waste incinerator: levels in breast milk. Chemosphere 2004; 57: 43–9.

4

Lactation

4.18 Industrial chemicals and environmental contaminants

Seidel HJ, Kaltenecker S, Waizenegger W. Rückgang der Belastung von Humanmilch mit ausgewählten chlororganischen Verbindungen. Umweltmed Forsch Prax 1998; 3: 83–9.

Sternowsky HJ, Wessolowski R. Lead and cadmium in breast milk. Arch Toxicol 1985; 57: 41–5.

Teufel M, Nissen KH, Sartoris J et al. Chlorinated hydrocarbons in fat tissue: analysis of residues in healthy children, tumor patients and malformed children. Arch Environ Contam Toxicol 1990; 19: 646–52.

Ursinyova M, Masanova V. Cadmium, lead and mercury in human milk from Slovakia. Food Addit Contam 2005; 22: 579–89.

Vieth B, Rüdiger T, Ostermann B et al. Rückstände von Flammschutzmitteln in Frauenmilch aus Deutschland unter besonderer Berücksichtigung von polybromierten Diphenylethern. Bericht des Umweltbundesamtes 2005.

Vreugdenhil HJ, Van Zanten GA, Brocaar MP et al. Prenatal exposure to polychlorinated biphenyls and breastfeeding: opposing effects on auditory P300 latencies in 9-year-old Dutch children. Dev Med Child Neurol 2004; 46: 398–405.

Walkowiak J, Wiener JA, Fastabend A et al. Environmental exposure to polychlorinated biphenyls and quality of the home environment: effects on psychodevelopment in early childhood. Lancet 2001; 358: 1602–7.

WHO. Polychlorinated Dibenzo-Paradioxins and Dibenzofurans; Environmental Health Criteria 88. Geneva: WHO, 1989.

Wolff S. Occupationally derived chemicals in breast milk. Am J Industr Med 1983; 4: 259–81.

1. North American Teratology Information Services collaborating in the Organisation of Teratogen Information Specialists (OTIS)
2. European, Israelian, and Latin American Teratology information centers collaborating in the European Network of Teratology Information Services (ENTIS)

North American Teratology Information Services collaborating in the Organisation of Teratogen Information Specialists (OTIS)

Additional information and addresses not presented below can be found at www.otispregnancy.org

Canada

Ontario
Safe Start Program
Hamilton Health Science Corporation
2100 Main Street West
L8N 3Z5 Canada
Tel.: (905) 521 2100 ext. 76788; serves Ontario; open M–F 8–4 EST; accepts calls from health care providers by referral only. Does not handle breastfeeding.

FRAME
Department of Pediatrics
c/o Dr Michael Rieder

Children's Hospital of Western Ontario
800 Commissioners Road East
London, Ontario N6C 2V5
Tel.: (519) 685 8293; serves Southwestern Ontario, Canada; open
M–F 8–4 EST; accepts calls from health care providers. Handles all
inquiries.

Motherisk Program
Hospital for Sick Children
555 University Avenue
Toronto, Ont. M5G 1X8 Canada
Tel.: (416) 813 6780; serves mostly Ontario, will take calls from
other areas; open M–F 9–5 EST; accepts calls from both public and
health care providers. Handles all inquiries.

Quebec
IMAGe: Info-Medicaments en Allaitement et Grossesse
3175 Cote Sainte Catherine
Montreal, Quebec, Canada H3T 1C5
Tel.: (514) 345 2323; serves Montreal; open M–F 9–4 EST, closed
daily from 12–1 pm; accepts calls from health care providers. Handles
all inquiries.

▶ USA

Arizona
Arizona Teratology Information Service
University of Arizona
Drachman Hall
1295 N. Martin
Room B308
PO Box 210202
Tucson, AZ 85721
Tel.: (888) 285 3410 or (520) 626 3410
Serves Arizona and national; open M–F 8:30–4:30 MST; accepts calls
from both public and health care providers. Handles all inquiries.

Arkansas
Arkansas Teratogen Information Service
University of Arkansas for Medical Sciences
Department of Obstetrics and Gynecology
Arkansas Genetics Program
4301 West Markham – Slot 506
Little Rock, AR 77205

Tel.: (800) 358-7229 or (501) 296 1700
Serves Arkansas and surrounding areas; open M–F 8–4: 30 CST; accepts calls from both public and health care providers. Handles all inquiries.

California
Gerald G. Briggs
9802 Saline Drive
Huntington Beach, CA 92646
Tel.: (714) 964 6937; serves national and international callers; open 24 hours; accepts calls from both public and health care providers. Handles all inquiries.

CTIS Pregnancy Risk Information
200 W. Arbor Drive
San Diego, CA 92103
Tel.: (800) 532 3749; serves California only; open M–F 9–5 PST; accepts calls from both public and health care providers. Handles all inquiries.

Connecticut
Connecticut Pregnancy Exposure Information Service
UCONN Health Partners Building
65 Kane Street
First Floor Genetics
West Hartford, CT 06119
Tel.: (800) 325 5391 CT only or (860) 523 6419; serves Connecticut only; open Monday, Tuesday, Thursday 8:30–3:30; Wednesday 12:30–3:30 EST; accepts calls from both public and health care providers. Handles all inquiries.

Illinois
Illinois Teratogen Information Service
680 N. Lake Shore Drive Suite #1230
Chicago, IL 60611
Tel.: (800) 252 4847 Illinois only or (312) 981 4354; serves Illinois only; open M–F 8:30–4:30 CST; accepts calls from both public and health care providers. Handles all inquiries.

Indiana
Indiana Teratogen Information Service
Indiana University
975 West Walnut Street 1B-130
Indianapolis, IN 46202
Tel.: (317) 274 1071; serves Indiana and surrounding areas; open M–F 8: 30–4: 30 EST; accepts calls from both public and health care providers. Handles all inquiries.

Massachusetts
Pregnancy Environmental Hotline
40 Second Avenue Suite #520
Waltham, MA 02451
Tel.: (800) 322 5014 or (781) 466 8474; serves Massachusetts and surrounding areas; open M–F 9–4 EST; accepts calls from both public and health care providers. Does not handle breastfeeding.

Nebraska
Nebraska TIS
University of Nebraska Medical Center
985440 Nebraska Medical Center
Omaha, NE 68198-5440
Tel.: (402) 559 5071; serves Nebraska and surrounding areas; open M–F 9–4 CST; accepts calls from both public and health care providers. Handles all inquiries.

North Carolina
NCTIS Pregnancy Exposure Riskline
14 Victoria Road
Ashville, NC 28801
Tel.: (800) 532 6302; serves North Carolina only; open M–F 8 30–4: 30 EST; accepts calls from both public and health care providers. Does not handle breastfeeding.

New Jersey
New Jersey Pregnancy Hotline
Southern New Jersey Perinatal Cooperative
2500 McClellan Avenue Suite 110
Pennsauken, NJ 08109-4613
Tel.: (888) 722-2903 (New Jersey); serves New Jersey only; open M–F 8:30–5 EST (returns calls on Tuesday and Thursday); accepts calls from both public and health care providers. Does not handle Hazardous Materials in the workplace.

New York
New York Pregnancy Risk Network
124 Front Street
Binghamton, NY 13905
Tel.: (800) 724 2454 (New York); serves New York only; open Monday, Wednesday, Thursday, Friday 10–1, and Tuesday 9–12 EST; accepts calls from both public and health care providers. Handles all inquiries.

PEDECS
University of Rochester Medical Center
Department of Obstetrics and Gynecology
601 Elmwood Avenue
Rochester, NY 14642-8668
Tel.: (585) 275 3638; serves New York only; open M–F 8–4 EST; accepts calls from both public and health care providers. Does not handle breastfeeding.

North Dakota
North Dakota Teratogen Information Service
Department of Pediatrics
UNDSMHS 501 Columbia Road stop 9037
Grand Forks, North Dakota 58202-9037
Tel.: (701) 777 4277; serves North Dakota; open M–F 8: 00–4: 30 CST; accepts calls from both public and health care providers. Handles all inquiries.

Texas
Texas Teratogen Information Service
UNT Department of Biology
PO Box 305220
Denton, TX 76203-5220
Tel.: (800) 733 4727 or (940) 565 3892; serves Texas and surrounding areas; open M–F 9–5 CST; accepts calls from both public and health care providers. Handles all inquiries.

Utah
Utah Pregnancy Riskline
Utah Department of Health
44 North Medical Drive
Box 144691
Salt Lake City, UT 84114-4691
Tel.: (801) 328 2229 or (800) 822 2229; serves Utah; open M–F 8:30–4:30 MST; accepts calls from both public and health care providers. Handles all inquiries.

Vermont
Vermont Pregnancy Risk Information
112 Colchester Avenue
Burlington, VT 05401
Tel.: (800) 932 4609 option 4; serves Vermont; open Tuesday and Thursday 8–4:30 EST; accepts calls from both the public and health care providers, prefers health care providers. Handles all inquiries.

Washington
CARE Northwest
University of Washington
Box 357920
Seattle, WA 98195-7920
Tel.: (888) 616 8484
Serves Washington, Idaho, Oregon and Alaska; open M–F 8–4 PST
accepts calls from both public and health care providers. Handle
all inquiries.

European, Israelian, and Latin American Teratology information centers collaborating in the European Network of Teratology Information Services (ENTIS)

Additional information and addresses not presented below can b
found at www.entis-org.com

Argentina
Línea Salud Fetal, Servicio de Información de Agentes Teratogénicos
Av. Las Heras 2670 3er piso
1425, Ciudad de Buenos Aires
Tel.: +54 011 4809 0799
Fax: +54 011 4801 4428
E-mail: sfetal@genes.gov.ar
Health care professionals and general public

Austria
Institut für Zellbiologie, Histologie und Embryologie
Harrachgasse 21/7
Medizinische Universität
8010 Graz
Tel.: +43 316 3804256
Fax: +43 316 3809625
E-mail: herbert.juch@meduni-graz.at
Health care professionals and general public

Brazil
Sistema de Informato sobre Agentes Teratogenicos (SIAT)
Servico de Genetica Medica
Hospital de Clinicas de Porto Alegre
Av. Ramiro Barcelos 2350
90035-003 Porto Alegre

Tel.: +55 51 2101 8008
Fax: +55 51 2101 8010
E-mail: lavinia.faccini@ufrgs.br
Health care professionals and general public

Servicio e Registro de Informatio Teratogenica do Rio de Janeiro
Dept. de Genetica – Universidade Federal de Rio de Janeiro
Caixa Postal 68.011
21.941-970 Rio de Janeiro
Tel.: +55 21 560 3432
Fax : +55 21 560 3432/2800994/2808043
E-mail: orioli@acd.ufrj.br

Czech Republic
Czech Teratology Information Service
Charles University
Institute of Histology and Embryology
3rd Faculty of Medicine
Ruská 87
100 00 Praha 10
Tel.: +420 267 102 310
Fax: +420 267 102 311
E-mail: lucie.heringova@lf3.cuni.cz
Health care professionals

Finland
Teratology information
Helsinki University Central Hospital
PO Box 340
00029 HUS, Helsinki
Tel.: +358 9 4717 6500
Fax: +358 9 4717 4702
E-mail: heli.malm@hus.fi
Health care providers and general public

France
Centre and Poisons/Info Agents Teratogenes
Centre Hospitalier Regional
Universitaire de Lille
5 Avenue Oscar Lambret
59037 Lille Cedex
Tel.: +33 320 444444
Fax: +33 320 445628
E-mail: mmathieu@chru-lille.fr

Centre de Pharmacovigilance de Lyon
162 Avenue Lacassagne

69424 Lyon, Cedex 03
Tel.: +33 472 116997
Fax: +33 472 116985
E-mail: thierry.vial@chu-lyon.fr
Health care professionals and general public

Centre Renseignement sur les Agents Teratogenes
Hopital Trousseau
26, Avenue Dr. Arnold Netter
75571 Paris, Cedex 12,
Tel.: +33 1 4341 2622
Fax: +33 1 4341 2622
E-mail: elisabeth.elefant@trs.ap-hop-paris.fr

Centre de Pharmacovigilance
Hôpital Saint-Vincent de Paul
82, Avenue Denfert Rochereau
75674 Paris Cedex 14
Phone +33 1 4048 8213
Fax +33 1 4335 4670
pvigilance.bavoux@svp.ap-hop-paris.fr

Laboratoire de Génétique Médicale
Faculté de Médecine
11 rue Humann
67085 Strasbourg Cedex
Tel.: +33 3 9024 3207
Fax: +33 3 8812 8125
E-mail: Claude.Stoll@medecine.u-strasbg.fr
Health care professionals and general public

Germany
Pharmakovigilanz- und Beratungszentrum Embryonaltoxikologie
Spandauer Damm 130, Haus 10
14050 Berlin
Tel.: +49 30 30308111
Fax: +49 30 30308122
E-mail: mail@embryotox.de
Health care professionals and general public

Krankenhaus St. Elisabeth
Elisabethenstr. 17
88212 Ravensburg
Tel.: +49 751872799
Fax: +49 751 872798
E-mail: paulus@reprotox.de
Health care professionals and general public

Greece
Teratology Information Service
Children's Hospital
P.A. Kyriakou
11527 Athens, Greece
Tel.: +3 010 7793777
Fax: +3 010 7486114
E-mail: tsamadoyathina@hotmail.com
poison_ic@aglaiakyriakou.gr
Health care providers and general public

Kentro Enimerosis Teratogonou Drasis Pharmakon-Information
Centre of Drug Teratogenic Actions
Laboratory of Histology-Embryology and Anthropology
Faculty of Medecine, Aristotle University of Thessaloniki
University Campus
Thessaloniki 54124
Tel.: +30 2310999148 , +30 2310999066
Fax: +30 2310999189 +30 2310999111
E-mail: emmanik@med.auth.gr

Israel
Israel Teratogen Information Service, Jerusalem Child Developmental
Center, Ministry of Health and Hebrew University Hadassah Medical
School
Rechov Yafo 157
Jerusalem
Tel.: +972 2 6243 663
Fax +972 2 6243 669
E-mail: ornoy@cc.huji.ac.il
arnon54@netvision.net.il
sveta54@netvision.net.il
diavcit@netvision.net.il
Health care providers and general public

Beilinson Teratology Information Service (BELTIS)
Rabin Medical Center
Beilinson Campus
49100 Petah Tikva
Tel.: +972 3 9377474 or +972 3 9376911
Fax: +972 3 922 0068
E-mail: merlobp@post.tau.ac.il
bstahl@clalit.org.il
Health care professionals and general public

Drug Information Center
Assaf Harofeh Medical Center
Zerifin 70300
Tel.: +972 8 9779309
Fax: +972 8 9779138
E-mail: mberkovitch@asaf.health.gov.il
General public

Italy
Servicio di Tossicologica Perinatale
U.O. Tossicologia Medica
Azienda Osperdaliera Careggi Firenze
Viale Morgagni 85
50134 Firenze
Tel.: +39 055794 6859 / 6713 / 6238
Fax: +39 055 794 6160
E-mail: toxper@ao-careggi.toscana.it
Health care professionals and general public

Telefona "Filo Rosso" ASM-Milano
c/o Clinica Obstetrica Ginecologica
San Paolo Hospital
Via a rudini 8
20142 Milano
Tel.: +39 2 891 0207
Fax: +39 2 8135662
E-mail: cinzia.paolini@libero.it

Servizio Informazione Terologica (SIT)
Genetica Medica Dipartimento di Pediatria
Via Giustiniani 3
35128 Padova
Tel.: +39 0 49 821 3513
Fax: +39 0 49 821 1425
E-mail: clementi@unipd.it

TelefonoRosso
Department of Obstetrics & Gyn
Catholic University of Sacred Heart
Largo A. Gemelli,
8 00168 - Rome
Tel.: +39 06 3050077
Fax: +39 06 30156572
E-mail: telefonorosso@rm.unicatt.it

Lithuania
Informacija apie Teratogenus/INFOTERA
Vilnius University Hospital
Human Genetics Center
Santariskiu 2
Vilnius 2021
Tel.: +3702 365 197
Fax: +3702 365 199
E-mail: autkus@hotmail.com
Health care professionals and general public

Netherlands
Teratology Information Service
National Institute of Public Health and Environment (RIVM)
Postbus 1, postbak 50
3720 BA Bilthoven
Tel.: +31 30 2742017
Fax: +31 30 2744460
E-mail: benedikte.cuppers@rivm.nl
bernke.te.winkel@rivm.nl
frans.los@rivm.nl
loes.de.vries@rivm.nl
marion.van.eijkeren@rivm.nl
netteke.wentges@rivm.nl
Health care professionals

Russia
IPMC (International Perinatal Medical Center)
Solidarnosti prosp. 6
193312 Saint-Petersburg

Spain
Servicio de Informacion sobre Teratogenos (SITTE). Sección de
Teratología Clínica
Centro de Investigacion sobre
Anomalias Congenitas (CIAC)
Instituto de Salud Carlos III
c/ Sinesio Delgado 6 (Pabellon 6)
28040 Madrid
Tel.: +34 91 8222435
Fax: +34 91 3877541
E-mail: mlmartinez.frias@isciii.es
e.rodriguez-pinilla@isciii.es

Fundació Institut Català de Farmacologia
Hospital Universitari Vall d'Hebron
Pg. Vall d'Hebron 119–129
Barcelona 08035
Tel.: +34 93 428 3029
Fax: +34 93 489 4109
Email: cam@icf.uab.es
ag@icf.uab.es
id@icf.uab.es

Switzerland
Swiss Teratogen Information Service
Division de Pharmacologie et Toxicologie Cliniques
Beaumont 06-624
Centre Hospitalier Universitaire Vaudois
1011 Lausanne
Tel.: +41 21 314 4267
Fax: +41 21 314 4266
E-mail: stis@chuv.ch

United Kingdom
The National Teratology Information Service
NHS Northern and Yorkshire Regional Drug & Therapeutics Centre
24 Claremont Place
Newcastle-upon-Tyne, NE2 4HH
Tel.: +44 191 2606183
Fax: +44 191 2606193
E-mail: Pat.McElhatton@nuth.nhs.uk
Health care professionals

Addresses for breastfeeding support

Appendix B

Additional addresses for countries not presented below can be requested from the IBLCE European Office, Austria and La Leche League International, USA.

Australia
Australian Lactation Consultant Association Limited.
13 Johnston Street
NARRABUNDAH ACT 2604
Tel./fax: +61 2 6295 0384
PO Box 4248
MANUKA ACT 2603.
Website: alca.asn.au
E-mail: info@alca.asn.au

Australian Breastfeeding Association
1818–1822 Malvern Road
East Malvern 3145 Victoria
PO Box 4000
Glen Iris 3146 Victoria
Tel.: +61 3 9885 0855
Fax: +61 3 9885 0866
Website: www.breastfeeding.asn.au
E-mail: info@breastfeeding.asn.au

Austria
IBLCE European Office
Regional Administrator
Ilse Bichler, IBCLC
Steinfeldgasse 11
A-25ll Pfaffstaetten
Tel.: +43 2252 20 65 95
Fax: +43 2252 20 64 87
E-mail: office@iblce-europe.org

Verband der Still- und Laktationsberaterinnen
Österreichs IBCLC; VSLÖ
(Austrian Lactation Consultant Association)
Lindenstraße 20
A-2362 Biedermannsdorf
Phone/Fax : +43 2236 72 336
E-mail: info@stillen.at

La Leche League Austria Maria Wiener
Zentagasse 6/13
1050 Wien
Tel.: +43 1 5458030

Belgium
IBLCE Coordinator Belgium
Dr Greet Stevens IBCLC
Beekstraat 42
2800 Mechelen
Tel. (home): +32 (0) 15 33 01 20
E-mail: be@iblce-europe.org

La Leche League Flanders
Koningin Astridlaan 155
2800 Mechelen
Tel. +32 (0) 56 20 00 51
E-mail: info@lalecheleague.be

Bosnia-Herzegovina
IBLCE Coordinator Bosnia-Herzegovina
Adisa Hotic IBCLC
Prvomajska 51
79260 Sanski Most
Tel. (work): +387 (0) 37 683 301
Fax (work): +387 (0) 37 683 301
Tel. (home): +387 (0) 37 685 117
E-mail: ba@iblce-europe.org

Canada
Canadian Lactation Consultant Association
10-3939 Indian River Drive
North Vancouver, BC, V7G 2P5
Tel.: +1 604 929 6751
E-mail: meb@unixg.ubc.ca
Madeleine Hegholz
Tel.: 780 467 4440
E-mail: mhegholz@telusplanet.net
Website: www.clca-accl.ca
E-mail: info@clca-accl.ca

La Leche League Canada
National Office
12050 Main St. W.
PO Box 700
Winchester, ON K0C 2K0
Tel.: +61 3 774 1842
Fax: +61 3 774 1840
E-mail: ofm@LLLC.ca

Croatia
IBLCE Coordinator Croatia
Irena Zakarija-Grkovic MD IBCLC
Krbavska 10
21000 Split
Tel.: +385 (0) 21 474 754
E-mail: hr@iblce-europe.org

Denmark
IBLCE Coordinator Denmark
Ingrid Nilsson IBCLC
Skovloebervangen 48
3500 Vaerlose
Tel. (work): +45 (0) 4075 3137
Tel. (home): +45 (0) 4448 4340
E-mail: dk@iblce-europe.org

Egypt
IBLCE Coordinator Egypt
Azza Abul-Fadl MD IBCLC
26B, ElGezira AlWosta
Zamalek, Cairo 11211
Tel. (work): +202 (0) 794 3932
Tel. (home): +202 (0) 735 2785
Mobile:+123494183
E-mail: eg@iblce-europe.org

Finland
IBLCE Coordinator Finland
Katja Koskinen IBCLC
Leppävaarankatu 19 A 5
02600 Espoo
Tel.: +358 (50) 57 31 677
E-mail: fi@iblce-europe.org

Appendix B

France
IBLCE Coordinators France
Chantal Audoin IBCLC
7, rue de Cherbourg
31300 Toulouse
Phone/fax: +33 (0) 5 61 42 96 95
E-mail: fr-exam@iblce-europe.org

Dr Marie-Claude Marchand, IBCLC
20, Rue des Acacias
F-91439 Ingy
Tel.: +33 1 69 85 34 73
Mobile: +33 6 16 74 64 42

La Leche League France
BP 18
78620 L'Etang-la-Ville
Tel.: +33 1 39 584 584
E-mail: contact@lllfrance.org

Germany
BDL-Sekretariat
(German Lactation Consultant Association)
Hildesheimer Straße 124 E
30880 Laatzen
Tel.: +49 511 87 64 98 60
Fax: +49 511 87 64 98 68
E-mail: sekretariat@bdl-stillen.de

La Leche League Germany
Dannenkamp 25
32479 Hille
Tel.: +49 571 48946
Phone (Hotline): +49 6851 2524
Fax: +49 571 4049480
E-mail: info@lalecheliga.de

Arbeitsgemeinschaft Freier Stillgruppen; AFS (Independent Breast-
feeding Support Groups)
AFS-Geschäftsstelle
Bornheimer Straße 100
53119 Bonn
Tel.: +49 228 35 038 71
Fax: +49 228 35 038 72
Hotline: 0180-5-STILLEN for 0.12 €/minute
E-mail: geschaeftsstelle@afs-stillen.de

Greece
IBLCE Coordinator Greece and Cyprus
Miloslava Ruzkova-Kosiari MD IBCLC
Sarantaekkklesion 3
671 00 Xanthi
Tel. (work): +30 (0) 25410 62 046
Fax (work): +30 (0) 25410 22 187
Tel. (home): +30 (0) 25410 93 904
E-mail: gr@iblce-europe.org

Hong Kong
Pan-Asian Lactation Consultant Association (PALCA)
Chee Yuet Oi, MEdSt, BAppSC, RN, RM, IBCLC
E-mail: yochee@navigator.com
Tel.: +85 2 2705 9322
Fax: +85 2 2719 0052

Hungary
IBLCE Coordinator Hungary
Ibolya Rozsa IBCLC
Petofi u. 16
2500 Pilisszentlelek
Tel.: +30 (0) 583 4877
E-mail: hu@iblce-europe.org

Iceland
IBLCE Coordinator Iceland
Björk Tryggvadóttir IBCLC
Hrisholt 9
210 Gardabaer
Simi/Tel.: +354 (0) 565 78 28
GSM/Mobile: +354 (0) 869 02 66
Fax: +354 (0) 544 8040
E-mail: is@iblce-europe.org

Iraq
IBLCE Coordinator Iraq
Dr Naira Al-Awqati IBCLC
Ministry of Health
PO Box 61246, Code 12114
Baghdad – Bab Al-Mutham
E-mail: iq@iblce-europe.org

Ireland
IBLCE Coordinator Republic of Ireland and Northern Ireland
Nicola Clarke IBCLC
26 Violet Hill Park
Glasnevin, Dublin 11
Tel.: +353 1 834 1883
E-mail: ie@iblce-europe.org

La Leche League of Ireland
Website: http://homepage.tinet.ie/~lalecheleague/
E-mail: mjbird@tinet.ie
lizquinn@tinet.ie
dpwhite@tinet.ie

Italy
IBLCE Coordinator Italy
Marina Baldocci IBCLC
Via Gravina di Puglia 44
00133 Roma
Phone/fax (home): +39 06 205 07 37
Mobile: +0338 31 123 39
E-mail: it@iblce-europe.org

La Leche League Italia
Casella Postale 1368
20100 Milano
Firenze
Tel. (Florence) +39 055 781737
Tel. (Rome): +39 065 258365
E-mail: lllinformazioni@supereva.it

Japan
Japanese Association of Lactation Consultants (JALC)
Tomoko Seo, MD, IBCLC
Fax: +81 11 733 3188
Website: http://www.jalc-net.jp/
E-mail: seo@jalc-net.jp

Jordan
IBLCE Coordinator Jordan
Dr Hanan Al-Najmi IBCLC
PO Box 850 909
11185 Amman
Tel. (work): +962 (0) 552 09 21
Fax (work): +962 (0) 552 09 21
Tel. (home): +962 (0) 553 337 92
E-mail: jo@iblce-europe.org

Kuwait
IBLCE Coordinator Kuwait
Dr Mona Al Sumaie IBCLC
PO Box 42432,
Food & Nutr. Adm. Shuwaikh – 70655
Tel. (work): +965 (0) 48 36 155 481 60 43
Fax (work): +965 (0) 481 3905
Tel. (home): +965 (0) 533 37 68 93 73 776
Fax (home): +965 (0) 53 33 768
E-mail: kw@iblce-europe.org

Lebanon
IBLCE Coordinator Lebanon
Iman Elzein IBCLC
PO Box 15-5005
1101 2010 Basta-Beirut
Tel. (home): +961 (0) 1 646729
E-mail: lb@iblce-europe.org

Lithuania
IBLCE Coordinator Lithuania
Daiva Sniukaite IBCLC
Pusu str. 32
08116 Vilnius
Tel./fax: +37 (0) 5 27 54 543
Mobile: +37 (0) 698 36 946
E-mail: lt@iblce-europe.org

Luxemburg
Initiativ Liewensufank
Marye Lehners, IBCLC
20, rue de Contern
5955 Itzig
Tel.: +352-360598/+352-36059 11
Fax: +352-366134
E-mail: maryse.lehners@ci.educ.lu
General E-mail: info@liewensufank.lu

La Leche League Luxemburg Rita Schroeder
29 Rue Raoul Follereau 1529 Luxembourg
Tel.: +352 437730
E-mail: schri@gmx.net

The Netherlands
IBLCE Coordinator Netherlands
Siemian Berghuijs-Krijger IBCLC
Turfberg 15

Appendix B

2716 LT Zoetermeer
Tel.: +31 (0) 79 329 0061
Mobile: +31 (0) 6 521 333 39
E-mail: nl@iblce-europe.org

Nederlandse Vereniging van Lactatiekundigen;
NVL
Postbus 1444
1300 BK Almere
Tel.: 0900 5228242
E-mail: e.m.krijnen@hetnet.nl

Stichting La Leche League Nederland
Postbus 212
4300 AE Zierikzee
Tel.: +31 11 1413189
E-mail: lll@borstvoeding.nl

Vereniging Borstvoeding Natuurlijk
Postbus 119
3960 BC Wijk bij Duurstede
Tel: 0343 – 57 66 26
E-mail: vbn@borstvoeding.nl
www.borstvoedingnatuurlijk.nl

New Zealand
Parents Centres NZ Inc. National Office
Unit 4, Bridgepoint
13 Marina View
PO Box 54 128
Mana
Tel.: +64 4 233 2022
Fax: +64 4 233 2063
Website: www.parentscentre.org.nz
E-mail: info@parentscentre.org.nz

New Zealand Lactation Consultant Association (NZLCA)
Jennifer Cox
Tel.: +64 4 801 5805
Website: http://www.lactcon.org.nz/
E-mail: mccox@xtra.co.nz

Norway
IBLCE Coordinator Norway
Elisabeth Tufte
Kjelsaasveien 69 C
0488 Oslo

Tel.: +47 2271 1184
Fax: +47 (0) 2271 1178
E-mail: no@iblce-europe.org

Mother to Mother Support Group
"Ammehjelpen"
P.b 112
2421 Trysil
Tel.: +47 62455251
Fax: +47 62455105
Website: www.ammehjelpen.no
E-mail: ammehjelpen@c2.net

Poland
IBLCE Coordinator Poland
Malwina Okrzesik, IBCLC
Ul. Przemysłowa 25
43-310 Bielsko-Biała
Mobile: 48502127588
E-mail: pl@iblce-europe.org

Qatar
IBLCE Coordinator Qatar
Dr Mohammed Ilyas Khan MBBS MPH IBCLC
Maternal & Child Health Section,
3050-Hamad Medical Corporation
Doha
Tel. (home): 0974 4687489
Fax: 0974 4681527
Mobile: 0974 5824859
E-mail: qr@iblce-europe.org

Saudi Arabia
IBLCE Coordinator Saudi Arabia
Mary J. Butterworth IBCLC
King Abdul Azziz Medical City
Mail Code 1213, PO Box 22 490
Riyadh 11426
Mobile: 0508 13 77 28
Tel. (work): +966 (0) 1 25 200 88 10 36
Tel. (home): +966 (0) 1 25 200 88 44 68
E-mail: sa@iblce-europe.org

Singapore
La Leche League of Singapore HELPLINE
7000-LLL-INFO

Tel.: 7000 555 4636
E-mail: sock_lll@yahoo.com.sg

Slovenia
IBLCE Coordinator Slovenia
Dr Andreja Tekauc-Golob, IBCLC
Splavarski prehod 6
2000 Maribor
Tel. (work): +386 (0) 2 321 2453
E-mail: si@iblce-europe.org

La Leche League Slovenia
E-mail: dojenje@yahoo.com

Spain
IBLCE Coordinator Spain
Adelina García Roldán IBCLC
c/s Ignacio N 4 – 4 B
48903 Barakaldo – Bizkaia
Tel. (home): +34 (0) 944 99 22 73
Mobile: +34 680 63 98 38
E-mail: es@iblce-europe.org

Federación Española de Asociaciones pro-Lactancia Materna
FEDALMA
(Spanish Federation of Pro-Breastfeeding Associations)
C/Pablo Neruda, 9, 1ºA
50018 Zaragoza
E-mail: contacto@fedalma.org

Sweden
IBLCE Coordinator Sweden
Ann Tiits IBCLC
Ilmars Väg 10
13792 Tungelsta
Tel.(work): +46 (0) 8 556 93 773
Fax (work): +46 (0) 8 500 111 12
Mobile: +46 (0) 708 235 977
E-mail: se@iblce-europe.org

Mother-to-Mother Support Group
Amningshjälpen
Amningshjälpen office:
Jutvik Krogsfall,
590 41 Rimforsa,
Tel./fax: 013 424 50
Website: www.amningshjalpen.se

Switzerland
IBLCE Coordinator Switzerland
Johanna Thomann Lemann IBCLC
Schulhausstrasse 26
3052 Zollikofen
Tel./fax: +41 (0) 31 911 35 36
E-mail: ch@iblce-europe.org

Berufsverband Schweizerischer
Stillberaterinnen; BSS/ASCL
(Swiss Lactation Consultant Association)
Postfach 696 (German)/Case postale 686 (French)
3000 Bern 25
Tel.: +41 41 6710173
Fax: +41 41 6710171
Website: www.stillen.ch
E-mail: office@stillen.ch

Verband europäische
Laktationsberaterinnen (VELB)
Sekretariat
Brünigstr. 12, Postfach 139
6055 Alpnach Dorf
Tel.: +41 41-671 01 73
Fax: +41 41-671 01 71
E-mail: velbsekretariat@gmx.net

La Leche League Switzerland
Sekretariat
La Leche Liga Schweiz
Postfach 197
8053 Zürich
Tel/fax: 081 943 33 00
E-mail: info@stillberatung.ch

South Africa
La Leche League South Africa
E-mail: mariliett@intekom.co.za

Syria
La Leche League Syria
Tel.: 332-5180
E-mail: saminaanthony@yahoo.com

United Arab Emirates
IBLCE Coordinator United Arab Emirates and Oman
Paula Miller IBCLC
Nasa Multiplex LLC
PO Box 1520
Dubai
Tel./fax: +971 4 34 80 774
Mobile: +50 65 011 89
E-mail: ae@iblce-europe.org

United Kingdom
IBLCE Coordinator United Kingdom
Carolyn Westcott IBCLC
19 Tadfield Crescent
Romsey SO 51 5AN
Tel.: 01 794 514 739
E-mail: uk@iblce-europe.org

Lactation Consultants of Great Britain
LCGB
PO Box 56,
Virginia Water,
GU25 4WB.
E-mail: info@lcgb.org

La Leche League Great Britain
PO Box 29
West Bridgford
Nottingham NG2 7NP
Tel.: +44 0845 456 1855
National Help Line: +44 0845 120 2918
Website: www.laleche.org.uk

USA
International Lactation Consultant Association
1500 Sunday Drive
Suite 102
Raleigh, North Carolina 27607
Tel.: +1 919 787 5181
Fax: +1 919 787 4916
Website: www.ilca.org
E-mail: info@ilca.org

La Leche League International
1400 N. Meacham Road
Post Office Box 4079

Schaumburg, Illinois 60173-4808
Tel.: +1 847 519 7730
Fax: +1 847 519 0035
Website: www.lalecheleague.org

Breastfeeding and Human Lactation Study Center
University of Rochester
School of Medicine and Dentistry
601 Elmwood Ave
Rochester, New York 14642-8321
Tel.: +1 585 275 0088
E-mail: lactation@urmc.rochester.edu
Available for information concerning drug and environmental exposures during lactation.

Subject Index

evening primrose oil, 493
everolimus, 321, 325, 739
exemestane, 357, 742
exercise and breastfeeding, 777
expectorants, 71–2, 644
eye drops, 459–60, 766–7
ezetimibe, 116, 655

H

I

M

Q

vitamin B$_6$, 86–7, 471
vitamin B$_{12}$, 14, 471–2, 775
vitamin C, 474–5
vitamin D, 475–6, 775–6
vitamin E, 476
vitamin K, 246–7
vitamin K antagonists, 242–6, 696
volume expanders, 249–51
vomiting *see* nausea

W

warfarin, 16, 242, 696
wart removal medications, 443, 449, 457, 769
water intoxication, 548–9
weight loss, 116–18
wheat bran, 652
Wilson's disease, 46

X

X-rays, 502–5, 779–80
xanthine oxidase, 635
xantinol nicotinate, 655
ximelagatran, 697

xipamide, 224, 690
xylene, 564
xylometazoline, 460

Y

yarrow, 496
yellow fever vaccine, 189

Z

zafirlukast, 70, 644
zalcitabine, 160, 671
zaleplon, 309, 731
zanamivir, 158, 671
zidovudine, 14, 160, 670, 792
zileuton, 70, 644
zinc, 481
ziprasidone, 302, 304, 726
zoledronic acid, 480
zolmitriptan, 43, 631
zolpidem, 309, 731
zonisamide, 280–1, 705
zopiclone, 309, 731
zotepine, 301, 723
zuclopenthixol, 301, 723